Removable Partial Dentures

Olcay Şakar
Editor

Removable Partial Dentures

A Practitioners' Manual

Second Edition

Springer

Editor
Olcay Şakar
Faculty of Dentistry, Department of Prosthodontics
İstanbul University
İstanbul, Türkiye

ISBN 978-3-031-47082-0 ISBN 978-3-031-47083-7 (eBook)
https://doi.org/10.1007/978-3-031-47083-7

This Springer imprint is published by the registered company Springer Nature Switzerland AG
The registered company address is: Gewerbestrasse 11, 6330 Cham, Switzerland

Foreword

Removable partial dentures (RPDs) have for long been a very common treatment option for subjects with partial edentulism, i.e., loss of some but not all teeth. Even if the prevalence varies considerably between countries, RPD treatment is in a global context still the most common prosthodontic option for partially edentulous patients. With the successful development of dental implants, many clinicians have come to believe that implant treatment can solve all problems related to tooth loss and substitute both RPDs and complete dentures. This is of course not true, not only because of often-unfavorable oral conditions but also of a number of nondental factors such as fear of surgery and suspicion of implant treatment. The most important obstacle is however economical. A majority of partially edentulous people belong to the poorest section of the population and can never be candidates for any implant treatment. For those, RPDs may be a realistic option. For others with positive experience of an RPD, it will remain an acceptable treatment.

During the last few decades, many dentists have considered RPDs an inferior treatment in the restoration of tooth loss when compared with fixed dental prostheses on natural teeth or on dental implants. It is true that the use of RPDs may involve a risk of potential harm to the oral tissues, probably greater than when using fixed restorations. However, this can be counteracted with proper planning and conduct of the treatment including individual instruction in oral hygiene, pre-prosthetic periodontal treatment, and maintenance of dental and periodontal health after the delivery of the RPD. A satisfactory prognosis for most RPD treatments can be obtained provided correct indications have been used, the dentist and the dental technician collaborate closely in the construction of the prosthesis, and the patient succeeds in maintaining good oral hygiene in the long run. These conditions and the fact that an RPD treatment is more rapidly performed and is less costly than other alternatives indicate that RPDs will remain a viable option in the rehabilitation of partially edentulous patients in the predictable future.

This impressive new textbook combines a straightforward description of well-established principles and methods for the treatment of partially edentulous patients with new and modern knowledge based on available scientific evidence. It contains basic information on the epidemiology of partial edentulism and its effect on the stomatognathic system as well as a detailed account and directions for the clinical and laboratory work in the fabrication of RPDs. There are interesting chapters on advanced RPD techniques using various attachments, double crown systems, and dental implants as well as a discussion on the role of partial edentulism and temporomandibular disorders.

The text is easy to read and supplemented with informative illustrations. The book will therefore be valuable both in undergraduate and postgraduate education. It deserves also to have a place in the office of any dentist treating adult and elderly patients.

Mölndal, Sweden
Gunnar E. Carlsson
LDS, Odont Dr/PhD, Dr Odont hc, Dr Dent hc, FDSRCS

Preface and Acknowledgments

The rapid increase in the population of elderly people all over the world and the economic crisis becoming more effective with the pandemic in recent years have caused difficulties in protecting the oral health and the need for prosthetic treatment. Thus, practical, relatively inexpensive and non-surgical restorations such as removable partial dentures have become more prominent, especially for the geriatric patients. These conditions formed the basis of the need for the second edition of our book.

In this edition, all chapters are updated according to current evidence-based literature with supplementary cases and visuals and four new chapters added.

Due to inevitable digitalization of not only clinical but also laboratory procedures of prosthodontic treatments, a new part "Digital Workflow of Removable Partial Dentures" is presented with rich illustrated content. Additionally, the pandemic once again emphasized the importance of infection control. The chapter "Disinfection and Hygiene Protocols" has been prepared as a guide that includes graphics that every clinician can refer to, starting from the preliminary impressions, materials used, exchange of the work between the laboratory and the clinic, to delivery of prostheses and office disinfection, all in detail. Finally, the "Prosthetic Treatment of Partially Edentulous Maxillofacial Defect Patients" chapter presents remarkable content such as etiology, classification, and surgical procedures as well as removable partial denture designs that can be applied to all types of defects, and these are described with illustrations over a wide range of cases.

I would like to reiterate the gratitude and appreciations that I mentioned in the first edition. Furthermore, I would like to thank all our previous authors who revised their chapters, the authors who have just joined our book family, Erkan Saraçoğlu for his contribution to the new illustrations, and our families for their support during this tough period.

I would like to thank our beloved readers who share and expand our knowledge and I believe this edition will further contribute to all the clinicians' professional practice.

İstanbul, Türkiye — Olcay Şakar

Preface and Acknowledgments to the First Edition

İstanbul University Faculty of Dentistry, which is located in the most crowded and socioeconomically cosmopolitan city of Türkiye, has a remarkable capacity regarding both the number of patients and students. Every year an average of 1800 complete and 1200 removable partial dentures are delivered in the department of prosthodontics.

As an academician, concentrated on removable dentures, my opinion is that with incomplete knowledge of removable dentures any prosthodontic treatment including intraoral appliances would fail to succeed.

Removable partial dentures appeal as complex structures mostly due to the components of the framework to both dental students and dentists. This is the main reason why a great part of the design process is left to dental technicians to be carried out. However, these dentures are simple and cost-effective solutions providing long-term service to a vast majority of patients when they are properly designed.

This book is designed as a guide to simplify basic knowledge and clinical procedures that are often regarded as complicated. It is therefore enriched with visual items like photographs, videos, and descriptive illustrations of selected cases, and clinical and desktop procedures as much as possible.

Even though this book is mainly meant for dentists, I hope it will also be an up-to-date handbook for both dental students and technicians.

Prosthodontic treatment may be considered to require the highest levels of artistic care combined with a wide curriculum of knowledge among all disciplines of dentistry. Therefore, I am thankful to my colleagues who contributed to the mutual effort of bringing this book to life with their valuable expertise and knowledge. I am also grateful to my senior tutors, especially to my mentor, Professor Mehmet S. Beyli, who showed me the way through my academic life, and to Professor Gunnar E. Carlsson, who led and inspired me with his knowledge and experience and honored me by writing the foreword.

I am also grateful to Springer for offering me the opportunity to publish this book and for their constant support.

I also thank our Ph.D. students Zeynep Mumcu, Ercan Yılmaz, Fatih Ayçiçek, Anıl Gürel, Pınar Şeşen, and Mehmet Berk Kaffaf who worked hard in every step of the book; Başak Çetinkaya on behalf of Profcat Interactive Media for preparing the illustrations; graphic designer Hakin Des for managing visual items; and our dental technicians Erbil Sümbüllü and Cihan Bozpınar for their valuable input.

I am much indebted to my family, especially to my daughter Doğa, my husband Semir, to my friends and to the families of all authors for their kind understanding and support.

"Knowledge grows when shared," so I am pretty sure that this book will mature with the precious feedback from our readers and new information will spring out for future generations. Therefore, I would like to thank all readers who share our knowledge in advance.

İstanbul, Türkiye Olcay Şakar

Contents

Part I

Introduction to Removable Partial Dentures

1 Current Status on Partial Edentulism and Removable Partial Dentures

Olcay Şakar

Abstract

What is the present status of total and partial edentulism and expectations for the future? What is the importance and validity of removable partial dentures (RPDs) in dental practice? Why do we need to update our knowledge on RPDs? This chapter allows us to find more answers and leads to further thinking about RPDs. It is in our best interest to provide a harvest of knowledge regarding the current, practical, scientific, and affordable ways to construct proper RPDs.

Oral health, certainly, plays a vital part in both general health and quality of life. According to a report by the World Health Organization (WHO) in 2022, approximately 50% of the world's population is suffering from oral diseases and 3 out of 4 people affected by these diseases are living in low- and middle-income countries. Among the major oral diseases, untreated caries of permanent teeth are the most prevalent with around 2 billion cases, severe periodontal diseases follow with around 1 billion cases, then untreated caries of deciduous teeth with about 510 million cases, and edentulism with 350 million cases. Although rates vary from country to country, the global average prevalence of edentulism is estimated at 22.7% for people older than 60 years.

Global untreated oral disease case numbers have increased by 1 billion over the past 30 years; this is a clear indication that many people do not have access to appropriate oral health care. For those who can receive treatment, the costs are often high and can lead to significant economic burdens. In other words, disadvantaged individuals with risk factors such as lack of education, low income, living in poor and rural areas, and physical or mental disabilities have more oral diseases. Inequalities in expenditure on oral health between countries are also striking. The average expenditure per capita in high-income countries is 500 times higher than in low-income countries. The COVID-19 pandemic also caused major disruptions in access to oral health care in all countries, regardless of the country's income level.

As the average lifespan of the global population is increasing rapidly, the oral health of elderly people is becoming more important. The average life expectancy worldwide, which was 72.8 years in 2019 is expected to rise to 77.2 years in 2050. Statistically, it is estimated that the number of elderly people aged 65 years and over, which was 771 million in 2022, will increase to 994 million by 2030, and 1.6 billion by 2050. As a result, there is a remarkable prediction that by 2050, the number of people aged 65 years and over worldwide will be twice the number of children under 5 years, and the number of children under 12 years will be approximately the same.

O. Şakar (✉)
Faculty of Dentistry, Department of Prosthodontics, İstanbul University, İstanbul, Türkiye
e-mail: osakar@istanbul.edu.tr

O. Şakar (ed.), *Removable Partial Dentures*, https://doi.org/10.1007/978-3-031-47083-7_1

Thus, the United Nations has created a global platform of cooperation to improve the lives of the rapidly aging world population and marked the years 2021–2030 as the "Decade of Healthy Aging" by emphasizing that the COVID-19 pandemic highlighted the current gaps in policies, systems, and services.

The rate of total and partial edentulous people in a population and relevant types of prosthetic restorations vary from one country to another. However, these parameters change even in a constant population over time. Socioeconomic status, attitude to dental care, dental anxiety, and smoking habits may be mentioned among many possible causes of these variations.

Total edentulism is in global decline and WHO declared a number of at least 20 teeth to define functional dentition but this goal of functional dentition has not yet been achieved for many dentate subjects over the age of 60 (Table 1.1). However, a campaign (8020) was launched in Japan in 1989 aimed at ensuring that people still have 20 teeth at the age of 80 so they can maintain their nutrition and social well-being. Studies in recent years have shown that half of the 80-year-old population is successful in meeting the goals of the "8020 Campaign", by preserving more than 20 natural teeth. WHO emphasizes that the success of this campaign offers an important model for promoting healthy and active aging.

The evident increasing elderly population versus decreasing total edentulism tendency indicates that we will be dealing with an escalating number of cases of partial edentulism in the following years. It is not hard to guess that this population will seek less complicated and more affordable treatment options when compared to young people who have higher incomes and motivation to cope with the exhausting, time-consuming, and expensive treatment alternatives.

It should not be ignored that even if a removable partial denture (RPD) is accepted as an economic treatment option for some parts of the world, the simplest basic applications of dentistry are still unaffordable for other less wealthy regions, because poverty is still the major issue that should urgently be addressed.

The United Nations Department of Economic and Social Affairs recently reported that (The World Economic Situation and Prospects 2023) the World is not on track to eliminate extreme poverty by 2030. The same report indicated that rising food and energy prices, severe climate crises, rising inflationary pressure, and especially the recent COVID-19 pandemic have eroded real incomes and exacerbated poverty. It is also emphasized that every 1% increase in food prices can push about ten million additional people into extreme poverty and that if the current trend continues, by 2030, 574 million people, or about

Table 1.1 In various countries, the percentages of total edentulism and the people with functional dentition in subjects 60 years old and over

Author (First name)	Publication Date	Country	Sample (*n*)	Age (years)	Prevalence of total edentulism (%)	People with functional dentition (%)
Ribeiro	2011	Brazil	5349	65–74	54.7	10.0[a]
Doğan	2012	Turkey	1545	65–74	48.0	12.4[b]
Urzua	2012	Chile	465	65–74	11.4	23.8[b]
Ribeiro	2016	Brazil	1451	≥ 60	39.3	17.3[b]
Guo	2018	China	4431	65–74	4.5	73.6[a]
Saito	2018	Japan	3163	75 or 80	4.4	56.8[a]
Musacchio	2021	Italy	3052	≥ 65	43.6	15.7[a]
Park	2021	South Korea	563	≥ 65	13.5	43.3[a]
Bof de Andrade	2021	Brazil	1021	≥ 60	35.6	20.9[a]

[a] *Min* 20 teeth
[b] *Min* 21 teeth

Table 1.2 The old-age dependency ratio is the ratio of the population aged 65 years or over to the population aged 15–64 years. They are presented as number of dependents per 100 people of working age (15–64 years)

Year	World	Sub-Saharan Africa	Africa	Asia	Europe	Latin America and the Caribbean	Northern America	Oceania
2000	11.0	5.6	6.1	9.1	21.8	9.1	18.6	15.3
2005	11.3	5.7	6.1	9.6	23.3	9.7	18.4	15.7
2010	11.7	5.8	6.2	10.1	23.9	10.4	19.6	16.4
2015	12.5	5.8	6.3	11.0	25.9	11.5	22.4	18.4
2020	14.2	5.8	6.5	12.9	29.0	13.3	25.9	20.4
2030	17.8	6.0	7.0	17.1	35.9	18.1	33.5	24.5
2050	24.7	8.0	9.5	27.0	46.6	30.5	36.2	29.0

7% of the World's population, will still be living on less than 2.15 USD a day (the extreme poverty cut-off value updated by World Bank in September 2022).

Another issue regarding the attainability of healthcare services is the ratio of elderly people who need, by various means, the care of the younger generation; this is called "the old age dependency ratio". The increase in this ratio indicates fewer working people taking care of more elderly dependent persons, which in turn complicates the availability of healthcare services socioeconomically (Table 1.2).

The type of treatment for partially edentulous patients varies according to local factors like the condition of remaining hard and soft tissues, systemic condition of the patient, socioeconomic status, and patient preferences.

Rehabilitation of complete or partial edentulism with fixed prostheses should indisputably be the first treatment alternative. Therefore, implant prostheses have been a choice of treatment for a long time and this trend is expected to continue. For example, it has been shown that if the trend in the United States continues at the current pace, the implant treatment rate can be expected to jump from 5.7% in 2016 to 17% by 2026. Recent studies show that the use of implants in people over the age of 65 years has also increased. However, due to the many risk factors involved in this type of treatment in elderly individuals, it is also emphasized that caution is required. Another clinical study revealed that even when the cost is ignored as a drawback, more than one-third of patients refused to have implants, even free of charge, to improve the comfort of their mandibular dentures. The main reason for refusal was the patients' concerns regarding surgery. These concerns included the thought of implants as unnecessary, drawbacks related to complications, negative feedback from unsatisfied people and not having enough time for the length of overall treatment. Due to socio-economic inequalities, the disadvantaged groups are the most vulnerable to having missing teeth and also do not seem to have access to implant-involved treatment options. On the other hand, there are studies showing that we are faced with the fact that there are elderly people in some low socio-economic regions of the world who still use acrylic RPDs because they cannot afford the metal-based RPDs or who have no knowledge about removable dentures and continue their lives without teeth at all. The idea of combining all mandibular complete dentures with two implants has gained wide acceptance, but even this may be limited to the wealthiest countries, which leaves most edentulous patients out of range. As the global dynamics of economics are not likely to change soon, treatment options involving implants seem to be restricted to a wealthy minority in the long term.

The term "appropriatech" has been created to describe a philosophy of treatment approach combining cheap yet effective materials and techniques to make the most cost-effective dentures without ignoring any basic principles of care. And, it has been emphasized that innovations in materials and techniques add many advantages to dental practice but may sometimes cause dentists to forget their humanistic priorities.

As a conclusion, the RPDs stand out as a less complicated and cost-effective alternative for achieving functional and esthetic goals of prosthetic rehabilitation. In the coming years, the need for RPD treatment will increase in parallel with the increase in the number of partially edentulous patients. Despite the lack of adequate information about the percentage of patients using RPDs all over the world, a limited number of studies from different countries reported varying proportions, such as Kazakhstan 54.6%, European countries at 10–19%, Taiwan 15.4%, and recently Sweden 6.1% and, China 11.1–26.7% have revealed that the RPD is a well-accepted treatment alternative and emphasized its indispensable status.

Therefore, people who are reluctant to have tooth preparation or who do not want to have their mobile teeth extracted, systemic conditions that jeopardize surgery, and extensive treatment periods may indicate an RPD treatment. In addition, whenever teeth-bound large edentulous spaces are present and flange support is inevitable due to extensively reduced alveolar ridges, an RPD is certainly the choice of treatment. Another indication is the maxillofacial defect patients, for whom an RPD can offer the fastest and satisfactory solution. When proper artificial teeth positions are hard to establish or implant positions turn the supra-structure design into a biomechanical challenge, an RPD can be the solution. Similarly, patients who need the reestablishment of occlusal vertical dimension and maximal intercuspal position are also candidates for both provisional and permanent overlay RPDs.

Through an evidence-based view, RPDs improve quality of life, and do not cause periodontal destruction and tooth loss if they are planned/maintained correctly, checked regularly, and relined when necessary. They can also be used during supportive periodontal treatment in periodontitis patients.

The long-term studies involving regular checkups showed the survival rates of properly designed clasp-retained RPDs to be 68.6% at 20 years, and 50.4% at 25 years, whereas double-crown-retained RPDs are 70.8% at 20 years.

It was also emphasized that the remaining tooth prognosis when the partially edentulous patients are treated with well-designed and rigid RPDs is similar to that of patients rehabilitated with implant-supported fixed prosthesis due to the appropriate occlusal force distribution to the remaining teeth.

Despite all these evidence-based advantages of RPDs, probably because of industrial pressure and the commercial campaigns of implant manufacturers, they are sometimes pronounced as out of circulation, even among dental practitioners. Actually, scientific research introduced interesting novelties to RPDs and treatment options for partial edentulism, like the shortened dental arch concept, non-metal clasp dentures, implant-assisted RPDs, and digital manufacturing of prostheses. However, even though both conventional RPDs and RPDs equipped with these innovations deliver premium service to patients, recent evaluations of denture services show that clinicians not only seem reluctant to update their knowledge with scientific and technological advances on RPDs but they also neglect their conventional knowledge as well. For example, according to several studies, the U-shaped major connector, which is known to have questionable rigidity and therefore should not randomly be chosen, was found to be the most preferred connector for maxillary frameworks. Too bulky major connectors and over-contoured rests may also be mentioned among frequently ignored issues. Neglecting rest seat preparation or improper rest seats are also frequently seen. Another reported issue is the use of flexible thermoplastic major connectors lacking metal frameworks which exert destructive forces to abutment teeth and periodontal tissues.

While performing our mission as healthcare professionals, we dentists should put great effort into preventive dentistry and avoid overtreatment. Of course, wherever possible, fixed prostheses should be the first choice of treatment, and hopefully one day, genetic engineering may provide us with the technology to prevent or replace tooth and tissue loss. However, the indications for fixed prostheses are still limited to a selected group of patients and, unfortunately, neither of these options is fully available today, nor will they be in the near future. Therefore, despite all scientific and technological advances, treatment of tooth loss will be continued by fixed prostheses, occasionally RPDs, or even complete dentures in the upcoming years.

It is up to us to choose the most cost-effective treatment option that will serve the needs of the patient for the longest possible time. RPDs have been and probably are still the most favorable treatment option for most partially edentulous patients; therefore, the routine prosthodontic practice and knowledge should be kept updated and supported by the developments in the field.

Further Reading

Al-Dwairi ZN. Partial edentulism and removable denture construction: a frequency study in Jordanians. Eur J Prosthodont Restor Dent. 2006;14:13–7.

Behr M, Zeman F, Passauer T, Koller M, Hahnel S, Buergers R, Lang R, Handel G, Kolbeck C. Clinical performance of cast clasp-retained removable partial dentures: a retrospective study. Int J Prosthodont. 2012;25:138–44.

Bof De Andrade F, de Oliveira C, de Oliveira Duarte YA, Sabbah W, Bernabé E. Tooth loss, dental prostheses use and cognitive performance in older Brazilian adults: The SABE cohort study. Geriatr Gerontol Int. 2021;21:1093–8.

Bohnenkamp DM. Removable partial dentures: clinical concepts. Dent Clin North Am. 2014;58:69–89.

British Society for the Study of Prosthetic Dentistry. The York consensus statement on implant-supported overdentures. Eur J Prosthodont Restor Dent. 2009;17:164–5.

Budtz-Jorgensen E, Bochet G. Alternate framework designs for removable partial dentures. J Prosthet Dent. 1998;80:58–66.

Bukleta MS, Bukleta D, Selmani M, Kuhar M. Frequency of complete and removable partial denture treatment in the primary health centres in three different regions of Kosovo from 2002 to 2013. Zdr Varst. 2019;58:104–11.

Bural C, Sülün T, Şakar O. What can be said about the future of complete edentulism and dentures? Dişhekimliğinde Klinik. 2008;25:148–51.

Campbell SD, Cooper L, Craddock H, Hyde TP, Nattress B, Pavitt SH, Seymour DW. Removable partial dentures: the clinical need for innovation. J Prosthet Dent. 2017;118:273–80.

Carlsson GE. Some dogmas related to prosthodontics, temporomandibular disorders and occlusion. Acta Odontol Scand. 2010;68:313–22.

Carlsson GE. Some issues related to evidence-based implantology. J Indian Prosthodont Soc. 2016;16:116–23.

Carlsson GE, Omar R. Trends in prosthodontics. Med Princ Pract. 2006;15:167–79.

Carlsson GE, Omar R. The future of complete dentures in oral rehabilitation. A critical review. J Oral Rehabil. 2010;37:143–56.

Charyeva OO, Altynbekov KD, Nysanova BZ. Kennedy classification and treatment options: a study of partially edentulous patients being treated in a specialized prosthetic clinic. J Prosthodont. 2012;21:177–80.

Chen Q, Lin S, Wu J, Lyu P, Zhou Y. Automatic drawing of customized removable partial denture diagrams based on textual design for the clinical decision support system. J Oral Sci. 2020;62:236–8.

Chung SY, Song KB, Lee SG, Choi YH. The strength of age effect on tooth loss and periodontal condition in Korean elderly. Arch Gerontol Geriatr. 2011;53:243–8.

Curtis DA, Curtis TA, Wagnild GW, Finzen FC. Incidence of various classes of removable partial dentures. J Prosthet Dent. 1992;67:664–7.

Dogan BG, Gokalp S. Tooth loss and edentulism in the Turkish elderly. Arch Gerontol Geriatr. 2012;54:e162–6.

Douglass CW, Watson AJ. Future needs for fixed and removable partial dentures in the United States. J Prosthet Dent. 2002;87:9–14.

Ehikhamenor EE, Oboro HO, Onuora OI, Umanah AU, Chukwumah NM, Aivboraye IA. Types of removable prostheses requested by patients who were presented to the University of Benin Teaching Hospital Dental Clinic. J Dent Oral Hyg. 2010;2:15–8.

Elani HW, Starr JR, Da Silva JD, Gallucci GO. Trends in dental implant use in the U.S., 1999-2016, and projections to 2026. J Dent Res. 2018;97:1424–30.

Ercoli C, Caton JG. Dental prostheses and tooth-related factors. J Periodontol. 2018;89(Suppl 1):S223–36.

Feine JS, Carlsson GE, Awad MA, Chehade A, Duncan WJ, Gizani S, Head T, Heydecke G, Lund JP, MacEntee M, Mericske-Stern R, Mojon P, Morais JA, Naert I, Payne AG, Penrod J, Stoker GT, Tawse-Smith A, Taylor TD, Thomason JM, Thomson WM, Wismeijer D. The McGill consensus statement on overdentures. Mandibular two-implant overdentures as first choice standard of care for edentulous patients. Gerodontology. 2002;19:3–4.

Fu T, Liu Y, Shen J, Shen H. Oral health status of residents in Jiangsu Province, China: an epidemiologic survey. Int Dent J. 2022;72:519–28.

GBD 2017 Oral Disorders Collaborators, Bernabe E, Marcenes W, Hernandez CR, et al. Global, regional, and national levels and trends in burden of oral conditions from 1990 to 2017: a systematic analysis for the global burden of disease 2017 study. J Dent Res. 2020;99:362–73.

Gotfredsen K, Rimborg S, Stavropoulos A. Efficacy and risks of removable partial prosthesis in periodontitis patients: a systematic review. J Clin Periodontol. 2022;49:167–81.

Guo J, Ban JH, Li G, Wang X, Feng XP, Tai BJ, Hu Y, Lin HC, Wang B, Si Y, Wang CX, Rong WS, Wang WJ,

Zheng SG, Liu XN, Wang SC. Status of tooth loss and denture restoration in Chinese adult population: findings from the 4th National Oral Health Survey. Chin J Dent Res. 2018;21:249–57.

Holm-Pedersen P, Lang NP, Müller F. What are the longevities of teeth and oral implants? Clin Oral Impl Res. 2007;18(Suppl. 3):15–9.

Ibiyemi O, Lawal FB. A short report on tooth replacement in an older suburban population in Nigeria. Gerodontology. 2017;34:508–11.

Inukai M, Baba K, John MT, Igarashi Y. Does removable partial denture quality affect individuals' oral health? J Dent Res. 2008;87:736–9.

Johansson AK, Omar R, Unell L, Sannevik J, Mastrovito B, Carlsson GE, Johansson A. Changes in conditions related to reported oral and general health over a ten-year period as reflected in two cohorts of 75-year-old subjects examined in 2007 and 2017. J Oral Rehabil. 2020;47:1382–93.

Jorge JH, Giampaolo ET, Vergani CE, Machado AL, Pavarina AC, Cardoso de Oliveira MR. Clinical evaluation of abutment teeth of removable partial denture by means of the Periotest method. J Oral Rehabil. 2007;34:222–7.

Keyf F. Frequency of the various classes of removable partial denture and selection of major connector and direct/indirect retainer. Turk J Med Sci. 2001;31:445–9.

Liebermann A, Erdelt K, Lente I, Edelhoff D, Schmitter M, Winter A. Oral health-related impact profile of patients treated with fixed, removable, and telescopic dental prostheses in student courses-a prospective bicenter clinical trial. Clin Oral Investig. 2021;25:2191–201.

Mojon P, Thomason JM, Walls AW. The impact of falling rates of edentulism. Int J Prosthodont. 2004;17:434–40.

Müller F, Naharro M, Carlsson GE. What are the prevalance and incidence of tooth loss in the adult and elderly population in Europe? Clin Oral Impl Res. 2007;18:2–14.

Musacchio E, Binotto P, Perissinotto E, Sergi G, Zambon S, Corti MC, Frigo AC, Sartori L. Tooth retention predicts good physical performance in older adults. PLoS One. 2021;16:e0255741.

Nicola M, Alsafi Z, Sohrabi C, Kerwan A, Al-Jabir A, Iosifidis C, Agha M, Agha R. The socio-economic implications of the coronavirus pandemic (COVID-19): a review. Int J Surg. 2020;78:185–93.

Owen P. Appropriatech:prosthodontics for the many, not just for the few. Int J Prosthodont. 2004;17:261–2.

Park T, Jung YS, Son K, Bae YC, Song KB, Amano A, Choi YH. More teeth and posterior balanced occlusion are a key determinant for cognitive function in the elderly. Int J Environ Res Public Health. 2021;18:1996.

Pellizzer EP, Almeida DA, Falcón-Antenucci RM, Sánchez DM, Zuim PR, Verri FR. Prevalence of removable partial dentures users treated at the Aracatuba Dental School-UNESP. Gerodontology. 2012;29:140–4.

Peres MA, Macpherson LMD, Weyant RJ, Daly B, Venturelli R, Mathur MR, Listl S, Celeste RK, Guarnizo-Herreño CC, Kearns C, Benzian H, Allison P, Watt RG. Oral diseases: a global public health challenge. Lancet. 2019;394:249–60.

Polychronakis N, Sotitiou M, Zissis A. A survey of removable partial denture casts and major connector designs found in commercial laboratories, Athens, Greece. J Prosthodont. 2013;22:245–9.

Pun DK, Waliszewski MP, Waliszewski KJ. Survey of partial removable dental prosthesis (partial RDP) types in a distinct patent population. J Prosthet Dent. 2011;106:48–56.

Rehmann P, Orbach K, Ferger P, Wöstmann B. Treatment outcomes with removable partial dentures: a retrospective analysis. Int J Prosthodont. 2013;26:147–50.

Ribeiro CG, Cascaes AM, Silva AE, Seerig LM, Nascimento GG, Demarco FF. Edentulism, severe tooth loss and lack of functional dentition in elders: a study in Southern Brazil. Braz Dent J. 2016;27: 345–52.

Ribeiro MT, Rosa MA, Lima RM, Vargas AM, Haddad JP, Ferreira E Ferreira E. Edentulism and shortened dental arch in Brazilian elderly from the National Survey of Oral Health 2003. Rev Saúde Pública. 2011;45:817–23.

Sadig WM, Idowu AT. Removable partial denture design: a study of a selected population in Saudi Arabia. J Contemp Dent Pract. 2002;15:40–53.

Saito M, Shimazaki Y, Nonoyama T, Tadokoro Y. Type of dental visit and number of remaining teeth in Japanese elders. J Oral Sci. 2018;60:611–7.

Schimmel M, Müller F, Suter V, Buser D. Implants for elderly patients. Periodontol 2000. 2017;73:228–40.

Shinsho F. New strategy for better geriatric oral health in Japan: 80/20 movement and healthy Japan 21. Int Dent J. 2001;51(3 Suppl):200–6.

Tsuneishi M, Sato T. The impact and future of Japan's 8020 campaign. Jakarta and Tokyo: Asian Health and Wellbeing Initiative (AHWIN); 2021. AHWIN Papers No. 2. https://www.ahwin.org/ahwin-papers-no-2-the-impact-and-future-of-japans-8020-campaign/. Accessed 18 Mar 2023.

Tuncer N, Gözler S, Şakar O. Evaluation of a group of dentists' opinion about partial denture design. Dişhekimliğinde Klinik. 1991;4:60–4.

United Nations. World economic situation and prospects 2023. New York: United Nations; 2023.

United Nations Department of Economic and Social Affairs, Population Division. World Population Prospects 2022: Summary of Results. UN DESA/POP/2022/TR/NO. 3. New York: United Nations; 2022.

Urzua I, Mendoza C, Arteaga O, Rodríguez G, Cabello R, Faleiros S, Carvajal P, Muñoz A, Espinoza I, Aranda W, Gamonal J. Dental caries prevalence and tooth loss in Chilean adult population: first national dental examination survey. Int J Dent. 2012;2012:810170.

Waliszewski MP. Turning points in removable partial denture philosophy. J Prosthodont. 2010;19:571–9.

Walton JN, Mac Entee MI. Choosing or refusing oral implants: a prospective study of edentulous volunteers for a clinical trial. Int J Prosthodont. 2005;18:483–8.

World Health Organization. Global oral health status report: towards universal health coverage for oral health by 2030. Geneva: World Health Organization; 2022. Licence: CC BY-NC-SA 3.0 IGO.

World Health Organization/Fédération Dentaire Internationale. Global goals for oral health in the year 2000. Int Dent J. 1982;32:74–7.

Wöstmann B, Budtz-Jørgensen E, Jepson N, Mushimoto E, Palmqvist S, Sofou A, Owall B. Indications for removable partial dentures: a literature review. Int J Prosthodont. 2005;18:139–45.

Xie Q, Ding T, Yang G. Rehabilitation of oral function with removable dentures-still an option? J Oral Rehabil. 2015;42:234–42.

Yamada R, Nogawa T, Takayama Y, Iwata K, Saito M, Yokoyama A. Comparison of the prognosis of the remaining teeth between implant-supported fixed prostheses and removable partial dentures in partially edentulous patients: a retrospective study. Clin Implant Dent Relat Res. 2022;24:83–93.

Yoshino K, Ito K, Kuroda M, Sugihara N. Survival rate of removable partial dentures with complete arch reconstruction using double crowns: a retrospective study. Clin Oral Investig. 2020;24:1543–9.

Yoshino K, Ito K, Kuroda M, Sugihara N. Survival rate of removable partial dentures with mandibular bilateral free end saddle: a retrospective study. Bull Tokyo Dent Coll. 2021;62:205–14.

Zitzmann NU, Hagmann E, Weiger R. What is the prevalence of various types of prosthetic dental restorations in Europe? Clin Oral Implants Res. 2007;18(Suppl 3):20–33.

The Effects of Partial Edentulism on the Stomatognathic System and General Health

2

Olcay Şakar

Abstract

Tooth loss is a very important phenomenon that affects both oral and systemic health. It may impair the functional stability of the stomatognathic system. The after-effects of tooth loss show individual differences that depend on local and systemic factors. The number and location of the missing teeth, occlusal relationships, the periodontal status of the remaining teeth, and the movement pattern or size of the tongue can be considered as local factors. The neuromuscular control mechanism, age, psychological status, and general resistance can be accepted as systemic factors. Dentists should be aware of the possible consequences or concomitant conditions of tooth loss and inform their patients or refer them to a physician when necessary. It is also vital to know which dentition and/or patient is at a greater risk due to tooth loss and to decide the treatment plan in light of these factors.

O. Şakar (✉)
Faculty of Dentistry, Department of Prosthodontics, İstanbul University, İstanbul, Türkiye
e-mail: osakar@istanbul.edu.tr

2.1 Definitions

Deflective occlusal contact: A contact that displaces a tooth, diverts the mandible from its intended movement or displaces a removable denture from its basal seat.

Interference: In dentistry, any tooth contact that interferes with or hinders harmonious mandibular movement; an undesirable tooth contact.

Occlusal interference: 1. any tooth contact that inhibits the remaining occluding surfaces from achieving stable and harmonious contacts; 2. any undesirable occlusal contact.

Residual ridge: The portion of the residual bone and its soft tissue covering that remains after the removal of teeth.

Residual ridge resorption: A term used for the diminishing quantity and quality of the residual ridge after the teeth are extracted.

Supraeruption: Movement of a tooth or teeth, along with the tooth-supporting structures, in discontinuity with the normal occlusal plane.

Dentition is completed by the eruption of the second molars. Thus, occlusion is achieved by the existence of 28 teeth. The absence of one or more third molars has been observed in approximately 25% of the population.

For the most part, posterior tooth loss is observed more than anterior tooth loss, and upper teeth are lost before lower teeth. Initially, the first molars are commonly lost. Afterward, second molars, second premolars, and first premolars

O. Şakar (ed.), *Removable Partial Dentures*, https://doi.org/10.1007/978-3-031-47083-7_2

may follow. Posterior tooth loss generally occurs bilaterally.

Due to individual differences in local and systemic factors, it has been concluded that it is not possible to predict the identical consequences of tooth loss for every patient, and it should also be noted that every partial edentulism does not have to be treated immediately (See Chap. 5).

2.2 Consequences of Tooth Loss

In spite of individual differences, one or more of the following consequences that might affect oral and systemic health can be observed after tooth loss:

1. Alveolar residual bone loss is the main result of tooth loss (Fig. 2.1a, b) and occurs rapidly in the first 3–6 months after the extraction; however, it continues lifelong at a slower rate. Various results from studies have shown that horizontal bone loss (average 3.87 mm) was greater than vertical bone loss (average 1.67 mm). Both horizontal and vertical bone loss have mainly been observed at the buccal part of the residual ridge that becomes narrower and shorter after the resorption process. Therefore, the alveolar ridge is relocated to a more posterior position. Relocation of the ridge is more noticeable in the maxilla, necessitating more lip and cheek support in the buccal region.

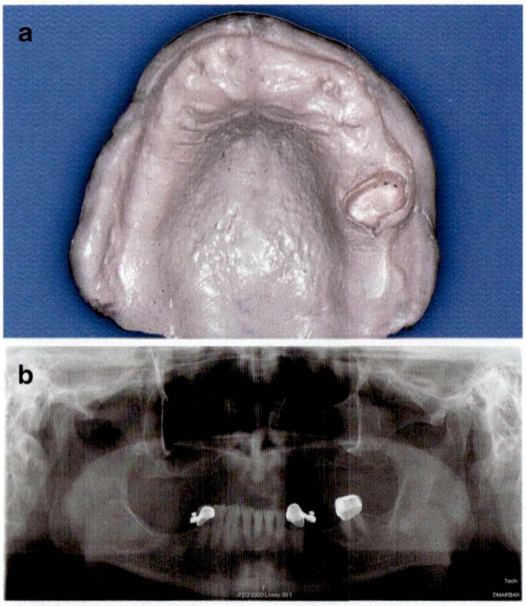

Fig. 2.1 (**a**, **b**) Tooth loss results in alveolar bone loss showing individual differences. Preserving of teeth is vital to protect the residual bone (**a**) and severe bone loss (**b**) can be prevented or slowed down by saving the teeth as long as possible with different prosthodontic treatment alternatives

2. Migration of the teeth in the form of tipping, extrusion, and rotation may occur, especially after the first year of the extraction. It has been demonstrated that supraeruption occurs in most of the unopposed teeth, resulting in periodontal attachment reduction, and is mostly observed in the upper arch (Fig. 2.2a, b). Supraeruption can be divided into active eruption (in which the tooth erupts out of its socket while the periodontium remains stable as seen in Fig. 2.2) and growth of the periodontium (growth in an occlusal direction of the periodontal tissues including the alveolar bone, together with the tooth as seen in Fig. 2.3a, b). The teeth adjacent to the extraction site tend to tip toward this side. While rotation of teeth mesial to the edentulous site has been more commonly observed in the mandible, rotation of teeth distal to the edentulous ridge is greater in the maxilla.

   This shift may continue until the tooth encounters an obstacle (such as other teeth or the residual ridge) and a new occlusal balance develops. After the migration of the teeth, premature contacts and interferences may occur. Thus, occlusal interferences/deflective occlusal contacts and pseudoprognathism (Fig. 2.4a, b) may develop or a pathway may be created by wearing between the opposite teeth (Fig. 2.5a–c). Further changes that could affect oral health may develop, such as traumatic occlusion, root and furcation exposure, soft tissue trauma, plaque retention, and loss of proximal contacts resulting in food impaction.

   There is no consensus regarding the negative effects of occlusal interferences on the stomatognathic system. Furthermore, it should be noted that the relationship between tooth loss or occlusal factors and temporomandibular disorders is controversial (see Chap. 20).

3. Enlargement of the tuberosities may be observed. When mandibular molars are lost, maxillary teeth may erupt together with the alveolar process, and as a consequence, excessive fibrous connective tissue may occur. If this tissue cannot be reduced surgically in the post-extraction phase, it may result in contact with the retromolar pad, an inappropriate occlusal plane, and/or lack of space for denture material (Fig. 2.6a, b). Although it is not observed in all cases, overgrowth of the tuberosities can also be observed in cases that have only anterior mandibular teeth and a maxillary complete denture. In addition, it has been revealed that these patients are at risk of the formation of hypermobile tissue in the anterior maxillary jaw region (Fig. 2.7a, b).

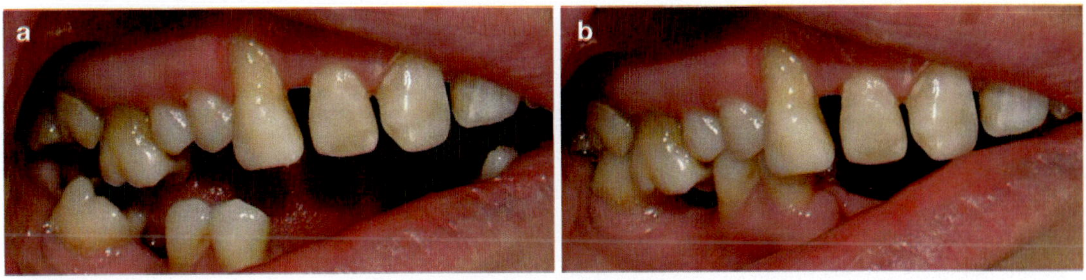

Fig. 2.2 (**a**, **b**) Active eruption can be observed in unopposed teeth. Periodontium remains stable in this supraeruption

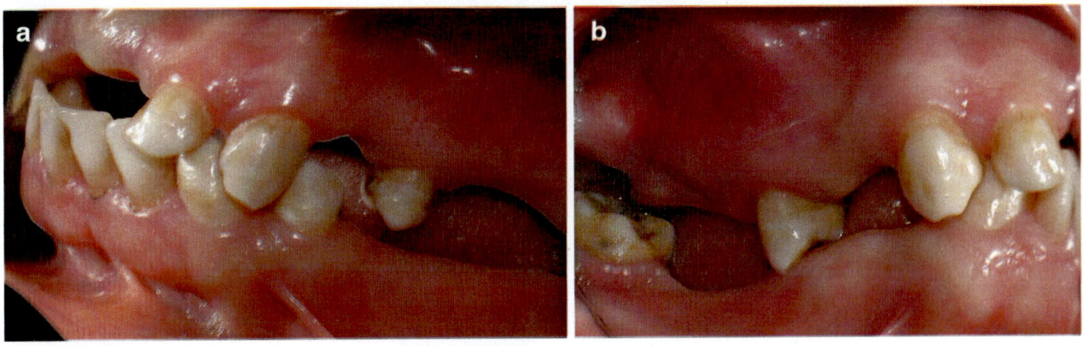

Fig. 2.3 (**a**, **b**) In some cases, supraeruption of the teeth occurs accompanied by the growth of the periodontal tissues and alveolar bone

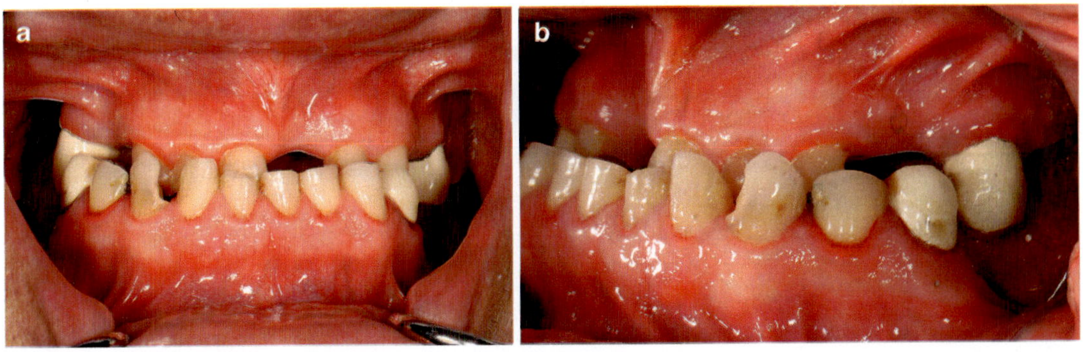

Fig. 2.4 (**a**, **b**) After tooth loss, migrated teeth may cause premature contacts and interferences

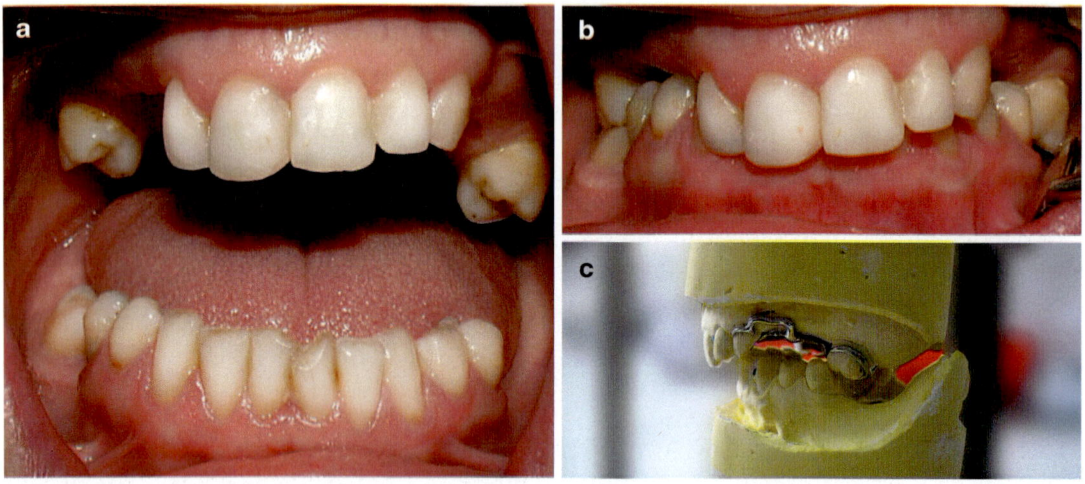

Fig. 2.5 (**a**–**c**) After 11 years of the partial edentulism without any prosthetic treatment, the patient is closing her mouth on a pathway formed by wearing on the second premolar

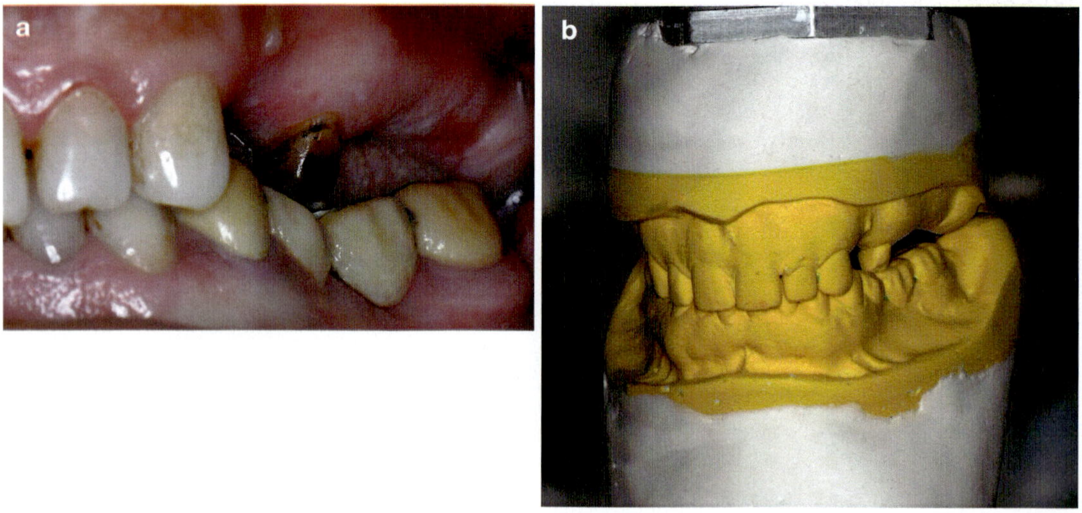

Fig. 2.6 (**a**, **b**) Overgrown tuberosity may contact with the retromolar pad leaving no space for a prosthetic restoration

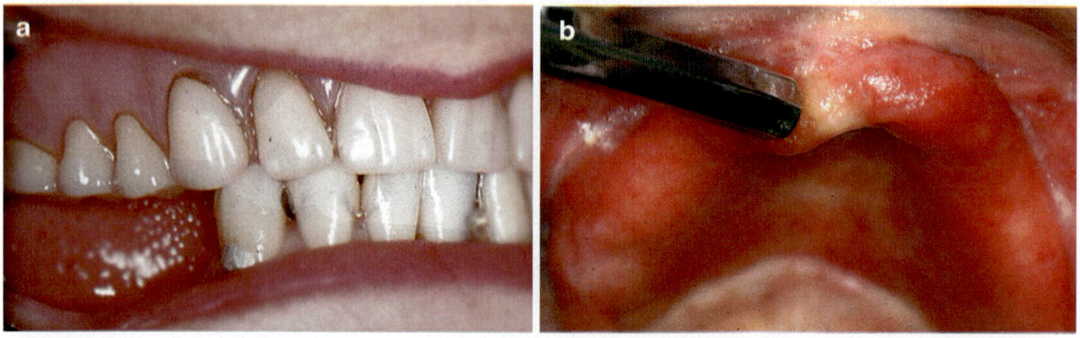

Fig. 2.7 (**a**, **b**) In cases having anterior mandibular teeth and maxillary complete denture, hypermobile tissue in the anterior region of the maxilla may be more likely to develop

4. A loss or decrease in occlusal vertical dimension may develop. Alterations of occlusal vertical dimension may occur due to loss of tooth contacts, displacement of the teeth, and uncompensated tooth wear (see Chap. 21).
5. When all posterior occlusal units have been lost, overloading of the anterior tooth region may occur (Fig. 2.8).
6. Masticatory function may be impaired and/or unilateral or anterior chewing may occur, especially in free-end saddle partially edentulous cases. Digestion begins in the mouth and many nutrients need chewing before swallowing. Patients with impaired dentition may encounter nutritional problems that may lead to systemic disorders and psychosocial difficulties. It has been revealed that chewing ability is significantly impaired when more than 7 teeth are missing and chewing ability is satisfactory with 20 or more teeth, especially if the teeth are well positioned as in the premolar dental arch. As a result, the numbers and types of occluding pairs of teeth are important to evaluate masticatory function (shortened dental arch- see Chap. 5). In cases having large or bilaterally tooth-bound edentulous areas, masticatory function may also be disturbed. Although these cases may be able to chew with most of the remaining occlusal contacts, they may need longer chewing time and swallow larger particles, which may lead to digestive problems, and this may cause them to prefer easy-to-chew food items.
7. Especially in the absence of anterior teeth and maxillary premolars, esthetics, speech, and physiognomy are affected (Fig. 2.9a, b). Psychosocial problems (such as loss of self-esteem and self-confidence) and disorders may develop. It has been shown that adults with depression and anxiety are more likely to have tooth loss. In other words, adults with depression, either long term or short term, were significantly more likely to have had at least one tooth removed than those without these disorders.

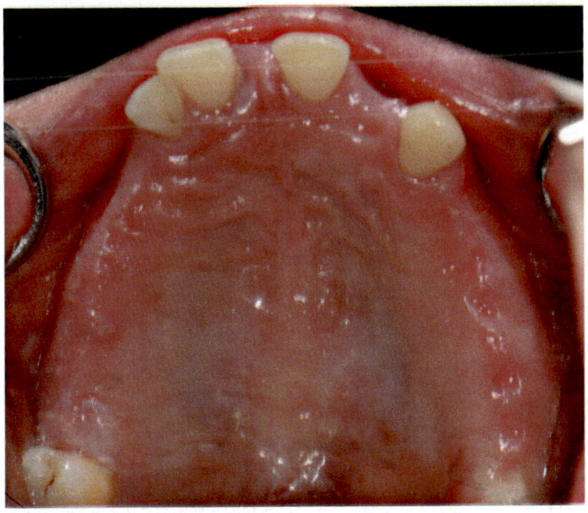

Fig. 2.8 Posterior tooth loss may result in overloading of the anterior tooth. This situation may be further exacerbated by the presence of periodontal problems

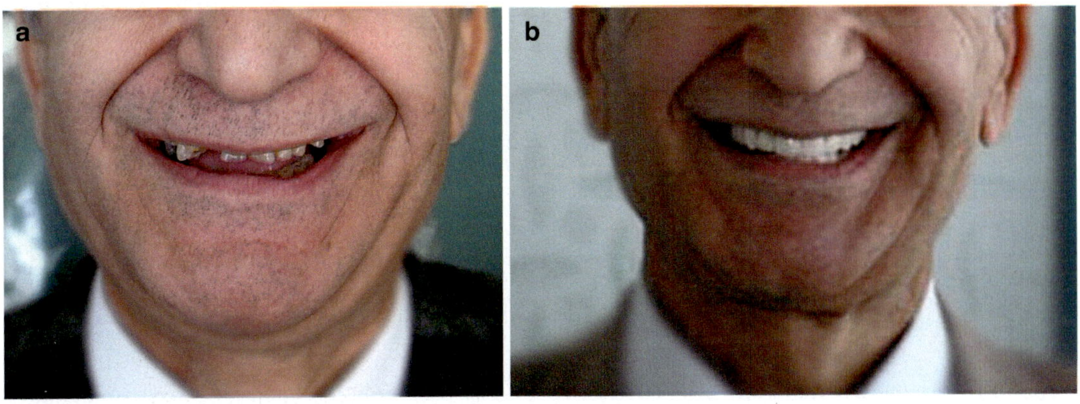

Fig. 2.9 (**a**, **b**) Loss of teeth can also cause psychological problems in addition to functional problems

8. Missing teeth may affect daily functions, physical fitness, cognitive function, and thus the quality of life.

   The above factors may be affected by the number, location, and distribution of missing teeth. It has been revealed that the number of occluding pairs is an important factor for oral health-related quality of life, that having fewer than 20 teeth increases the prevalence of negative impacts, and that having 9 or fewer teeth also has a significant effect on the physical index of general health-related quality of life. Remarkably, it has been found that reduced dentition, if not treated with a removable or fixed denture, reduces the physical index of quality of life to the same degree as cancer or renal diseases. A longitudinal study revealed that in individuals aged 65 years and over, having 20 teeth or more is associated with healthy aging defined by the criteria of the absence of functional disability and depression and having high health-related quality of life and life satisfaction.

9. Tooth loss may be associated with systemic diseases/chronic conditions or increase the risk of these conditions.

   It is known that tooth loss is caused by periodontal disease and caries. A partially edentulous individual with one or two teeth can be described as fully edentulous. For this reason, this factor should be considered when examining the effects of partial edentulism on the stomatognathic system and general health. Many studies have assessed the relationship between poor oral health (tooth loss/periodontal disease/caries) and systemic diseases or general health. The results of the studies emphasize that tooth loss may be associated with many systemic diseases or constitute a risk factor for these diseases. In addition, tooth loss can lead to the progression of some systemic diseases, and restoring tooth loss or treating periodontal disease that may cause tooth loss may have a positive effect on systemic disease; for example, it has been shown that timely prosthetic treatment may reduce the progression of dementia and cognitive decline, and that treatment of severe periodontal disease may lead to improvements in diabetes status.

   Recently, an umbrella review reported that tooth loss is correlated with cardiovascular and cerebrovascular diseases, diabetes mellitus, chronic obstructive pulmonary disease, and dementia. It has been emphasized that periodontitis is predominantly correlated with diabetes mellitus, cardiovascular and cerebrovascular diseases, as well as chronic obstructive pulmonary disease, dementia, psoriasis, and lung cancer. Finally, it has been reported that caries is correlated with diabetes mellitus, and cardiovascular and cerebrovascular diseases.

   In addition, associations of tooth loss with other diseases or conditions have also been found: weight changes (obesity or weight loss); sarcopenia caused by decreased muscle mass and osteopenia/osteoporosis caused by decreased bone mass; gastrointestinal disorders; pneumonia; rheumatoid arthritis; chronic kidney disease; atherosclerotic cardiovascular diseases; cognitive decline; and orodigestive, gastrointestinal/pancreatic cancers.

   Although it is recognized that the nature of associations between poor oral health and systemic diseases is not necessarily causal and is generally weak compared to other underlying risk factors, a potential cause–effect link has been assessed and attempted to be explained by various mechanisms:

   (a) Poor diet: As patients with impaired dentition tend to eat soft foods containing more carbohydrates, less proteins, and micronutrients and avoid vegetables or fruit which are hard, this diet may negatively affect the overall health and may result in weight changes. Although links have been observed between tooth loss/edentulism and obesity in some studies, there is also a longitudinal study which stated that tooth loss is associated with increased weight loss in older adults and that the use of a removable or fixed prosthesis reduces the risk of weight loss.
   (b) Biological mechanisms (Infection, inflammation, and adaptive immunity): Sustained inflammation in periodontal

tissues may be linked to general health or may trigger the initiation of a systematic inflammatory response that may contribute to the pathogenesis of some systemic conditions. The immune response may display individual differences that are affected by many factors such as nutritional habits, physical health, and socioeconomic status.

(c) Psychosocial and/or common risk factors: Lack of teeth can cause psychological problems such as loss of self-confidence, social isolation, and depression. In addition, conditions such as increased smoking and alcohol consumption accompanying psychological problems are risk factors that have a direct negative effect on both general health and oral health. In other words, caries and periodontal problems that cause tooth loss share common risk factors with systemic diseases. As mentioned above, apart from smoking and alcohol consumption accompanying poorer socioeconomic conditions, stress and trauma, poor diet, obesity/weight loss, and hygiene have also been reported as common risk factors for dental and chronic systemic conditions. Age is one of the other most important common risk factors. Elderly individuals may have difficulty performing basic dental care, such as brushing their teeth. The risk of chronic conditions increases with age, and medications taken to treat them can have side effects such as dry mouth that leads to cavities and tooth loss. In addition, older people's access to dental treatment may be much more difficult due to both financial and physical limitations. This may require them to choose treatment options such as tooth extraction, which can be performed in a shorter time and is cheaper.

Hence, it should be considered that tooth loss or poor oral health may be an early indicator of many systemic diseases and good oral health is crucial to healthy aging. The examination of oral condition, especially during regular health check-ups of geriatric patients, is not a time-consuming situation, on the contrary, it can facilitate early diagnosis by providing useful information for general health. Bearing in mind the rapid increase in the elderly population all over the world, preventive care can be considered a cost-effective method. As a result, in terms of its effects on public health, it is stated that the main aim is to improve the oral condition, which can be considered as a marker of fragility, and to achieve "successful aging" criteria. In addition, it is emphasized that ensuring timely and appropriate prosthetic treatment for people with tooth loss will play an important role not only in restoring oral function but also in maintaining general health.

Further Reading

Abnet CC, Qiao YI, Dawsey SM, Dong W, Taylor PR, Mark SD. Tooth loss is associated with increased risk of total death and death from upper gastrointestinal cancer, heart disease, and stroke in Chinese population-based cohort. Int J Epidemiol. 2005;34:467–74.

Agerberg G, Carlsson GE. Chewing ability in relation to dental and general health. Acta Odontol Scand. 1981;39:147–53.

Ahmadinia AR, Rahebi D, Mohammadi M, Ghelichi-Ghojogh M, Jafari A, Esmaielzadeh F, Rajabi A. Association between type 2 diabetes (T2D) and tooth loss: a systematic review and meta-analysis. BMC Endocr Disord. 2022;22:100.

Ansai T, Takata Y, Yoshida A, Soh I, Awano S, Hamasaki T, Sogame A, Shimada N. Association between tooth loss and orodigestive cancer mortality in an 80-year-old community-dwelling Japanese population: a 12-year prospective study. BMC Public Health. 2013;13:814.

Badr SE, Unger JW. Some treatment alternatives for dealing with the enlarged maxillary tuberosity. Quintessence Int. 1987;18:465–8.

Batty GD, Jung KJ, Mok Y, Lee SJ, Back JH, Lee S, Jee SH. Oral health and later coronary heart disease: cohort study of one million people. Eur J Prev Cardiol. 2018;25:598–605.

Beukers NGFM, Su N, Loos BG, van der Heijden GJMG. Lower number of teeth is related to higher risks for ACVD and death-systematic review and meta-analyses of survival data. Front Cardiovasc Med. 2021;8:621626.

Bramantoro T, Hariyani N, Setyowati D, Purwanto B, Zulfiana AA, Irmalia WR. The impact of oral health on physical fitness: a systematic review. Heliyon. 2020;6:e03774.

Cleary TJ, Hutton JE. An assessment of the association between functional edentulism, obesity, and NIDDM. Diabet Care. 1995;18:1007–9.

Compagnon D, Woda A. Supraeruption of the unopposed maxillary first molar. J Prosthet Dent. 1991;66:29–34.

Craddock HL. Occlusal changes following posterior tooth loss in adults. Part 3. A study of clinical parameters associated with the presence of occlusal interferences following posterior tooth loss. J Prosthodont. 2008;17:25–30.

Craddock HL, Youngson CC, Manogue M, Blance A. Occlusal changes following posterior tooth loss in adults. Part 1: a study of clinical parameters associated with the extend and type of supraeruption in unopposed posterior teeth. J Prosthodont. 2007;16:485–94.

Craddock HL, Youngson CC, Manogue M, Blance A. Occlusal changes following posterior tooth loss in adults. Part 2. Clinical parameters associated with movement of teeth adjacent to the site of posterior tooth loss. J Prosthodont. 2007;16:495–501.

Emami E, de Souza RF, Kabawat M, Feine JS. The impact of edentulism on oral and general health. Int J Dent. 2013;2013:498305.

Fisher MA, Taylor GW, Shelton BJ, Jamerson KA, Rahman M, Ojo AO, Sehgal AR. Periodontal disease and other nontraditional risk factors for CKD. Am J Kidney Dis. 2008;51:45–52.

Gerritsen AE, Allen PF, Witter DJ, Bronkhorst EM, Creugers NH. Tooth loss and oral health-related quality of life: a systematic review and meta-analysis. Health Qual Life Outcomes. 2010;8:126.

Griffin SO, Jones JA, Brunson D, Griffin PM, Bailey WD. Burden of oral disease among older adults and implications for public health priorities. Am J Public Health. 2012;102:411–8.

Hag Mohamed S, Sabbah W. Is tooth loss associated with multiple chronic conditions? Acta Odontol Scand. 2023;12:1–6.

Holmlund A, Holm G, Lind L. Number of teeth as a predictor of cardiovascular mortality in a cohort of 7,674 subjects followed for 12 years. J Periodontol. 2010;81:870–6.

Hung HC, Joshipura KJ, Colditz G. The association between tooth loss and the self-reported intake of selected CVD-related nutrients and foods among US women. Community Dent Oral Epidemiol. 2005;33:167–73.

Hung HC, Joshipura KJ, Colditz G, Manson JE, Rimm EB, Speizer FE, Willett WC. The association between tooth loss and coronary heart disease in men and women. J Public Health Dent. 2004;64:209–15.

Iwasaki M, Kimura Y, Ogawa H, Wada T, Sakamoto R, Ishimoto Y, Fujisawa M, Okumiya K, Ansai T, Miyazaki H, Matsubayashi K. The association between dentition status and sarcopenia in Japanese adults aged ≥75 years. J Oral Rehabil. 2017;44:51–8.

Kelly E. Changes caused by a mandibular removable partial denture opposing a maxillary complete denture. J Prosthet Dent. 1972;27:140–50.

Kusama T, Kiuchi S, Umehara N, Kondo K, Osaka K, Aida J. The deterioration of oral function and orofacial appearance mediated the relationship between tooth loss and depression among community-dwelling older adults: a JAGES cohort study using causal mediation analysis. J Affect Disord. 2021;286:174–9.

Kusama T, Nakazawa N, Kiuchi S, Kondo K, Osaka K, Aida J. Dental prosthetic treatment reduced the risk of weight loss among older adults with tooth loss. J Am Geriatr Soc. 2021;69:2498–506.

Käyser AF. Teeth, tooth loss and prosthetic appliances. In: Öwall B, Käyser AF, Carlsson GE. Prosthodontics: principles and management strategies. London: Mosby-Wolfe; 1996.

Mack F, Schwahn C, Feine JS, Mundt T, Bernhardt O, John U, Kocher PT, Biffar R. The impact of tooth loss on general health related to quality of life among elderly Pomeranians: results from the study of health in Pomerania (SHIP-O). Int J Prosthodont. 2005;18:414–9.

Manabe K, Tanji F, Tomata Y, Zhang S, Tsuji I. Preventive effect of oral self-care on pneumonia death among the elderly with tooth loss: the Ohsaki cohort 2006 study. Tohoku J Exp Med. 2019;247:251–7.

Matsuyama S, Lu Y, Aida J, Tanji F, Tsuji I. Association between number of remaining teeth and healthy aging in Japanese older people: the Ohsaki cohort 2006 study. Geriatr Gerontol Int. 2022;22:68–74.

Musacchio E, Binotto P, Perissinotto E, Sergi G, Zambon S, Corti MC, Frigo AC, Sartori L. Tooth retention predicts good physical performance in older adults. PLoS One. 2021;16:e0255741.

Naka O, Anastassiadou V, Pissiotis A. Association between functional tooth units and chewing ability in older adults: a systematic review. Gerodontology. 2014;31:166–77.

Nascimento GG, Leite FRM, Conceição DA, Ferrúa CP, Singh A, Demarco FF. Is there a relationship between obesity and tooth loss and edentulism? A systematic review and meta-analysis. Obes Rev. 2016;17:587–98.

Okoro CA, Strine TW, Eke PI, Dhingra SS, Balluz LS. The association between depression and anxiety and use of oral health services and tooth loss. Community Dent Oral Epidemiol. 2012;40:134–44.

Österberg T, Dey DK, Sundh V, Carlsson GE, Jansson JO, Mellström D. Edentulism associated with obesity: a study of four national surveys of 16 416 Swedes aged 55-84 years. Acta Odontol Scand. 2010;68:360–7.

Qi X, Zhu Z, Plassman BL, Wu B. Dose-response meta-analysis on tooth loss with the risk of cognitive impairment and dementia. J Am Med Dir Assoc. 2021;22:2039–45.

Schmalz G, Bartl M, Schmickler J, Patschan S, Patschan D, Ziebolz D. Tooth loss is associated with disease-related parameters in patients with rheumatoid arthri-

tis and ankylosing spondylitis-a cross-sectional study. J Clin Med. 2021;10:3052.
Seitz MW, Listl S, Bartols A, Schubert I, Blaschke K, Haux C, Van Der Zande MM. Current knowledge on correlations between highly prevalent dental conditions and chronic diseases: an umbrella review. Prev Chronic Dis. 2019;16:E132.
Stolzenberg-Solomon RZ, Dodd KW, Blaser MJ, Virtamo J, Taylor PR, Albanes D. Tooth loss, pancreatic cancer, and helicobacter pylori. Am J Clin Nutr. 2003;78:176–81.
Sülün T, Şakar O, Bilhan H, İspirgil E. The effect of mandibular anterior teeth on the hypermobile tissue in the anterior part of the maxilla. Arch Gerontol Geriatr. 2012;55:12–5.
Takeda M, Matsuda Y, Ikebuchi K, Takeda M, Abe T, Tominaga K, Isomura M, Nabika T, Kanno T. Relationship between oral health status and bone mineral density in community-dwelling elderly individuals: a cross-sectional study. Healthcare (Basel). 2021;9:432.
Tan WL, Wong TLT, Wong MCM, Lang NP. A systematic review of postextractional alveolar hard and soft tissue dimensional changes in humans. Clin Oral Implants Res. 2012;23(suppl 5):1–21.
Techapiroontong S, Limpuangthip N, Tumrasvin W, Sirotamarat J. The impact of poor dental status and removable dental prosthesis quality on body composition, masticatory performance and oral health-related quality of life: a cross-sectional study in older adults. BMC Oral Health. 2022;22:147.
The glossary of prosthodontic terms: ninth edition. J Prosthet Dent. 2017;117(5S):e1–e105.
Van der Weijden F, Dell'Acqua F, Slot DE. Alveolar bone dimensional changes of post-extraction sockets in humans: a systematic review. J Clin Periodontol. 2009;36:1048–58.
World Health Organization. Global oral health status report: towards universal health coverage for oral health by 2030. Geneva: World Health Organization; 2022. Licence: CC BY-NC-SA 3.0 IGO.

Classification of Partially Edentulous Arches

3

Olcay Şakar

Abstract

Classification of partially edentulous arches is vital to ensure effective communication between dental professionals and to discuss the most suitable treatment plan for patients. Partially edentulous arches have been classified according to several methods. The Kennedy classification proposed by Dr. E. Kennedy is the most widely accepted and used classification method due to its simplicity and ease of application, with nearly 65,000 possible combinations of partially edentulous arches. Although this system does not give information about the condition of the teeth and periodontal tissues, it allows easy visualization of the arches, differentiates between free-end and tooth-bounded partially edentulous arches, and gives a logical approach to design. Therefore, only Kennedy classification is described in this book. In addition, a classification system (Implant-Corrected Kennedy/ICK) for partially edentulous arches incorporating implants placed or to be placed for a removable partial denture (RPD) is described and used. It is proposed by Al-Johany SS. and Andres C. and based, with modifications, on the Kennedy classification system.

O. Şakar (✉)
Faculty of Dentistry, Department of Prosthodontics, İstanbul University, İstanbul, Türkiye
e-mail: osakar@istanbul.edu.tr

3.1 Kennedy Classification

Partially edentulous arches are divided into four classes:

Class I: Bilateral edentulous areas located posterior to the remaining natural teeth (Fig. 3.1).

Class II: Unilateral edentulous area located posterior to the remaining natural teeth (Fig. 3.2).

Class III: A unilateral edentulous area with natural teeth both anteriorly and posteriorly (Fig. 3.3).

Class IV: A single but bilateral (crossing the midline) edentulous area anterior to the remaining natural teeth (Fig. 3.4).

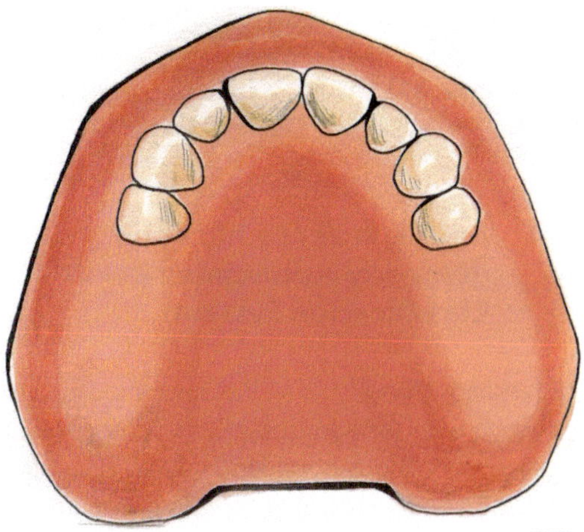

Fig. 3.1 Kennedy Class I

O. Şakar (ed.), *Removable Partial Dentures*, https://doi.org/10.1007/978-3-031-47083-7_3

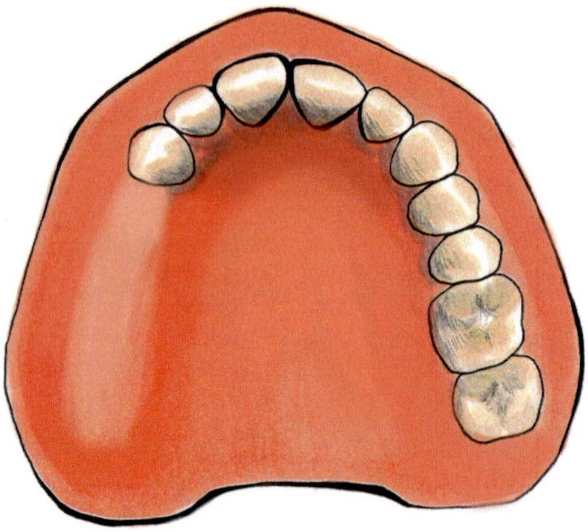

Fig. 3.2 Kennedy Class II

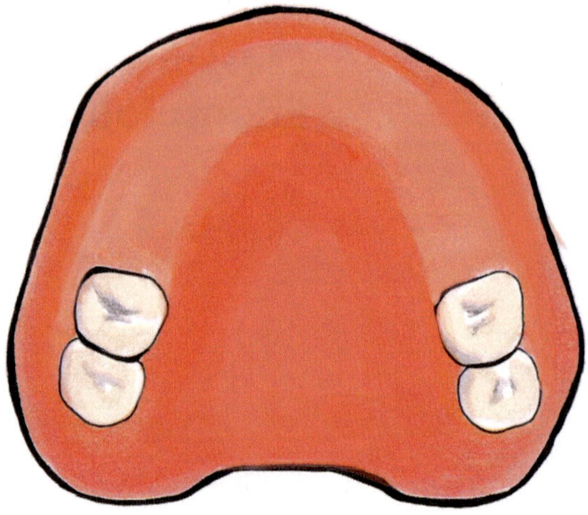

Fig. 3.4 Kennedy Class IV

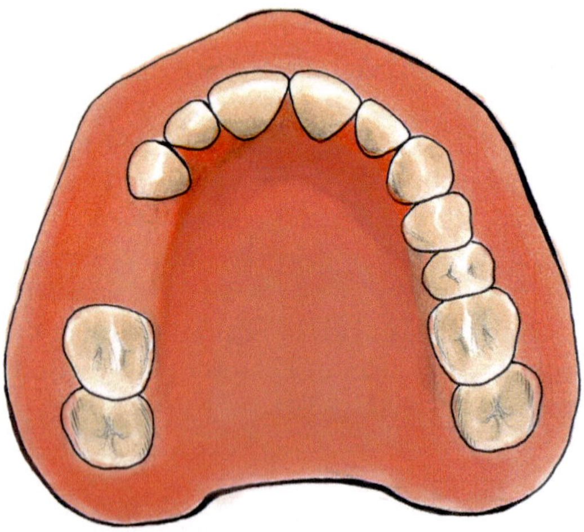

Fig. 3.3 Kennedy Class III, at the same time, this case can be named as Kennedy- Applegate Class VI according to Applegate's modification

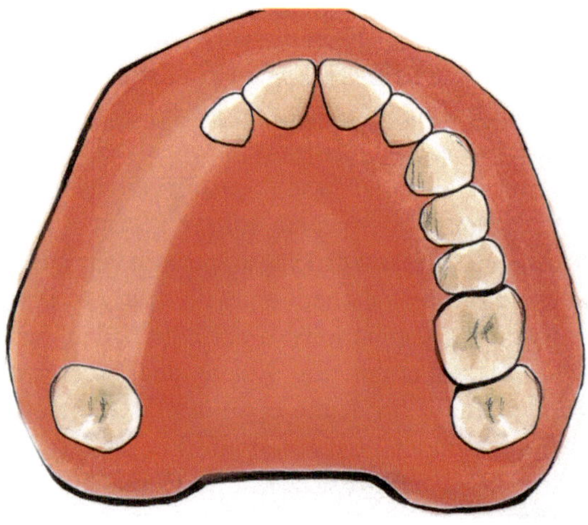

Fig. 3.5 Kennedy-Applegate Class V

3.1.1 Applegate's Modification (Kennedy-Applegate Classification System)

The Kennedy classification has been modified by Applegate with the addition of two more groups.

Class V: Tooth-bounded edentulous area where the anterior abutment is a weak abutment (e.g., lateral incisor) that is incapable of providing support for a conventional RPD and edentulous space is long (Fig. 3.5).

Class VI: Tooth-bounded edentulous area but restoration can be a fixed partial denture because the edentulous space is short and abutments are capable of providing support for a denture (Fig. 3.3).

3.1.2 Applegate's Rules

Certain rules have been provided by Applegate to govern the application of the Kennedy classification.

1. The classification should include only natural teeth involved in the definitive dentures and should follow rather than precede extraction (Classification is identified after extraction(s)).

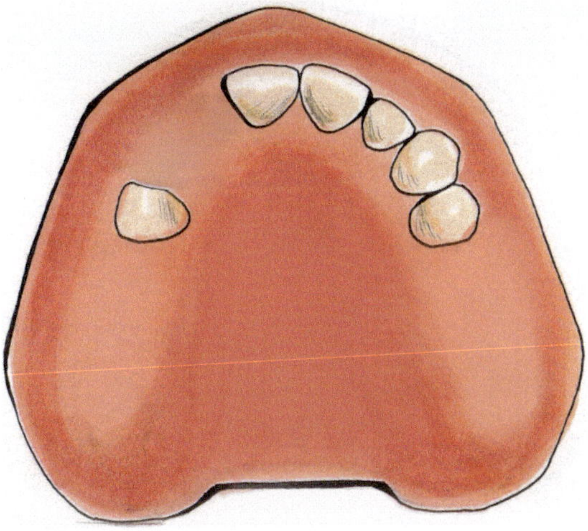

Fig. 3.6 Kennedy Class I, mod. 1

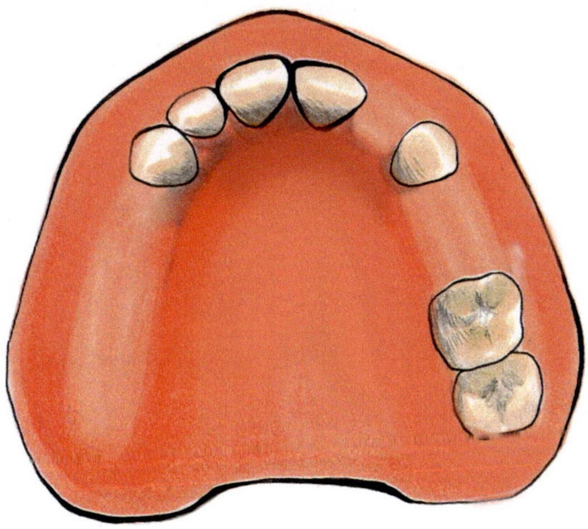

Fig. 3.7 Kennedy Class II, mod. 2

2. If the third and second molars are missing and not to be replaced, they are not considered in the classification.
3. The main classification is determined by the most posterior area (or areas).
4. Edentulous areas other than those determining classification are called "modification" and the number of modification spaces is considered, not their extent (Figs. 3.6, 3.7, and 3.8).
5. Modification spaces can be included in Class I, II, and III. Class IV can have no modification.

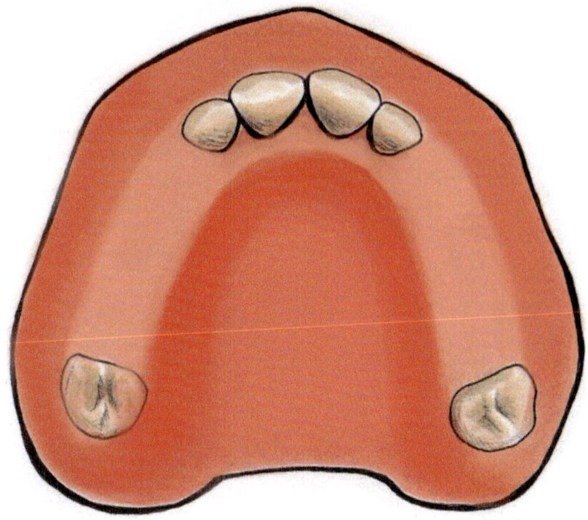

Fig. 3.8 Kennedy Class III, mod.1

3.2 Implant-Corrected Kennedy Classification System

The new classification system was named the Implant-Corrected Kennedy (ICK) Classification System to be differentiated from other partially edentulous arch classification systems.

This system is used with the following guidelines:

1. If the edentulous space needs to be restored with an implant-supported fixed partial denture, it is not included in the classification.
2. The maxillary arch is drawn as a half circle facing up and the mandibular arch as a half circle facing down. The orientation of the drawing is "doctor's view," so the left and right sides correspond to the patient's right and left, respectively.
3. The classification begins with the phrase "Implant-Corrected Kennedy (class)," followed by the description of the classification. It is abbreviated as follows:
   (a) ICK I, for Kennedy Class I situations (Fig. 3.9),
   (b) ICK II, for Kennedy Class II situations (Fig. 3.10),
   (c) ICK III, for Kennedy Class III situations (Fig. 3.11), and
   (d) ICK IV, for Kennedy Class IV situations (Fig. 3.12).

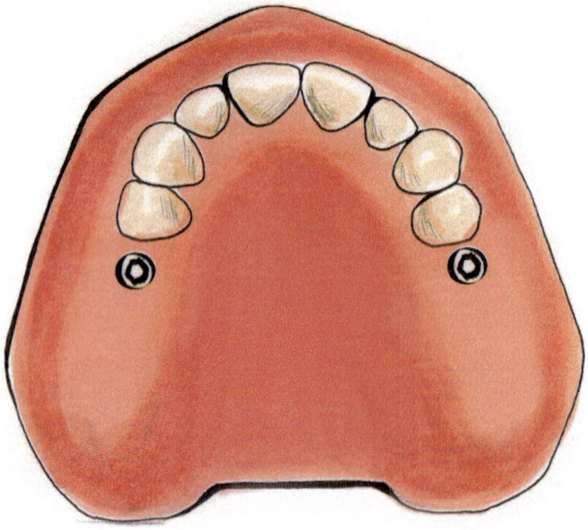

Fig. 3.9 ICK I (#15, 25)

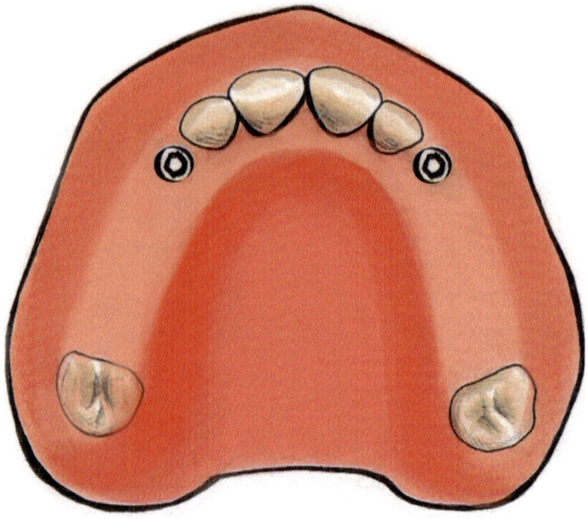

Fig. 3.11 ICK III mod 1 (#13, 23)

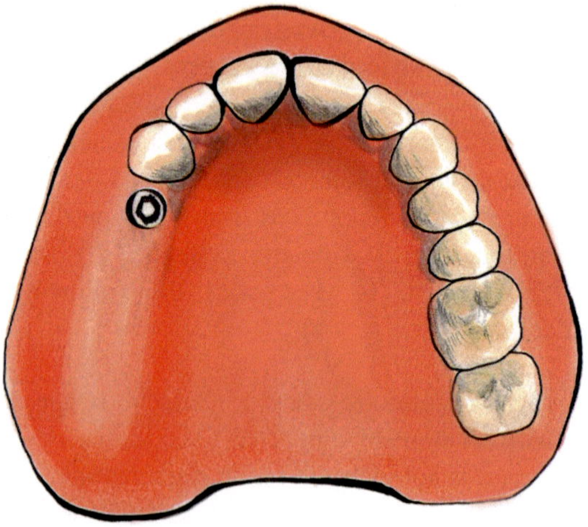

Fig. 3.10 ICK II (#14)

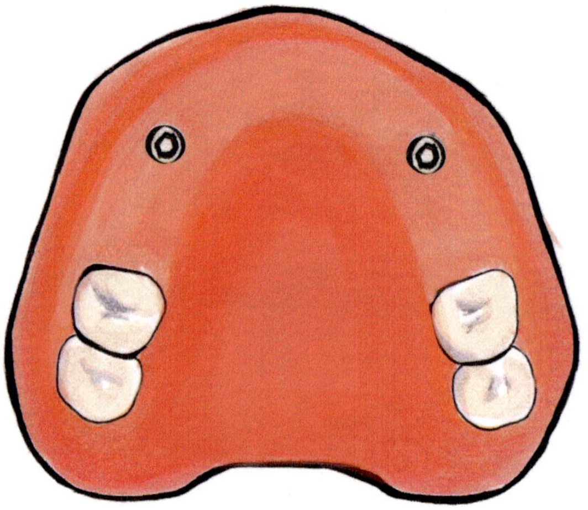

Fig. 3.12 ICK IV (#13, 23)

4. The abbreviation “max” for maxillary and “man” for mandibular can precede the classification.
5. The word “modification” is abbreviated as “mod” and follows the abbreviation of “ICK”.
6. Roman numerals are used for the classification, and Arabic numerals are used for the number of modification spaces and implants.
7. All tooth numbering systems can be used to give the number and exact position of the implant in the arch. The “Fédération Dentaire Internationale (FDI)” system is used in this book.
8. The classification is presented according to the following order:
   (a) The abbreviation of maxilla or mandible as “max” and “man”, respectively, where the drawing is absent.
   (b) Main classification.
   (c) The number of modification spaces as “mod”.
   (d) The number of implants in parentheses according to their position in the arch (according to the FDI numbering system) preceded by the number sign (#) (e.g., ICK I mod. 2 (# 16, 27).

9. The classification can be used both before and after placement of implants to discuss the treatment plan or to indicate the number and position of implants to be placed for implant-assisted RPDs.

Further Reading

Al-Johany SS, Andres C. ICK classification system for partially edentulous arches. J Prosthodont. 2008;17:502–7.

Applegate O. Essentials of removable partial denture prostheses. 1st ed. Philadelphia, PA: Saunders; 1954.

Galagali G, Mahoorkar S. Critical evaluation of classification systems of partially edentulous arches. Int J Dent Clin. 2010;2:45–52.

Kennedy E. Partial denture construction. Dent Items Interest. 1928;1:3–8.

Miller EL. Systems for classifying partially dentulous arches. J Prosthet Dent. 1970;24:25–40.

Nallaswamy D. Textbook of prosthodontics. 1st ed. New Delhi: Jaypee Brothers Medical Publishers Ltd; 2003.

Shifman A, Ben-Ur Z. Prosthodontic treatment for the Applegate-Kennedy class V partially edentulous patient. J Prosthet Dent. 1996;76:212–8.

The glossary of prosthodontic terms: ninth edition. J Prosthet Dent. 2017;117(5S):e1–e105.

Part II

Treatment Planning, Mouth Preparation and Impression Procedures

Biomechanics of Removable Partial Dentures

4

Canan Bural Alan

Abstract

Biomechanics is the study of the structure and function of biological systems by means of mechanics. Functional mandibular movement is defined as all the normal, proper, or characteristic of three-dimensional movements of the mandible during speech, mastication, swallowing, and other associated movements. Most functional movement occurs during mastication and speech. A removable partial denture (RPD) is not rigidly attached to the teeth, and therefore, there is a potential for movement of the denture when these functional movements create forces on the teeth and denture. The practitioner should begin with the understanding of how these three-dimensional functional forces (mechanics) act on the biological environment (abutment teeth, residual ridges, and alveolar mucosa). During treatment planning of the RPD, the clinician must also consider the biomechanical behavior of the RPD as well as providing patient's comfort, esthetics, and the prognosis of the abutments to withstand the functional forces.

C. Bural Alan (✉)
Faculty of Dentistry, Department of Prosthodontics, İstanbul University, İstanbul, Türkiye
e-mail: cbural@istanbul.edu.tr

4.1 Definitions

Abutment: 1. That part of a structure that directly receives thrust or pressure; an anchorage 2: a tooth, a portion of a tooth, or that portion of a dental implant that serves to support and/or retain a prosthesis.

Biomechanics: 1. The application of mechanical laws to living structures, specifically the locomotor systems of the body **2:** the study of biology from the functional viewpoint **3:** an application of the principles of engineering design as implemented in living organisms.

Dental biomechanics: The relationship between the biologic behavior of oral structures and the physical influence of a dental restoration.

Denture supporting structures: The tissues (teeth and/or residual ridges) that serve as the foundation for removable partial or complete dentures.

Fulcrum line: 1. A theoretical line passing through the point around which a lever functions and at right angles to its path of movement **2:** an imaginary line, connecting occlusal rests, around which a partial removable dental prosthesis tends to rotate under masticatory forces the determinants for the fulcrum line are usually the cross arch occlusal rests located adjacent to the tissue borne components.

Fulcrum line of a removable dental prosthesis: A theoretical line around which a removable dental prosthesis tends to rotate.

O. Şakar (ed.), *Removable Partial Dentures*, https://doi.org/10.1007/978-3-031-47083-7_4

Rotation: 1. The action or process of rotating on a mechanical center or on an axis. **2**: the movement of a rigid body in which the parts move in circular paths with their centers on a fixed line called the axis of rotation the plane of the circle in which the body moves is perpendicular to the axis of rotation.

Stress: Force per unit area; a force exerted on one body that presses on, pulls on, pushes against, or tends to invest or compress another body; an internal force that resists an externally applied load or force; it is normally defined in terms of mechanical stress, which is the force divided by the perpendicular cross sectional area over which the force is applied.

Biomechanics is the study of the structure and function of biological systems by means of mechanics. Functional mandibular movement is defined as all the normal, proper, or characteristic of three-dimensional movements of the mandible during speech, mastication, swallowing, and other associated movements. Most functional movement occurs during mastication and speech. A removable partial denture (RPD) is not rigidly attached to the teeth, and therefore, there is a potential for movement of the denture when these functional movements create forces on the teeth and denture. The practitioner should begin with the understanding of how these three-dimensional functional forces (mechanics) act on the biological environment (abutment teeth, residual ridges, and alveolar mucosa). During treatment planning of the RPD, the clinician must consider the biomechanics of the RPD as well as the patient's comfort, esthetics, and the prognosis of the abutments to withstand the forces.

4.2 Understanding Biomechanical Aspects

The functional forces acting on the oral cavity are to be considered in terms of direction, duration, frequency, and magnitude. The abutment teeth and the residual alveolar ridges are the supporting structures that are subjected to these functional forces. When considering the biomechanical aspects of the treatment planning of the RPD, the clinician should criticize the resistance capacity of the supporting structures against the functional forces.

4.2.1 Rotational Movement

The mastication is not merely a vertically oriented function and occurs in three dimensions. Although it seems that the food is vertically chewed, the mastication occurs on the sloped cusps or planes; therefore, the resultant forces that cause the RPD to potentially move are the combination of the forces that occur in multiple planes. The magnitude and the loading direction of the multiple vectors and the possible movement of the RPD should be taken into consideration when designing RPD. It is not possible to completely prevent the movement of the RPD, but it is possible to minimize the possible movement during RPD design planning so that the remaining teeth and the tissues would be least affected by the functional forces and their vectors.

Movement in the human body can occur in any of three planes

1. Sagittal plane.
2. Frontal plane.
3. Horizontal plane.

The potential movement of the RPD may occur in any of these planes, which intersect each other at right angles and the intersection of any two planes forms a linear axis. These axes are:

1. Horizontal axis.
2. Vertical axis.
3. Sagittal axis.

The RPD rotates around any of the three axes within a plane that is perpendicular to that axis.

4.2.1.1 Rotational Movement in the Sagittal Plane Around the Horizontal Fulcrum Line

A horizontal fulcrum line will extend through the rests on the most distally placed abutment teeth and the rotational movement will be around the mediolateral axis, which will cause the distal

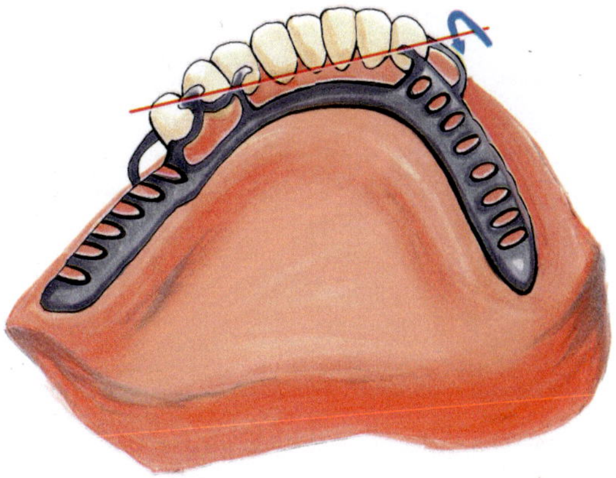

Fig. 4.1 A horizontal fulcrum line will extend through the rests on the most distally placed abutment teeth and the rotational movement will be around the mediolateral axis, which will cause the distal extension move away or towards the tissue in the sagittal plane. This fulcrum line is called as the principal fulcrum line. The resultant force on the abutment tooth due to the rotational movement is mesioapically or distoapically directed

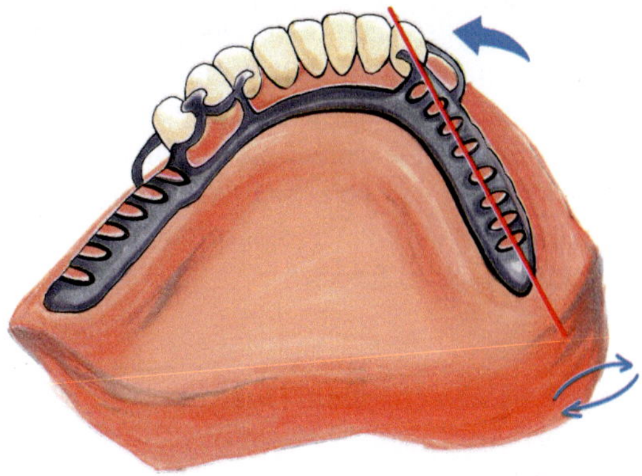

Fig. 4.2 An anteroposterior horizontal fulcrum line will extend through the one of the rest on the most distal abutment tooth to the edentulous ridge on one side of the dental arch. The rotational movement around the anteroposterior rotational axis will cause the denture to dislodge or flip from one side to the other in the frontal plane. The resultant force on the abutment tooth due to the rotational movement is mostly horizontally directed

extension to move away or toward the tissue in the sagittal plane. This fulcrum line is called the principal fulcrum line. The resultant force on the abutment tooth due to the rotational movement is mesioapically or distoapically directed (Fig. 4.1).

4.2.1.2 Rotational Movement in the Frontal Plane Around the Anteroposterior Horizontal Fulcrum Line

An anteroposterior horizontal fulcrum line will extend through one of the rest on the most distal abutment tooth to the edentulous ridge on one side of the dental arch. The rotational movement around the anteroposterior rotational axis will cause the denture to dislodge or flip from one side to the other in the frontal plane. In bilaterally distal extension cases, there will be two anteroposterior horizontal fulcrum lines. The resultant force on the abutment tooth due to the rotational movement is mostly horizontally directed (Fig. 4.2).

4.2.1.3 Rotational Movement in the Horizontal Plane around the Vertical Fulcrum Line

The third fulcrum line is the vertically extending fulcrum line on the midline of the anterior teeth. This rotational movement around the vertical fulcrum line will also cause the denture to move relative to the edentulous alveolar ridge (mediolateral movement) in the horizontal plane (Fig. 4.3).

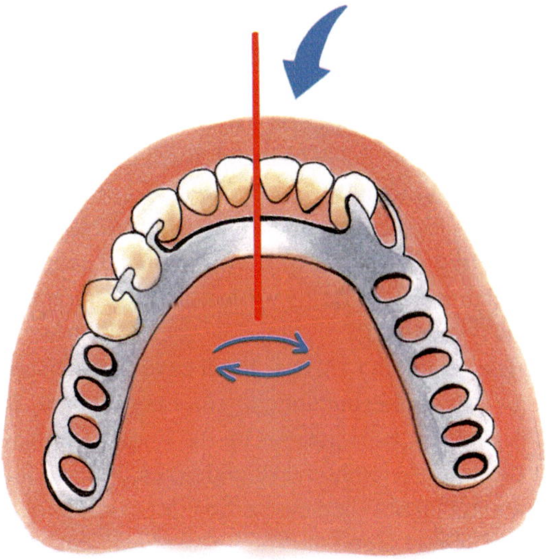

Fig. 4.3 The fulcrum line is the vertically extending fulcrum line on the midline of the anterior teeth. This rotational movement around the vertical fulcrum line will also cause the denture to move relative to the edentulous alveolar ridge (mediolateral movement) in the horizontal plane

Although these rotational movements and the resulting displacement of the RPD cannot be completely eliminated, minimum rotation as possible and minimum trauma to the supporting structures of the denture (abutment teeth and residual ridges) can be considered during treatment planning and RPD design solutions to avoid off-axially directed forces.

4.2.2 Biomechanical Design Principles

The design of the RPD necessitates the knowledge and the understanding of the working principles of two of the six simple machines, such as the lever, and the inclined plane may be helpful when designing an RPD to function properly under the functional forces.

4.2.2.1 The Inclined Plane

The inclined plane is simply a flat surface raised at an angle, like a ramp. The inclined plane can easily lift a load along the ramp that would be more difficult to lift the same amount of load straight up. The angle of the inclined plane determines the amount of effort that is needed to lift the load. The higher the angle, the more effort is required. The force of movement also exerts a lateral force both on the object and the inclined plane (Fig. 4.4).

The remaining anterior teeth have lingual surfaces, which are anatomically inclined shaped. If a lingual rest is positioned on the lingual surface of the anterior tooth, the sloped surface acts as an inclined plane. When the vertical force is applied to the object along the inclined plane, the two vectors of this force can cause the movement of the rest and a lateral force exertion on the tooth. A proper rest seat should be prepared to transmit the forces along the vertical axis of the teeth to prevent lateral forces. It would be better to prepare a cingulum rest seat on the lingual surface of the canine instead of anterior teeth, because canines are more resistant to the lateral forces because of its greater root surface. In clinical practice, a proper lingual or cingulum rest seat preparation on the lingual surfaces can be provided with the aid of a bonded composite resin (see Chap. 10).

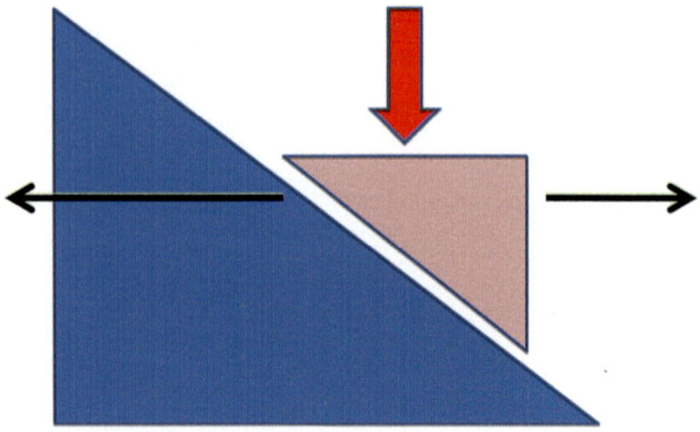

Fig. 4.4 The inclined plane. When an effort (occlusal load) is applied on the object (the occlusal rest), the object is moved along the plane (lingual surface of the abutment teeth). The angle of the inclined plane determines the amount of effort that is needed to lift the load. The higher the angle, the more effort is required. The force of movement also exerts a lateral force both on the object and the inclined plane

4.2.2.2 The Lever

A lever is a simple mechanical machine that consists of a rigid rod, which is pivoted at a fixed fulcrum. The lever rotates around the fulcrum and amplifies an input force (effort) to provide a greater output force (resistance), which is called the leverage. In terms of dental biomechanics, the denture rotates around a fulcrum when it is displaced from the basal seat. During the rotational movement, the resistance is provided by a direct retainer or a guiding plane surface, whereas the fulcrum is the tooth surface, such as an occlusal rest and the input force is the occlusal force or the gravity itself.

In mechanics, levers have three types according to the positions of the fulcrum, effort, and resistance forces. The function of the lever varies according to these three types.

In Class I lever, fulcrum is located in the middle in between the load and the exerted effort (Fig. 4.5). A typical seesaw movement occurs with this type of leverage. A pair of scissors is another example of Class I levers. Class I lever type is the most efficient lever when a great output force (resistance) load is to be lifted with little effort (occlusal effort).

In Kennedy Class I and II cases, Class I type lever is formed when a distoocclusal rest (fulcrum) is placed on the most distal abutment tooth with a circumferential clasp (resistance) (Fig. 4.6). When an occlusal load is applied on the extension base, the retentive tip of the circumferential clasp will move along the undercut area that will result in a distally tipping movement of the abutment tooth. With the great efficiency of the class I lever system, the higher torque will be applied on the abutment tooth with distoocclusal rest, which will negatively affect the prognosis of the abutment tooth. Another type of class I leverage formed in RPD design is to get support only from one tooth in one side of the arch that acts like a cantilever in Kennedy Class I and II cases. This design should always be avoided. To eliminate or reduce the possible torque on the abutment teeth, Class II type leverage system is to be formed during treatment planning.

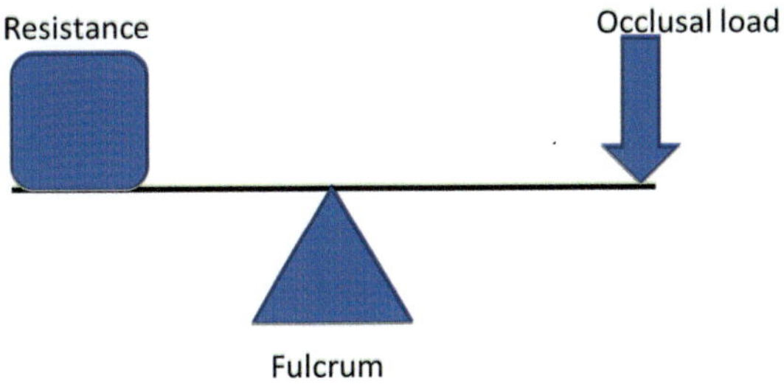

Fig. 4.5 Class I type leverage system. Fulcrum is located in the middle in between the load and the exerted effort

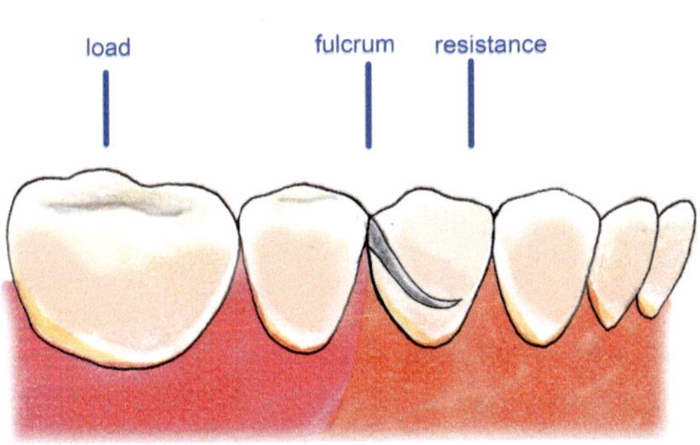

Fig. 4.6 In Kennedy Class I and II cases, Class I type leverage is formed when a distoocclusal rest (fulcrum) is placed on the most distal abutment tooth with a circumferential clasp (resistance)

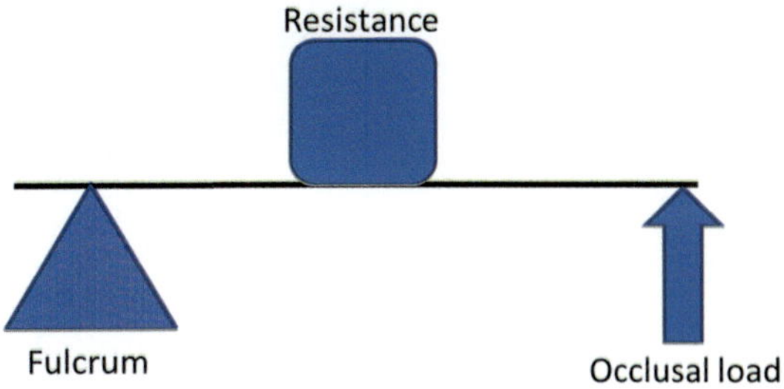

Fig. 4.7 Class II type leverage system. Resistance is positioned in the middle in between the fulcrum and the exerted effort

In Class II type lever, resistance is positioned in the middle in between the fulcrum and the exerted effort (Fig. 4.7). A wheelbarrow or a nutcracker is a typical example of this type of lever. With a less movement, Class II type lever is less efficient lever than Class I.

In Kennedy Class I and II cases, Class II type lever is formed when a mesioocclusal rest (fulcrum) is placed on the most distal abutment tooth with a bar clasp (resistance) under occlusal or gravitational forces (Fig. 4.8). In this design, the efficiency of the lever is reduced with the smaller movement of the extension base that will apply less torque on the abutment tooth.

In Class III levers, exerted effort is applied in the middle in between the fulcrum and the resistance (Fig. 4.9). The human mandible or tweezers are examples of Class III levers. Class III levers are the least efficient type of lever, where the movement is at a minimum with the same exerted force. Class III type lever system is formed in tooth-supported RPDs, where a disto-occlusal rest (fulcrum) is placed on the mesial abutment tooth and a circumferential clasp on the distal abutment tooth (Fig. 4.10).

4.2.2.3 Mechanical Advantage

The effectiveness of the lever is calculated by the mechanical advantage (MA) that is the ratio of the distance between the fulcrum and the load that is called the load arm (a) to the distance between the fulcrum and the resistance that is called the effort arm (b) (Fig. 4.11).

The greater the MA, the less effort is required to provide a bigger movement. Clinically speaking, in Kennedy Class I, II, and Kennedy IV class

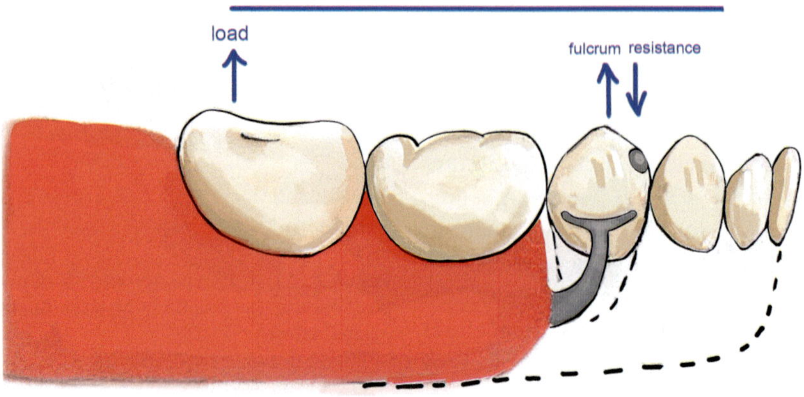

Fig. 4.8 In Kennedy Class I and II cases, Class II type lever is formed when a mesioocclusal rest (fulcrum) is placed on the most distal abutment tooth with a bar clasp (resistance) under occlusal or gravitational forces. In this design, the efficiency of the lever is reduced with the smaller movement of the extension base that will apply less torque on the abutment tooth

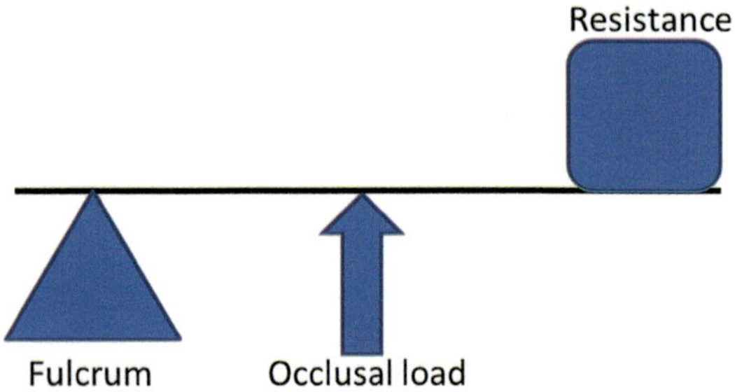

Fig. 4.9 Class III type leverage system. Exerted effort is applied in the middle in between the fulcrum and the resistance

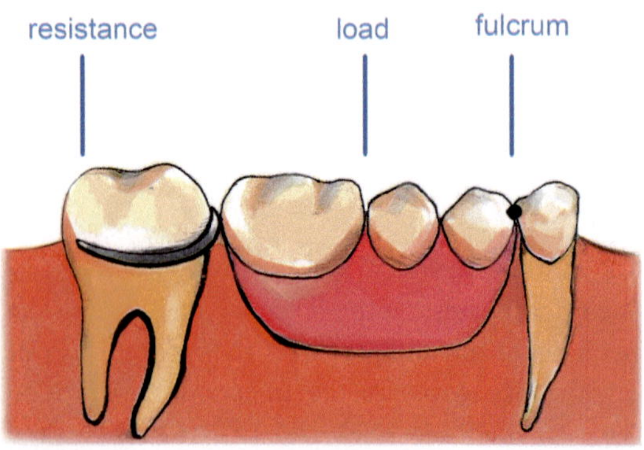

Fig. 4.10 In Kennedy Class III cases, Class III type lever system is formed, where a disto-occlusal rest (fulcrum) is placed on the mesial abutment tooth and a circumferential clasp on the distal abutment tooth

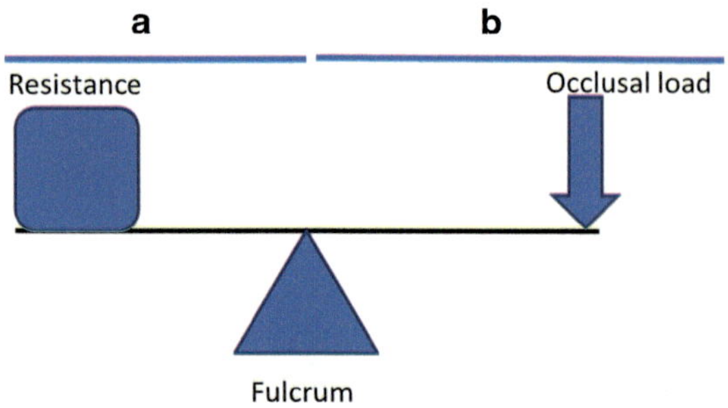

Fig. 4.11 The mechanical advantage is the ratio of the distance between the fulcrum and the effort that is called the effort arm (**a**) to the distance between the fulcrum and the load that is called the load arm (**b**). In Kennedy Class I, II and Kennedy IV class with long edentulous span cases, the mechanical advantage is the ratio of the distance between the rest and the edentulous span (**b**) to the distance between the rest and the retentive tip of the clasp (**a**). The greater the mechanical advantage, the longer the edentulous span and the greater displacement of the denture base (an undesirable condition for an RPD). The displacement of the denture is the result of a rotational movement of the RPD around the horizontal fulcrum line extending through the rests on the most distally placed abutment teeth

with long edentulous span cases, the MA is the ratio of the distance between the rest and the edentulous span (the most distal point of the denture base to the rest) to the distance between the rest and the retentive tip of the clasp. The greater the MA, the longer the edentulous span and the greater displacement of the denture base, which is an undesirable condition for an RPD. The displacement of the denture is the result of a rotational movement of the RPD around the horizontal fulcrum line extending through the rests on the most distally placed abutment teeth.

4.3 The Displacement of the Removable Partial Denture

Rotational movement causes the RPD to displace in two directions:

1. Movement toward the tissue.
2. Movement away from the tissue.

4.3.1 Movement Toward the Tissue

In Kennedy Class I and II cases, the rotational movement of the RPD is complex and dynamic. This rotational movement must be controlled but cannot be completely eliminated. In these cases, the denture rotates around the most distal abutment teeth. If the chewing force is applied on the denture base, the major connector and the retentive tip of the clasp will move in the opposite direction to provide a balance for Class I type lever, acting like a seesaw. The retentive tip of the clasp will move upwards along the survey line while the proximal part will move toward anterior. The movement of the clasp assembly will create torque on the abutment teeth, which are laterally subjected to the vectors of the forces. In other words, during the movement toward the tissue, the rest will act as a fulcrum and all the components of the RPD posterior to the rest (fulcrum) will move toward the tissue while all the components of the RPD anterior from the rest, including the tip of the direct retainer will move away from the tissue. The tip of the clasp in the undercut will apply lateral force to the abutment tooth. In addition, the lateral forces may also be compensated if an adjacent tooth contacting the abutment teeth at the mesial side is present. A Class II type leverage system is to be formed to minimize the displacing movement of the denture base. If a rest is placed on the mesial of the abutment teeth, Class II type lever is formed where the retentive tip of the direct retainer (resistance) is located in between the rest (fulcrum) and the chewing force. When the chewing force is applied on the denture base, the RPD rotates around the mesially positioned fulcrum. If a distoocclusal rest is placed on the most distally positioned abutment tooth, the greater displacement of the denture base should be expected due to Class I type leverage. This type of lever causes the denture base easily to displace, apply torque on the abutment teeth and cause possible traumatization on the residual ridges.

4.3.2 Movement Away from the Tissue

When a sticky food is consumed, the denture will tend to move away from the tissue (Fig. 4.12). During the movement of the RPD away from the tissue, the fulcrum line passes from the tips of the direct retainers but not the rests. In other words, all the components of the RPD posterior to the tip of the direct retainer (fulcrum) will move away from the tissue while all the components of the RPD anterior from the tip of the direct retainer will impinge to the tissue. To prevent the movement of the RPD away from the tissue, indirect retainers should be added to the RPD design so that the indirect retainer will act as a fulcrum and

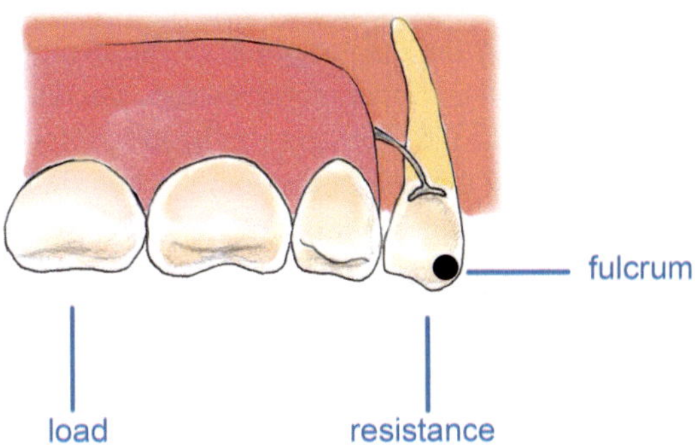

Fig. 4.12 When a sticky food is consumed, the denture will tend to move away from the tissue. During the movement of the RPD away from the tissue, the fulcrum line passes from the tips of the direct retainers but not the rests. All of the components of the RPD posterior to the tip of the direct retainer (fulcrum) will move away from the tissue while all the components of the RPD anterior from the tip of the direct retainer will impinge to the tissue

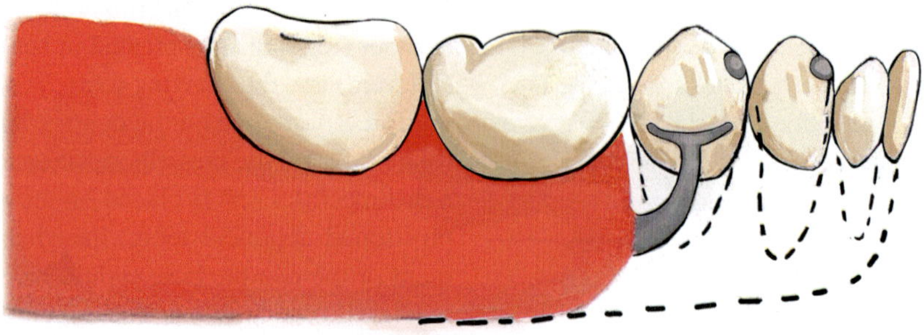

Fig. 4.13 To prevent the movement of the RPD away from the tissue, indirect retainers should be added to the RPD design so that the indirect retainer will act as a fulcrum and limit movement of the anterior part of the RPD by serving as a class II type leverage system. To balance the displacement of the denture base, indirect retainers should be positioned as much farther to the most distal abutment

limit movement of the anterior part of the RPD by serving as a class II type leverage system. To balance the displacement of the denture base, indirect retainers should be positioned as much farther to the most distal abutment (see Chap. 11) (Fig. 4.13).

In tooth-tissue supported cases, such as Kennedy Class I, II cases, and Kennedy IV classes with long edentulous span, forces will be transmitted to the edentulous soft tissue and the periodontal ligament of the abutment tooth. Because the soft tissue is more displaceable than the adjacent teeth, Class I type of levers should be converted to Class II and III types of levers by adding additional components, such as indirect retainers, placing posterior dental implants. In clinical practice, the choice of the altered cast impression technique may also be effective in the minimization of the displacement of the denture by increasing the support for the base, decreasing the forces on the abutment tooth, and protecting the gingival mucosa of the abutment tooth. In addition, maximum coverage of the soft tissues to distribute the forces is also effective in protecting the supporting structures. It should be noted that the ideal design of an RPD should focus on protecting both the abutment teeth and the residual ridge in an attempt to distribute the occlusal forces on them.

Class III type of lever is formed in tooth-supported Kennedy Class III and Kennedy Class IV with short-span classified cases. In tooth-supported cases, the rotational movement depends on the resiliency of the periodontal ligament. In tooth-supported RPDs, movement toward the tissue is primarily prevented by the rests on the abutment teeth. In these cases, the rigid portion of the framework and rigid component of the direct retainer are also helpful in the prevention of this movement. The movement of the tooth-supported RPDs away from the tissue is prevented by the action of direct retainers.

A biomechanically alternative solution to prevent the rotational movement of the RPD is to place dental implants to the distal extension sites so that the case can be converted from tooth-tissue-supported to implant-supported RPDs. The placement of the free-standing dental implant at the distal region of the edentulous ridge can prevent the rotational movement of the distally extended RPD and reduce the pressure on the edentulous molar region. To obtain maximal support and stability, the implant should be positioned as distally as possible for Kennedy I and II classes; while in Kennedy IV class partial edentulous cases implants should be located as medially as possible. The use of implant support in Kennedy III classes can only be considered in cases with extended edentulous span or with the need for the elimination of the undesirable appearance of the clasps. In these cases, the implants should be placed adjacent to the abutment teeth as much as possible. The use of stress-breaking attachments, such as ERA or locator attachmens has been suggested to protect the implants from excessive forces. It has also been reported that implant placement at the distal region of the mandibular edentulous ridge can prevent the displacement of the denture, regardless of the denture supporting area. This finding suggests that a shorter denture periphery with no need for maximal coverage of the edentulous ridge is not necessary for implant-assisted RPDs. Although this treatment modality could represent a low-cost, biomechanically beneficial approach with improved patient satisfaction for distal-extension RPDs, further studies are strictly needed to validate the clinical outcomes (see Chap. 17).

4.4 Factors that Are Related to the Force Transfer to the Abutment Teeth and the Residual Ridges

Stress transmitted to the abutment teeth and the residual ridges may cause clinical problems such as periodontal damage, irritation of the mucosa, and patient discomfort.

Pain-pressure threshold data for different regions of the oral mucosa indicates stresses in the range of 0.25 MPa in the buccal regions of the mandible and around 1 MPa in the palatal regions. The pressure-pain threshold limits the stress in patients wearing RPD during functional movements to protect the oral mucosa contacting the denture base from pain. In distally extending partial edentulous cases, basic biomechanical variables such as occlusal loading, rotational movements, and denture foundation area are key factors in preventing detrimental forces higher than the pain pressure threshold. It should be remembered that most of the RPD patients continue to wear their dentures despite discomfort and pain resulting in irreversible changes in alveolar bone and oral mucosa.

The understanding of the factors related to the stress transmission to the denture supporting structures is important for treatment planning for RPDs.

4.4.1 The Residual Ridge Support

Maximal support and well adaptation of the denture base in distal-extension RPDs are the most important clinical factors regarding the residual ridge support. The occlusal load on the RPD, especially in Kennedy Class I and II cases, is shared between the abutment teeth and the residual ridge. When compared to a fixed partial denture with a cantilever design, lower stress intensity with uniform stress distribution on the abutment teeth with the RPD is formed due to the shared loads between the residual ridge and the abutment teeth.

The resiliency of the abutment teeth and the edentulous mucosa has been the subject of many studies in the literature. The difference in resiliency causes a rotational displacement of the distal extension of the RPD around the most distal abutment teeth. The thickness and the resiliency of the edentulous mucosa play a role in the load transfer to the abutment teeth. A mucosal thickness of approximately 1 mm can bear a functional occlusal force while a thin, atrophic, or flabby characterized edentulous mucosa may not provide sufficient vertical support; thus increased displacement of the denture and stress transmission to the abutment teeth should be expected. It seems clinically important that functional impression techniques should be applied to reflect the resiliency of the supporting structures. A clinical study reported a 0.19 mm of vertical displacement, as being the lowest value, of the RPDs fabricated using the altered-cast impression technique compared to the impressions with border molded custom tray and a stock tray with irreversible hydrocolloid. The same trend was observed in another study that suggested no superior influence of the altered-cast impression technique that produced a 0.15 mm of discrepancy between the denture base and the mucosa. Nevertheless, the clinical significance of only a 0.15–0.19 mm difference in the vertical direction obtained with the altered-cast impression technique should be questioned.

Another factor related to the residual ridge support is the form of the alveolar ridges. Large, parallel-sided, broad-sectioned ridges can provide vertical ridge support than the thin, knife-edged, or resorbed ridges to resist lateral forces and thus the transmission of the lateral forces to the abutment teeth. In distally extended maxillary RPDs, large vertical movement of the maxillary denture base was also associated with a large buccal movement of the abutment tooth.

4.4.2 The Length of the Edentulous Span

The rotational movement of the denture base will lead to the transmission of the load to the abutment teeth. As mentioned above under the mechanical advantage title, as the edentulous span gets longer, the greater displacement of the denture base should be expected.

4.4.3 The Periodontal Support of the Abutment Teeth

An in-vivo 3D study showed that the force on the abutment teeth was lowered with wearing the RPD than without wearing the RPD. The resultant forces with both lateral and vertical vectors arising from the displacement of the denture will be applied on the abutment teeth. When it comes to the context of periodontal support to withstand the resultant forces, many periodontal considerations in addition to periodontal therapy should be evaluated by a prosthodontist. A 35% loss of periodontal support has been shown to increase the stress concentration in bilaterally distal extension maxillary RPDs. In a photoelastical study, it was shown that the highest stress concentrations were observed with the model that had the least periodontal support. In addition, fixed splinting of the distal abutment teeth was more pronounced when the amount of the periodontal support decreased. On the other hand, it was also reported that the number of the splinting was not directly proportional to the stress transmitted. However, it was also reported that when an additional tooth was splinted to the most distal two abutment teeth, the force was transmitted to the most distal abutment tooth more axially in a uniform distributed characteristic. Splinting more than three teeth around the arch may be beneficial as it can provide a curve for resistance for the buccolingual rotational movement. Although it is conventionally believed that the number of fixed splinted teeth will proportionally reduce the stress transmitted to the abutment teeth, the literature seems to be lacking evidence about the effect of splinting of abutment teeth either with normal or reduced periodontal support.

4.4.4 The Design of the Removable Partial Denture

The common material of choice in RPD framework has been chrome–cobalt alloy for a long time. With the introduction of commercially available alternative materials as well as new manufacturing techniques has led to new horizons in RPD framework studies. The design of the RPD has always been the subject of many studies regarding the biomechanics. Many previous studies suggested that the rigid major connectors can reduce the stress concentration on the abutment teeth and the residual ridges by distributing the occlusal forces across the denture arch and decreasing the load on the ipsilateral to the loading side. RPD designed with a highly rigid major connector is related to less deflection during function. The deflection of the denture results in unequal distribution of the stress in the underlying tissues and might cause inflammation and resorption of the residual ridge. Finite element analysis (FEA) studies have indicated that a cast metal framework RPD transferred the maximum amount of load to the terminal abutment, while the edentulous ridge and mucosa were secured with lower levels of stresses evident in the edentulous region. A recent 3D FEA study compared the stress distribution and load transfer created by cast metal and polyacetal resin-based flexible RPD and indicated 5 times more stress with the flexible polyacetal resin on the edentulous region while 9 times more stress on the abutment teeth with rigid cast RPD. Just the opposite to this finding, in a Kennedy class II mod 1 scenario, higher stress in the abutment teeth and on the residual ridge was observed with an RPD design with polyacetal resin framework (due to the non-rigid characteristics of the polyacetal resin) than an RPD design with a conventional cast metal framework. The same trend in stress distribution was observed in another study that reported the decreased movement of abutment teeth and denture base with the conventional cobalt–chrome framework than the metal-reinforced acrylic resin framework. These controversial findings need clinical assessments by directing randomized studies. The rigidity of the RPD design seems to positively affect the dynamics of the denture as a very well-known factor.

Although the use of mesial rests is a theoretically established point of view regarding the leverage effects, the findings of some studies indicated no superior advantage with mesial rests over distal rests. A FEA study indicated that a distally placed rest on the terminal abutment improved the stress distribution and stiffened the metal frameworks and acrylic resin denture bases by 66% when compared with the mesially placed rest. On the other hand, an RPD design without the rests turns up with the poor biomechanical results.

There is still no clear consensus about the ideal RPD design on the stress distribution to the abutment teeth and the residual ridge.

4.4.5 The Design of the Direct Retainer

The design of a direct retainer is considered an important factor on the force transmitted to the abutment teeth and the residual ridges.

The rigidity of the direct retainers has a significant effect on the transmission of the force to the abutment teeth and the vertical displacement of the RPD.

When compared to rigid designs of the distal-extension based RPD's, such as conical telescopic crowns, a wrought wire clasp conducts less stress to the abutment teeth while Akers type clasp is in the between of these two retainers in stress transmission. In a 6-month clinical follow-up, no significant changes were observed in the mobility of the abutment teeth with a T-clasp for unilateral and bilateral distal extension cases and cast circumferential clasp for tooth-supported cases. A clasp-retained design applies less torque on the abutment teeth than the intracoronal precision attachments. The reason for the reduction of the stress concentration on the residual ridges for the rigid design was related due to the transmission of the force along the long axis of the abutment teeth. Moreover, an RPI clasp design (with mesial rest seat and buccal I-bar) has been shown to produce less torque on the abutment teeth than the circumferential clasp. In addition, in experimental model studies, non-rigid wire clasp was found to have an association with an increased buccal movement of the abutment tooth than the rigid-designed retainers. A randomized clinical trial reported that there was no significant difference between the circumferential and bar clasps on the periodontal health of abutment teeth and success rates and maintenance of RPDs.

It seems that the rigid-type direct retainer is better for residual ridge maintenance with minimal need for tissue support. On the other hand, stress transfer to the abutment tooth seemed to increase with the rigidity of the direct retainer, showing that the stress-releasing type of direct retainer theory does not work.

These findings suggest the consideration of maintenance of the denture-supporting structures during treatment planning. It should be noted that further controlled clinical trials and randomized studies are required regarding the effect of the design of the direct retainer.

4.4.6 The Antagonist Dentition

The antagonist occluding forces acting on the denture base of the RPD may influence the load transmission to the abutment teeth. The amount of the load transferred varies from being intact to completely edentulous.

The findings of these studies suggest that if correct treatment planning is done with an understanding of the biomechanical aspects, high success rates and patient comfort should be expected with a well-constructed RPD with a logical design.

Further Reading

Akaltan F, Kaynak D. An evaluation of the effects of two distal extension removable partial denture designs on tooth stabilization and periodontal health. J Oral Rehabil. 2005;32:823–9.

Aridome K, Yamazaki M, Baba K, Ohyama T. Bending properties of strengthened Ti-6Al-7Nb alloy major connectors compared to Co-Cr alloy major connectors. J Prosthet Dent. 2005;93:267–73.

Berg T, Caputo AA. Maxillary distal-extension removable partial denture abutments with reduced periodontal support. J Prosthet Dent. 1993;70:245–50.

Bohnenkamp DM. Removable partial dentures: clinical concepts. Dent Clin N Am. 2014;58:69–89.

Budtz-Jorgensen E, Bochet G. Alternate framework designs for removable partial dentures. J Prosthet Dent. 1998;80:58–66.

Carr AB, Brown DT. McCracken's removable partial prosthodontics. 13th ed. St. Louis, MO: Elsevier; 2016.

Chou TM, Caputo AA, Moore DJ, Xiao B. Photoelastic analysis and comparison of force-transmission characteristics of intracoronal attachments with clasp distal-extension removable partial dentures. J Prosthet Dent. 1989;62:313–9.

Chou TM, Eick JD, Moore DJ, Tira DE. Stereophotogrammetric analysis of abutment tooth movement in distal-extension removable partial dentures with intracoronal attachments and clasps. J Prosthet Dent. 1991;66:343–9.

de Freitas RF, de Carvalho DK, da Fonte Porto Carreiro A, Barbosa GA, Ferreira MA. Mandibular implant-supported removable partial denture with distal extension: a systematic review. J Oral Rehabil. 2012;39:791–8.

DeBoer J. The effects on function of distal-extension removable partial dentures as determined by occlusal rest position. J Prosthet Dent. 1988;60:693–6.

Grossmann Y, Nissan J, Levin L. Clinical effectiveness of implant-supported removable partial dentures: a review of the literature and retrospective case evaluation. J Oral Maxillofac Surg. 2009;67:1941–6.

Hosman HJ. Influence of clasp design of distal extension removable partial dentures on the periodontium of the abutment teeth. Int J Prosthodont. 1990;3:256–65.

Igarashi Y, Ogata A, Kuroiwa A, Wang CH. Stress distribution and abutment tooth mobility of distal-extension removable partial dentures with different retainers: an in vivo study. J Oral Rehabil. 1999;26:111–6.

Itoh H, Baba K, Aridome K, Okada D, Tokuda A, Nishiyama A, Miura H, Igarashi Y. Effect of direct retainer and major connector designs on RPD and abutment tooth movement dynamics. J Oral Rehabil. 2008;35:810–5.

Itoh H, Caputo AA, Wylie R, Berg T. Effects of periodontal support and fixed splinting on load transfer by removable partial dentures. J Prosthet Dent. 1998;79:465–71.

Jiao T, Chang T, Caputo AA. Load transfer characteristics of unilateral distal extension removable partial dentures with polyacetal resin supporting components. Aust Dent J. 2009;54:31–7.

Jorge JH, Giampaolo ET, Vergani CE, Machado AL, Pavarina AC, Cardoso de Oliveira MR. Clinical evaluation of abutment teeth of removable partial denture by means of the Periotest method. J Oral Rehabil. 2007;34:222–7.

Kapur KK, Deupree R, Dent RJ, Hasse AL. A randomized clinical trial of two basic removable partial denture designs. Part I: comparisons of five-year success rates and periodontal health. J Prosthet Dent. 1994;72:268–82.

Kawata T, Kawaguchi T, Yoda N, Ogawa T, Kuriyagawa T, Sasaki K. Effects of a removable partial denture and its rest location on the forces exerted on an abutment tooth in vivo. Int J Prosthodont. 2008;21:50–2.

Kono K, Kurihara D, Suzuki Y, Ohkubo C. Pressure distribution of implant-supported removable partial dentures with stress-breaking attachments. J Prosthodont Res. 2014;58:115–20.

Kumar N, Koli DK, Jain V, Nanda A. Stress distribution and patient satisfaction in flexible and cast metal removable partial dentures: finite element analysis and randomized pilot study. J Oral Biol Craniofac Res. 2021;11:478–85.

Lee HE, Wu JH, Wang CH, Lan TH, Du JE. Biomechanical analysis of distal extension removable partial dentures with different retainers. J Dent Sci. 2008;3:133–9.

Leupold RJ, Flinton RJ, Pfeifer DL. Comparison of vertical movement occurring during loading of distal-extension removable partial denture bases made by three impression techniques. J Prosthet Dent. 1992;68:290–3.

Mousa MA, Abdullah JY, Jamayet NB, El-Anwar MI, Ganji KK, Alam MK, Husein A. Biomechanics in removable partial dentures: a literature review of FEA-based studies. Biomed Res Int. 2021;2021:5699962.

Ogata K, Miyake T, Okunishi M. Longitudinal study on occlusal force distribution in lower distal-extension removable partial dentures with circumferential clasps. J Oral Rehabil. 1992;19:585–94.

Petridis H, Hempton TJ. Periodontal considerations in removable partial denture treatment: a review of the literature. Int J Prosthodont. 2001;14:164–72.

Phoenix RD, Cagna DR, Defreest CF. Stewart's clinical removable partial prosthodontics. 4th ed. Chicago: Quintessence Publishing; 2008.

Ramakrishnan AN, Röhrle O, Ludtka C, Varghese R, Koehler J, Kiesow A, Schwan S. Numerical study of the stress state on the oral mucosa and abutment tooth upon insertion of partial dentures in the mandible. Int J Numer Method Biomed Eng. 2022;38:e3604.

Sahin V, Akaltan F, Parnas L. Effects of the type and rigidity of the retainer and the number of abutting teeth on stress distribution of telescopic-retained removable partial dentures. J Dent Sci. 2012;7:7–13.

Sato M, Suzuki Y, Kurihara D, Shimpo H, Ohkubo C. Effect of implant support on mandibular distal extension removable partial dentures: relationship between denture supporting area and stress distribution. J Prosthodont Res. 2013;57:109–12.

Taylor DT, Pflughoeft FA, McGivney GP. Effect of two clasping assemblies on arch integrity as modified by base adaptation. J Prosthet Dent. 1982;47:120–5.

Tebrock OC, Rohen RM, Fenster RK, Pelleu GB Jr. The effect of various clasping systems on the mobility of abutment teeth for distal-extension removable partial dentures. J Prosthet Dent. 1979;41:511–6.

The glossary of prosthodontic terms: ninth edition. J Prosthet Dent. 2017;117(5S):e1–e105.

Wismeijer D, Tawse-Smith A, Payne AG. Multicentre prospective evaluation of implant-assisted mandibular bilateral distal extension removable partial dentures: patient satisfaction. Clin Oral Implants Res. 2013;24:20–7.

Diagnosis and Treatment Planning in Partially Edentulous Patients

5

Tonguç Sülün and Olcay Şakar

Abstract

Diagnosis and treatment planning in partially edentulous patients is a complex process that involves evaluating the patient's dental and medical history, performing a thorough clinical examination, and assessing the patient's functional and esthetic needs. This process requires the dentist to consider various treatment options, such as removable or fixed partial dentures, implant-supported restorations, or combinations of these approaches. The ultimate goal is to restore the patient's ability to chew, speak, and smile with confidence while maintaining the health and integrity of the remaining dentition. A successful diagnosis and treatment plan requires close collaboration between the patient and the dental team, as well as careful consideration of the patient's financial and psychological factors.

5.1 Definitions

Canine protected articulation: A form of mutually protected articulation in which the vertical and horizontal overlap of the canine teeth disclude the posterior teeth in the excursive movements of the mandible; (synonym, **anterior protected articulation**, **canine guidance**)

Centric relation: A maxillomandibular relationship, independent of tooth contact, in which the condyles articulate in the anterior-superior position against the posterior slopes of the articular eminences; in this position, the mandible is restricted to a purely rotary movement; from this unstrained, physiologic, maxillomandibular relationship, the patient can make vertical, lateral or protrusive movements; it is a clinically useful, repeatable reference position.

Centric stop: Opposing cuspal/fossae contacts that maintain the occlusal vertical dimension between the opposing arches.

Contralateral: Occurring on or acting in conjunction with similar parts on an opposite side.

Cross-arch stabilization: Resistance against dislodging or rotational forces obtained by using a partial removable dental prosthesis design that uses natural teeth on the opposite side of the dental arch from the edentulous space to assist in stabilization.

Definitive cast: A replica of the tooth surfaces, residual ridge areas, and/or other parts of the dental arch and/or facial structures used to fabricate a dental restoration or prosthesis; (synonym, **final cast, master cast**)

Deflective occlusal contact: A contact that displaces a tooth, diverts the mandible from its intended movement or displaces a removable

T. Sülün (✉)
Faculty of Dentistry Department of Prosthodontics, İstanbul University, İstanbul, Türkiye
e-mail: tsulun@istanbul.edu.tr

O. Şakar (✉)
Faculty of Dentistry Department of Prosthodontics, İstanbul University, İstanbul, Türkiye
e-mail: osakar@istanbul.edu.tr

O. Şakar (ed.), *Removable Partial Dentures*, https://doi.org/10.1007/978-3-031-47083-7_5

denture from its basal seat; (synonym, **premature contact**).

Diagnostic cast: A life-size reproduction of a part or parts of the oral cavity and/or facial structures for the purpose of study and treatment planning.

Eccentric interocclusal record: A registration of any maxillomandibular position other than centric relation.

Group function: Multiple contact relations between the maxillary and mandibular teeth in lateral movements on the working side whereby simultaneous contact of several teeth acts as a group to distribute occlusal forces.

Interim prosthesis: A fixed or removable dental prosthesis, or maxillofacial prosthesis, designed to enhance esthetics, stabilization and/or function for a limited period of time, after which it is to be replaced by a definitive dental or maxillofacial prosthesis. Often such prostheses are used to assist in determination of the therapeutic effectiveness of a specific treatment plan or the form and function of the planned for definitive prosthesis.

Laterotrusion: Condylar movement on the working side in the horizontal plane. This term may be used in combination with terms describing condylar movement in other planes, for example, laterodetrusion, lateroprotrusion, lateroretrusion, and laterosurtrusion.

Maximal intercuspal position: The complete intercuspation of the opposing teeth independent of condylar position, sometimes referred to as the best fit of the teeth regardless of the condylar position; comp, centric occlusion.

Mediotrusion: A movement of the condyle medially.

Mounting: (1) The laboratory procedure of attaching a cast to an articulator or cast relater. (2) The relationship of dental casts to each other and the instrument to which they are attached.

Nonworking side: That side of the mandible that moves toward the medial line in a lateral excursion. The condyle on that side is referred to as the nonworking side condyle.

Occlusal reshaping: Any change in the occlusion intended to alter the occlusal surfaces of the teeth or restorations to change their form; (synonym, **occlusal adjustment, selective grinding**).

Occlusal analysis: A systematic examination of the occlusion with special consideration to the interocclusal relations of mounted casts.

Preliminary cast: A cast formed from a preliminary mpression for use in diagnosis and/or the fabrication of a custom impression tray (synonym, **study cast**).

Retrusion: Movement toward the posterior.

Shortened dental arch: Having an intact anterior region but a reduced number of occluding pairs of posterior teeth or a dentition with a reduction of teeth starting posteriorly.

Splint: (1) A rigid or flexible device that maintains in position a displaced or movable part; also used to keep in place and protect an injured. (2) A rigid or flexible material used to protect, immobilize, or restrict motion in a part.

Supraeruption: Movement of a tooth or teeth, along with the tooth-supporting structures, in discontinuity with the normal occlusal plane.

Supporting cusps: Those cusps of teeth that contact in and support maximal intercuspal position; usually facial cusps of the mandibular posterior teeth and the maxillary palatal cusps.

Syneresis: The separation of water from its component base, for example, a gel or impression material.

Working side: The side toward which the mandible moves in a lateral excursion.

Patients generally visit a dental office not to receive a removable partial denture (RPD) but to resolve the functional and/or esthetic problems or pain. Thus, the primary challenge of the clinician is to understand the needs and the expectations of the patient. In order to obtain a unique treatment plan, evaluation of the patient's medical and dental history, financial capability, behavioral and socioeconomic profiles, a full-mouth series of periapical and panaromical radiographs, a complete clinical examination and proper diagnostic casts that have been transferred to a semi-adjustable articulator using face bow (when necessary) and interocclusal records are required (Fig. 5.1a–e).

However dental students and new graduates often find it extremely difficult to register the assembled diagnostic data for patients with complex problems and develop a logical treatment plan that will correspond to the patient's

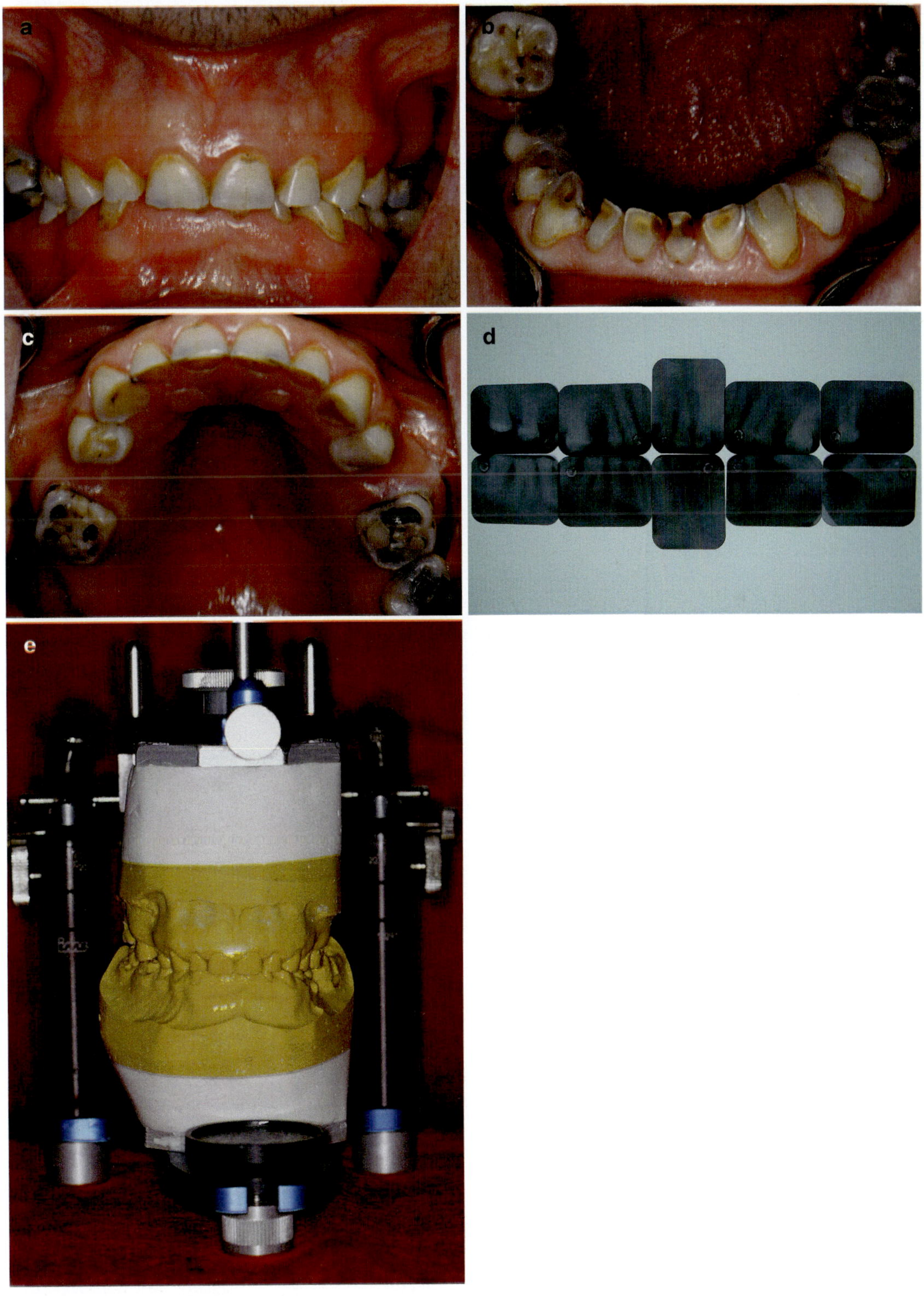

Fig. 5.1 (**a**) A patient with severely worn dentition in maximal intercuspal position. (**b**) Occlusal view of the mandibular arch. (**c**) Occlusal view of the maxillary arch. (**d**) The periapical radiographs of the patient. (**e**) The diagnostic casts are mounted to a semi-adjustable articulator

needs. This is a very well-known story: an extremely supraerupted tooth of a partially edentulous patient is treated endodontically and periodontally, followed by a metal-ceramic restoration that is made, all in order to receive a final RPD. The above-mentioned clinical procedures take too much time and money, yet at the end when designing an RPD, it is "surprisingly" observed that the tooth could not be used as an abutment for the prosthesis. Needless to say, all the pretreatment stages applied to the patient turned out to be unnecessary. This tooth had to be extracted in the first place. Such a situation is very disappointing for the patient and a waste of time and money for both the doctor and the patient. Therefore, the treatment plan and decision-making have to be established prior to any treatment, including even a simple filling or an extraction (Fig. 5.2a–d).

There are two basic questions to answer when planning a treatment for a partially edentulous patient:

- What to do with the existing teeth of the patient?
- What does the patient expect from us?

The treatment of edentulous areas with fixed prostheses, when possible, is one of the basic principles of prosthetic treatments. Alternatives can be evaluated due to systemic diseases, economic problems, need for complex treatment, geriatric patients, or defects. Therefore, for both young and old patients, the RPD option (or necessity thereof) needs to be explained thoroughly by using demonstration casts. To explain the patients the possible treatment alternatives at hand, diagnostic casts transferred to an articulator appear to be the most rational way.

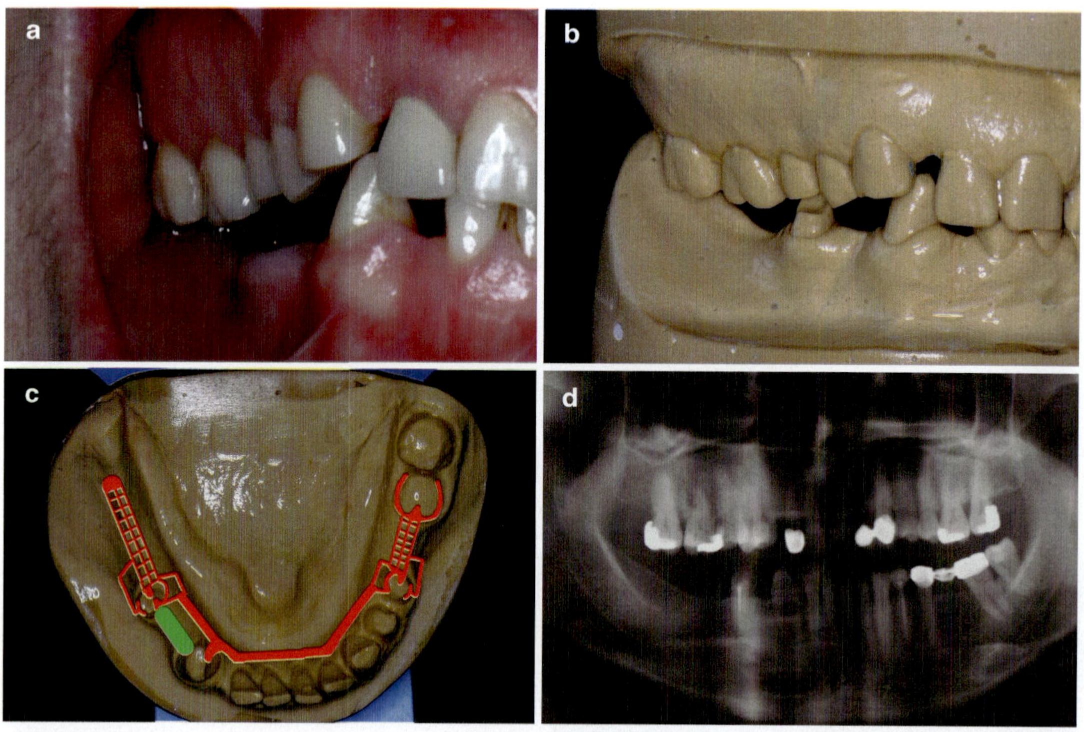

Fig. 5.2 (**a**) A patient with extreme growth of the periodontal tissues in an occlusal direction including the alveolar bone, together with the teeth. (**b**) The diagnostic casts are mounted to a semi-adjustable articulator. However there is no place for the prosthesis' posterior part. (**c**) The planning of the mandibular RPD design. (**d**) The panoramic radiograph of the patient

5.2 Diagnostic Casts and Occlusal Analysis

5.2.1 The Importance of Diagnostic Casts

There are certain limits to the information that can be accumulated through clinical examination and radiographs. So diagnostic casts give us valuable additional information about the clinical status. To start with, diagnostic casts reveal a three-dimensional representation of the oral situation alongside with a lingual view of the occlusion (Fig. 5.3a, b). A patient who visits a dental clinic with partial edentulism may just seek the treatment of the painful tooth/teeth. At times, the patient may have esthetic and/or functional complaints that require a complex treatment. In such cases, diagnostic casts transferred to a semi-adjustable articulator are needed in order to plan a treatment for the patient in question. These casts are useful not only for decision-making but also for communicating and consulting with several other specialists (e.g., periodontists, orthodontists, dental surgeons, or dental technician), not to mention the ease of demonstrating the oral status and the treatment options to the patient (Fig. 5.4a–f).

Once the casts are prepared, they can be mounted to some form of an articulator or can be held by hand in an intercuspal position without using any device. Out of these options, the choice for how to proceed can be made according to the following data on the needs of the patient:

Unmounted diagnostic casts
When

- To assess static interarch relationships where there are sufficient occluding teeth.
- To assess single arch problems.

Mounted diagnostic casts on a hinge-type articulator
When

- To assess static interarch relationships where there are insufficient occluding teeth.
- To analyze cases with small unit fixed partial dentures (FPD) within an acceptable occlusion.

Mounted diagnostic casts on a semi-adjustable articulator
Where

- Any major prosthodontic treatment is required.
- Any increase of occlusal vertical dimension is required.
- A significant discrepancy in maximum intercuspal position (MIP) and centric relation (CR) is present.
- There is a need to create a new occlusal relationship.

5.2.2 The Impression and Casts for Diagnostic Models

Most of the clinicians have a tendency to believe that the primary impressions and diagnostic casts can be prepared without too much effort and attention. They believe a diagnostic cast

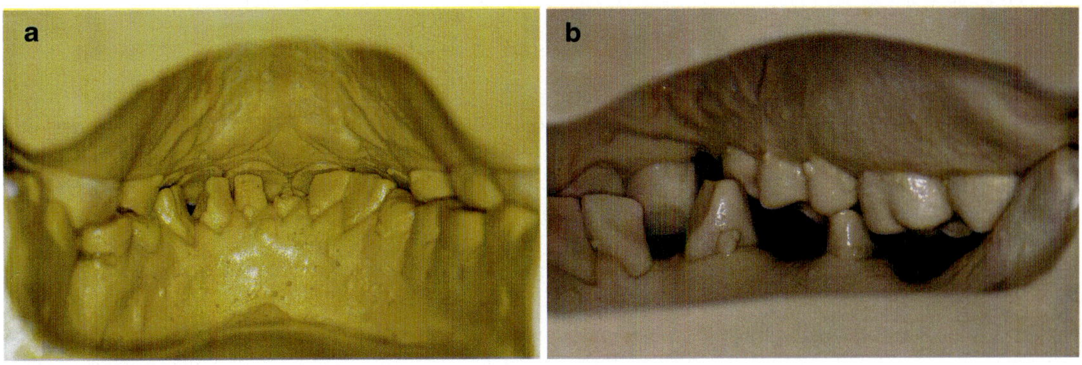

Fig. 5.3 (**a**) The lingual view of the casts of the patient mentioned in Fig. 5.1. (**b**) The lingual view of the casts of the patient

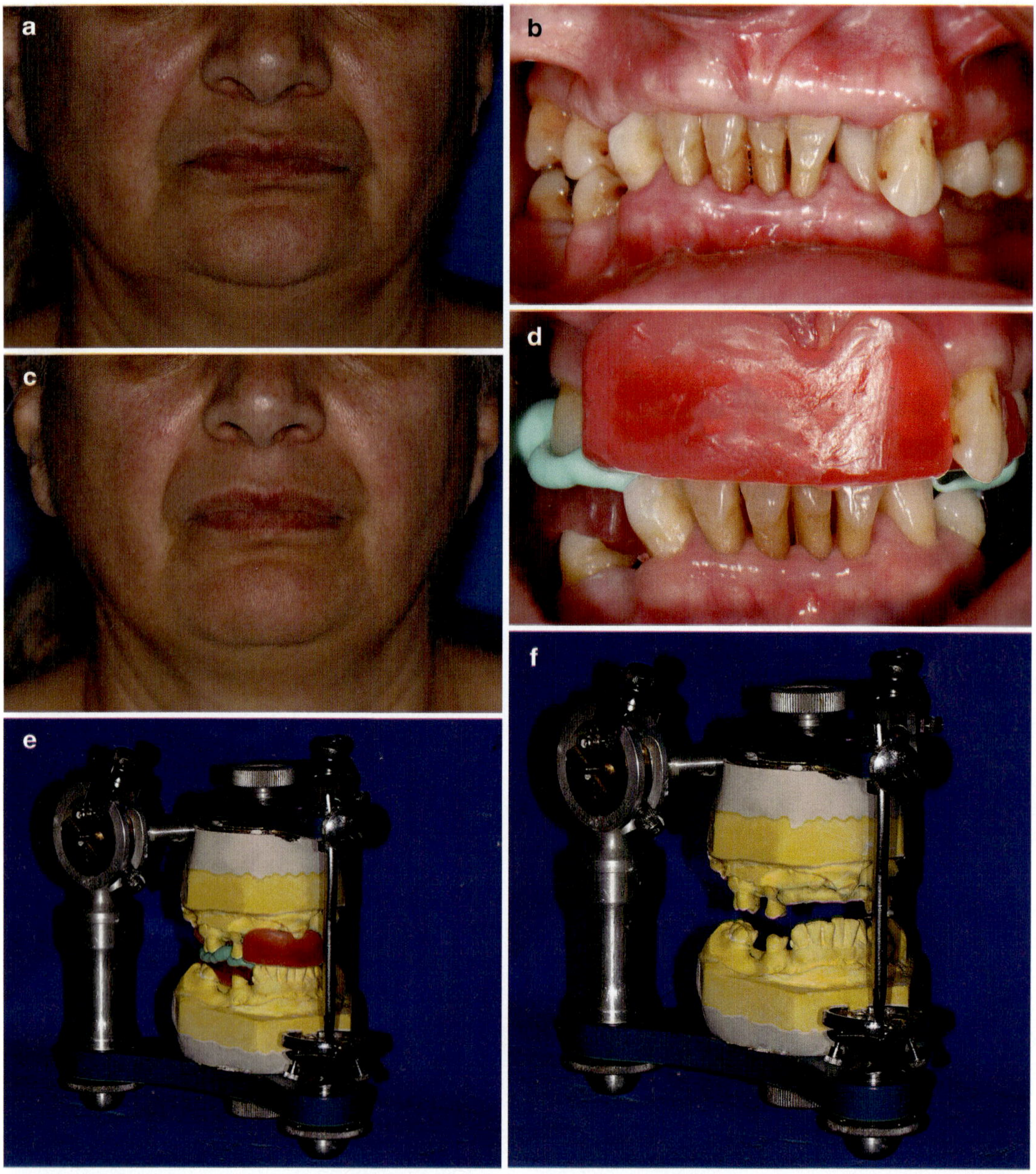

Fig. 5.4 (**a**) The facial view of the patient with severely decreased occlusal vertical dimension. (**b**) The intraoral view of the patient in maximum intercuspal position. (**c**) The facial view of the patient with increased occlusal vertical dimension. (**d**) An increased occlusal vertical dimension and centric relation record are completed using base plates and occlusion rims. (**e**) The records are transferred to a semi-adjustable articulator. (**f**) The casts mounted to the articulator are ready to analyze and plan the new prosthodontic work. Please notice the enormous interocclusal distance

does not need to be as correct as a master cast, which is absolutely wrong. Without any exception, these diagnostic casts have to reflect all the details of the hard and soft tissue. For example, in order to decide between an RPD and FPD, we need to examine both the dentition and the residual ridges. Therefore, it is definitely incorrect to assume that only the evaluation of the dentition or a part of the dentition or only the residual ridges are sufficient to make a treatment planning. A diagnostic cast should contain the following:

- Sufficient occlusal surfaces for an occlusal analysis.
- Sufficient axial surfaces and soft tissue parts for making an analysis on a parallelometer (surveying) to find the path of insertion and the undercuts.
- Sufficient residual ridges for preparing a well-fitting interim prosthesis (a temporary FPD, RPD, or an immediate denture).

It is usually enough to use a metal stock tray and an alginate for the primary impression of a partially edentulous patient. But sometimes the stock trays should be modified using wax or impression compound. To have a satisfactory impression of occlusal surfaces, non-perforated rim-lock trays with tray adhesive should be preferred. Finally, a bubble-free impression that contains all parts of the dentition and residual ridges should be poured with Class III dental stone by the clinician him/herself to avoid a potential syneresis phenomenon.

5.2.3 Using the Diagnostic Casts for Decision Making

As an additional option, the diagnostic casts transferred to the semi-adjustable articulator may well be used with other diagnostic tools like radiographs, anamnesis, and clinical examination. But first of all the clinician has to decide to either extract the tooth/teeth or restore it. Therefore, we need to analyze the periodontal and coronal status of the teeth, the relationship of each tooth to the occlusal plane, and the existing occlusion in detail. Thereafter, to arrive at a rational treatment planning all these data should be combined and checked against the expectations, financial condition, general health, and age of the patient.

5.2.3.1 Periodontal Status

A proper clinical and radiographic examination is needed to decide on periodontal therapy or extract the tooth/teeth. This decision, however, is mostly dependent on the following:

- The periodontal destruction level of the tooth/teeth (In case of a hopeless tooth we need to consider that an RPD will aggravate the periodontal status of the teeth).
- Do we use the tooth/teeth as an abutment for RPD? (in which case a better periodontal health is required.)
- Is the tooth/teeth inevitable for the RPD? (e.g., a single maxillary or mandibular anterior tooth with a moderate periodontal status is not necessarily useful.)
- The motivation of the patient toward his/her oral hygiene (if the patient is not able or not motivated to his/her oral hygiene the periodontal therapy should be reconsidered.)

5.2.3.2 Coronal Status

A proper clinical and radiographic examination is needed to decide for making a restoration or extracting the tooth/teeth. This decision is also dependent on the following:

- Are the tooth/teeth restorable? (e.g., a severely damaged tooth is not useable as an abutment where a ferrule effect is impossible.)
- Do we use the tooth/teeth as an abutment for RPD? (An abutment tooth for a bridge or RPD should comprise sufficient resistance. To name an example, a tooth which can only be restored with apical resection may otherwise be well held in the mouth for years, will not lend itself a good choice as an abutment.)
- Is the tooth/teeth inevitable for the RPD? (e.g., a restorable, single maxillary second molar tooth could better be extracted and a complete denture may be preferred.)
- The oral habits of the patient (if the patient has bruxism, etc.) over-sized restorations are questionable.
- Supra-erupted or tilted teeth (This kind of teeth should be analyzed on an articulator in both centric and eccentric positions. When analyzed only in centric occlusion, a tilted or supra-erupted tooth may sometimes seem utilizable after some preparations. However, if analyzed in eccentric occlusion, especially in protrusive and/or mediotrusive movement it comes out that the premature contacts are not correctable with occlusal equilibration or not even with FPD. Thus, one or more orthodontic,

endodontic, and periodontal treatment modalities need to be applied before the definitive prosthodontic treatment. Even seldomly, the extraction of the tooth may remain as the only choice.)

On the diagnostic cast, the tooth is grinded until it attains a proper occlusal clearance both in centric and eccentric occlusion. After that, the tooth should be adjusted to have a perpendicular axis. To make the clinical decision for an FPD, the amount of the preparation should only be analyzed afterward. These pretreatment modalities will be discussed in Chaps. 20 and 21 in detail.

5.2.3.3 Analysis of the Existing Occlusion

Prior to any kind of extensive restorative procedure, occlusal analysis and if necessary an occlusal adjustment should be prepared, with the general exemption (not a rare case) of a healthy masticatory system which is free of any kind of dysfunctional signs and/or symptoms. The pre-treatment modalities will be discussed in Chaps. 20. There are two basic reasons why the occlusal adjustments need to be done primarily in diagnostic casts transferred to a semi-adjustable articulator:

- To observe if just an occlusal equilibration is sufficient or should we better restore the teeth.
- To create an appropriate chart ahead of any occlusal adjustment in the mouth of the patient.

5.2.3.4 Deciding the Type of the Prosthesis

To make a proper treatment planning in a partially edentulous patient, the clinician needs to analyze a wide range of physical variations and health conditions. Therefore using an organized guideline for diagnostic criteria will be very helpful for the dental professionals. The American College of Prosthodontists (ACP) has developed a Classification System for Partial Edentulism in 2002. This system is constructed basically on four issues:

- Location and extent of the edentulous areas.
- Condition of the abutment teeth.
- Occlusal scheme.
- Residual ridge characteristics.

These issues are then classified as ideal or minimal, moderately, substantially, and severely compromised.

Classification System for Partial Edentulism

Location and Extent of the Edentulous Areas

A. Ideal or minimal compromised (The edentulous span is confined to a single arch and one of the following)
- Any anterior maxillary edentulous area that does not exceed 2 incisors.
- Any anterior mandibular edentulous area that does not exceed 4 incisors.
- Any posterior maxillary or mandibular edentulous area that does not exceed 2 premolars, or 1 premolar and 1 molar.

B. Moderately compromised (Edentulous areas in both arches and in one of the following)
- Any anterior maxillary edentulous area that does not exceed 2 incisors.
- Any anterior mandibular edentulous area that does not exceed 4 incisors.
- Any posterior maxillary or mandibular edentulous area that does not exceed 2 premolars, or 1 premolar and 1 molar.
- A missing maxillary or mandibular canine.

C. Substantially compromised
- Any posterior maxillary or mandibular edentulous area greater than 3 teeth or 2 molars.
- Any edentulous areas including anterior and posterior areas of 3 or more teeth

D. Severely compromised
- Any edentulous area or combination of edentulous areas requiring a high level of patient compliance.

Condition of the Abutment Teeth

A. Ideal or minimal compromised
- No pre-prosthetic therapy is indicated

B. Moderately compromised
- Abutments in 1 or 2 sextants have insufficient tooth structure to retain or support intracoronal or extracoronal restorations.

- Abutments in 1 or 2 sextants require localized adjunctive therapy (ie, periodontal, endodontic, or orthodontic procedures).

C. Substantially compromised

- Abutments in 3 sextants have insufficient tooth structure to retain or support intracoronal or extracoronal restorations.
- Abutments in 3 sextants require more substantial localized adjunctive therapy (i.e., periodontal, endodontic, or orthodontic procedures).

D. Severely compromised

- Abutments in 4 or more sextants have insufficient tooth structure to retain or support intracoronal or extracoronal restorations.
- Abutments in 4 or more sextants require extensive adjunctive therapy (ie, periodontal, endodontic, or orthodontic procedures).
- Abutments have guarded prognoses.

Occlusal Scheme

A. Ideal or minimal compromised

- No preprosthetic therapy is required.
- Class I molar and jaw relationships are seen.

B. Moderately compromised

- Occlusion requires localized adjunctive therapy (e.g., enameloplasty on premature occlusal contacts).
- Class I molar and jaw relationships are seen.

C. Substantially compromised

- Entire occlusion must be re-established but without any change in the occlusal vertical dimension.
- Class II molar and jaw relationships are seen.

D. Severely compromised

- Entire occlusion must be re-established, including changes in the occlusal vertical dimension.
- Class II division 2 and Class III molar and jaw relationships are seen.

Residual Ridge Characteristics

A. Ideal or minimal compromised.

- The residual bone height of 21 mm measured at the least vertical height of the mandible on a panoramic radiograph.
- Residual ridge morphology resistant to horizontal and vertical movement of the denture base; type A maxilla.
- Location of muscle attachments conducive to denture base stability and retention; type A or B mandible.

B. Moderately compromised

- Residual bone height of 16 to 20 mm measured at the least vertical height of the mandible on a panoramic radiograph.
- Residual ridge morphology resistant to horizontal and vertical movement of the denture base; type A or B maxilla.
- Location of muscle attachments with limited influence on denture base stability and retention; type A or B mandible.

C. Substantially compromised

- Residual alveolar bone height of 11 to 15 mm measured at the least vertical height of the mandible on a panoramic radiograph.
- Residual ridge morphology with minimum influence to resist horizontal or vertical movement of the denture base; type C maxilla.
- Location of muscle attachments with moderate influence on denture base stability and retention; type C mandible.

D. Severely compromised

- Residual vertical bone height of 10 mm measured at the least vertical height of the mandible on a panoramic radiograph.
- Class I, II, or III maxillomandibular relationships.
- Residual ridge offering no resistance to horizontal or vertical movement; type D maxilla.
- Muscle attachment location that can be expected to have a significant influence on denture base stability and retention; type D or E mandible.

This guideline is very helpful for an FPD, an RPD, or the combination of both. Naturally, Ante laws, root shape, and angulations of abutment teeth, etc., can also be utilized in making this decision. As a rule, an RPD is then indicated when the following circumstances are there:

Removable Partial Denture Indications

- In the absence of distal abutment tooth. The question is which tooth in the posterior region is sufficient for an FPD and in which situation should we make an RPD. To answer these questions, we should discuss here the "shortened dental arch concept".

Shortened Dental Arch Concept

The shortened dental arch (SDA) concept was first introduced by Arnd Käyser in 1981. Despite the SDA concept taking a long time to gain acceptance among traditionalists, today's dental literature agrees that the SDA concept should be considered as an alternative to any prosthetic treatment in partially edentulous arches. Käyser proposed that the four occlusal units/pairs, preferably in a symmetrical position, are sufficient for the functioning of the dentition (Fig. 5.5a, b).

The World Health Organization recommends that a functional, esthetic, natural dentition consists of at least 20 teeth (10 pairs of antagonistic or functional units/as from premolars to premolars). Likewise, the dental literature indicates that dental arches, including the anterior and premolar regions (premolar arch), meet the requirements of a functional dentition. It has also been shown that SDAs having 3–4 posterior occluding pairs can last for 27 years or more when lost teeth are restored with fixed restorations.

There have been many studies evaluating the SDA concept in terms of different factors such as occlusal stability, chewing ability, temporomandibular disorders (TMD), tooth loss, periodontal problems, oral function and comfort, and quality of life. The results obtained from the remarkable studies are summarized below:

1. In cases having 0–2 pairs of occluding premolars (extreme SDA), occlusal instability may occur. On the other hand, no evidence exists showing that occlusal instability occurs in cases having 3–4 pairs of occluding premolars. Clinically insignificant migration may occur. When compared to full dentition, more interdental gaps between the premolars and anterior teeth contact and less alveolar bone support have been observed in SDA cases having 3–5 occluding pairs. However, it has been shown that all the parameters remained stable in the long-term period.
2. Premolar arches and at least one occluding pair of molars provide satisfactory masticatory efficiency. Only extreme SDA cases present severely reduced chewing ability.
3. It has been observed that the lack of molar support did not cause TMD. However, when all premolar and molar teeth were unilaterally or bilaterally lost, the risk of pain and joint sounds seemed to increase. There is no evidence that the replacement of molars with an RPD is superior when compared to SDA regarding TMD pain over the 5-year period. Sufficient mandibular stability can be provided by the presence of bilateral premolar support. It has been shown that SDA has no significant effect on the progression of temporomandibular joint internal derangement.
4. In cases having three to five occluding pairs, it has been shown that the oral function and com-

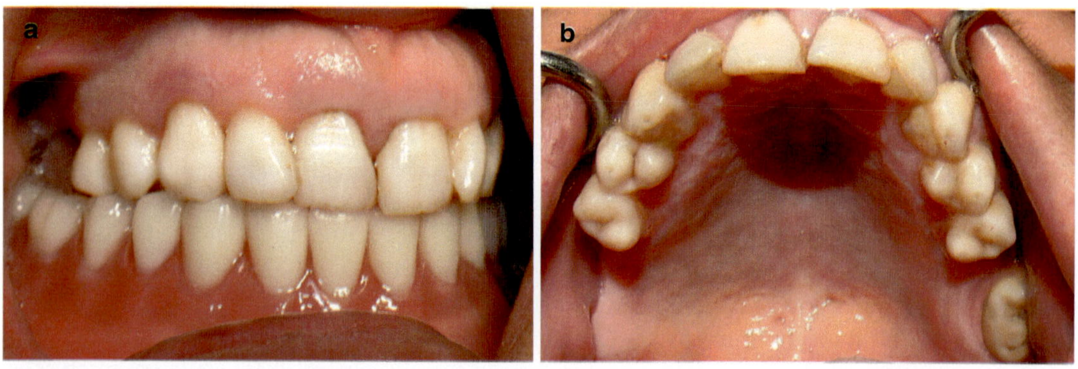

Fig. 5.5 (**a**) Shortened dental arch in MIP. (**b**) Shortened dental arch. Occlusal view of the maxillary arch

fort were not evidently enhanced by a free-end RPD. It has been also revealed that survival of premolars was higher in full dentitions when compared to SDAs, but in SDA cases no difference has been found between those with or without an RPD. Therefore, it has been recommended that patients having SDA have to be evaluated in high-risk groups, and special care should be given to avoid further tooth loss. In addition, in a multicenter study, it has been shown that there were no differences regarding tooth loss and periodontal health over a 10-year period between patients treated with precision attachment-retained RPDs and according to the SDA concept, conserving or restoring a premolar arch with cantilever-fixed prosthesis. It has been concluded that both treatment options are feasible and the SDA patient's opinion will become more important when choosing the fixed or removable restorations. However, a 3-year follow-up study revealed that resin-bonded bridge restorations were more successful than conventional RPDs in SDA cases. The results emphasize that the use of conventional RPDs in SDA cases should not be recommended. On the other hand, in-vitro results have shown that as the number of missing teeth from posterior to anterior in the mandible increases, the forces applied by the mandibular anterior teeth to the maxillary anterior teeth also increases and the use of mandibular RPD decreases these forces. More studies especially conducted in clinical situations are needed to conclude this issue.
5. No significant differences have been found between the SDA patients (having teeth with or without restoration from premolars to premolars) and the patients treated with precision attachment-retained RPDs regarding oral-health-related quality of life.

Although the anterior teeth and premolars can together compensate for the function (such as biting, chewing, speech, esthetics, temporomandibular joint, and dental arch stability) of the molars, the molars cannot compensate for the function of the anterior teeth and premolars. Thus, it clearly emerges that anterior teeth and premolars are indispensable for the stomatognathic system. From this perspective, prosthetic dentistry has been focused on the patient's subjective oral functional needs and has emphasized that the following "physiological or healthy occlusion principles" should be considered essential: (1) absence of pathologic symptoms and signs; (2) presence of satisfactory function, esthetics, and comfort; (3) existence of mandibular stability and variability in form and function of the stomatognathic system; and (4) presence of adaptive capacity of the stomatognathic system to changing situations.

If a patient with only a premolar dental arch is satisfied with the esthetic appearance, masticatory function, psychosocial comfort, and other functions including phonetics, tactile perception, and taste without feeling pain, restoration of the missing molars is not necessary. In fact, a treatment approach that insists on restoring all missing teeth has been called "28-tooth syndrome" and "overtreatment" in dental literature. In the light of the above research results, it is recommended that the patients should be informed about all restorations, including the SDA alternative, and their consent should be obtained and a joint decision should be made.

In SDAs, it is not recommended to extract healthy non-opposed posterior teeth due to their esthetic and functional contribution to the stomatognathic system. Thus, alveolar bone loss can also be prevented, and possible abutment can be preserved.

In the SDA concept, it is important to remember that some contraindications exist, such as severe Class III and Class II malocclusions, indication of parafunction, anterior open occlusal relationship, noticeable alveolar bone loss, excessive tooth wear, and pre-existing TMD.

The presence of periodontal diseases, caries, and occlusal instability should be carefully evaluated in SDAs. Such SDAs or dentitions are considered "complicated impaired dentitions." After eliminating complicating factors, prosthetic treatment can be an alternative, or patients should be monitored more frequently. The use of an occlusal splint may also be recommended. It has also been shown that the SDA cases with or without RPDs in the mandible had more mobile teeth and lower alveolar bone scores compared to full dentition cases. This highlights also the importance of regular follow-ups in SDA cases without complicating factors.

It has been emphasized that extending the SDAs by a cantilever-fixed prosthesis, RPDs, or implant-assisted prostheses may lead to a positive outcome in the presence of the following situations: chewing difficulties, esthetic problems, patient's preference for restoration, and extreme and asymmetric SDAs. It has also been shown that replacing the first molar with an implant-assisted prosthesis improved the bite force and masticatory efficiency in SDAs. This treatment option additionally prevents the alveolar bone resorption.

- Where resistance to a lateral movement is needed from contralateral teeth and soft tissues (cross-arch stabilization).
- When there is a considerable bone loss in the visible anterior region.

It is well known that multiple edentulous gaps mostly are best restored with a combination of FPDs and RPDs. However, all this information is still not sufficient to decide where a confusing question remains unanswered: Which edentulous gap should be restored with an FPD and which gap should be left as a modification for an RPD in combined planned prosthetic therapy? The rules for making this decision can be summarized as follows:

- If possible, anterior edentulous spaces should be restored with FPDs.
- In cases of missing canine tooth together with 2 or more adjacent teeth, it is impossible to restore this gap with an FPD.
- A single premolar tooth is a weak abutment for an RPD. The clinician should seek alternatives to include this tooth into the FPD. For example, the gap between the second premolar and canine tooth (maxillary or mandibular) should best be restored with an FPD.
- In Kennedy Class II cases with contralateral modification spaces, at least one modification space should be left for the purpose of bilateral stabilization. If not, the situation is changed to a pure Kennedy Class II case which has well-documented prosthodontic difficulties (Fig. 5.6a–e).

5.2.3.5 Using the Diagnostic Casts for Pretreatment

Indications of Occlusal Equilibration

- The patient has a TMD and occlusal problems (always after occlusal splint therapy) (see Chaps. 20).
- The patient has no TMD, but only occlusal problems and the occlusion needs to be reestablished by constructing extensive restorations.
- The occlusal problems in which occlusal equilibration is indicated are mostly:
- A prominent (bigger than 2.5 mm) with a lateral component (asymmetric slide-in-centric) (Pullinger-Seligman) discrepancy between CR and MIP.
- The lack of anterior or canine guidance without a prominent attrition in incisors and/or canine teeth. The premature occlusal contacts in eccentric movements of the mandible are mostly a result of supra–erupted or tilted molar teeth. In such cases, the most frequently seen occlusal problem is an premature nonworking side occlusal contact in the second or third molar teeth; the premature contact between the mandibular third molar and maxillary second molar teeth during protrusive movement being the second.

The Rules of Occlusal Equilibration

- Patient should be aware of the treatment procedures and should have no objections. Patients with psychosomatic disorders are not good candidates for occlusal treatments.
- The procedure should be tested in mounted casts before applying any treatment to the mouth of the patient.
- An occlusal adjustment diagram should be finished before grinding the teeth.
- The adjustments on the mounted casts should be done by the clinician himself/herself maximum 30 min before the treatment in the mouth of the patient, adding to the hand memory of the clinician.

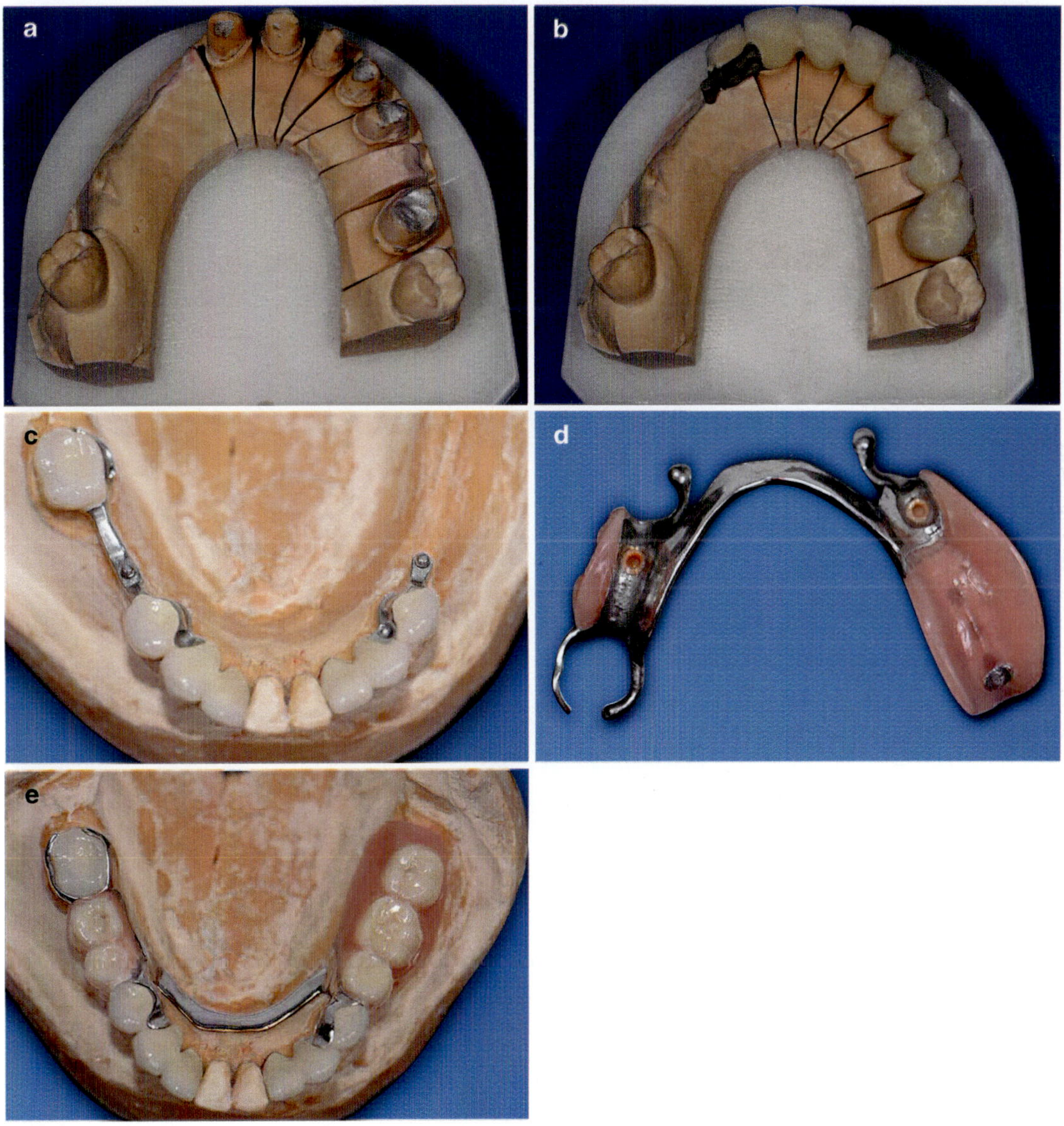

Fig. 5.6 (**a**) A Kennedy Class III Modification 1. (**b**) A wrong treatment planning of the case. The smaller edentulous gap should be left as a modification space for cross-arch stabilization. (**c**) A Kennedy Class II Modification 1. In this case, the treatment planning is logical. The edentulous gap is splinted with a bar attachment. (**d**) The RPD. Mucosal view. (**e**) The RPD. Occlusal view

- Given the choice, the restorative material should be chosen against a natural tooth surface.
- The centric premature contacts should be adjusted first, followed by working side contacts, protrusive contacts, and non-working side contacts.
- The centric premature contact should be grinded from fossa, not from the cusp.
- Once the centric adjustment is finished, the centric stops should be preserved during the eccentric adjustments.
- Ideally occlusal adjustments should not exceed the enamel boundaries.
- For the occlusal adjustments to be precisely and securely made, proper instruments should be selected to generate a smooth surface texture while not overheating the teeth. After the

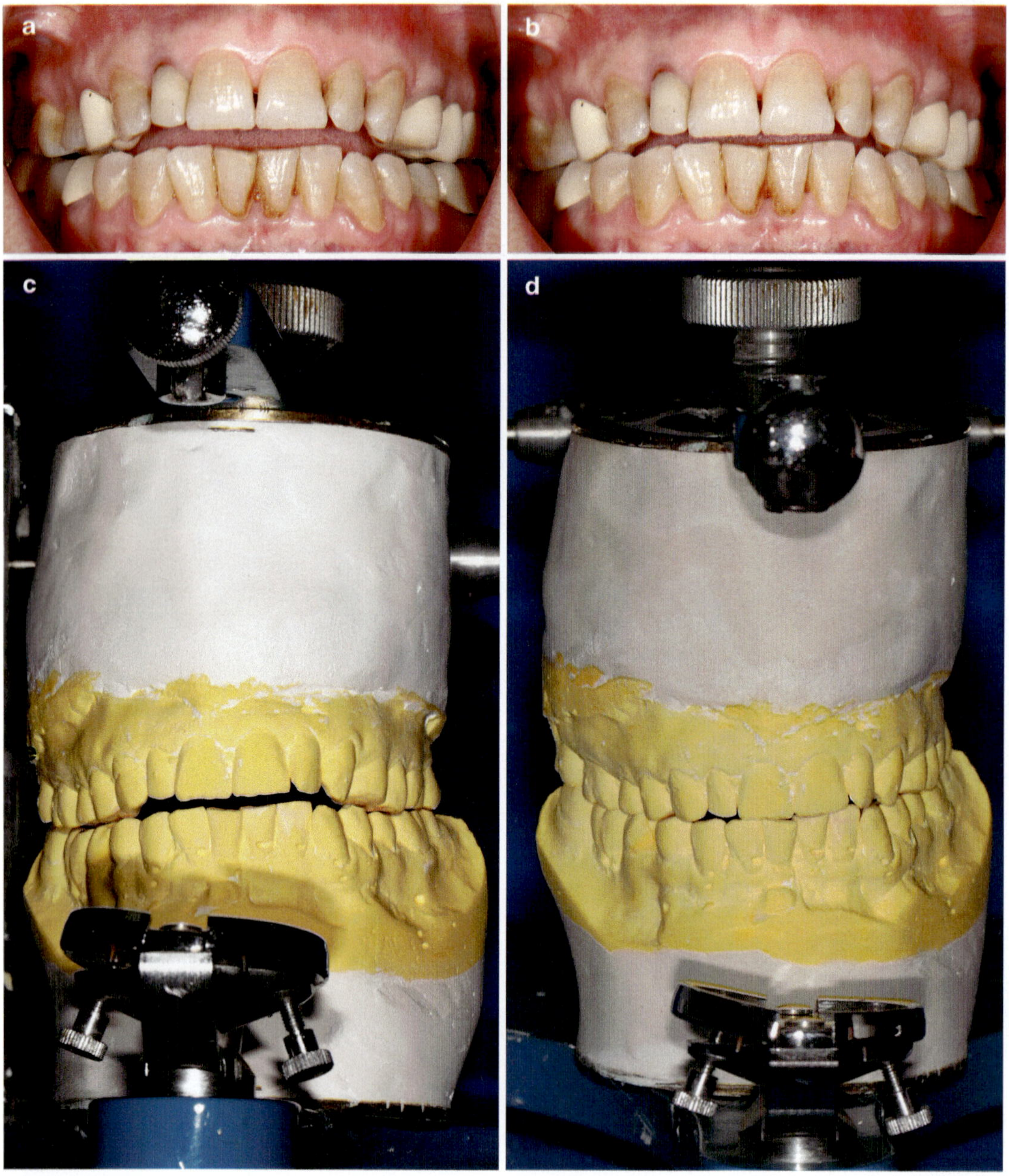

Fig. 5.7 A patient with extremely long slide-in-centric. (**a**) CR. (**b**) MIP. (**c**) CR in articulator. (**d**) The occlusal adjustment is prepared on study casts. Yet maximum occlusal contacts are created in both mandibular positions

grinding and polishing procedures, fluoride application over the teeth is recommended.

Maximal Intercuspal Position-Centric Relation Adjustments

Regardless of which centric record has been preferred for the prosthodontic restoration, the important point is to achieve a smooth and symmetrical slide between MIP and CR. A slight decrease in occlusal vertical dimension (about 1 mm) from CR to MIP is acceptable (Fig. 5.7a–d). These dynamic contacts should be prepared on each posterior tooth, although in nature these contacts only appear in the first premolar or second molar teeth. If it is possible, the adjustment should be applied only on central or marginal grooves. In cases that the cusp also needs to be grinded, it is important to avoid touching the tips of the supporting cusps. Premature contacts are marked and removed with a sharp blade continuously until a slightly curved platform is created at the depth of the occlusal fossa in order to supply a centric stop for the opposing supporting cusp. It is important to note that the articulator's incisal pin is always in contact with the curved (10–15 grad) incisal table during the small movement between MIP-CR. An articulating paper with 20–60 microns will serve the purpose. The clinician should be careful not to grind down or break the cusps of the gypsum cast. For hardening the gypsum, it is advisable to apply a proper solution on the occlusal surface of the cast.

Eccentric Adjustments

In a natural dentition for the eccentric occlusion almost always canine guidance is chosen. Accordingly, following the centric adjustments, the working side contacts are analyzed in the articulator. The upper buccal and lower lingual cusps should be eliminated. In cases in which a canine guidance is impossible to attain, group function occlusion is the next preferred option. The non-working side contacts are undesirable and should be adjusted accordingly. The main problem of equilibrating this kind of premature contacts is the risk of destroying the harmony of the centric stops. In a normal occlusion, the mediotrusive contacts are established between the upper palatinal and lower buccal cusps, collectively named supporting cusps. Thus, by eliminating these contacts, clinicians might easily grind the centric stops. If this happens, in order to re-establish the centric occlusion, the occluding antagonist fossa should be restored.

Further Reading

Amorim VC, Laganá DC, de Paula Eduardo JV, Zanetti AL. Analysis of the condyle/fossa relationship before and after prosthetic rehabilitation with maxillary complete denture and mandibular removable partial denture. J Prosthet Dent. 2003;89:508–14.

Arita S, Gonda T, Togawa H, Maeda Y, Ikebe K. Influence of mandibular free-end partial edentulism on the force exerted on maxillary anterior teeth. J Prosthodont Res. 2020;64:454–9.

Bain C. Treatment planning in general dental practice. Edinburgh: Churchill Livingstone; 2003.

Bessadet M, Nicolas E, Sochat M, Hennequin M, Veyrune JL. Impact of removable partial denture prosthesis on chewing efficiency. J Appl Oral Sci. 2013;21:392–6.

Carlsson GE, Omar R. Trends in prosthodontics. Med Princ Pract. 2006;15:167–79.

Carr AB, Brown DT. McCracken's removable partial prosthodontics. 13th ed. St. Louis, MO: Elsevier; 2016.

Davies SJ, Gray RM, McCord JF. Good occlusal practice in removable prosthodontics. Br Dent J. 2001;191:491–502.

Dhingra K. Oral rehabilitation considerations for partially edentulous periodontal patients. J Prosthodont. 2012;21:494–513.

Gernet W, Beuer F. Zahnärztliche Prothetik. Stuttgart: Thieme; 2007.

Gerritsen AE, Witter DJ, Bronkhorst EM, Creugers NH. Increased risk for premolar tooth loss in shortened dental arches. J Dent. 2013a;41:726–31.

Gerritsen AE, Witter DJ, Bronkhorst EM, Creugers NH. An observational cohort study on shortened dental arches clinical course during a period of 27–35 years. Clin Oral Investig. 2013b;17:859–66.

Graber G, Besimo C, Wiehl P, Rateitschak K. Farbatlanten der Zahnmedizin. Stuttgart: Thieme; 1992.

Grossmann Y, Sadan A. The prosthodontic concept of crown-to-root ratio: a review of the literature. J Prosthet Dent. 2005;93:559–62.

Jones JD, Turkyilmaz I, Garcia LT. Removable partial dentures-treatment now and for the future. Tex Dent J. 2010;127:365–72.

Käyser AF. Shortened dental arches and oral function. J Oral Rehabil. 1981;8:457–62.

Kanno T, Carlsson GE. A review of the shortened dental arch concept focusing on the work by the Käyser/Nijmegen group. J Oral Rehabil. 2006;33:850–62.

Loney RW. Removable partial denture manual. Halifax, NS: Dalhousie University Faculty of Dentistry; 2011. http://removpros.dentistry.dal.ca/ewExternalFiles/RPD%20Manual%2011.pdf

Mazurat NM, Mazurat RD. Discuss before fabricating: communicating the realities of partial denture therapy. Part I: patient expectations. J Can Dent Assoc. 2003a;69:90–4.

Mazurat NM, Mazurat RD. Discuss before fabricating: communicating the realities of partial denture therapy. Part II: clinical outcomes. J Can Dent Assoc. 2003b;69:96–100.

McGarry TJ, Nimmo A, Skiba JF, Ahlstrom RH, Smith CR, Koumjian JH, Arbree NS. Classification system for partial edentulism. J Prosthodont. 2002;11:181–93.

McKenna G, Tada S, McLister C, DaMata C, Hayes M, Cronin M, Moore C, Allen F. Tooth replacement options for partially dentate older adults: a survival analysis. J Dent. 2020;103:103468.

Meena A, Jain V, Singh N, Singh N, Arora N, Jha R. Effect of implant-supported prosthesis on the bite force and masticatory efficiency in subjects with shortened dental arches. J Oral Rehabil. 2014;41:87–92.

Miller E, Grasso J. Removable partial prosthodontics. 2nd ed. Baltimore: Williams & Wilkins; 1981.

Nassani MZ, Tarakji B, Baroudi K, Sakka S. Reappraisal of the removable partial denture as a treatment option for the shortened dental arch. Eur J Dent. 2013;7:251–6.

Neto AF, Duarte AR, Shiratori FK, de Alencar e Silva Leite PH, Rizzatti-Barbosa CM, Bonachela WC. Evaluation of senior Brazilian dental students about mouth preparation and removable partial denture design. J Dent Educ. 2010;74:1255–60.

Öwall B, Käyser AF, Carlsson GE. Prosthodontics: principles and management strategies. London: Mosby-Wolfe; 1996.

Preti G. Prosthetic rehabilitation. London: Quintessence Pub; 2008.

Ramfjord SP, Ash MM. Occlusion. 4th ed. Philadelphia: WB Saunders; 1995.

Reissmann DR, Anderson GC, Heydecke G, Schiffman EL. Effect of shortened dental arch on temporomandibular joint intra-articular disorders. J Oral Facial Pain Headache. 2018;32:329–37.

Reissmann DR, Heydecke G, Schierz O, Marré B, Wolfart S, Strub JR, Stark H, Pospiech P, Mundt T, Hannak W, Hartmann S, Wöstmann B, Luthardt RG, Böning KW, Kern M, Walter MH. The randomized shortened dental arch study: temporomandibular disorder pain. Clin Oral Investig. 2014;18:2159–69.

Rosenstiel SF, Land MF, Walter R. Contemporary fixed prosthodontics. 6th ed. Philadelphia: Elsevier; 2022.

Santos JJ. Occlusion. Chicago: Quintessence Pub. Co.; 2007.

Sarita PT, Kreulen CM, Witter D, Creugers NH. Signs and symptoms associated with TMD in adults with shortened dental arches. Int J Prosthodont. 2003;16:265–70.

Sarita PT, Kreulen CM, Witter DJ, Van't Hof M, Creugers NH. A study on occlusal stability in shortened dental arches. Int J Prosthodont. 2003;16:375–80.

Sarita PT, Witter DJ, Kreulen CM, Matee MI, Van't Hof MA, Creugers NH. Decayed/missing/filled teeth and shortened dental arches in Tanzanian adults. Int J Prosthodont. 2004;17:224–30.

Sarita PT, Witter DJ, Kreulen CM, Van't Hof MA, Creugers NH. Chewing ability of subjects with shortened dental arches. Community Dent Oral Epidemiol. 2003;31:328–34.

Sasse M, Kern M, Marré B, Walter MH. Clinical performance of cantilevered fixed dental prostheses abutments in the shortened dental arch. J Dent. 2014;42:373–6.

Schierz O, Reissmann DR, Rauch A, John MT, Marré B, Luthardt RG, Mundt T, Hannak W, Kohal R, Kern M, Nothdurft F, Hartmann S, Böning K, Boldt J, Stark H, Edelhoff D, Wöstmann B, Wolfart S, Jahn F, Walter MH. Impact of shortened dental arch on oral health—related quality of life. J Evid Based Dent Pract. 2021;21:101622.

Schwass DR, Lyons KM, Purton DG. How long will it last? The expected longevity of prosthodontic and restorative treatment. N Z Dent J. 2013;109:98–105.

Silverman SI. Differential diagnosis. Fixed or removable prosthesis. Dent Clin N Am. 1987;31:347–62.

The glossary of prosthodontic terms: ninth edition. J Prosthet Dent. 2017;117(5S):e1–e105.

Togawa H, Gonda T, Karino T, Maeda Y, Ono T, Ikebe K. Force exerted on maxillary anterior teeth in mandibular unilateral and bilateral distal extension partial edentulous situation. Odontology. 2023;111:451–60.

Walter MH, Dreyhaupt J, Hannak W, Wolfart S, Luthardt RG, Stark H, Pospiech P, Mundt T, Kern M, Böning KW, Wöstmann B, Scheller H, Jahn F, Reinhardt W, Strub J, Marré B, Heydecke G. The randomized shortened dental arch study: tooth loss over 10 years. Int J Prosthodont. 2018;31:77–84.

Walter MH, Dreyhaupt J, Mundt T, Kohal R, Kern M, Rauch A, Nothdurft F, Hartmann S, Böning K, Boldt J, Stark H, Edelhoff D, Wöstmann B, Luthardt RG, Hannak W, Wolfart S, Heydecke G, Jahn F, Pospiech P, Marré B. Periodontal health in shortened dental arches: a 10-year RCT. J Prosthodont Res. 2020;64:498–505.

Walter MH, Marré B, Dreyhaupt J, Heydecke G, Rauch A, Mundt T, Hannak W, Kohal RJ, Kern M, Nothdurft F, Hartmann S, Böning K, Boldt J, Stark H, Edelhoff D, Wöstmann B, Wolfart S, Jahn F, Luthardt RG. Rehabilitation of shortened dental arches: a fifteen-year randomised trial. J Oral Rehabil. 2021;48:738–44.

Walther W. The concept of a shortened dental arch. Int J Prosthodont. 2009;22:529–30.

Witter DJ, Van Elteren P, Käyser AF, van Rossum MJ. The effect of removable partial dentures on the oral function in shortened dental arches. J Oral Rehabil. 1989;16:27–33.

Witter DJ, Van Elteren PH, Käyser AF. Migration of teeth in shortened dental arches. J Oral Rehabil. 1987;14:321–9.

Witter DJ, van Palenstein Helderman WH, Creugers NH, Käyser AF. The shortened dental arch concept and its implications for oral health care. Community Dent Oral Epidemiol. 1999;27:249–58.

Wostmann B, Budtz-Jorgensen E, Jepson N, Mushimoto E, Palmqvist S, Sofou A, Öwall B. Indications for removable partial dentures: a literature review. Int J Prosthodont. 2005;18:139–45.

Yuan JC, Sukotjo C. Occlusion for implant-supported fixed dental prostheses in partially edentulous patients: a literature review and current concepts. J Periodontal Implant Sci. 2013;43:51–7.

Preparation of the Mouth for Removable Partial Dentures

6

Hakan Bilhan

Abstract

The long-term prognosis of removable partial dentures should rely on optimal tissue and tooth support. A good technical work is not the only factor bringing clinical success. Denture-bearing areas, abutment teeth, and all surrounding tissues should be adequately prepared before any impression for initialization of denture fabrication is attempted. A reliable preprosthetic preparation will not only guarantee a more comfortable patient use but also a better esthetic result. Preprosthetic interventions generally need a multidisciplinary approach since a couple of the treatment methods belong in the scope of specialized dental fields and be better exercised by experienced hands. Preprosthetic oral surgery, periodontal, and orthodontic preparations do not belong to the daily clinical practice of a dental professional. The different treatment modalities to be considered are presented and explained briefly in this chapter. It should be remembered that these interventions classified as periodontal, oral surgical, soft tissue conditioning, and orthodontic preparations will ensure a long-term success for the planned prosthesis.

H. Bilhan (✉)
Faculty of Dentistry, Department of Periodontology, University of Witten/Herdecke, Witten, Germany
e-mail: hakan.bilhan@uni-wh.de
http://www.ruhrweiss.de

6.1 The Importance of Preprosthetic Preparations

The preparation of the mouth plays a key role in the long-term success and patient satisfaction of a removable partial denture (RPD). Preprosthetic procedures involve methods for the preparation or improvement of patients' ability to wear removable dentures. Most procedures are centered around soft or hard tissue corrections to allow prosthetic devices to fit more securely and function more comfortably. However, dental arrangements are indispensable, too. Except for crown and bridge work (see Chap. 7), periodontal, endodontic, restorative, and orthodontic preparations are important in the long-term success of an RPD. For the evaluation of whether a tooth is to be kept or extracted, factors such as the mobility, condition of the crown, the endodontic status, and radiographic assessment play a key role. A good root canal treatment is vital, especially if the tooth will be used as an abutment. If an existing root canal filling seems unreliable, a retreatment should be considered. In the same manner, decayed or damaged teeth should be restored before the prosthetic treatment is initiated.

In the era when dental implants were not a rescuer yet, bony augmentation was incorporated in severe cases and included very invasive procedures such as cartilage grafts, rib grafts, alloplastic augmentation, visor osteotomies as well as sandwich grafts. Patients who had been considered poor candidates for that kind of extensive

O. Şakar (ed.), *Removable Partial Dentures*, https://doi.org/10.1007/978-3-031-47083-7_6

surgery were often left with less satisfactory results both functionally and esthetically. The goal of preprosthetic surgery in this century is to establish a functional biological platform that will support prosthetic restoration without contributing to further bone or tissue loss. In this manner, it will be possible to achieve a denture that restores function, is stable and retentive, preserves the associated structures, and satisfies esthetics.

The supporting hard, soft as well as the dental tissues must be in excellent form to be able to provide a problem-free adaptation and usage period. The procedures should commence with a detailed anamnesis followed by a proper examination. The anamnesis consists of information about dental and medical history giving the clinician a global view of the patient. During the oral examination, soft and hard tissues likewise the remaining dentition are inspected. The color, thickness, consistency, and surface of the mucosa should be healthy. The bony base should provide solid, but smooth support. The status of the teeth will be a substantial hint for the planning of the denture. Missing teeth, angulated, rotated, or inclined teeth, teeth needing additional restorative procedures, and teeth being candidates for extraction should be jotted down. A radiographic evaluation is vital in the prosthetic planning of any kind of prosthesis. On radiographs, the clinician can see impacted teeth, hidden chronic infections, cysts, residual roots, the real bony (periodontal) support of abutment teeth and other important findings. Study casts are an efficacious way to evaluate the patients' oral condition and propose subsequent treatment such as extractions, orthodontics, or design of tooth restorations. By the assessment of the casts mounted to the articulator, details from jaw relation to interarch distance may be visualized. On the other hand, the casts should be surveyed to determine the path of insertion and tissues interfering. This approach will ease the detection of many preprosthetic intervention needs and help with the treatment planning. The oral preparation principles will be explained here by the following order:

The purpose of these procedures is to attain an oral status with optimum health and to eliminate any unfavorable conditions. The initial prosthetic treatment consisting of tooth preparation as well as the adaptation or modification of an interim prosthesis should follow the other preparation steps listed above. Being faithful to the philosophy of this book, the prosthetic arrangement should be the last step and is the subject of the next chapter. In this manner, the impression procedures will follow the accomplished mouth preparation. Surgical and periodontal preparation should be completed in a certain time interval in advance, if at all possible, at least 6 weeks and preferably 3–6 months, allowing the necessary healing period before abutment tooth preparation.

6.2 Periodontal Preparation

It is meanwhile well known that RPDs may favor plaque accumulation and it is of great importance to maintain or reach a status with stable periodontal conditions and tissues free of inflammation before any prosthodontic approach is attempted. It is clinically vital to ensure an established periodontal health condition for a long-term successful RPD treatment. Patients should receive detailed instructions on oral hygiene procedures to keep plaque around abutment teeth and RPD components to a minimum. Periodontal preparation, however, not only includes sub- and supragingival debridement, scaling, and root planing, or attainment of oral hygiene but also various minor surgical interventions. Crown lengthening procedures to obtain better pink esthetics or a biomechanically more stable crown height in some instances may be a very valuable treatment choice. On the contrary, from time to time, lateral or coronal sliding flaps can be necessary to cover recessions.

Elimination of extreme occlusal interferences is essential to avoid overloading any teeth in the arch. Depending on the strength of the early contact and position of the related tooth, elimination measures from simple grinding to tooth extraction may be considered. Teeth with slight-to-moderate mobility should be judged for splinting or by fixed prostheses. If there are several teeth of that kind, an occlusal splint is recommended. Using a splint, occlusal forces are more evenly distributed and the probability of occlusal trauma for individual teeth is reduced. Intermittent repeating occlusal forces may cause a jiggling trauma, resulting in rapid bone loss around the exposed tooth. In clinical cases where the posterior support have been lost due to missing molars, the most distal premolars are under the threat of being overloaded.

The introduction of dental implants has changed the look at periodontal efforts in partially edentulous patients drastically. The attempt to keep teeth with an indefinite prognosis is rather considered risky and instead of doing complicated and uncomfortable respective or invasive osseous surgery, teeth are rather extracted. Interventions such as furcation involvement, guided tissue regeneration, or flap operation may endanger the long-term success of the planned denture by a possible unplanned early tooth loss. If it is an abutment candidate, the extraction of a compromised tooth should always be regarded as an option, since it is known that teeth provided with clasps should have at least 70% of bony support. In periodontally compromised patients, the recall sessions should be scheduled more frequently, and those patients should be clinically checked at least every 6 months.

6.2.1 Oral Hygiene Motivation and Ensuring Hygiene Ability

The elimination of inflammation around the abutment teeth as well as the rest of the dentition plays a key role in the preprosthetic oral preparation. The main reason for the inflammation is the biofilm that must be removed professionally. In this phase of the approach, the patient will be motivated and educated meticulously about hygiene habits, methods of better cleaning, and helpful instruments such as the interdental brushes. In the meantime, a plaque-free environment should be targeted and at the end of this period, a possible gingivitis is treated successfully if there is no other reason behind it. There are oral hygiene indices such as the approximal plaque indices (API) or the MAPI (modified API) and the papilla bleeding index (PBI) for evaluating the degree of the reached clinical situation. They are a good instrument for measuring the achievement. The professional cleaning and motivation/education of the patients are crucial in regaining and maintaining gingival health. However, the role of the clinician is not limited to this approach. Factors such as poorly adapted crown margins (Fig. 6.1) and/or fillings, or bridge pontics hindering access for the interdental brushes, making the oral hygiene difficult, should

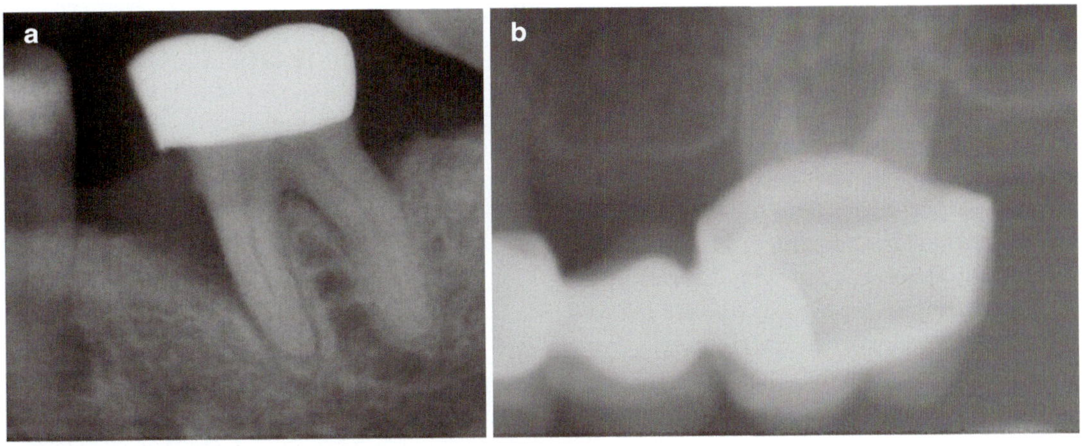

Fig. 6.1 Poorly adapted, overlapping crown margins making the oral hygiene difficult, (**a**) lower molar, (**b**) upper molar

be detected and eliminated. The patient should be informed that the cause of gingival bleeding or generally gingival problems is the biofilm. The patient should be aware of the consequences of insufficient oral hygiene and rare dental visits.

A gingivitis is diagnosed with bleeding on probing (BOP), and signs of inflammation in the gingiva, such as slight swelling, and change in texture and color, whereas the pocket probing depth (PPD) should not exceed 3 mm. In the case of higher pocket depths, which points out to a bone loss, it should be taken as a periodontitis, where the treatment strategy will be different.

It is a helpful policy to see a patient at least once a year for a routine check-up, including the periodontal screening index (PSI), which gives the clinician an idea about the PPD and thus the periodontal status. The presence of deep pockets, if not pseudo such as in the case of gingival hyperplasia, indicates a periodontitis that must be treated to slow down or even stop bone loss.

During the prephase of the periodontal therapy, following steps must be considered:

(a) *Dental hygiene performed by professional staff.*
(b) *Patient motivation/education and working on patient compliance:* revision of oral hygiene habits by elucidating patients about tools and techniques. The clinician must be convinced of the patients' determination before going to the next level and observe the perfect oral hygiene motivation. In this manner, it is the clinician's duty to inform the patient about the relationship of periodontitis and smoking habits. The patient should be well informed and aware of the importance of reducing/quitting the smoking habit. Another important factor behind periodontitis is the uncontrolled hyperglycemia. Patients with diabetes mellitus, either type 1 or type 2, who are not well controlled and have an HbA1c value (giving information about the long-term status) of over 6.5% are more prone to periodontitis. For this reason, the consultation with the patients' physician and the motivation of the patient to comply will positively influence the therapy outcome.
(c) *Clinical examination of the occlusion* and elimination of overloading of individual teeth and preventing jiggling trauma. An overloaded tooth will show clinical mobility and is easily recognized radiographically by the widened periodontal gap (Fig. 6.2). At this stage, slight grinding and/or splinting may be applied. The splinting can be easily performed by using a composite filling material to fix the mobile tooth to its neighbor to enable immobilization and distribution of occlusal forces. In more severe situations, a light polymerized glass fiber material may be used, as well, for more stable and reliable splinting (Fig. 6.3). If this will be an abutment tooth of the planned RPD, being subject to vertical and horizontal loading via retainers and rests, it is advisable to use this kind of more stable splinting methods. It

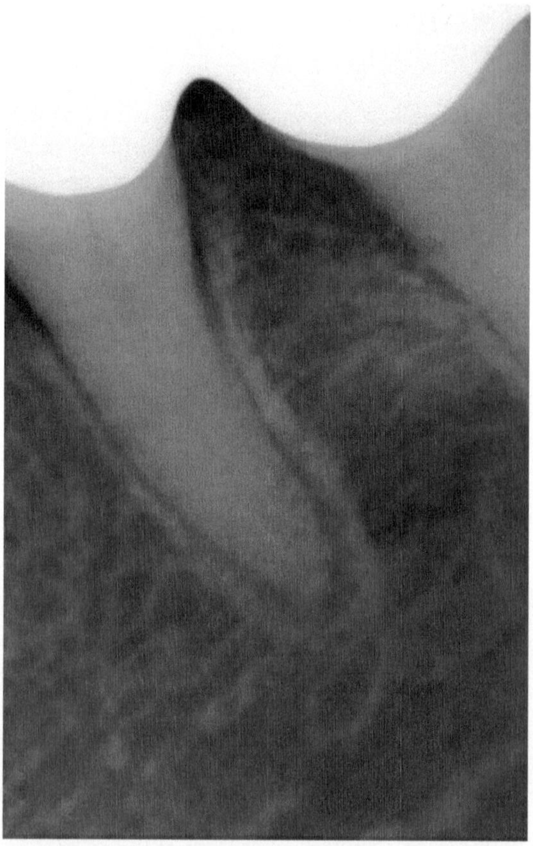

Fig. 6.2 An overloaded tooth is easily recognized radiographically by the widened periodontal gap

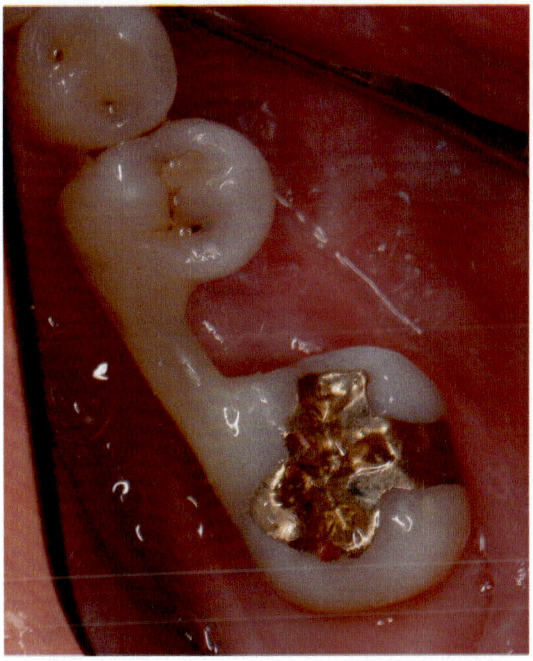

Fig. 6.3 A more stable and reliable splinting can be performed by using a glass fiber material such as everStick®Perio to fix the mobile tooth to its neighbor to enable immobilization and distribution of occlusal forces

should always be kept in mind that a tooth with a bone loss exceeding 30% of the root length is an abutment tooth candidate with a poor prognosis. In case of weakened abutment teeth neighboring the free-end situation, the alternative planning with dental implants may be considered (see Chap. 17).

(d) *Restorative procedures supporting the periodontal therapy:* Clinical examination and treatment of cavities, completion of endodontic therapies, elimination of poor margins of old fillings, and improvement of interdental contact points are crucial parts of the periodontal preparation phase. Restorative measures at coronal level, easing the hygiene procedures, eliminating rough surfaces, and indentations favoring plaque accumulation are crucial for a good gingival health; insufficient fillings should be exchanged. Weak contact points and badly shaped embrasures of neighboring fillings may result in food impaction, thus periodontal problems and deep localized pockets. The check of vitality of all teeth is a very important clinical step. It is known that there may be a relation between a deep pocket and an apical lesion, caused by an endodontic problem: an endo-perio lesion (Fig. 6.4). To ensure a successful periodontal therapeutic strategy, the endodontic treatment must be accomplished meticulously, parallel to the other preparation steps before scaling and root planing (SRP).

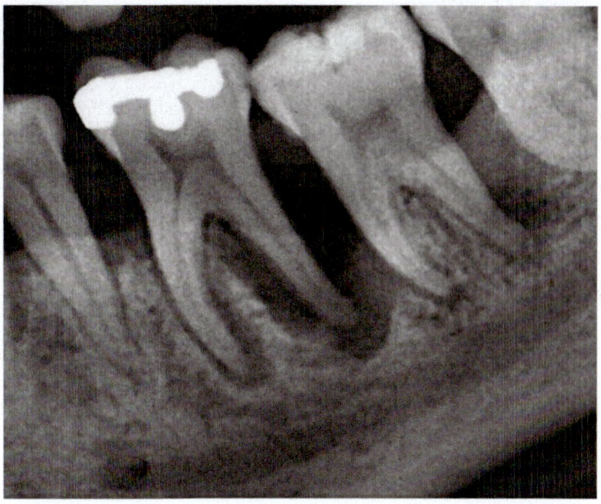

Fig. 6.4 Endo-perio lesion making a root canal treatment necessary

(e) *Inspection of crown margins and bridge pontics for cleanability:* Poor margins and inaccessible pontics may give the reason for renewal of the prosthetic work. In patients who are in a periodontitis therapy planning phase, it is advisable to proceed with long-term provisional restorations, fabricated in the laboratory (for precision reasons and a good marginal fit). During this period, it is possible to observe the response of periodontal tissues to the new situation. For the definitive prosthetic planning, the ideal time point seems to be when stable periodontal conditions are recorded during the supporting periodontal therapy (SPT) phase.

At the end of the prephase of the periodontal therapy, the PPDs, recessions and furca involvements are measured and noted and the diagnosis following the new periodontitis classification with staging and grading is determined. At this stage, the patient may be informed extensively about the status, therapy goals, therapy process, and anticipated prognosis. An important point will be, to explain that the primary goal is to reduce PPDs, thus the inflammation process, causing bone loss. The patient should be aware of the expected recessions and the consequences, such as sensitive teeth and esthetic drawbacks.

6.2.2 Scaling and Root Planing (SRP)

Following the preparation phase, the anti-infectious therapy phase may begin. Scaling and root planing constitute the central element in the periodontal component of this phase, where bacteria are removed mechanically and the immune system is activated. Specific purposes for scaling and root planing mainly include:

(a) removing plaque and calculus,
(b) conservatively removing endotoxin-infected root cementum,
(c) determining the extent of healing and pocket reduction with nonsurgical therapy.

Most of the time, the use of local anesthetics is inevitable since the whole procedure may be painful. In the absence of pain or discomfort, the patient is better able to tolerate the procedure and the clinician can accomplish a better instrumentation. Superficial instrumentation may be efficient to heal the gingiva that can return to a normal contour and texture, thus giving the patient and clinician the false sense that the periodontal disease is now under control and a reinstrumentation is unnecessary. If calculus somehow cannot be removed by non-surgical therapy, it is advisable to plan a later open flap debridement. Once the SRP is completed, the supporting periodontal therapy (SPT) sessions are planned, and the appointments are scheduled. Generally, in patients younger than 40 years, the treatment is additionally supported by adjunctive systemic antibiotics. The antibiotics regimen applied in these cases is the so-called "Winkelhoff Cocktail" that is named after van Winkelhoff. A combination of Amoxycillin and Metronidazol (3 × 375–500 mg/day Amoxycillin +3 × 250–500 mg Metronidazol) is administered for 8 days. During SPT, the treatment outcome is evaluated and if necessary further interventions such as regenerative periodontal therapies (Fig. 6.5a, b), open flap debridement, tunnelling, or premolarization/hemisections are planned and scheduled. It should be kept in mind that a resected tooth, where an amputation, hemisection or a premolarization had been performed, is not a suitable abutment tooth. These teeth are weakened and splinting by prosthetically combining them in a bridge work with neighboring teeth is always recommended; in this manner, it should not be expected that these teeth are good candidates to show the capacity to bear the load of clasps and rests.

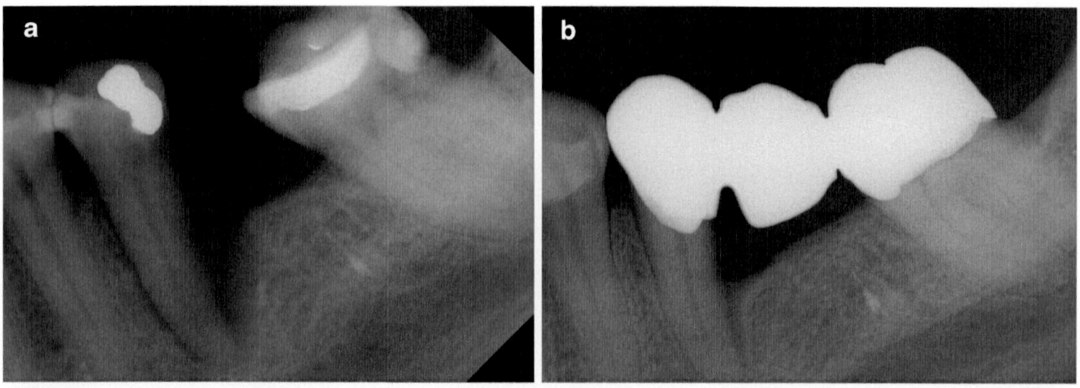

Fig. 6.5 Periodontal regeneration—guided tissue regeneration (GTR) for reducing PPD without a recession: (**a**) before intervention, (**b**) after 7 months

6.2.3 Respecting the Biological Width and Surgical Crown Lengthening

The biological width is important in maintaining gingival health, avoiding inflammation and going for a predictable outcome. Biological width, its maintenance, and applications of crown lengthening in cases of biological width violation (Fig. 6.6) are very important concepts ensuring long-term gingival and periodontal health. There is a close relationship between the restoration margins and gingival health. Too subgingivally placed restoration margins are a source of biological width violation.

The biological width is defined as the dimension of the soft tissue, which is attached to the portion of the tooth coronal to the crest of the alveolar bone. Ectodermal tissues serve as protection against the penetration of bacteria and other foreign materials into inner parts of the body. This natural seal that exists around teeth, protecting the alveolar bone from infection and disease, is known as the biological width. It is crucial for preserving the periodontal health and preventing irritation that might damage the periodontium The distance from the margin of the restoration to the marginal bone must be at least 2 mm. In the ideal scenario, the margins should remain supragingivally or epigingivally and 3 mm from the surrounding bone. This 3 mm is composed of 1 mm supracrestal connective tissue attachment, 1 mm junctional epithelium, and 1 mm for gingival sulcus on an average. If subgingival margins are desired, the clinician must not disrupt the junctional epithelium or connective tissue apparatus during preparation or impression-taking. It should be recommended to limit the subgingival margin extension to 0.5–1.0 mm because it is impossible for the clinician to detect where the sulcular epithelium ends and the junctional epithelium begins.

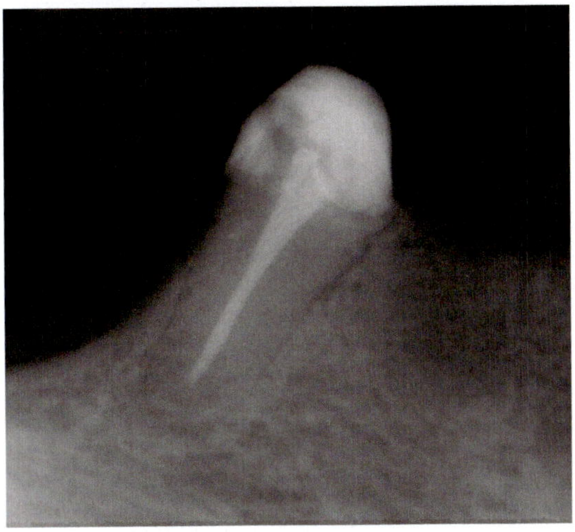

Fig. 6.6 Radiographic view of a tooth with a violated biological width

The biological width violation is clinically and radiologically easy to diagnose. Mostly, it is observed as a chronic progressive gingival inflammation around the restoration (Fig. 6.6), bleeding on probing or localized gingival hyperplasia with minimal bone loss. During the radiographic evaluation on conventional radiography impingement of the width on the mesial and distal aspects of the teeth may be illusive, while the X-ray anglulation may play a decisive role in the decision-making process. A radiograph taken with the parallel or the bite-wing technique bears information that is more representative.

The suitable treatment to regain the biological width may be either surgically removing from surrounding bone away to distance the restoration margin, or orthodontic extrusion of the tooth and thus moving the margin away from the bone.

The first above-mentioned alternative is "crown lengthening" which is a surgical procedure where clinical crown height is increased by removing marginal bone.

Clinical crown lengthening may be indicated in 3 different situations:

(a) Clinical crown length is too short - one of the reasons may be tooth wear. Nevertheless, teeth may be short without being worn. Especially in the anterior region, where the golden proportions are desired to be reached in an esthetic planning, teeth may be lengthened by clinical crown lengthening.
(b) The biological width is violated and it is necessary to gain a security zone of at least 2 mm, but if possible 3 mm. Clinical conse-

quences (Fig. 6.7) in case of ignoring are inflamed, swollen gingiva with bleeding. The real cause may sometimes be overlooked. Often the clinical findings are mixed up with allergies to the restorative material and the restorations are exchanged several times in a futile attempt to no avail.

(c) When a filling restoration margin is, due to whatever reason, too subgingival, so that an adhesive cementation is not possible. This happens especially in the posterior region, after the removal of large restorations with the purpose of restoring with a full ceramic partial crown, onlay, or an overlay. For the adhesive cementation, the restoration margins must be epi- or supragingival, to ensure dry conditions, without the leakage of gingival fluid or other humidity sources. The prosthetic treatment may only begin after a complete cure of the region, which is not earlier than 4–8 weeks.

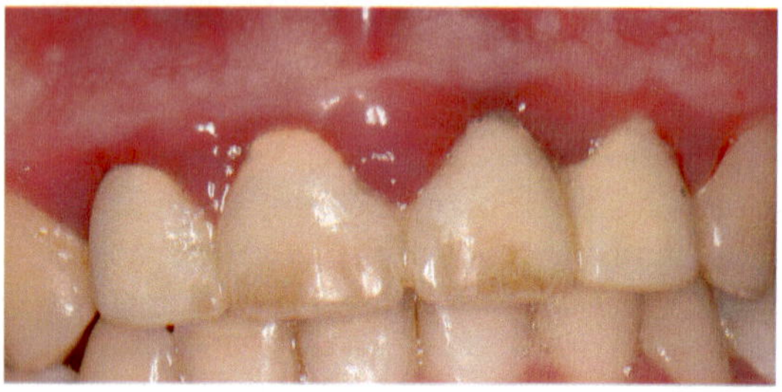

Fig. 6.7 Clinical appearance of restorations with biological width violation: inflammation in surrounding gingiva

6.2.4 The Importance of Keratinized Gingiva and Free Gingival Grafts

It is meanwhile a well-known fact that the presence of attached gingiva is very important for the maintenance of gingival health. In the absence of attached and keratinized gingiva, carrying out the oral hygiene becomes painful for the patient; thus, it is neglected. The result is inflamed, bleeding gingiva. The missing attached gingiva may be augmented. The gingival augmentation by surgery has the aim to establish a zone of gingiva that is not mobile. Generally, a free gingival graft (FGG) is very useful in creating the desired zone of attached keratinized gingiva and hinders the progression of gingival recession. The FGG procedures performed in sites with an absence of attached gingiva (Fig. 6.8a, b), probably associated with recessions, provide regaining of attached keratinized gingiva (Fig. 6.9a, b). In successful cases, a so-called "creeping attachment" may develop and cover a part of the existing

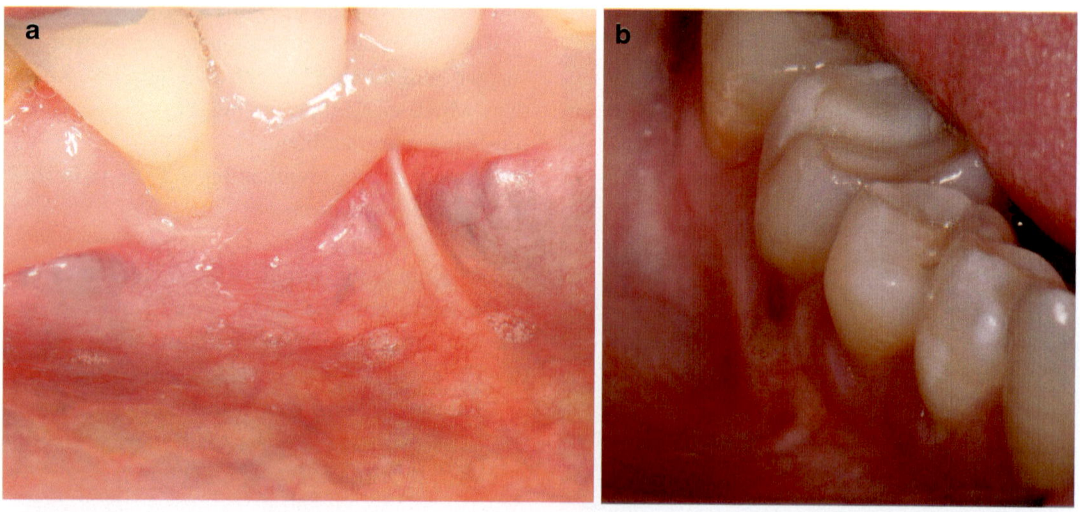

Fig. 6.8 Free gingival grafts (FGGs) are indicated in sites with absent attached gingiva that probably already ended up in recessions: (**a**) front, (**b**) molar region

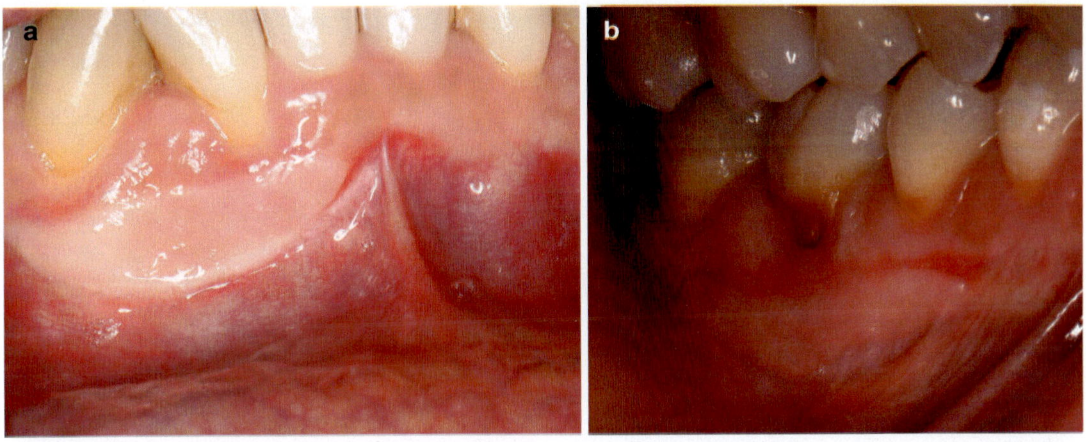

Fig. 6.9 FGG assures a certain amount of keratinized tissue which is helpful in stopping recessions: (**a**) front, (**b**) molar region

recession. In routine, however, at least a recession reduction over a long period of time can be expected.

6.3 Oral Surgical Interventions

6.3.1 Preparation of the Bony Base

It may be necessary to intervene surgically before RPD construction in several situations. As a general principle, in all bony interventions, a full mucoperiosteal flap is reflected to expose all the bony area. Vertical releasing incisions may be necessary if adequate exposure cannot be obtained since trauma of the soft tissue flap may occur. Recontouring of bone may require the use of a rotary instrument in large areas or a hand file in smaller areas. Once the bony correction is complete and visualization confirms that no irregularities or undercuts exist, surgery may be finished.

Bony prominences or spikes (Fig. 6.10) that could cause ulcerations or sore spots under the denture base should be smoothed (Fig. 6.11). Too prominent bony undercuts could create difficulties in the establishment of the path of placement of the planned denture and should be eliminated before an alveoloplasty. An easy bidigital pressure may prevent most alveoloplasties after tooth extraction (Fig. 6.12), which is the simplest alve-

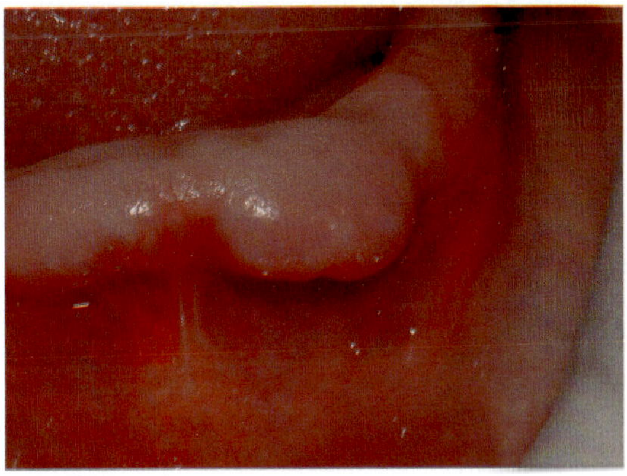

Fig. 6.10 Bony prominences or spikes that could cause ulcerations or sore spots under the denture base or even complicate the path of insertion

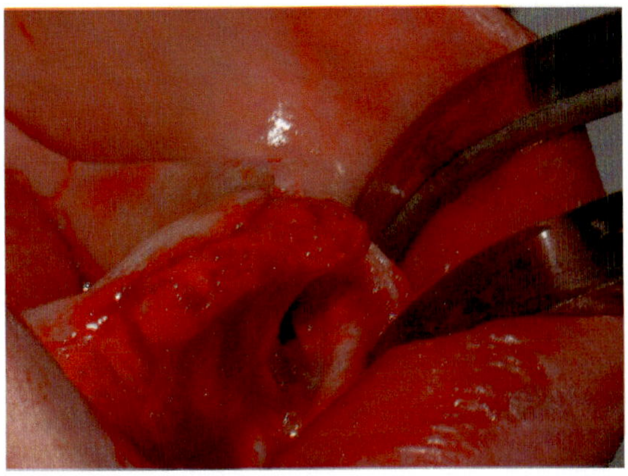

Fig. 6.11 A simple surgical procedure could help obtaining a smooth mucosal surface for denture base support

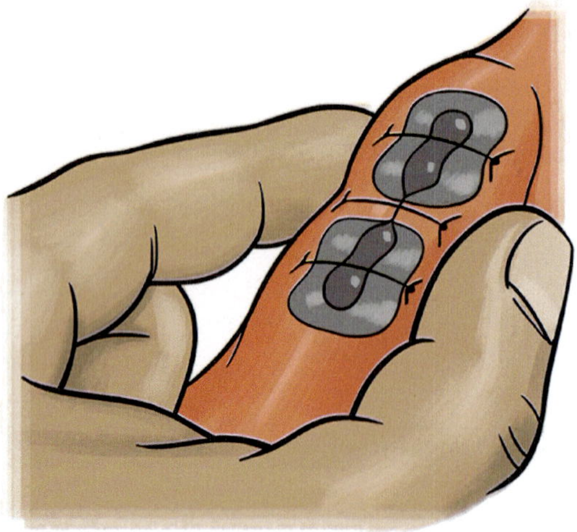

Fig. 6.12 An easy bidigital pressure after tooth extraction, which could be considered as the simplest alveoloplasty procedure, may prevent most of alveoloplasties

oloplasty procedure. However, overcompression and overreduction of irregularities should be avoided. The only exception for the need of bidigital pressure after tooth extraction would be a planned future implantation at the same site since it could reduce the necessary bucco-lingual width of the alveolar crest. If there are several irregularities, these may cause undercuts hindering the path of insertion for RPDs. These need more complex alveoloplasties and in many cases, the elevation of mucoperiosteal flaps using a crestal incision with vertical releases is necessary to prevent tears and to produce the best access to the alveolar ridge, thus increased pain and discomfort for the patient and a longer healing period before prosthetic restoration can proceed may be expected.

An exostosis or a torus is found either on the lingual side of mandibular premolars (Fig. 6.13) or on the palatal midline (Fig. 6.14). In both cases, it is a hindrance to denture construction and should be resected surgically. The etiology is unknown and an incidence of up to 40% in males and 20% in females is reported. Tori may appear as a big single or multilocular bony mass either unilaterally or bilaterally. They are rarely removed if a patient is not a candidate for a removable denture. Nevertheless, they may be a

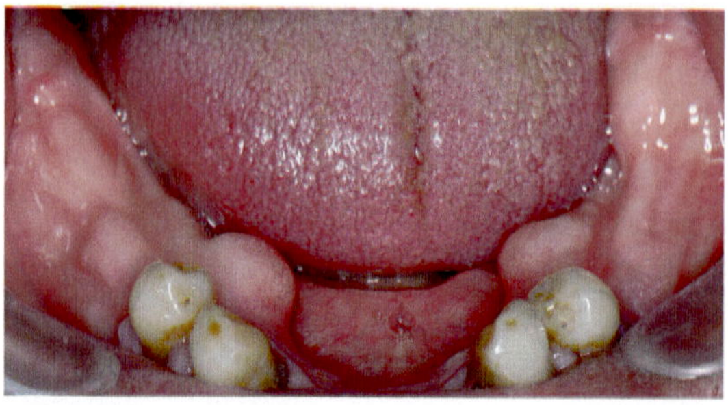

Fig. 6.13 An exostosis or a torus on the lingual side of mandibular premolars

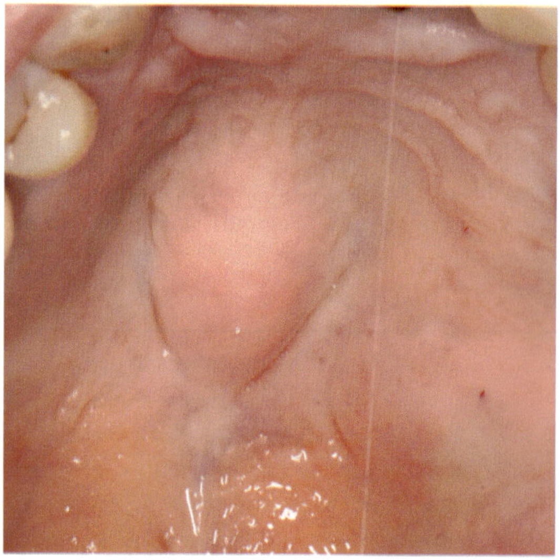

Fig. 6.14 Palatal torus is found in the midline of the maxilla and may be a great obstacle for denture seating

significant bulk to insertion, interfering with the overall comfort, fit, and function of the planned prosthesis. As usual in bony interventions, rotary instrumentation with a round bur may be used for small areas, whereas the treatment of choice for large tori should be rather sectioning with a fissure bur. Once sectioned into several pieces, the torus is easily removed with a chisel. Care must be taken not to expose the floor of the nose. Final contouring may be done with an egg-shaped or a larger round bur or a hand file. The same principles are valid for mandibular tori. Small protuberances can be taken away with a mallet and chisel. Large tori should be divided superiorly from the adjacent bone with a fissure bur parallel to the medial axis of the mandible and treated as

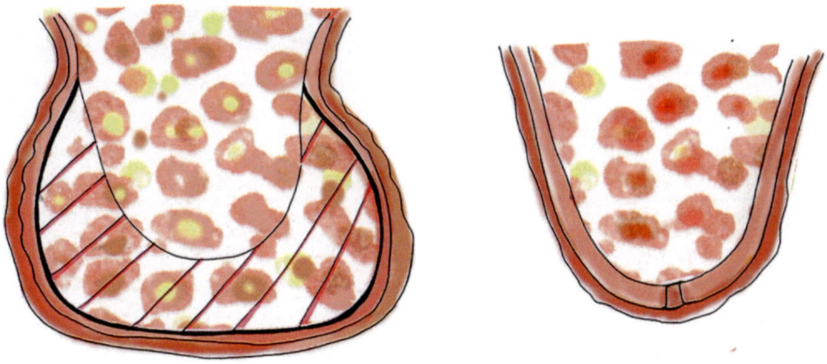

Fig. 6.15 A tuberostosis occupies bucco-lingually too much space and should be reduced

in small protuberances with a mallet and chisel. It is not important that the bony protuberance is totally removed if the goals of the procedure are achieved.

Excesses in the maxillary tuberosity, also named tuberostosis, may consist of soft tissue, bone, or both. Sounding with a needle or a panoramic radiography can help differentiate between the tissues. However, the most certain way to identify bony irregularities and variations in anatomy is to visualize during surgery when mucoperiosteal flap is raised and the level of the maxillary sinuses should be ascertained radiographically before the operation. Excesses in the maxillary tuberosity may encroach on the interarch space and decrease the overall freeway space needed for proper prosthetic function. It is of great value that the necessary interarch distance is regained before denture planning. In addition, a tuberostosis occupies bucco-lingually too much space, too (Fig. 6.15). In many cases, this may create a bilateral undercut situation being an obstacle to a decent path of denture insertion. The level of the maxillary sinus should be carefully evaluated before any bony intervention is attempted in the tuberosity. Although small sinus perforations are generally reported to require no treatment if the membrane remains intact and only large perforations must be treated with a tension-free tight closure, it is advisable to keep a greater distance to the sinus to avoid later complications. The overlying soft tissue may be removed in a wedge-shaped fashion to thin the overall soft tissue bulk overlying the bony tuberosity. Excess overlying soft tissue may be trimmed in an elliptic fashion from the edges of the crestal incision to allow a tension-free passive closure. Genioglossus and mylohyoid muscle attachments can interfere with the stability and function of conventional mandibular prostheses from time to time and should be relieved. In cases of mandibular atrophy, especially the mylohyoid muscle contributes significantly to the displacement of conventional dentures. Compared to a few decades ago, there are fewer indications for the reduction of the mylohyoid ridge, especially with the availability of dental implants. Nevertheless, in severe cases of mandibular atrophy, the external oblique and mylohyoid ridges may be a significant source of discomfort as the overlying mucosa is thin and easily irritated by denture flanges. This book is designed to give clinicians recommendations for daily practice. Some of these procedures are rarely indicated and need a serious surgical background. There are additionally some other titles being part of the preprosthetic surgery list, such as "Treatment of Skeletal and Alveolar Ridge Discrepancies", "Alveolar Distraction Osteogenesis", or "Mandibular Augmentation". However, these treatment modalities are severe surgical interventions, needing oral and maxillofacial surgery cooperation in a multidisciplinary approach.

6.3.2 Soft Tissue Interventions

With the eventual bony remodeling following tooth loss, muscle, and frenulum attachments initially not being in a problematic position, can start to create complications in prosthetic reconstruction and to pose increasing problems about prosthetic comfort, stability, and fit. From time to time, these attachments should be altered before removable dentures can be attempted. Inflammatory fibrous hyperplasia of the vestibule called epulis fissuratum and inflammatory hyperplasia of the palate should be addressed before any type of prosthetic reconstruction can proceed. Frenulum attachments consist of thin bands of fibrous tissue covered with mucosa extending from the lip, cheek, or floor of the mouth to the alveolar periosteum. The height of this attachment varies from individual to individual. Although in dentates, frenulum attachments rarely cause a problem, in individuals using removable dentures they may interfere with fit, stability, and retention of the prostheses. A pronounced frenulum can additionally weaken the denture and cause fractures. Several surgical methods have been introduced for the excision of these attachments. While simple excision and Z-plasty are effective for narrow frenulum attachments, a vestibuloplasty is often indicated for frenulum attachments with a wide base. Although vestibular frenectomies are less associated with complications, careful attention is advised to Wharton's ducts and superficial blood vessels in the floor of the mouth and ventral tongue for lingual frenectomy interventions. The severity of the frenulum interaction may be identified by eversion of the lip or cheek or by tongue movement.

Hyperplastic soft tissues such as epulis fissuratum or fibrous ridge (flabby ridge) or fibromae caused by chronic trauma are subject to soft tissue surgery before any prosthodontic planning can be accomplished. In general, a 3- to 4-week period to allow for soft tissue remodeling is adequate before impressions for prosthesis fabrication may be taken. Fibrous inflammatory hyperplasia is often the result of ill-fitting dentures producing inflammation of the underlying mucosa and eventual fibrous proliferation. The adjustment of the offending denture flange with an associated soft reline of the prosthesis is mostly an insufficient measure. Most of the time, a surgical excision is necessary, and some sources even suggest laser ablation, too.

Vestibuloplasty operations are ridge extension procedures in the maxilla and mandible and once have been very important in obtaining better vertical height of the alveolar ridge. They have lost their significance after the introduction of dental implants. However, in combination with removable dentures, the importance of a safe distance without mobile soft tissue, from alveolar crest to sulcus is not neglectable. In cases where the sulcus depth is lost, vestibuloplasty operations can be necessary. In some situations, even free connective tissue grafts and/or free gingival grafts may be necessary. The use of rearranged dentures with elongated denture flanges after vestibuloplasty operations is vital to reduce the shrinkage and keep the tissues and regained sulcus depth in place. If there is no existing denture, a preoperatively prepared plate may be used. The plate can be used with or without tissue conditioners. However, it is advisable to fixate the plate to assist in a healthy healing of the wound. If retention cannot be maintained conventionally with the tissue conditioner a screw fixation may be considered.

6.3.3 Removal of Teeth or Tooth Remnants

Before RPD production, retained roots or impacted teeth should be surgically removed, especially when they are located very superficial in edentulous parts. Any pathology associated with teeth or dental remnants is to be extracted. Exceptions would be a not operable patient due to systemic conditions, a tooth with a strategic position, such as the canine, where the left root may serve to delay alveolar atrophy and keep the crestal height. In systemically or financially compromised patients, where the use of dental implants cannot be considered, a decent root canal-treated tooth remainder can be useful. Keeping the root with a root cap can be helpful in the bone height maintenance and if the root is strong enough, an attachment retained in the root could help to increase patient comfort, thus patient compliance. A tooth occupying a strategically false position may be considered as candidate for extraction, even if it is free of decay and periodontally healthy, if an orthodontic treatment is not a choice. In this chapter, interventions such as apicectomies, bi- or hemisections are not appreciated for abutment teeth since the surgical weakening of abutment teeth may mislead the readers.

6.4 Restorative Approach: Fillings and Root Canal Treatment

An important aspect of preprosthetic planning is the determination of the need for restorative treatment, among others the indication for a root canal treatment. An important reason why radiographic evaluation during prosthetic planning is compulsory is to see the intrabony situation including the roots and apical parts of especially the abutment teeth. In the case of a suspicious radiolucency, the vitality of that tooth should be checked. An apical lesion is in some cases confounded with a widened periodontal gap. An apical lesion should not be ignored since it bears the potential of flaring up as an infection and endangering the prognosis of the denture. If the tooth is devital, it is advisable to treat it endodontically. If the tooth is already treated endodontically and shows a periapical lesion, there are two treatment options: (a) a revision of the root canal filling or (b) an apicectomy.

Old fillings that have the potential to cause leakage, fractures, or various problems should also be exchanged. Particularly in abutment teeth, care should be taken about the choice of material. The rest seats could create a problem, if not a suitable filling material is used. The material must ensure good retention of the tooth and show sufficient compressive strength.

An important indication for adhesive restorations is the creation of a height of contour where a retentive area for the clasp is missing. In this manner, a composite material addition to the part where the retentive area is not present may help create an undercut, giving the clasp a chance for retention (see Chap. 7).

6.5 Preprosthetic Soft Tissue Conditioning Procedures

From time-to-time, patients, who are candidates for a new denture, need conditioning of supporting tissues in edentulous areas before the final impression phase of treatment begins. An inflammation or irritation of the mucosa at denture-bearing sites (Fig. 6.16) or distortion of normal anatomic structures, such as incisive papillae, rugae and retromolar pads make a pretreatment inevitable. If not a systemic disease or bruxism is the etiology, in general, ill-fitting, or poorly occludings are the causative factor for these conditions. The allergic stomatitis as a differential diagnosis must be always kept in mind. Early stages are easily treated by an improvement of hygiene practices. In the case of denture-related stomatitis, a well-defined home care program should implement the denture and tissue conditioning. The brushing of the palate and the dorsum of the tongue should be meticulously explained and ordered to the patients as it strictly belongs to the hygiene program. Tissue conditioning materials are elastopolymers that continue to flow for an extended period, permitting in amounts sufficient to provide a cushioning effect to distorted tissues, and thus, to recover, probably through more evenly distributed occlusal forces.

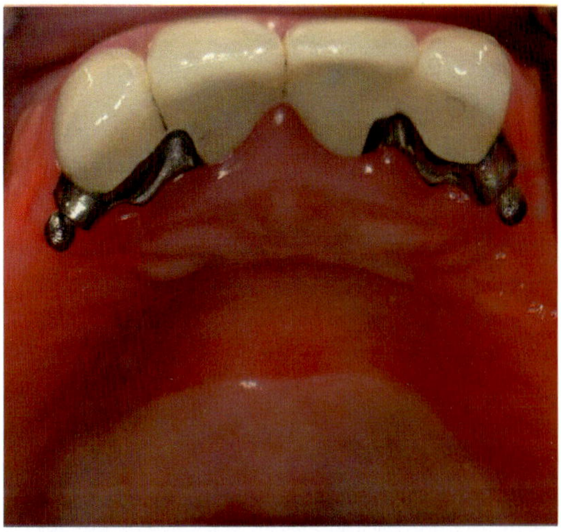

Fig. 6.16 Sight of inflamed mucosa at denture-bearing sites

The tissue conditioner is more beneficiary when deflective or interfering occlusal contacts of old dentures are eliminated or the denture base is extended to enhance support, retention, and stability. The conditioning period should be long enough to allow tissues to recover. Although generally change of the provisional relining material in 4–7-day intervals is considered clinically acceptable, the authors of this book recommend a maximal 3-day interval for a faster relief. Most of the time, the clinician will notice a dramatic change within a few visits. In resistant situations where no improvement in irritated and inflamed tissues is seen, a consultation with a physician would be advisable. Differential diagnosis would include a candida-induced denture stomatitis, where drug administration following microbiological analysis is indispensable. In the case of an inflammatory papillary hyperplasia that is also called Newton III after Newton's classification, the latest stage of an untreated denture stomatitis, the lesion appears as multiple proliferative nodules underlying a mandibular prosthesis likely colonized with *Candida*, mainly *Candida albicans*. In addition to systemic drugs, soaking of the prosthesis in a chosen antifungal solution or in a very dilute sodium hypochlorite solution helps decrease the overall colonization of the prosthesis, in case there is no alloy part of the partial denture, since it would initialize an undesired corrosion. In addition, the oral disinfection with a chlorhexidine rinse is advisable (see Chap. 25). It must be addressed that in comparison to lesions such as the epulis fissuratum, inflammatory papillary hyperplasia reacts in a positive way to denture adaptation and tissue conditioning. In proliferative and persistent cases necessitating surgical treatment, excision should be the method of choice. Many methods including sharp excision with a scalpel, rotary debridement, loop electrocautery, and laser ablation with a carbon dioxide laser are acceptable. Treatment precedes supraperiosteally to prevent exposure of underlying palatal bone. Subsequently, the use of a tissue conditioner is helpful to minimize patient discomfort and stabilize the result. Although very often patients do not comply, a good way for tissue conditioning could be to let the tissues rest. If the patient agrees, the best way for tissue healing is to quit wearing the dentures for a certain time. Systemic drug administration is inevitable if a microbiological smear test gives a positive result. After a critical search of the latest articles about the modern treatment of oral candidiasis, it could be concluded that although nystatin and amphotericin B can be classified as the drugs most often used locally, fluconazole oral suspension has been proven to be a very effective drug. Owing to its good antifungal properties, its high acceptance of the patient, and its efficacy compared with other antifungal drugs, fluconazole was found to be worldwide the drug of choice as a systemic treatment of oral candidiasis. In cases when Candida strains resist to fluconazole, other drugs like itraconazole or ketoconazole may be considered as alternatives.

6.6 Orthodontic Preparation

There may be different indications for preprosthetic orthodontic preparations. A common indication is that the neighboring teeth are mesialized or distalized into the gap, or an unsupported tooth from the opposing jaw may have elongated into the space, where a tooth was lost earlier. The orthodontic treatment has the goal of repositioning this kind of teeth (Fig. 6.17) to improve the path of insertion and avoid future food-trapping undercuts. Another helpful orthodontic interven-

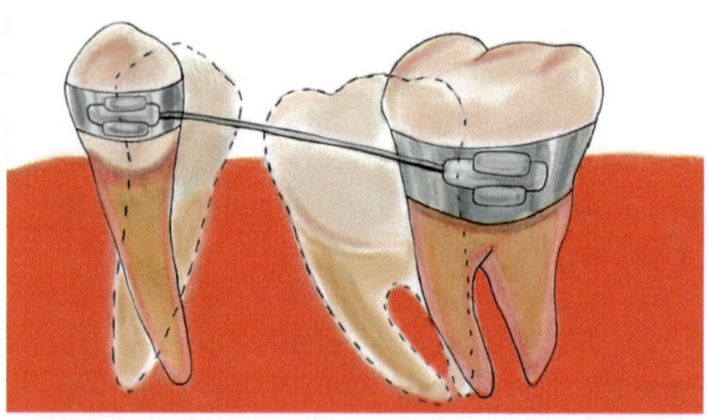

Fig. 6.17 Neighboring teeth which are mesialised or distalised into the gap where a tooth was lost earlier, may be orthodontically repositioned, to improve the path of insertion and avoid future food trapping undercuts

tion is the preparation of the edentulous gap for exact mesio-distal width. Mainly for esthetic reasons, it is important that the gap of missing teeth overlaps the teeth to be set up in the denture. Mostly, a mesialization or distalization of neighboring teeth can be a compulsive measure to enhance esthetics.

Another indication for orthodontic treatment may be the vertical movement of teeth. In cases where elongated teeth interfere with the planned occlusion, an intrusion can be beneficial. Extrusion may be indicated in certain conditions, too, such as violation of the biological width due to too subgingival positioning of the preparation margins or the necessity for longer clinical crowns. It was already in the 1970s when forced orthodontic eruption was recommended for "nonrestorable" or previously "hopeless" teeth. Forced eruption is an alternative to ostectomy. It is contraindicated in cases of inadequate crown-to-root ratio and lack of interocclusal space. However, this technique may be more advantageous over a surgical approach, especially in situations where bone removal would compromise adjacent teeth.

Further Reading

Agudio G, Nieri M, Rotundo R, Cortellini P, Pini Prato G. Free gingival grafts to increase keratinized tissue: a retrospective longterm evaluation (10 to 25 years) of outcomes. J Periodontol. 2008;79:587–94.

Al Jabbari YS. Frenectomy for improvement of a problematic conventional maxillary complete denture in an elderly patient: a case report. J Adv Prosthodont. 2011;3:236–9.

Bensimon GC. Surgical crown-lengthening procedure to enhance esthetics. Int J Periodontics Restorative Dent. 1999;19:332–41.

Bidra AS, Uribe F. Preprosthetic orthodontic intervention for management of a partially edentulous patient with generalized wear and malocclusion. J Esthet Restor Dent. 2012;24:88–100.

Bilhan H, Geckili O, Ergin S, Erdogan O, Ates G. Evaluation of satisfaction and complications in patients with existing complete dentures. J Oral Sci. 2013;55:29–37.

Bilhan H, Sulun T, Erkose G, Kurt H, Erturan Z, Kutay O, Bilgin T. The role of Candida albicans hyphae and lactobacillus in denture-related stomatitis. Clin Oral Investig. 2009;13:363–8.

Bilhan H, Sulun T, Kutay Ö. The prevalence and aetiology of denture related stomatitis in patients wearing removable dentures. Balk J Stom. 2005;9:191–7.

Cilingir A, Bilhan H, Baysal G, Sunbuloglu E, Bozdag E. The impact of frenulum height on strains in maxillary denture bases. J Adv Prosthodont. 2013;5:409–15.

Cohen ES. Atlas of cosmetic and reconstructive periodontal surgery. 3rd ed. Hamilton: BC Decker Inc.; 2007.

Costello BJ, Betts NJ, Barber HD, Fonseca RJ. Preprosthetic surgery for the edentulous patients. Dent Clin North Am. 1996;40:19–38.

Cunliffe J, Grey N. Crown lengthening surgery—indications and techniques. Dent Update. 2008;35:29–35.

Davenport JC, Basker RM, Heath JR, Ralph JP, Glantz PO. Preparation of mouth. In: A clinical guide to removable partial dentures. London: BDJ Books; 2000. p. 69–75.

Drisko CH. Nonsurgical periodontal therapy. Periodontol 2000. 2001;25:77–88.

Ford DE. Commentary. Preprosthetic orthodontic intervention for management of a partially edentulous patient with generalized wear and malocclusion. J Esthet Restor Dent. 2012;24:101–2.

Fragiskos DF. Preprosthetic surgery. In: Oral surgery. 15th ed. Berlin: Springer; 2007. p. 243–79.

Garcia-Cuesta C, Sarrion-Pérez MG, Bagán JV. Current treatment of oral candidiasis: a literature review. J Clin Exp Dent. 2014;6:e576–82.

Goncalves TM, de Oliveira JA, Sanchez-Ayala A, Rodrigues Garcia RC. Surgical resection and prosthetic treatment of an extensive mandibular torus. Gen Dent. 2013;61:65–8.

Hillerup S. Preprosthetic surgery in the elderly. J Prosthet Dent. 1994;72:551–8.

Ingber JS. Forced eruption: part II. A method of treating nonrestorable teeth—periodontal and restorative considerations. J Periodontol. 1976;47:203–16.

Jameson LM, Malone WF. Crown contours and gingival response. J Prosthet Dent. 1982;47:620–4.

Lindhe J, Lang NP, Karring T. Clinical periodontology and implant dentistry. 6th ed. Oxford: Blackwell Munksgaard; 2008.

Loukas M, Hulsberg P, Tubbs RS, Kapos T, Wartmann CT, Shaffer K, Moxham BJ. The tori of the mouth and ear: a review. Clin Anat. 2013;26:953–60.

Morrison MD, Tamimi F. Oral tori are associated with local mechanical and systemic factors: a case-control study. J Oral Maxillofac Surg. 2013;71:14–22.

Motamedi MH, Motamedi MK. Technique to manage the enlarged maxillary tuberosity in elderly edentulous patients requiring dentures. J Oral Maxillofac Surg. 2011;69:1283–5.

Nevins M, Skurow HM. The intracrevicular restorative margin, the biologic width, and the maintenance of the gingival margin. Int J Periodontics Restorative Dent. 1984;4:30–49.

Nugala B, Kumar BS, Sahitya S, Krishna PM. Biologic width and its importance in periodontal and restorative dentistry. J Conserv Dent. 2012;15:12–7.

Padbury A Jr, Eber R, Wang HL. Interactions between the gingiva and the margin of restorations. J Clin Periodontol. 2003;30:379–85.

Rezavandi K. Periodontal factors. In: Levine JB, editor. Design integrating esthetics and function - essentials of esthetic dentistry, vol. 2. Missouri: Mosby; 2016. p. 123–48.

Şakar O, Bilhan H, Sülün T, Çalışır F, Ispirgil E, Erturan Z, Erköse G. Denture related stomatitis and candida counts of a rest home population: an epidemiologic pilot study in patients wearing upper full removable dentures. Balk J Stom. 2008;12: 98–102.

Spagnoli DB, Gollehon SG, Misiek DJ. Preprosthetic and reconstructive surgery. In: Peterson's principles of Oral and maxillofacial surgery. New York: Third Edition, BC Decker Inc.; 2012. p. 159–87.

Stefanac S, Nesbit S. The disease control phase of treatment. In: Diagnosis and treatment planning in dentistry. 3rd ed. Amsterdam: Elsevier; 2015. (eBook ISBN: 9780323287319).

Thomas GA. Denture-induced fibrous inflammatory hyperplasia (epulis fissuratum): research aspects. Aust Prosthodont J. 1993;7:49–53.

van Winkelhoff AJ, Rodenburg JP, Goené RJ, Abbas F, Winkel EG, de Graaff J. Metronidazole plus amoxycillin in the treatment of Actinobacillus actinomycetemcomitans associated periodontitis. J Clin Periodontol. 1989;16:128–31.

Yeh S, Andreana S. Crown lengthening: basic principles, indications, techniques, and clinical case reports. N Y State Dent J. 2004;70:30–6.

Preparation of the Abutment Teeth for Removable Partial Dentures

7

Muzaffer Ateş

Abstract

One of the important steps of the mouth preparation is the preparation of the abutment teeth. Before starting preparations, the dentist should make sure that the other stages of the mouth preparation are completed. Usually, tooth decay and periodontal destruction on the abutment teeth of removable partial denture (RPD) wearers are observed. However, studies show that a well-planned removable denture does not cause any damage to the abutment teeth and the periodontal tissues. Actually, the space between the denture and the supporting teeth is a favorable place for food retention. Therefore, dentists claim that the patients are also responsible for tooth loss since they do not pay enough attention to their oral hygiene. Although this assertion may hold true in many instances, should the dentist not be held accountable if they fail to take appropriate precautions? This chapter focuses on providing the necessary information to the dentist who will fabricate the RPD regarding the preparation of supporting teeth.

M. Ateş (✉)
Faculty of Dentistry, Department of Prosthodontics, İstanbul Medipol University, İstanbul, Türkiye
e-mail: mates@medipol.edu.tr

7.1 Definitions

Guiding planes: Two or more vertically parallel surfaces on abutment teeth and/or fixed dental prostheses oriented so as to contribute to the direction of the path of placement and removal of a removable partial denture, maxillofacial prosthesis, and overdenture.

Reciprocation: The mechanism by which lateral forces generated by a retentive clasp passing over a height of contour are counterbalanced by a reciprocal clasp passing along a reciprocal guiding plane.

Rest: A rigid extension of a removable partial denture that contacts the occlusal, incisal, cingulum, or lingual surface of a tooth or restoration, the surface of which is commonly prepared to receive it.

Rest seat: The prepared recess in a tooth or restoration developed to receive the occlusal, incisal, cingulum, or lingual rest.

The principle of "protection of healthy remaining tissues", which is one of the basic rules when preparing abutment teeth for RPDs is occasionally ignored. This situation causes various problems, especially on abutment teeth in RPD wearers. Due to these problems, abutment teeth loss occurs and, hence, additional treatments need to be performed on prosthesis. To avoid such probable problems, for an RPD wearer patient, primarily a diagnostic cast model should be formed, and treatment plan should be carefully evaluated on this model. Following surgical,

O. Şakar (ed.), *Removable Partial Dentures*, https://doi.org/10.1007/978-3-031-47083-7_7

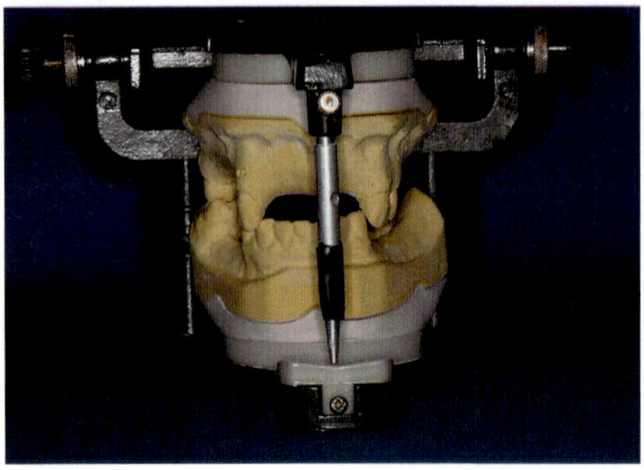

Fig. 7.1 Fixing of diagnostic casts to articulator by split cast mounting

periodontal, and endodontic treatments, the model should be placed into a surveyor to examine the guide surfaces and to determine which teeth will be used as abutment teeth. In order to ensure parallelism, the teeth which require grinding, and the teeth which will be crowned, should be determined. The order and scheme of these treatments and the necessary precautions required to be taken for crowned teeth are discussed below.

In order to decide for the preparation of the supporting teeth, a diagnostic cast should be first obtained. After determining the vertical dimension of occlusion and centric relation, the diagnostic models are attached to the articulator using the split cast (Fig. 7.1). Then the model is studied by the surveyor to determine which teeth could be used as an abutment and decide the preparations needed to be done.

These preparations can be performed in the following order:

1. Forming (creating) the guide planes.
2. Preparation of rest seat.
3. Forming a retentive area.
4. Crowning abutment tooth/teeth.

The first three steps are completed on the supporting tooth/teeth.

These preparations should not go beyond the enamel borders. If performing of grinding is within the borders of the enamel, a crown restoration might not be necessary. Following the grinding, the tooth surfaces should be polished, and afterward topical fluoride should be applied. If the adjustments by grinding goes beyond the enamel, and penetrates dentine tissue, then crown restorations would be necessary.

7.2 Relationship of Guide Surface and Guide Plate

An important consideration in RPD fabrication is the region where the teeth and gums meet. This area is often associated with gum recession and dental caries in people who wear RPDs. When a tooth is extracted, there will be soft and hard tissue loss, but no change will be observed in the teeth adjacent to this soft tissue. As a result, an undercut area forms between the tooth and the soft tissues. When an RPD is fabricated under certain circumstances, there is often a gap between the tooth and the prosthesis in the gingival zone. In such cases, possible problems arising are (1) food accumulation in this area, (2) hypertrophy of the tissues adjacent to the gap, (3) decrease in support of teeth, and (4) gingival recession due to food impaction.

In order to prevent these problems, metal framework should be adapted precisely to the interproximal surface of the abutment teeth. The part of the metal framework, which contacts the proximal surface of the supporting teeth, is called guide (proximal) plate, and the proximal surface of the supporting tooth is called the guide surface (plane).

The advantages of the accurate maintenance of the guide plate-guide surface relationship are as follows:

1. Food impaction is prevented.
2. Hypertrophy of the soft tissue between the tooth and the prosthesis is prevented.
3. The friction force in these areas supports the retention and stability of the prosthesis in great proportion.
4. Controlling of the movement of the teeth by supporting in antero-posterior direction.
5. The parts that are extended along the lingual/palatinal surfaces maintain reciprocation by compensating the pressure that the retentive

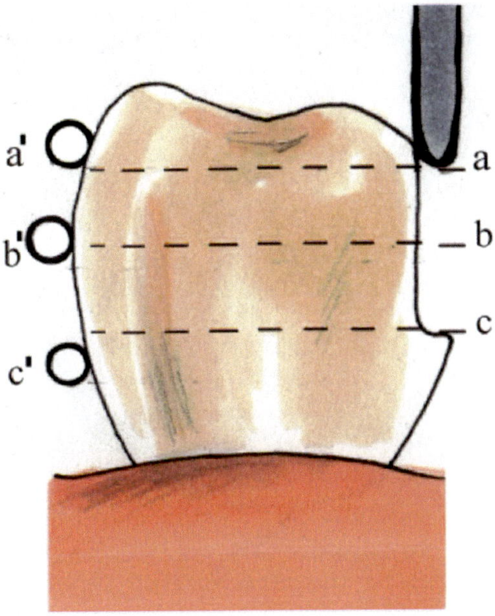

Fig. 7.2 To achieve the real reciprocation; reciprocal arm should contact *a* at the moment retentive arm contacts *a*' and reciprocation arm should contact point *c* while retentive arm is moving towards *c*'. Namely, the reciprocation arm should keep its contact to tooth during retentive arm's trace route from first contact to tooth until the end; thus, it should compensate particularly the pressure applied by the retentive arm while passing the survey line

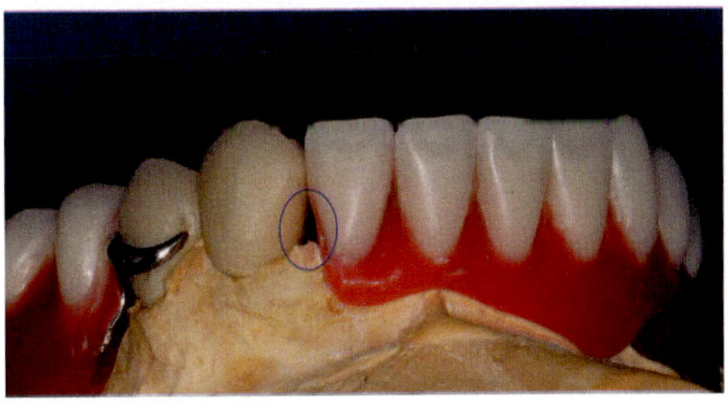

Fig. 7.3 The case that a gap (*stated oval shape*) remains between metal framework and supporting tooth

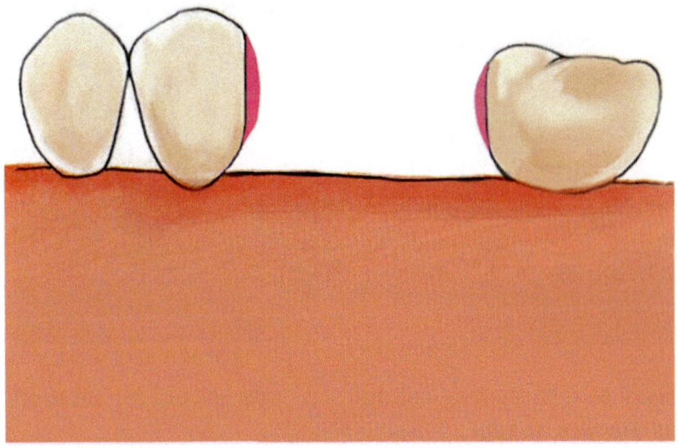

Fig. 7.4 Surfaces that are required to be abraded on guide planes (marked as red)

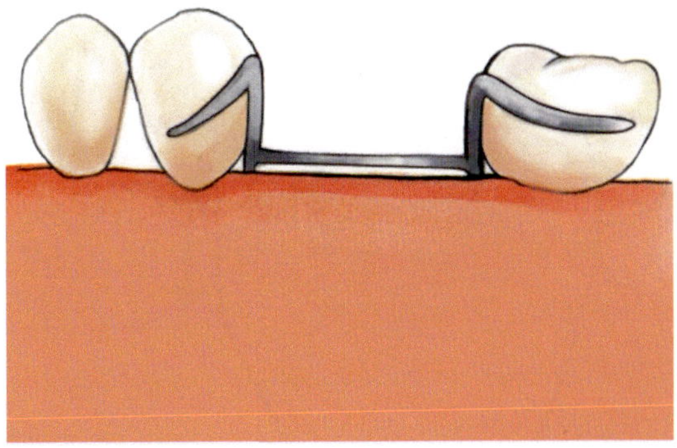

Fig. 7.5 Settled form of metal framework after abrasions is completed. In this way, guide plate and guide plane relationship and path of insertion of prosthesis (insertion/dislodgement) is determined

arm applies while wearing and removing the prosthesis (Fig. 7.2).

6. A natural appearance is obtained by full contact of tooth and RPD without any space in between. Otherwise, the area between the teeth and the prosthesis will appear as a dark space, which will cause esthetic problems (Fig. 7.3).
7. Guide surfaces mean making proximal surfaces of two or more supporting teeth parallel to each other and determining only one path of insertion for the RPD (Figs. 7.4 and 7.5).

By maintaining an accurate guide plate–guide surface relationship for all the abutment teeth, only one path of insertion for the prosthesis is designated. Otherwise, different paths of insertion will be formed and while the patient is wearing and removing the prosthesis, forces from multiple directions will be exerted on the abutment teeth with the clasps exceeding the elastic-

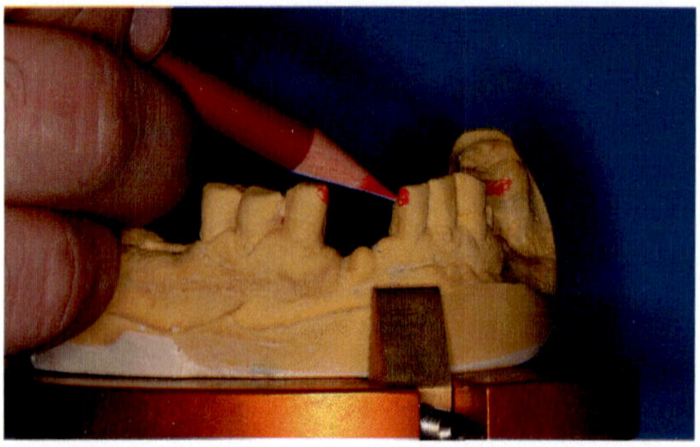

Fig. 7.6 Marking of the surfaces that should be abraded on diagnostic cast

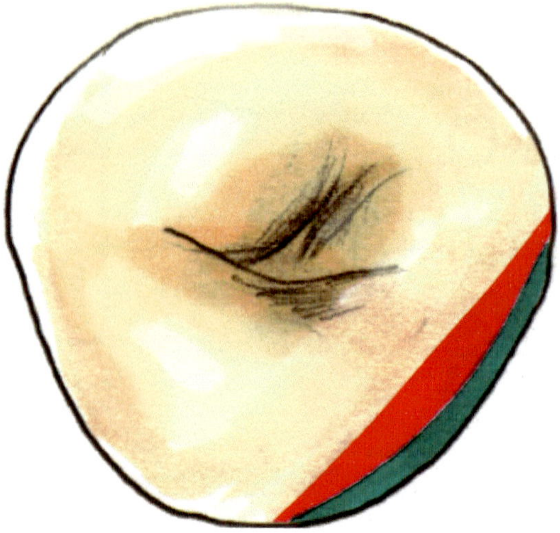

Fig. 7.7 The preparation on the guide planes should follow the teeth's curvature (Green is right)

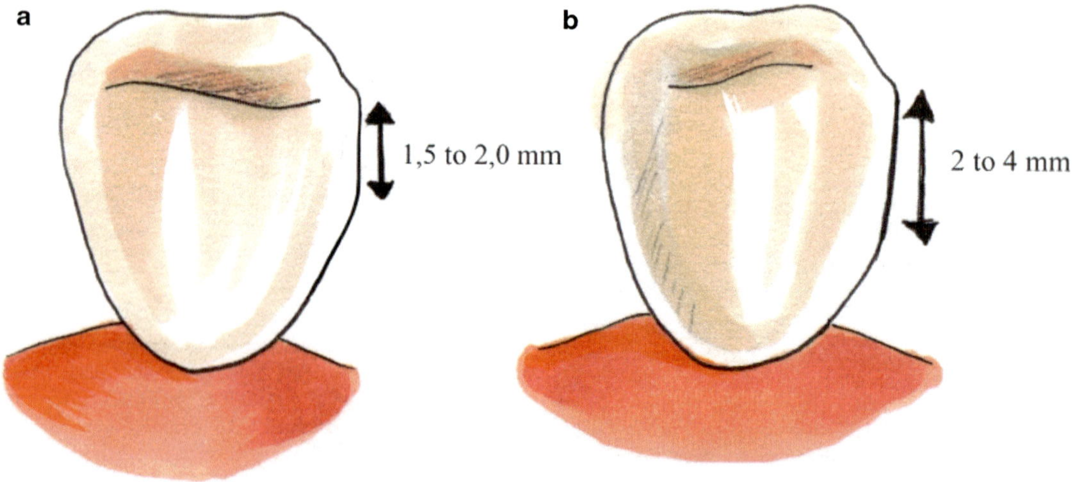

Fig. 7.8 (**a**)Amount of preparation for free-end prosthesis, (**b**) amount of preparation for tooth-supported prosthesis

ity (proportional limits) and resulting in an eventual deformation.

To maintain an accurate guide plate–guide plane relationship, the study model is examined on a surveyor, and the proximal surfaces that need to be grinded are determined depending on the path of insertion. These surfaces are marked with a red pen and necessary grinding is completed in the mouth according to these marks (Fig. 7.6). The grinding abrasions on the guide planes should not be plain and follow the teeth's curvature (Fig. 7.7). Guide planes should be prepared as 1.5–2.0 mm wide/height for the distal extension RPD and 2–4 mm height for the tooth supported RPD (Fig. 7.8).

7.3 Preparation of Rest Seats

After guide plate–guide plane relationship is maintained, rest seats should be prepared according to the rules mentioned in Chap. 10. As mentioned before, the rest seats should be prepared within the enamel borders and should be polished

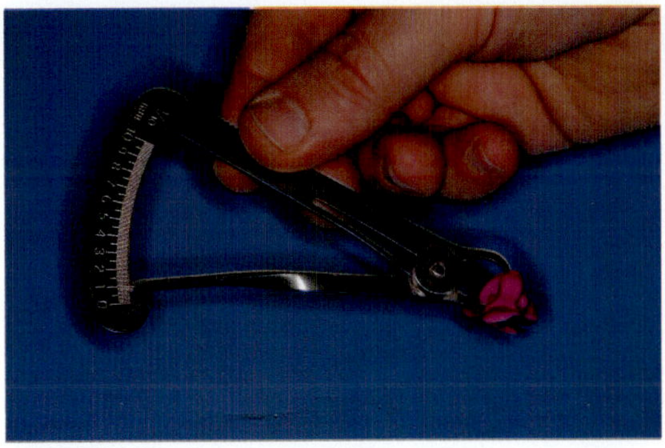

Fig. 7.9 Measuring whether the rest seat thickness is sufficient or not

with various rubbers and fluoride should be applied then. If enamel borders are exceeded, inlay/onlay restorations may be helpful. In some cases, rest seats can be prepared on amalgam or composite resin. To obtain a sufficient sturdiness, the rests should have minimum thickness of 1 mm, and it should not cause occlusal interferences.

To comprehend if the rest seats have sufficient depth or not, it should be checked by making the patient bite a piece of baseplate wax. Silicone-based bite registration materials may also be used for this purpose (Fig. 7.9). Rests should never be placed on inclined planes, such as the anterior teeth, when a rest is to be designed on a canine tooth, a cingulum rest should be prepared (Fig. 7.10). The fact that the lingual surfaces of the anterior teeth in the lower jaw is very plain in general, usually it is not possible to prepare rest seats without exceeding enamel borders. In this case, either tooth should be crowned and a cingulum rest seat should be prepared on crown or a cingulum rest seat should be formed with composite resin. If a cingulum rest is to be prepared with composite resin, the rests should be planned on more than one tooth to ensure the distribution of the forces.

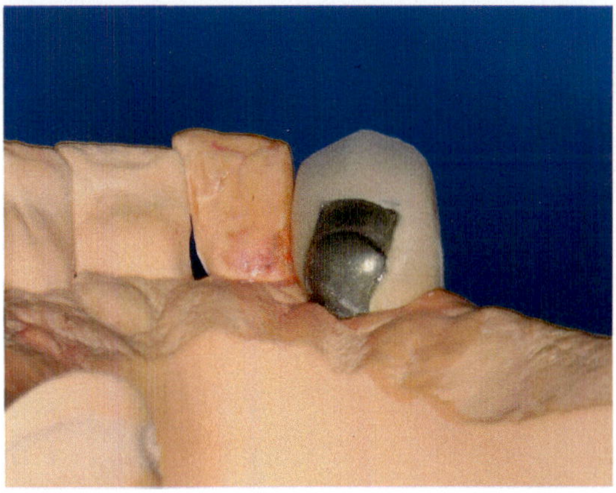

Fig. 7.10 Cingulum rest seat

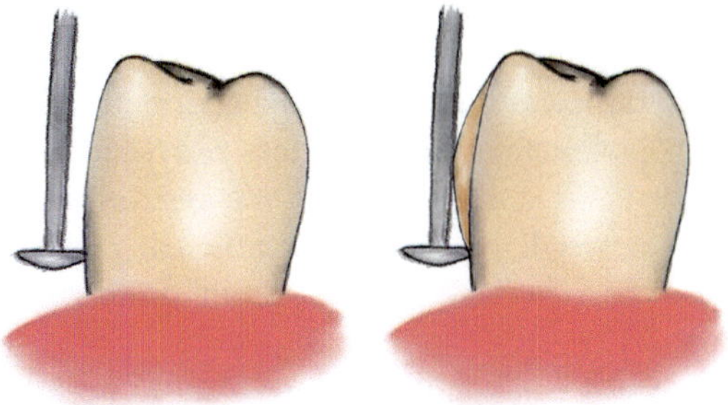

Fig. 7.11 Forming of undercut by composite in case of insufficient presence of undercut

7.3.1 Forming of the Retentive Area

In some cases, despite not having sufficient undercut on the abutment tooth, with little abrasions, a sufficient undercut area can be formed. However, because enamel is thin in the gingival third, it may be hard to prepare a retentive area without exceeding the enamel borders. In such cases, forming the undercut area with the composite resin material is possible (Fig. 7.11). If these methods are not sufficient, a crown restoration would be necessary. Height of contour can be quite high on some abutment teeth. The clasps on such teeth might be so close to the occlusal surface that they may cause occlusal interference. Because this situation will also cause deformation of the clasp and esthetic problems, this part of the tooth should be grinded to lower the height of contour toward gingivae.

7.4 Crowning the Supporting Tooth/Teeth

Determination of crowning the abutment teeth is usually performed in such cases that requires repositioning of crown or occlusion, especially when the rest seats should be prepared on anterior

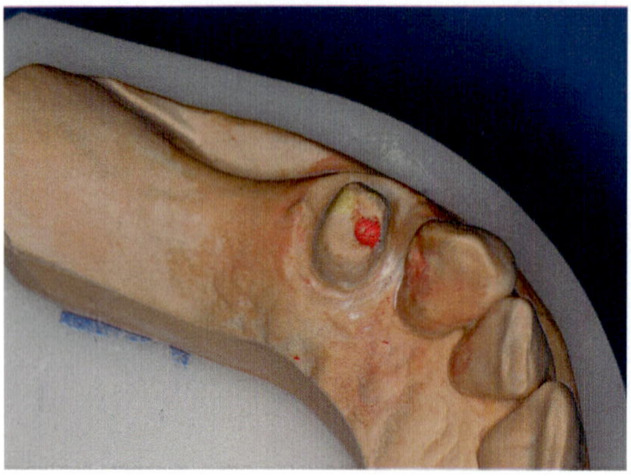

Fig. 7.12 Deeper preparation of insertion area of rest seat while tooth preparation (red area)

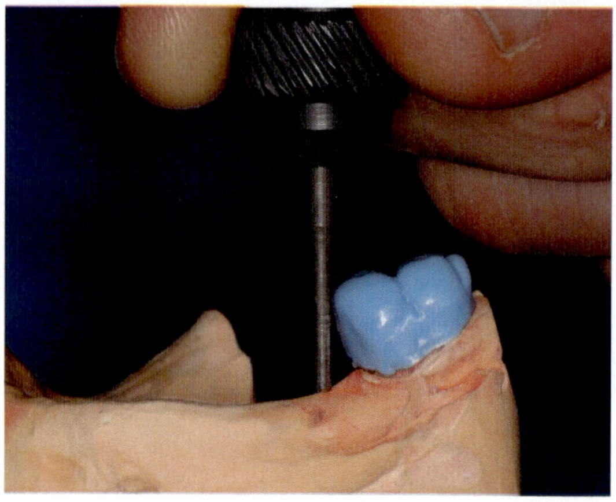

Fig. 7.13 Checking of the parallelism of guide surfaces on wax pattern

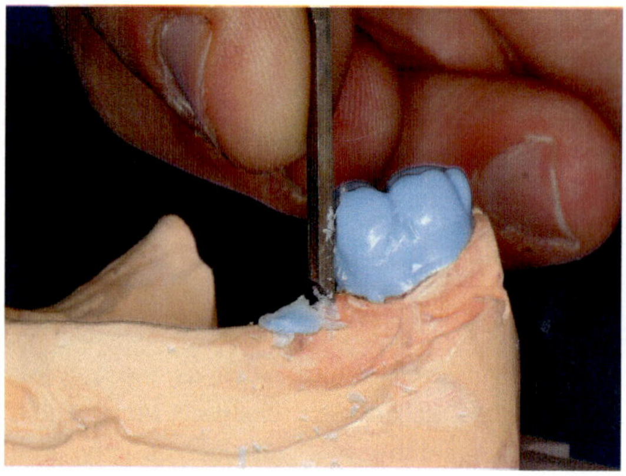

Fig. 7.14 Adjusting of non-parallel surfaces by the use of surveyor's cutting tip

teeth and/or when a clinical crown is fractured. After the decision of crowning the abutment teeth, sufficient space should be allocated during tooth preparation for esthetics, rest seats, and planned clasps. Especially on the area, in which rest seats will be prepared, sufficient distance must be checked during tooth preparation (Fig. 7.12).

Since it is much more convenient to perform abrasions on the wax pattern, crowning of the abutment teeth should be initially controlled in the waxing stage. Otherwise, these processes will be much harder to perform on metal.

If more than one crown will be prepared, all of the crowns should be replaced on the same cast and then controlled by a surveyor.

While checking the wax pattern, the parallelism of the guide planes should be ensured and all of the proximal surfaces should be made parallel to each other by using the surveyor's cutting tip (Figs. 7.13 and 7.14).

Therefore, the metal framework will be seated appropriately according to the way of path of insertion. Food accumulation between the guide plane and the guide plate will be prevented, as there will not be any space in this area. It should be kept in mind that the guide plane/surface on the crown restoration should be prepared only with metal. After all of the guide planes are prepared, rest seats and retention should be reconsidered. If a full metal crown will be fabricated, the height of contour should be marked with surveyor's marker tip, and undercut's sufficiency should be checked by undercut measuring tip. To easily see the height of contour on wax pattern, a fine layer of powder can be applied on wax surfaces (Fig. 7.15a, b). If metal-ceramic crown will be constructed for the abutment teeth, these processes should be done in dentine try-in (Fig. 7.16a, b).

To maintain the stabilization and reciprocation, a step should be prepared on lingual/palatinal surface of the crown. Clasp reciprocation will provide both horizontal stabilization and indirect retention. Reciprocal arm is necessary to compensate for the horizontal force that the retentive

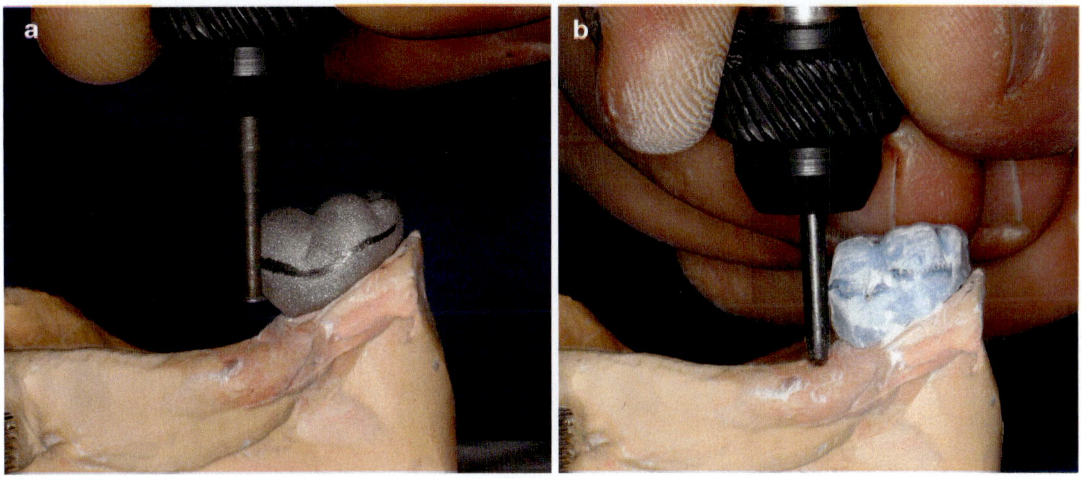

Fig. 7.15 Marking of height of contour on full metal crown (**a**) and wax pattern (**b**)

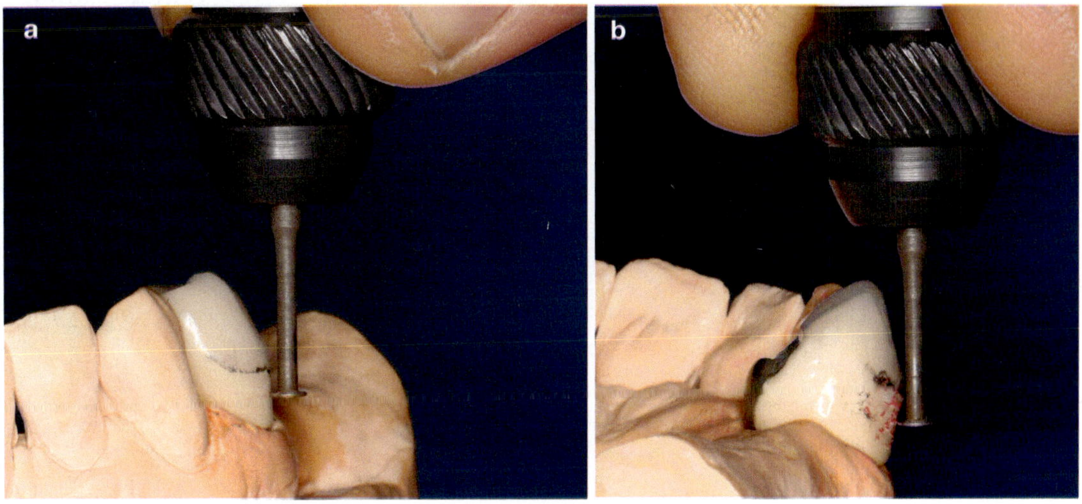

Fig. 7.16 Determining whether sufficient undercut is present or not, during dentine try-in. (**a**) insufficient undercut, (**b**) sufficient undercut

arm applies while wearing and removing the prosthesis. The force that the retentive arm applies during wearing and removal is temporary but strong, so it can cause orthodontic movement and periodontal destruction. Real reciprocation cannot be achieved with a retentive arm that is on the height of contour of the tooth, because when the retentive arm moves away, it loses contact with the tooth or when the retentive arm passes the height of contour and is seated on the tissues completely, it cannot compensate the horizontal force that the retentive arm applies to the tooth. Real reciprocation can be achieved only if it is appropriate for the path of insertion, parallel to the guide planes, and if a step for reciprocation arm is prepared. Thus, reciprocal arm can contact the tooth and compensate for the force that retentive arm applies on the tooth from when it contacts the tooth until the prosthesis is seated on the tissues. Guide plane that is prepared for the reciprocal arm, in this way, can compensate for the forces that are applied during the wearing and removal of prosthesis. The step that is prepared on the crown also acts as a stop for the reciprocal

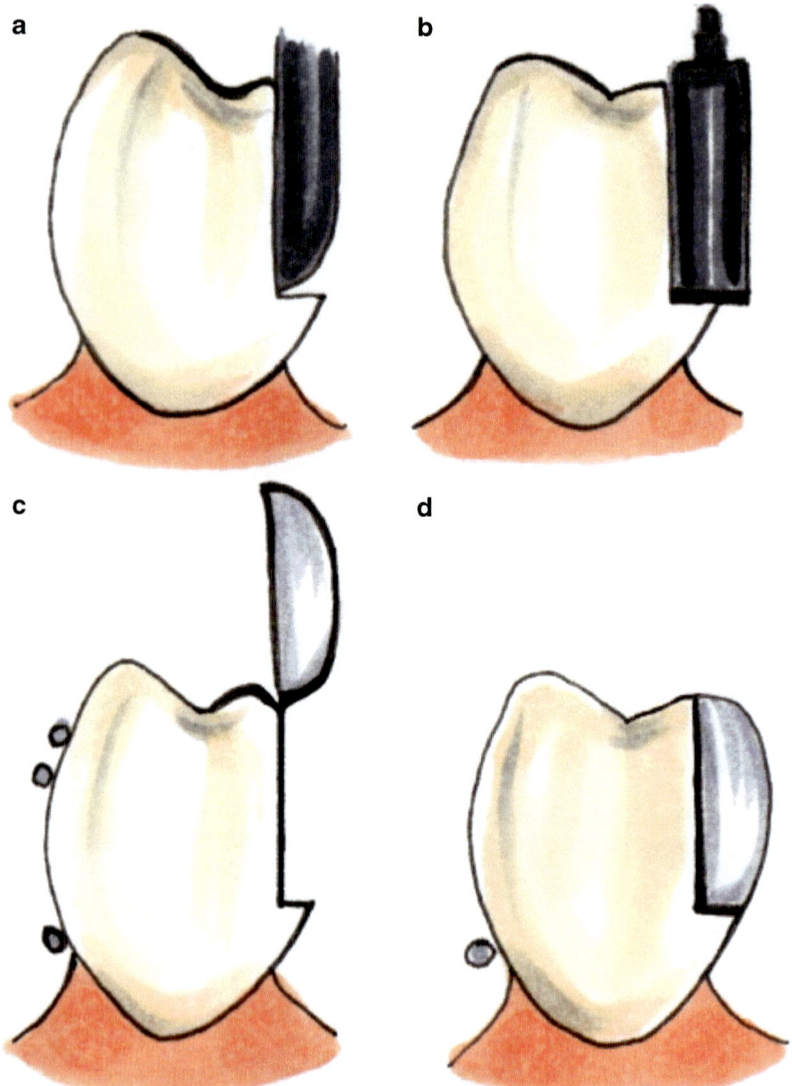

Fig. 7.17 (**a**, **b**) Adjustment of step according to prosthesis' path of insertion by surveyor's knife. (**c**) Appropriate contact of reciprocal arm to prosthesis' path of placement and removal when the step is adjusted in this manner. (**d**) Accurately seated position of reciprocal arm

arm and it supports occlusal rest and indirect retention (Fig. 7.17).

Another advantage of such a step is that it does not make a bulge on the tooth. Thus, the patient feels comfortable as tooth's natural contour is not destroyed and does not disturb the tongue. This step for the reciprocal arm is generally used on premolar and molar teeth, but it can be used on canine teeth, if necessary. The step should follow gingival inclination and it should have sufficient durability. The step that is prepared on lingual surface should be carved by the surveyor's cutting tip after path of insertion is determined and proximal guide planes and rest seats are prepared. Thus, proximal guide plates can continue to lingual surface and the step will be formed according to the path of insertion. Preparations that are made in the waxing stage should be checked on the cast metal crown. To do this, all of the parallelism that is mentioned above should be controlled with a dental handpiece, which is attached to a surveyor.

Rest seats on the crown should have sufficient depth. During the tooth preparation, a deeper rest seat should be prepared where the rest will be seated. If this preparation is not accomplished

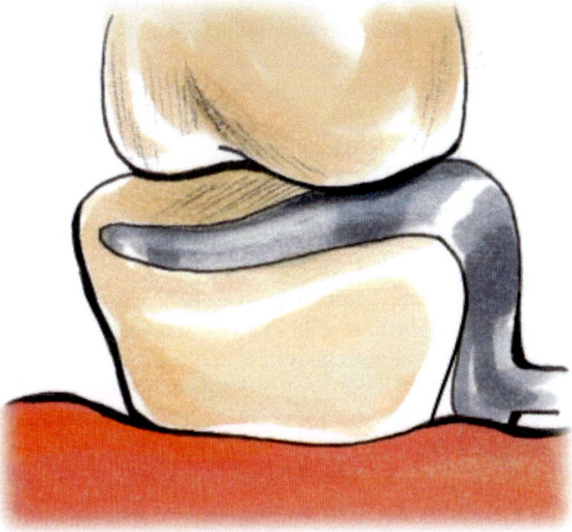

Fig. 7.18 Occlusal interferences may occur in case of insufficient depth of rest seats prepared

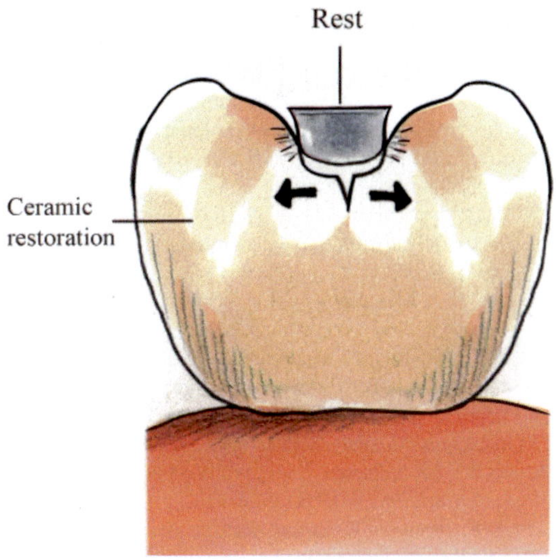

Fig. 7.19 Since rests may cause chipping and fracture on porcelain, the proper fit of the rest to the rest seat is very critical to avoid possible fractures

during tooth preparation, it may not be possible to make rest seats with appropriate depth (Fig. 7.18). In addition, a rest that is seated on an inappropriate rest seat cannot completely achieve its function.

The location of rest seats should be decided in advance during tooth preparation.

While the crown is being constructed, if there is not sufficient space at waxing stage, this may cause various problems, such as occlusal interferences or fracture of the thin rest. Rest seats should always be prepared on metal, and they should be at least 1 mm away from the porcelain.

An alternative to metal-ceramic restorations for supporting RPDs is all-ceramic crowns. However, before engaging all-ceramic crowns as RPD support for non-vital teeth, careful clinical evaluation is recommended due to their increased susceptibility to fracture. The design of the rest seat in all-ceramic restorations is a critical factor affecting their fracture resistance. The axial surfaces should be arranged according to the path of insertion in conventional manner, particularly the guiding surfaces. For the rest seat design for all-ceramic fixed restorations, the following guidelines should be followed: the occlusal rest seat should be narrower in the bucco-lingual direction and should have a more rounded shape than traditional rest seat designs. The proper fit of the rest to the rest seat is very critical to avoid possible fractures (Fig. 7.19). In addition, the base of the cingulum rest seat should have a rounded shape with a radius of approximately 0.5 mm.

Further Reading

Bergman B, Hugoson A, Olsson CO. A 25 year longitudinal study of patients treated with removable partial dentures. J Oral Rehabil. 1995;22:595–9.

Bezzon OL, Mattos MG, Ribeiro RF. Surveying removable partial dentures: the importance of guiding planes and path of insertion for stability. J Prosthet Dent. 1997;78:412–8.

Brudvik JS. Advanced removable partial dentures. Chicago: Quintessence; 1999.

Burns DR, Unger JW. The construction of crowns for removable partial denture abutment teeth. Quintessence Int. 1994;25:471–5.

Carr AB, Brown DT. McCracken's removable partial prosthodontics. 13th ed. St. Louis, MO: Elsevier; 2016.

Chaiyabutr Y, Brudvik JS. Removable partial denture design using milled abutment surfaces and minimal soft tissue coverage for periodontally compromised teeth: a clinical report. J Prosthet Dent. 2008;99:263–6.

Chaturvedi S, Alqahtani T, Alsolami S, Alqahtani A, Das G, Alsubaiy E. Fracture resistance of CAD-CAM all-ceramic surveyed crowns with different occlusal rest seat designs. J Adv Prosthodont. 2021;13:36–45.

Davenport JC, Basker RM, Heath JR, Ralph JP. A colour atlas of removable partial dentures. 1st ed. London: Wolfe Medical Publications Ltd; 1988.

Graber G. Color atlas of dental medicine. Removable partial dentures. 2nd ed. Stuttgart: Thieme Medical; 1988.

Grant AA, Johnson W. An introduction to removable denture prosthetics. Edinburgh: Churchill Livingstone; 1983.

Jepson NJA. Removable partial dentures.1th ed.London: Quintessence Publishing; 2004.

Kancyper S, Sierraalta M, Razzoog ME. All-ceramic surveyed crowns for removable partial denture abutments. J Prosthet Dent. 2000;84:400–2.

Kern M, Wagner B. Periodontal findings in patients 10 years after insertion of removable partial dentures. J Oral Rehabil. 2001;28:991–7.

Kratochvil FJ. Partial removable prosthodontics. Philadelphia, PA: W.B. Saunders Co; 1988.

Loney RW. Removable partial denture manual. Halifax, NS: Dalhousie University Faculty of Dentistry; 2011. http://removpros.dentistry.dal.ca/ewExternalFiles/RPD%20Manual%2011.pdf.

Manchester JA, Chung KH, Brudvik JS, Ramos V Jr, Chen YW. Fracture resistance of cingulum rest seats in CAD-CAM tooth-colored crowns for removable partial denture abutments. J Prosthet Dent. 2019;121:828–35.

Oh WS, Oh JY, May K. Loss of nonvital abutment teeth for removable partial dentures: a systematic review and meta-analysis. Quintessence Int. 2021;52: 210–9.

Phoenix RD, Cagna DR, DeFreest CF. Stewart's clinical removable partial prosthodontics. 4th ed. Chicago: Quintessence Publishing; 2008.

Pihlaja J, Näpänkangas R, Kuoppala R, Raustia A. Veneered zirconia crowns as abutment teeth for partial removable dental prostheses: a clinical 4-year retrospective study. J Prosthet Dent. 2015;114:633–6.

Rudd RW, Bange AA, Rudd KD, Montalvo R. Preparing teeth to receive a removable partial denture. J Prosthet Dent. 1999;82:536–49.

Saito M, Notani K, Miura Y, Kawasaki T. Complications and failures in removable partial dentures: a clinical evaluation. J Oral Rehabil. 2002;29:627–33.

Shifman A, Ben-Ur Z. Prosthodontic treatment for the Applegate-Kennedy class V partially edentulous patient. J Prosthet Dent. 1996;76:212–8.

Stratton RJ, Wiebelt FJ. An atlas of removable partial denture design. Chicago: Quintessence Publishing; 1988.

The glossary of prosthodontic terms: ninth edition. J Prosthet Dent. 2017;117(5S):e1–e105.

Uchikura K, Murakami N, Yamazaki T, Lyu H, Nagata K, Ona M, Iwasaki N, Takahashi H, Wakabayashi N. Fracture resistance of CAD/CAM restorative materials in mismatched removable partial denture rests: an in vitro experimental and finite element analysis. Dent Mater J. 2022;41:466–72.

Waghorn S, Kuzmanovic DV. Technique for preparation of parallel guiding planes for removable partial dentures. J Prosthet Dent. 2004;92:200–1.

Impression Materials and Procedures for Removable Partial Dentures

8

Burç Gençel

Abstract

An impression basically is the negative replica of oral tissues. In the case of removable partial dentures (RPDs), these tissues are the remaining teeth, residual ridge, and the surrounding mucosa. Among these three, the teeth are the easiest to capture. Any elastic impression material can easily mold the shape of the remaining teeth satisfactorily. The tricky part of an RPD impression is to record the edentulous spaces so that they can deliver additional support to the denture base if necessary. The denture base of an RPD certainly helps the retention and stability, however especially for Kennedy Class I and II cases with long free-end saddles the main input of the denture base is in terms of support. The amount of support from the distal extension bases is directly proportional to the amount of covered area. This area is functionally bounded by the surrounding tissues. Determining the shape of this area under functional load also increases the amount of support by compressing the mucosa within the limits of its resilience.

Before final impressions, a preliminary impression is always made with a stock tray, commonly with an alginate impression material. There are more sophisticated alternatives to alginate like polyethers or improved silicones. None of these alternatives serve better for diagnostic impressions.

B. Gençel (✉)
Dental Laboratory Technology Program, İstanbul University-Cerrahpaşa, İstanbul, Türkiye
e-mail: bgencel@iuc.edu.tr

8.1 Definitions

Alginate: Synonym, **Irreversible hydrocolloid**. A hydrocolloid consisting of a sol of alginic acid having a physical state that is changed by an irreversible chemical reaction forming insoluble calcium alginate.

Altered Cast: A final cast that is revised in part before processing a denture base. Synonym, **Corrected cast or Modified cast**.

Altered Cast Removable Partial Denture Impression: A negative likeness of a portion or portions of the edentulous denture bearing area made independent of and after the initial impression of the natural teeth; this technique uses an impression tray(s) attached to the framework of the removable partial denture, or its likeness.

Border Molding: 1. The shaping of impression material along the border areas of an impression tray by functional or manual manipulation of the soft tissue adjacent to the borders to duplicate the contour and size of the vestibule. 2. Determining the extension of a prosthesis by using tissue function or manual manipulation of the tissues to shape the border areas of an impression material.

O. Şakar (ed.), *Removable Partial Dentures*, https://doi.org/10.1007/978-3-031-47083-7_8

Boxing an Impression: The enclosure (box) of an impression to produce the desired size and form of the base of the cast and to preserve desired details.

Custom Tray: An individualized impression tray made from a cast recovered from a preliminary impression; it is used in making a final impression.

Custom Tray Relief: An agent applied onto a preliminary cast in fabrication of a custom tray to aid in reduction or elimination of undesirable pressure or force from a specific region while making a definitive impression.

Custom Tray Spacer: An agent applied onto a preliminary cast in fabrication of a custom tray in order to provide space for the impression material in order to make a definitive impression.

Dental Impression: A negative imprint or a positive digital image display of intraoral anatomy; used to cast or print a 3D replica of the anatomic structure that is to be used as a permanent record or in the production of a dental restoration or prosthesis.

Digital Scan: In dentistry, capturing the optical image directly of the patient's anatomy or indirectly of a definitive cast of the anatomy.

Elastomeric Impression Material: A group of flexible chemical polymers that are either chemically or physically cross-linked; Generally, they can be easily stretched and rapidly recover their original dimensions when applied stresses are released.

Final Impression: The impression that represents the completion of the registration of the surface or object.

Imbibition: The act or process of imbibing or absorbing; In dentistry, an example is the absorption of water in hydrocolloid impression materials when stored in water and the resultant dimensional change that occurs.

Impression Tray: A device that is used to carry, confine, and control impression material while making an impression.

Intaglio Surface: The portion of the denture or other restoration surface that has its contour determined by the impression; the interior or reversal surface of an object.

Land Area: The portion of a dental cast that extends beyond the impression's replica surface laterally that defines the area between the end of the replica's surface and the cast base.

Master Impression: The negative likeness made for the purpose of fabricating a prosthesis.

Maximal Intercuspal Position: The complete intercuspation of the opposing teeth independent of condylar position, sometimes referred to as the best fit of the teeth regardless of the condylar position.

Modeling Plastic Impression Compound: A thermoplastic dental impression material composed of wax, rosin, resins, and colorants. Synonym, **Impression compound or Modeling compound**.

Partial Denture Impression: A negative likeness of all supporting teeth and/or dental implants and tissues of a partially edentulous arch.

Pick-up Impression: An impression that incorporates a prosthesis, framework, copings, or attachments for the purpose of making a cast as a relationship record within the arch; comp, COPING PICK-UP IMPRESSION, transfer impression.

Polyether: An elastomeric impression material of ethylene oxide and tetra-hydrofluro copolymers that polymerizes under the influence of an aromatic ester.

Poly(vinyl siloxane): An addition reaction silicone elastomeric impression material of silicone polymers having terminal vinyl groups that cross-link with silanes on activation by a platinum or palladium salt catalyst.

Preliminary Cast: A cast formed from a preliminary impression for use in diagnosis and/or the fabrication of a custom impression tray. Synonym, **Diagnostic cast or Study cast**.

Preliminary Impression: A negative likeness made for the purpose of diagnosis, treatment planning, and/or the fabrication of a custom impression tray.

Rebase: The laboratory process of replacing the entire denture base material on an existing prosthesis.

Reline: The procedures used to resurface the intaglio of a removable dental prosthesis with new base material, thus producing an accurate adaptation to the denture foundation area.

Remount Procedure: Any method used to relate restorations to an articulator for analysis and/or to assist in development of a plan for occlusal equilibration or reshaping.

Resilient: Characterized or noted by resilience, as (1) capable of withstanding shock without permanent deformation or rupture or (2) tending to recover from or easily adjust to change.

Sectional Impression: A negative likeness that is made in sections.

Stability (Denture): 1. The quality of a complete or removable partial denture to be firm, steady, or constant, to resist displacement by functional horizontal or rotational stresses; 2. Resistance to horizontal displacement of a prosthesis.

Stock Tray: A metal or plastic prefabricated impression tray typically available in various sizes and used principally for preliminary impressions.

Support: The foundation area on which a dental prosthesis rests; with respect to dental prostheses, the resistance to forces directed toward the basal tissue or underlying structures.

Syneresis: The separation of water from its component base, for example, a gel or impression material.

Tissue Displacement: The change in the form or position of tissues as a result of pressure; frequently used to describe gingival tissue placement prior to impression making.

Tissue Registration: 1. the accurate registration of the shape of tissues under any condition by means of a suitable (impression) material.

8.2 Material and Tray Selection for Preliminary Impressions

Alginate impressions are conventionally made with perforated or non-perforated, rim-lock metal trays (Fig. 8.1a, d). The accuracy of an alginate impression is not only dependent on the surface detail but also on the strength of the bond between the material and the tray. The mechanical bond between the impression material and the tray is provided either by the rim-lock design at the borders of the stock tray and/or perforations on the tray surface. Tray adhesives for alginate materials help the impression material to stick on the tray surface. These adhesives are available in spray or liquid form. If the impression is separated, even slightly, from the tray, then it should be repeated. Trays without mechanical retentions may need additional retentive modifications for proper impressions. Modeling plastic impression compound (impression compound),

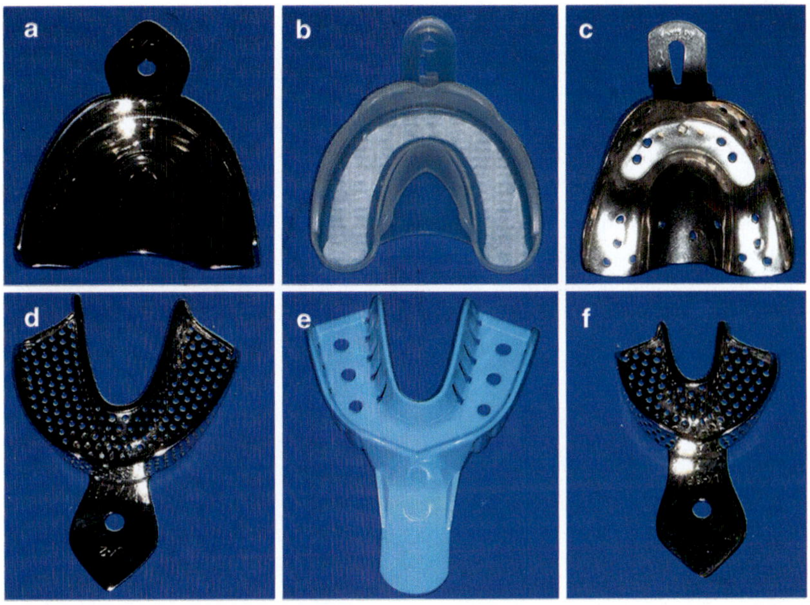

Fig. 8.1 Stock impression trays for preliminary impression. (**a**) Rim-Lock non-perforated metal stock impression tray. (**b**) Rim-Lock, non-perforated, rigid plastic stock impression tray. (**c**) Maxillary metal stock tray for Kennedy Class I cases with perforations and without Rim-Lock borders. (**d**) Rim-Lock, perforated metal stock tray. (**e**) Plastic perforated tray with flat borders. Flexible and not suitable for RPD impressions. (**f**) Pediatric size impression tray

wax, and acrylic resin are commonly used materials to customize stock trays, both to improve coverage area and to create mechanical areas of retention (Fig. 8.2a, b). Adding perforations and applying the adhesive to the extended borders of the custom tray will also help to keep the impression material–tray interface intact.

There are non-metal trays, similar in shape with regular metal stock trays. These trays can be safely used if they are rigid enough to keep their shape during impression-making, otherwise, they should be avoided even for diagnostic impressions (Fig. 8.1b, e).

Stock trays are present in assorted sizes. Besides regular small, medium, and large sizes, there are extra-small pediatric trays and extra-large trays (Fig. 8.1f). It is commercially impossible to fabricate stock trays for every possible type of partial edentulism, so they are available in the shape to fit fully dentate jaws. However, there are stock trays for Kennedy Class I cases with dentate anterior and anatomic posteriors (Fig. 8.1c). A few manufacturers also produce stock trays for Kennedy Class II cases.

Before making the impression, the tray should be checked for fit in the mouth. It should cover all the relevant structures and the impression material should be supported by the tray over the whole impression surface. When the stock tray doesn't fit properly, the borders must be corrected with wax, acrylic resin, or impression compound. The unsupported impression material may possibly deform during plaster pouring and that would result in a corrupt cast.

There should be sufficient space between the tray and the oral tissues for an accurate impression. The amount of required space changes according to the impression material chosen (Fig. 8.2). For alginate, it should be 4–5 mm as it shows plastic deformation beyond 50% elastic deformation. Other elastomeric alternatives like polyether and silicones have superior elastic recovery properties, therefore they are less prone to deform during the removal of the impression from the mouth.

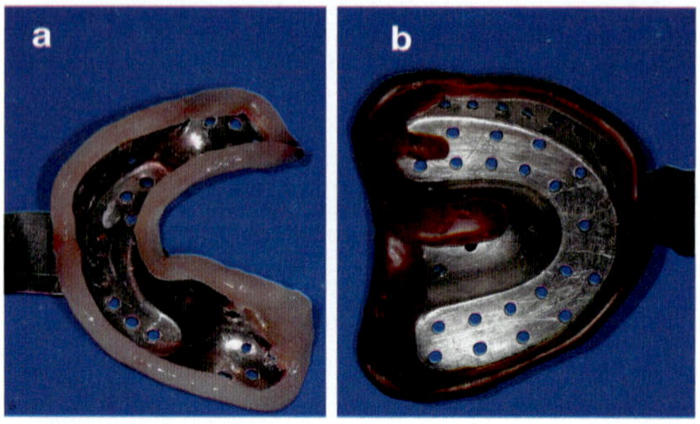

Fig. 8.2 Customization of stock impression trays. (**a**) Mandibular stock metal tray for Kennedy Class I case. Disto-lingual borders are extended, and mechanical retention is provided with utility wax. Alginate adhesive is applied for alginate to stick on the-tray surface. (**b**) Maxillary tray is modified to cover tuber area and periphery is borderlocked with utility wax. The clearance between the tray and the impression area is also adjusted

8.3 Final Impressions

Once the diagnostic cast is analyzed and pre-prosthetic preparations are completed, a new impression should be made. This is referred to as "the final impression" or "master impression" as it is the recording of the final state of the mouth with all the altered tissues before proceeding with denture construction.

Final impression can be a single-step procedure as a current version of the preliminary impression. It may also be a multistep procedure, when free-end saddles of a Kennedy Class I or Kennedy Class II case are desired to be finished on an altered cast. The aim is not only to precisely determine the functional borders of the distal extension denture base(s) but also to provide additional support by compressing the mucosa under functional loads. This is referred to as "*functional impression*" if it is made at chair-side in the control of the clinician. If a long-term corrective impression during function after the RPD is delivered to the patient is made, then this is called a "muco-dynamic impression".

8.3.1 Tray Selection for Single-Step Final Impressions

Stock trays can also be used for final impressions if the selected tray has proper clearance from tissues for the selected impression material and a satisfactory fit to the impression area. However, unless a conventional RPD is meant to be constructed without any pre-prosthetic preparations with a single impression, it is best to use a custom tray that is prepared on the diagnostic cast. These are conventionally produced with autopolymerizing polymethylmethacrylate or light-curing urethane-dimethacrylate resins (Fig. 8.3).

***Advantages of custom trays:**

- They are rigid and dimensionally stable. They provide excellent support for the impression material.
- They are tailored to have a superior fit to the impression area. They usually need little to no adjustments before impression-making.
- The position of the tray on the diagnostic model can be transferred to the mouth with acrylic stops (Fig. 8.4).
- The space between the tray and the tissues can be adjusted by applying a custom tray spacer before fabrication. Material-specific adjustment delivers the best possible results. Functional borders can be molded and surface details can be precisely captured (Fig. 8.4).
- They can provide mechanical retention and/or chemical adhesion to the impression material with custom perforations and adhesive agents, therefore impressions can be removed safely from deep undercuts and other retentive areas without damaging the integrity of the impression.

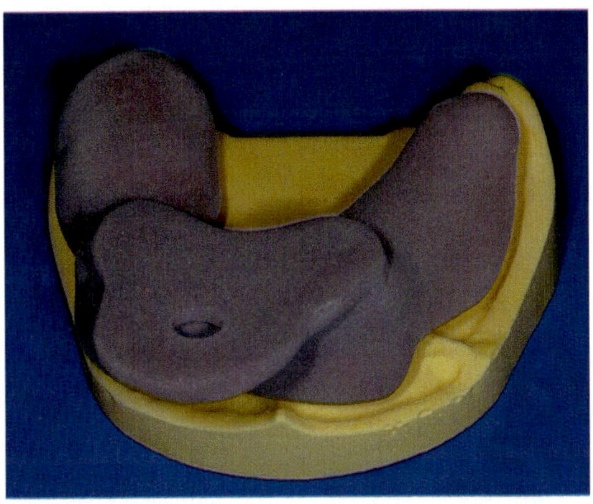

Fig. 8.3 Custom tray for a Kennedy Class II RPD. Material is light-cure urethane dimethacrylate

8.3.2 Impression Materials for Single-Step Final Impressions

Alginate is still an accepted choice for final impressions. It was reported to be in the curriculum of more than 60% of dental schools in the United States and 70% in Turkey. It delivers a single-step, mucostatic impression with fair surface detail which is satisfactory for most RPD cases. However, the expansive borders, weak tear resistance, and limited surface resolution are a few drawbacks. Post-impression needs of the material may also cause problems. Particularly, the plaster should be poured immediately once the alginate is set, and this mostly requires a

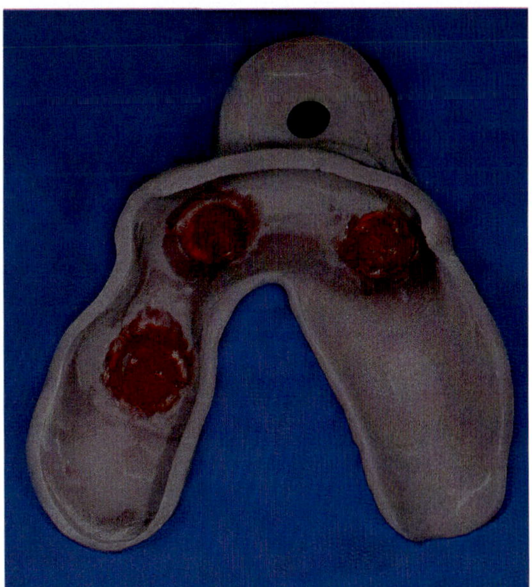

Fig. 8.4 Acrylic stops transfer the position of the tray from the diagnostic cast to the mouth. Borders and the clearance of the tray are also adjusted according to the materials chosen for impression-making

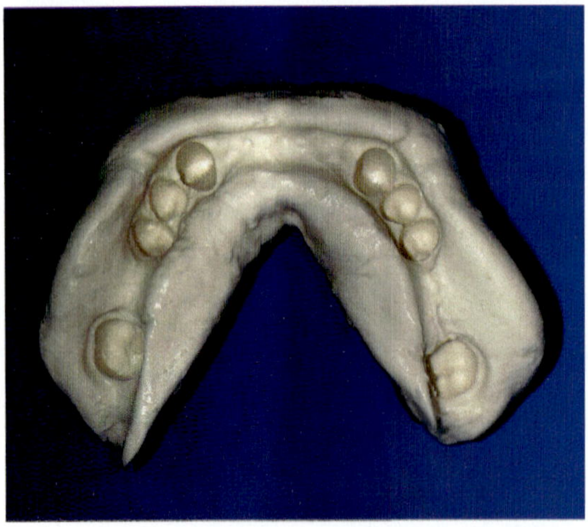

Fig. 8.5 Final impression made with alginate and stock tray

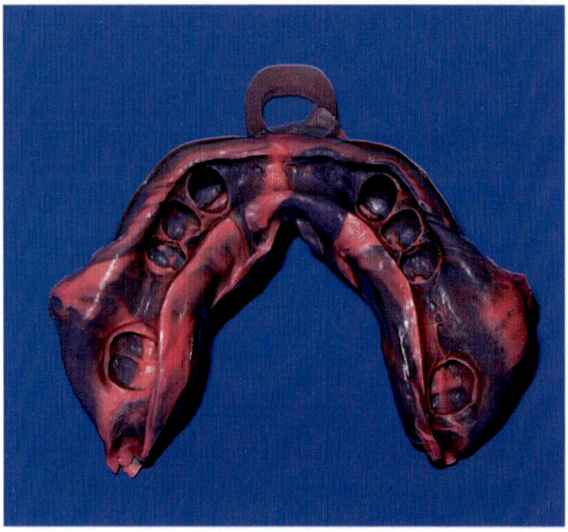

Fig. 8.6 Final impression made with a custom tray and polyether

skilled assistant if the dental laboratory is not nearby. However, there are extended pour-type alginates that may allow the transfer of the impression to the dental laboratory without dimensional changes. Alginate is also not suitable for the transfer of implant positions with either closed or open tray impressions.

The final impression procedure for a tooth-supported RPD is very much like the preliminary impression. These are mostly Kennedy III and IV cases. However, when the distal free-end edentulous space is short and the support from the free-end saddle is not crucial, then the same procedure is also valid for Kennedy Class I and II cases as well. The whole impression surface is captured with a single-step impression made with a stock tray if it fits the arch sufficiently (Fig. 8.5).

When implants are involved, surface detail is important and the preparation of the cast is not possible almost immediately then A-type silicones, polyether reinforced A-type silicones, and polyether impression materials are available. Some of these materials are improved to have hydrophilic properties but this is a little misleading. It doesn't come to mean that they work as precisely in wet environments like irreversible hydrocolloids. To achieve better results, the impression area should be dried before impression-making. The hydrophilic property of these materials actually makes them friendly with dental stones. They can be applied with non-perforated stock trays or for further precise impressions custom trays can be used. Regardless of the type of tray, these materials should always be used with an appropriate tray adhesive. They serve perfectly with open and closed tray techniques in implant-involved cases. They can also mold functional borders almost precisely with superior surface detail. They are more resistant to disinfectants, and they can be safely transported to the dental laboratory without any dimensional changes (Fig. 8.6).

8.4 Handling the Impression

There are specific hints for each impression material and there are commons of impression-making:

- Tray selection and modifications, as well as the amount of relief space for the impression should be prepared according to the material chosen.
- All measures to secure the impression-tray integrity should be taken. Providing mechanical retention and/or using an appropriate adhesive are important.
- Care must be given not to entrap air in the impression material while loading the tray.

Alginate should firmly be stuffed in with a stiff spatula. Dough-type materials should be well kneaded, rolled, and stuffed in the tray with finger pressure. When loading auto-mix materials, tray should be filled from one side to another and the impression tip should always be kept in the flowing paste. It may be useful to wet undercut areas and teeth surfaces with the impression material before inserting the tray. This is done by simply rubbing a small amount of impression material to desired areas with fingers.

- Rima oris should be avoided with the help of a diagnostic mirror while inserting the tray to prevent the lips from sweeping the impression material off the tray.
- The tray should be positioned with mild finger pressure giving the material time to make its thixotropic flow.
- The tray should be kept still with fingers on the premolar area during the setting of the material. Any movement of the tray during setting may result in a defective impression.
- The tray should be pulled parallel to the long axis of teeth for easy and safe removal. A small initial movement will release the adhesion of the impression. The lips should be pulled to allow air to the impression–tissue interface.
- Once removed, the impression must be checked for material-tray integrity, surface details, and borders.
- After proper cleaning and disinfection, an appropriate type of dental stone should be poured. If an alginate impression is taken, it should be poured immediately.

8.5 Functional Impressions

The idea of making an impression of the functioning mucosa goes back a while. The aim is not only to cover as much area as possible but also to record the shape of the ridge within the limits of its resilience and fully employ the primary stress-bearing areas to provide mucosa support for the free-end saddle. It is mostly meant for mandibular Kenney Class I and II cases where mucosa support is weak. The maxillary coverage of an average RPD is much wider and the hard palate provides a firm support to the denture eliminating the need for a functional impression.

Several methods are introduced to clinical practice, yet there are basically three methods of making functional impressions. After diagnostic cast is analyzed and mouth preparations are complete, the conventional technique, originally introduced by Applegate, describes a multi-step sectional impression in which a stock or occasionally a custom tray is used to make an overall impression only to design and construct the metal framework. The functional part of the impression is carried out after the framework is cast and the subsequent procedures are carried out on the new or modified cast. Another approach makes the use of a custom tray, which is prepared to make the final impression of all structures at a single appointment. In this concept, the master cast is poured and all following procedures, including construction of the metal framework, are carried out on this final cast. Another option is to finish the denture without making a functional impression and then make an early reline.

8.5.1 The Altered Cast and Its Modifications

The classic altered cast technique was the first effective clinically applicable method that found ground in dental practice. The popular derivative of the technique is a multi-step procedure starting with a conventional impression, which is used to construct the metal framework. The metal framework is then utilized to make the impression of the free-end edentulous space(s) with the help of acrylic saddles built on the retentive gridwork. The saddles are treated like an individual tray for a complete denture, first border-molded then surface impression is made (Fig. 8.7a, b).

The alignment of the framework in each insertion is critical for the success of this procedure. To prevent any clinic born errors, during border molding and wash surface impression, the frame-

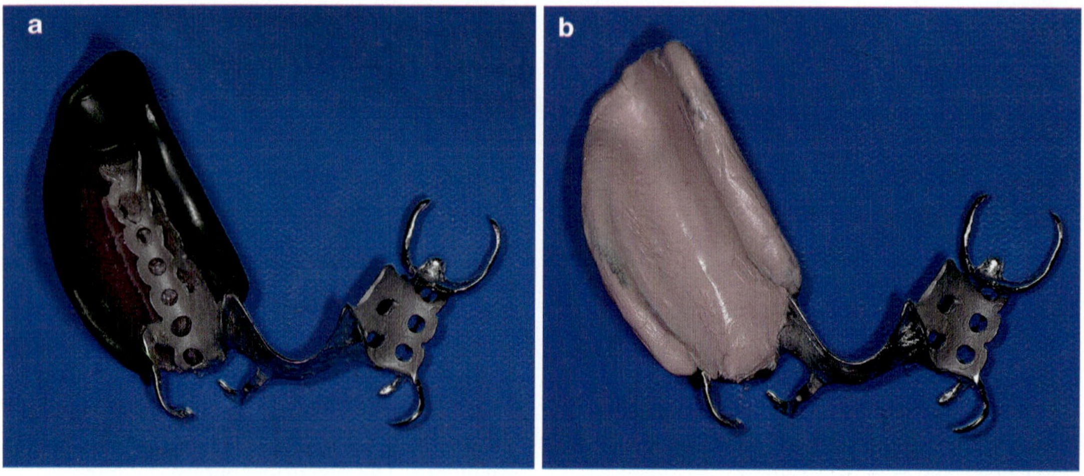

Fig. 8.7 (**a**) Acrylic saddle is border-molded for functional impression. (**b**) Functional impression is completed with zinc oxide and eugenol paste

work should be fixed in its position on the abutment teeth by pressing at least 3 supporting points at each insertion. These supporting points can be occlusal, cingulum or incisal rests and the part of the major connector that provides support like a lingual plate or a cingulum bar but not the stops under the retentive gridwork. In other words, while holding the framework in "position" pressure should not be applied on the saddles as the resilience of the mucosa, which we are trying to capture, may probably cause a rotational movement around fulcrum axis (Fig. 8.8). This will eventually lead to a faulty impression.

Once the functional impression is complete, the relevant parts of the initial cast are cut away and the final cast is prepared by replacing the removed parts with the help of the new functional impression. The framework is seated and fixed on the grinded cast. The borders of the impression are boxed and dental stone is poured as supplementary to the former cast. The final hybrid cast is then used for consecutive procedures (Figs. 8.9a–c).

This is a sophisticated method that needs delicate work even in the hands of an experienced clinician. The laboratory work is also critical not only when preparing the altered cast but also at previous stages. Any slight difference in the seating of the framework between the mouth and the cast, which is possible due to numerous reasons, may result in a defective cast as the alignment of the saddles would not have been transferred correctly.

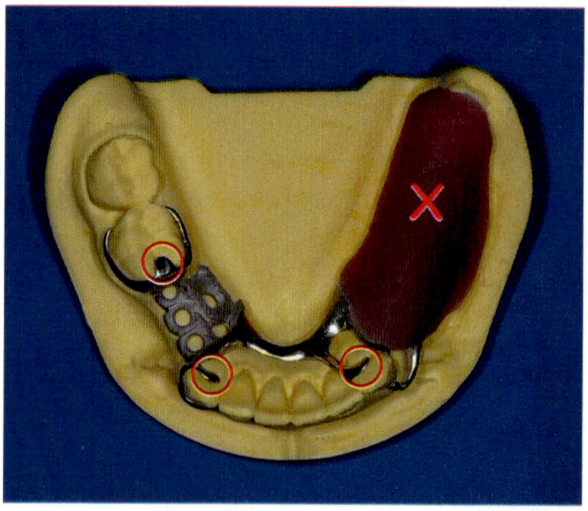

Fig. 8.8 Pressure points when the framework is seated. Pressure should not be applied on the acrylic saddle

Once a defective cast is produced, it becomes complicated to proceed with the following steps. A new impression must be made while the framework is seated in the mouth to provide a fresh working cast after which you can either choose to repeat the functional impression or to skip the step and make an early functional reline after the prosthesis is finished.

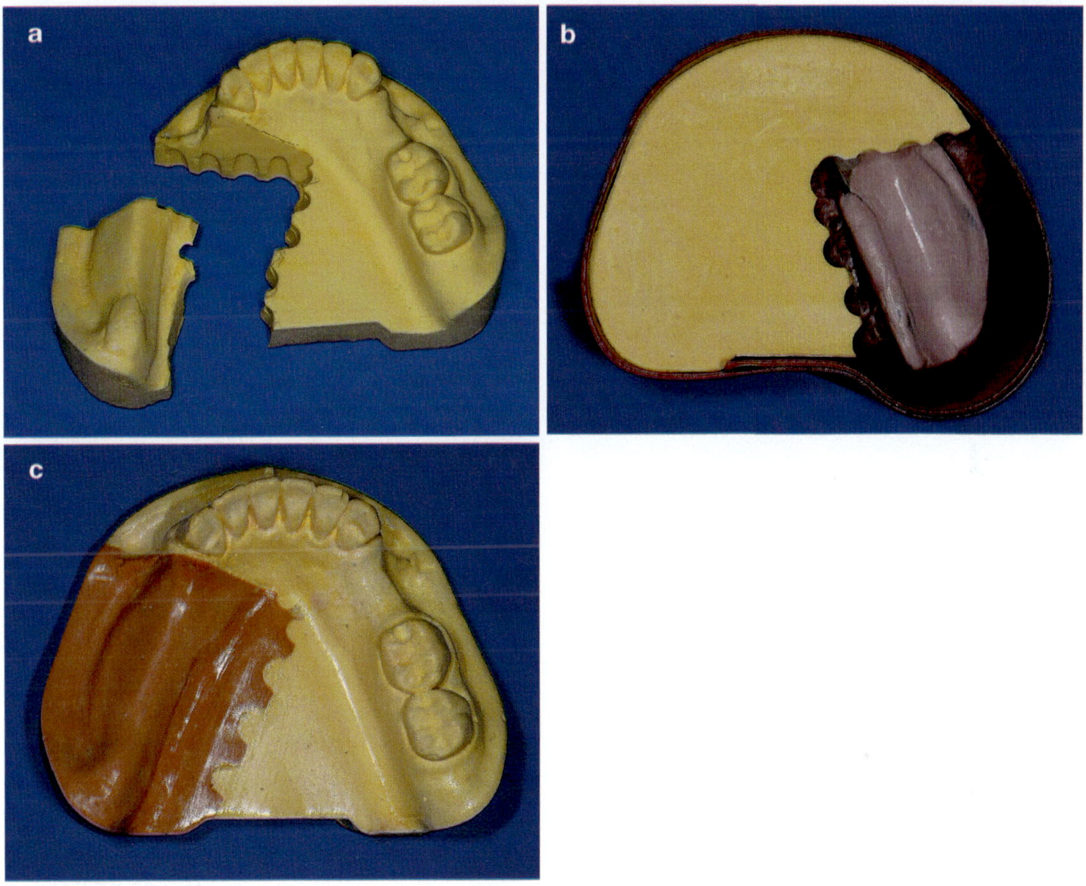

Fig. 8.9 (**a**) The cast is cut before transferring the final impression. The edentulous free-end ridge is cut away and retentive grooves for the supplementary dental stone are prepared. (**b**) Functional impression and the framework is fixed on the remaining cast and boxed. (**c**) The supplementary dental stone is poured, and the altered cast is ready

There is a wide spectrum of modifications made to simplify, shorten, and secure the outcomes of the process both regarding the materials used and the procedures applied. The corrective Korecta waxes used in the original method have almost been abandoned. The modeling impression compound stands out as the most popular border-molding material available. Almost 80% of dental schools in the United States and 100% in Turkey are reported to be using impression compounds for functional borders. Alternatives to impression compounds are light-cured composite resin, utility wax, zinc-oxide and eugenol paste, and tissue conditioners. The materials used for final surface impression are polysulfide, polyether, polyvinylsiloxane, zinc-oxide and eugenol paste and tissue conditioners.

The laboratory procedure of making a hybrid cast is also a sensitive work that can ruin the delicately made clinic work. To eliminate the risks in the process of cast altering, an overall pick-up impression over the finished functional impression in place can be made, thus the position of the framework, as it is in the mouth, can be transferred to the new cast along with the functionally shaped surfaces. This can be done with stock trays and one of any elastic impression materials available (Fig. 8.10). Care must be given to prevent any movement of the framework while making the pick-up impression. If the impression material leaks to the functional impression–mucosa interface, this indicates a hyper-expansive impression, the framework has moved from its place, and the saddles are displaced during the procedure. The pick-up impression should either be short of the functional impression borders, or it should flawlessly continue expansively. If the impression is short of the borders, the borders are boxed before pouring plaster, if it is expansive and masking the borders then the expansive material is cut away to expose functional borders before pouring the cast (Figs. 8.11a, b).

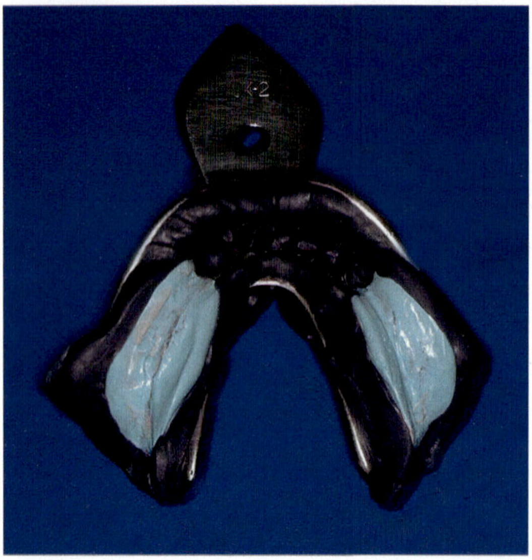

Fig. 8.10 Pick-up impression to transfer the functional impression to the final cast

8.5.2 Single Tray Functional Impressions

This is actually a derivative of single-step final impression with a custom tray. The custom tray is shaped like the acrylic saddles in the altered cast technique over the free-ending edentulous ridge and the dentate area is produced conventionally. The clearance between the tray and the cast is adjusted according to the impression material to be used. Acrylic stops over teeth keeps the tray position during impression making.

The clinical procedure is first to make the functional part of the impression with one of the border-molding materials and then to make an overall wash impression with one of the elastomeric impression materials (Figs 8.12a, b). This single-piece impression is relatively simple, time-saving, and easy to process. All parts of the RPD including the metal framework are constructed on this final cast. Furthermore, the clinical outcomes of the altered cast technique and single-step functional impressions are reported to be similar (Fig. 8.13).

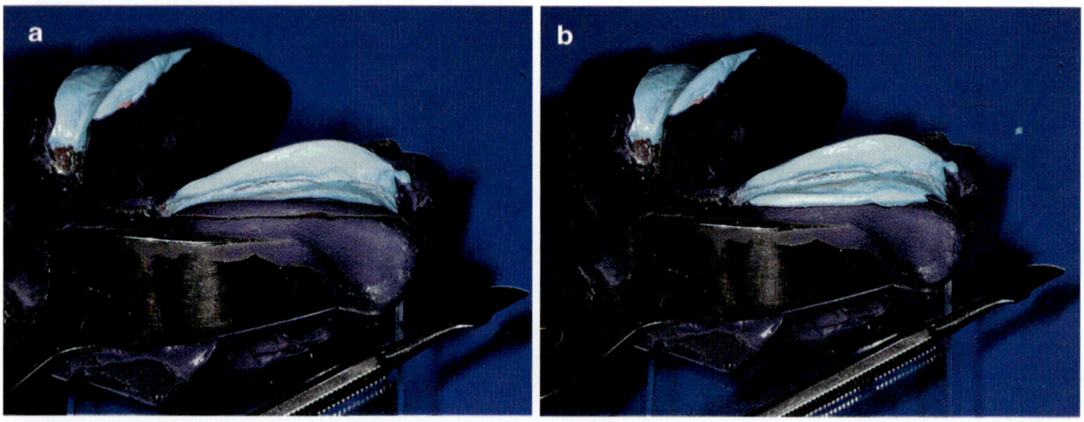

Fig. 8.11 (**a**, **b**) The overextended borders of the pick-up impression is cut at the boxing level to clear the functional borders; thus the borders can be seen and the land area around functional borders is provided on the master model

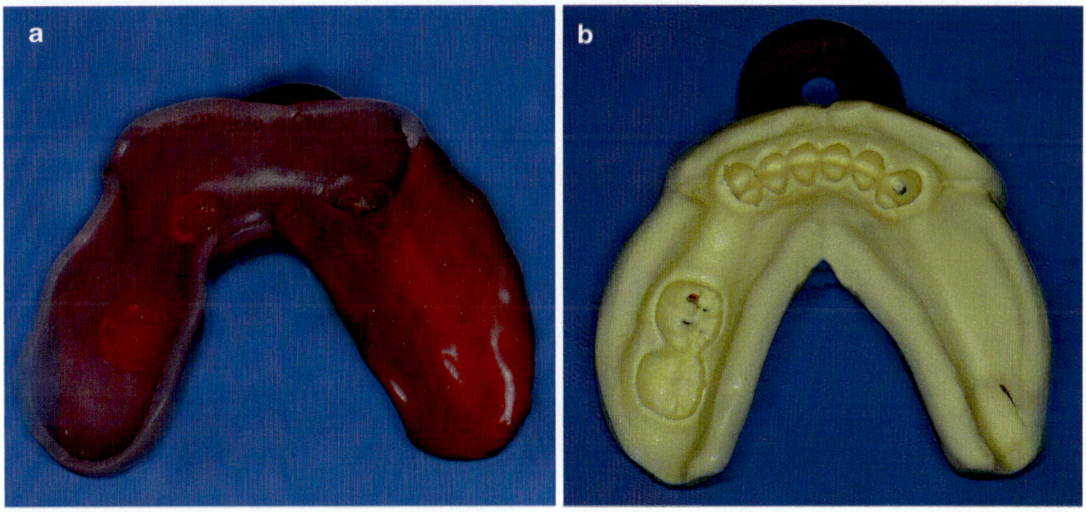

Fig. 8.12 (**a**) Border molding of the custom tray. Tray adhesive is applied on both the tray and the impression compound. (**b**) Impression completed with polyvinyl siloxane

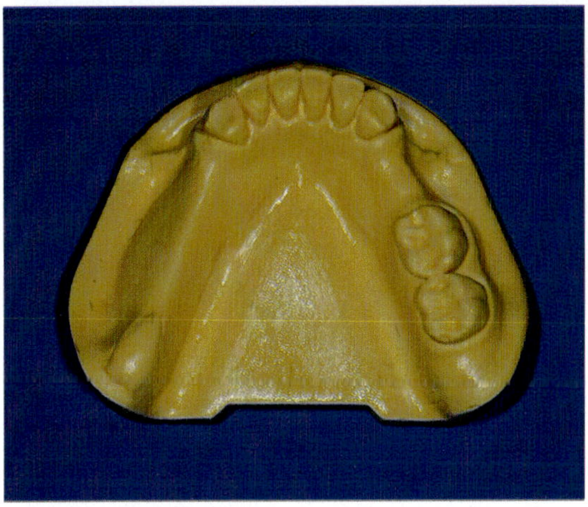

Fig. 8.13 Single piece cast from the single-tray functional impression

8.6 Impressions for Relining and Rebasing

The intaglio surface of an RPD in service may lose its adaptation to the bearing mucosa due to several reasons. The resorption of the alveolar ridge is a well-known cause for the failure of support from the denture foundation area. Errors in laboratory procedures may also result in ill-fitting denture bases. Improper handling of sore spots after the delivery of an RPD may also end in destructed intaglio surfaces and

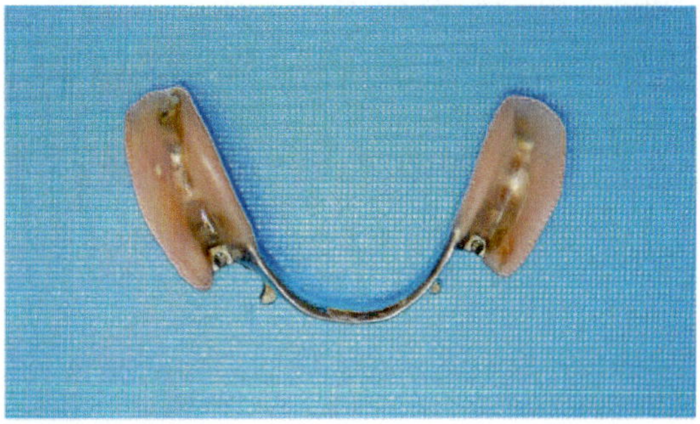

Fig. 8.14 Buccal, lingual, and posterior borders are too short

faulty borders of the denture base. After the extraction of an abutment tooth, the re-establishment of the intaglio surface may also be reasonable to provide further service ability to an existing RPD. It may also be the clinician's choice or plan to make an early reline to improve the functional efficiency of the denture base (Figs. 8.14, 8.15 and 8.16). Whatever the reason is, the solution to the lack of satisfactory denture bases is either resurfacing the existing denture base by relining its intaglio surface or replacing the whole base by rebasing (Figs. 8.17, 8.18, 8.19 and 8.20).

The clinical procedures of both relining and rebasing are almost identical. An impression with the denture base, which is treated as the acrylic saddles of the altered cast technique, is made and

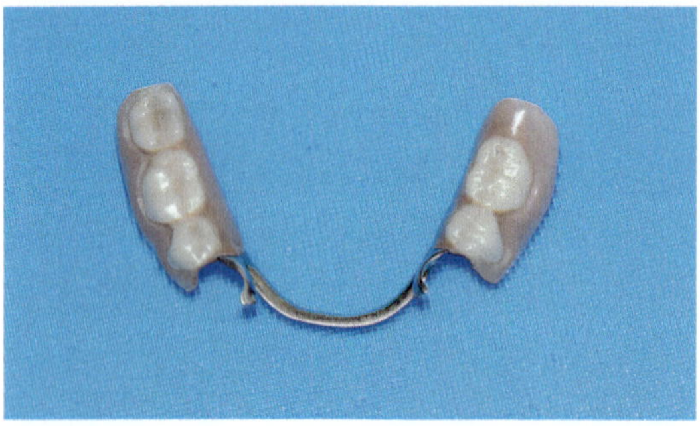

Fig. 8.15 Denture base is not capable of covering supporting structures

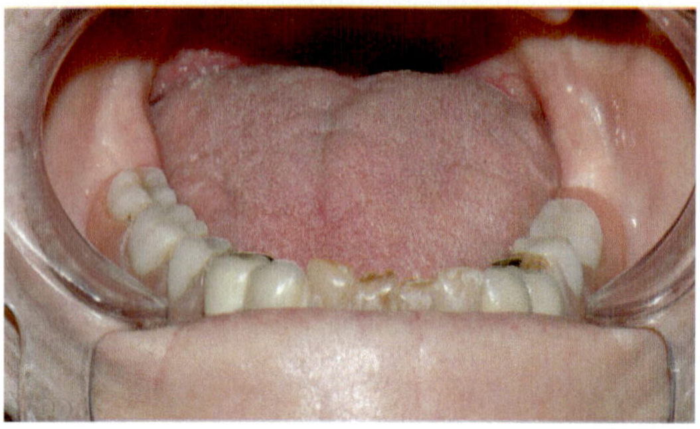

Fig. 8.16 Posterior border is too short. Retromolar pad is completely exposed

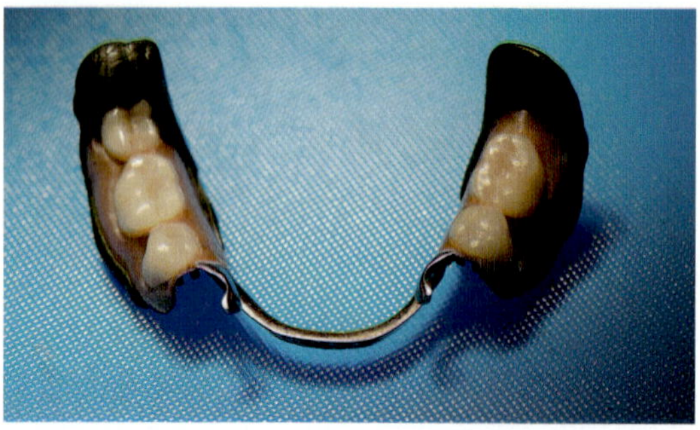

Fig. 8.17 Short borders are molded before wash surface impression

the dental laboratory will complete the procedure as ordered. For most of the cases, relining will provide satisfactory results. However, it is better to replace the whole acrylic in case it is discolored and worn out extensively which is the situation for most RPDs that are in service for a prolonged time. Another indication for rebasing is the porous finish of the acrylic where relining is not an option.

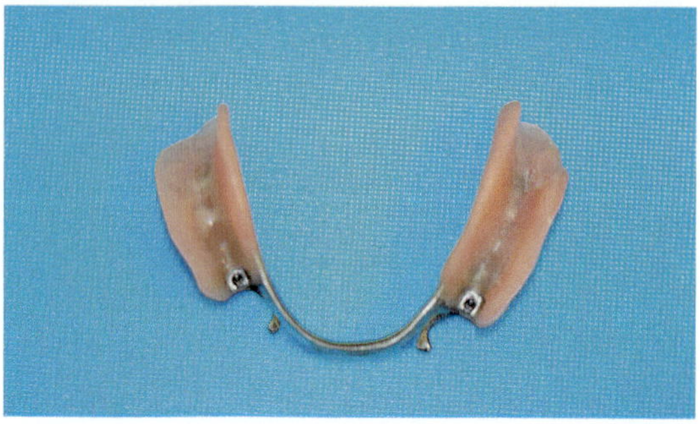

Fig. 8.18 Intaglio surface after rebasing. Denture base covers molded borders

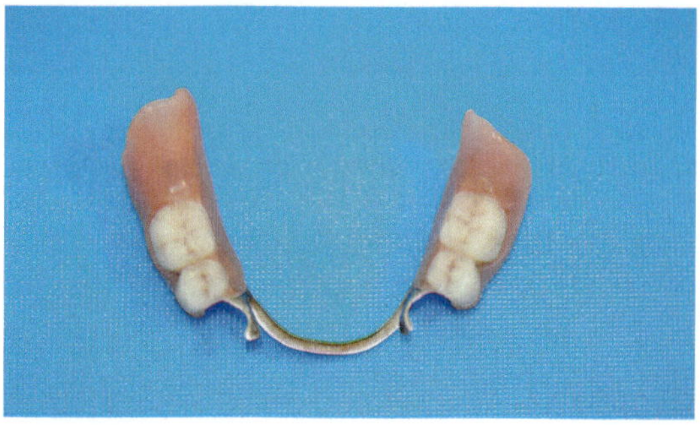

Fig. 8.19 Denture base with extended borders after rebasing

The success of a reline/rebase impression mostly depends on the preparation of the acrylic surfaces and the handling of the denture during impression making. The borders of the acrylic parts, particularly the free-end saddles, should be checked for over-extension or being too short. The over-extended borders should first be trimmed to 2 mm short of possible functional borders except for the area covering the retromolar pad for a mandibular RPD and the tuber area for a maxillary RPD. It is best to mold the borders before the surface impression to achieve the volumetric shape of the functional borders (Fig. 8.17). Acrylic volume filling deep tissue undercuts should be removed. The impression should be completed with either zinc oxide eugenol paste or a polyether impression material as it is basically a soft tissue impression (Fig. 8.7b). The tricky clue is to refrain from making closed-mouth impressions and treat the denture like a framework with custom saddles for an altered cast technique. The opposing

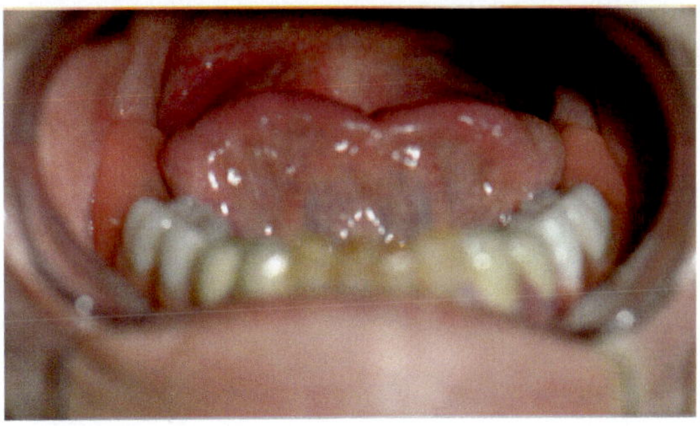

Fig. 8.20 Posterior border covers the retromolar pad

teeth might have moved occlusally to compensate for the lost teeth contacts due to alveolar resorption. This causes the metal framework to rotate around the fulcrum axis and indirect retainers diverge from supporting teeth during function. A missed premature tooth contact may cause the same error. Therefore, the reline/rebase impressions for dentures with free-end saddle(s) should be made with the open mouth technique described above for altered cast impressions (Figs. 8.7, 8.8, 8.9, 8.10 and 8.11). The impression is relatively simple in the absence of free-end saddles. After the preparation of acrylic surfaces, the denture with impression material applied on the intaglio surface is inserted in the mouth, and rests are firmly seated on abutment teeth. During the setting of the impression material, rests should be kept in their seats with finger pressure while the patient is making tongue movements. For the rest of the borders, the patient can make functional movements with his/her lips and cheeks when teeth are in contact at maximum intercuspal position.

It is highly recommended to make a remounting for occlusal adjustments before delivering the denture to the patient.

Further Reading

Carlsson GE. Critical review of some dogmas in prosthodontics. J Prosthodont Res. 2009;53:3–10.

Carlsson GE, Ortorp A, Omar R. What is the evidence base for the efficacies of different complete denture impression procedures? A critical review. J Dent. 2013;41:17–23.

Carr AB, Brown DT. McCracken's removable partial prosthodontics. 13th ed. St. Louis, MO: Elsevier; 2016.

Donovan TE, Chee WW. A review of contemporary impression materials and techniques. Dent Clin North Am. 2004;48:445–70.

Dumbrigue HB, Esquivel JF. Selective-pressure single impression procedure for tooth-mucosa-supported removable partial dentures. J Prosthet Dent. 1998;80:259–61.

Faria AC, Rodrigues RC, Macedo AP, Mattos Mda G, Ribeiro RF. Accuracy of stone casts obtained by different impression materials. Braz Oral Res. 2008;22:293–8.

Feit DB. The altered cast impression technique revisited. J Am Dent Assoc. 1999;130:1476–81.

Frank RP, Brudvik JS, Noonan CJ. Clinical outcome of the altered cast impression procedure compared with use of a one-piece cast. J Prosthet Dent. 2004;91:468–76.

Jayaraman S, Singh BP, Ramanathan B, Pazhaniappan Pillai M, MacDonald L, Kirubakaran R. Final-impression techniques and materials for making complete and removable partial dentures. Cochrane Database Syst Rev. 2018;4:CD012256.

Kilfeather GP, Lynch CD, Sloan AJ, Youngson CC. Quality of communication and master impressions for the fabrication of cobalt chromium removable partial dentures in general dental practice in England, Ireland and Wales in 2009. J Oral Rehabil. 2010;37:300–5.

Kitamura A, Kawai Y. Basic investigation of the laminated alginate impression technique: setting time, permanent deformation, elastic deformation, consistency, and tensile bond strength tests. J Prosthodont Res. 2015;59:49–54.

Loney RW. Removable partial denture manual. Halifax, NS: Dalhousie University Faculty of Dentistry; 2011. http://removpros.dentistry.dal.ca/ewExternalFiles/RPD%20Manual%2011.pdf.

Mandikos MN. Polyvinyl siloxane impression materials: an update on clinical use. Aust Dent J. 1998;43:428–34.

Millstein P, Maya A, Segura C. Determining the accuracy of stock and custom tray impression/casts. J Oral Rehabil. 1998;25:645–8.

Nallaswamy D. Textbook of prosthodontics. 1st ed. New Delhi: Jaypee Brothers Medical Publishers Ltd; 2003.

Nassar U, Aziz T, Flores-Mir C. Dimensional stability of irreversible hydrocolloid impression materials as a function of pouring time: a systematic review. J Prosthet Dent. 2011;106:126–33.

Ozkurt Z, Dikbas I, Kazazoglu E. Predoctoral prosthodontic clinical curriculum for complete dentures: survey in Turkish dental schools. J Dent Educ. 2013;77:93–8.

Petropoulos VC, Rashedi B. Removable partial denture education in U.S. dental schools. J Prosthodont. 2006;15:62–8.

Phoenix RD, Cagna DR, Defreest CF. Stewart's clinical removable partial prosthodontics. 4th ed. Chicago: Quintessence Publishing; 2008.

Radhi A, Lynch CD, Hannigan A. Quality of written communication and master impressions for fabrication of removable partial prostheses in the Kingdom of Bahrain. J Oral Rehabil. 2007;34:153–7.

Rajapur A, Dixit S, Hoshing C, Raikar SP. The influence of tray space and repeat pours on the accuracy of monophasic polyvinylsiloxane impression. J Contemp Dent Pract. 2012;13:824–9.

Rathee S, Eswaran B, Eswaran MA, Prabhu R, Geetha KR, Krishna GP, Jagadeshwari. A comparison of dimensional accuracy of addition silicone of different consistencies with two different spacer designs in-vitro study. J Clin Diagn Res. 2014;8:ZC38–41.

Rubel BS. Impression materials: a comparative review of impression materials most commonly used in restorative dentistry. Dent Clin North Am. 2007;51:629–42.

The glossary of prosthodontic terms: ninth edition. J Prosthet Dent. 2017;117(5S):e1–e105.

Thongthammachat S, Moore BK, Barco MT 2nd, Hovijitra S, Brown DT, Andres CJ. Dimensional accuracy of dental casts: influence of tray material, impression material, and time. J Prosthodont. 2002;11:98–108.

Todd JA, Oesterle LJ, Newman SM, Shellhart WC. Dimensional changes of extended-pour alginate impression materials. Am J Orthod Dentofacial Orthop. 2013;143:S55–63.

Part III

Clasp Retained Removable Partial Dentures

Major and Minor Connectors

9

Olcay Şakar

Abstract

Although design is a very important stage in the fabrication of the removable partial dentures (RPDs), unfortunately, dentists have a minimal input on this issue and they generally leave it to the dental technician. This results in the common usage and preference of the technician's familiar designs (like the U-shaped maxillary major connector, considered the least preferable option). RPDs will not have any harmful effects on the remaining teeth and periodontal tissues if they are well-designed and oral hygiene checked regularly. This chapter summarizes the metal major and minor connector designs, giving lots of samples for every Kennedy classification. Thus, dentists can easily create the most suitable design for their patients.

9.1 Definitions

Cross arch stabilization: Resistance against dislodging or rotational forces obtained by using a fixed or removable partial denture design that uses natural teeth on the opposite side of the dental arch from the edentulous space to assist in stabilization.

Guiding planes: Two or more vertically parallel surfaces on abutment teeth and/or fixed dental prostheses oriented so as to contribute to the direction of the path of placement and removal of a removable partial denture, maxillofacial prosthesis, and overdenture.

Major connector: The part of a removable partial denture that joins the components on one side of the arch to those on the opposite side.

Minor connector: The connecting link between the major connector or base of a removable partial denture and the other units of the prosthesis, such as the clasp assembly, indirect retainers, occlusal rests, or cingulum rests.

Path of placement: The specific direction in which a prosthesis is placed on the residual alveolar ridge, abutment teeth, dental implant abutment(s), or attachments; synonym: Path of insertion.

9.2 Major Connectors

A removable partial denture (RPD) framework includes five components: major connector, minor connectors, rests, direct retainers, and indirect retainers (in distal extension RPDs) (Fig. 9.1). RPDs should be designed according to biomechanical and hygienic principles (see Chap. 4).

O. Şakar (✉)
Faculty of Dentistry, Department of Prosthodontics, İstanbul University, İstanbul, Türkiye
e-mail: osakar@istanbul.edu.tr

O. Şakar (ed.), *Removable Partial Dentures*, https://doi.org/10.1007/978-3-031-47083-7_9

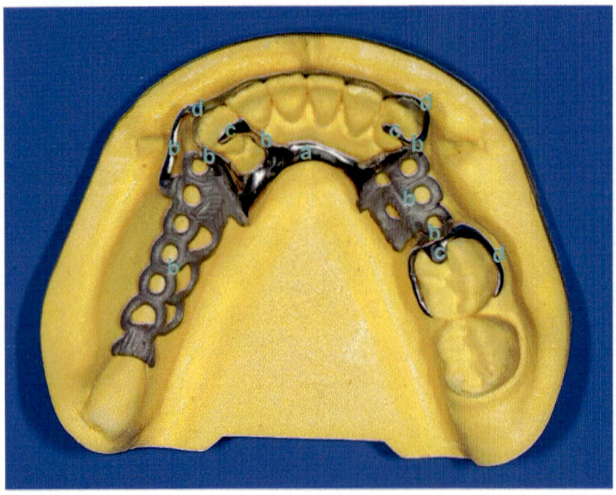

Fig. 9.1 The components of a removable partial denture framework: (**a**). Major connector; (**b**).Minor connectors; (**c**). Rests, (rest and minor connector on the right canine serve as indirect retainer); (**d**). Direct retainers

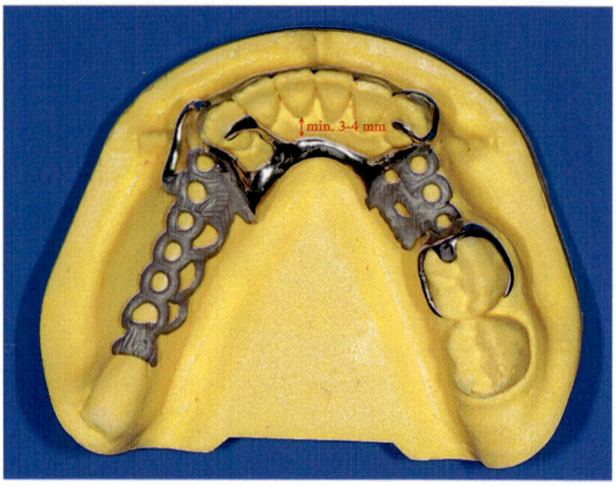

Fig. 9.2 All major connectors' borders should run parallel to the gingival margins of the remaining teeth. Borders of a mandibular major connector should be placed at least 3–4 mm away from the free gingival margins

A major connector combines all other components of an RPD so that the partial denture acts as one unit. Thus, functional loads can be distributed to all abutment teeth, and cross-arch stabilization can be provided. In addition, in distal extension RPDs, forces can be distributed between both the abutment teeth and the mucosa by the unification of the direct retainers with the denture base.

RPD frameworks can be produced with metal alloys and polymer materials by using traditional (see Chap. 14), as well as digital techniques (see Part V) but the principles of a major connector design will remain the same no matter what materials are used.

9.2.1 General Aspects of Major Connectors

All major connectors should have the following characteristics to function effectively and to protect the teeth and soft tissues:

1. Major connectors should:
   (a) be rigid,
   (b) have smooth and rounded line angles,
   (c) conform to anatomic structures,
   (d) not interfere with movable tissues,
   (e) not allow food entrapment,
   (f) not cover more tissue than necessary,
   (g) not use marginal gingiva for support,
   (h) not impinge on soft and hard tissue prominences or gingival tissue during placement, removal, or function.
2. Borders of a major connector should:
   (a) run parallel to the gingival margins of the remaining teeth in both arches (Figs. 9.2 and 9.3).
   (b) be placed at least 3–4 mm away from the free gingival margins *in the mandibular arch* (Fig.9.2). Otherwise, the major connector should cover the lingual surfaces of the teeth as a plate. On the anterior teeth, the plate should cover the cingula but not be higher than the middle third of the teeth, except to cover the interproximal spaces at the contact points. On the posterior teeth, the plate should end at the height of contour *in both arches.*
   (c) be placed at least 6 mm away from the free gingival margins *in the maxillary arch.* Otherwise, the major connector should cover the lingual surfaces of the teeth as a plate (Fig. 9.3).
   (d) not end on the crest of rugae or at the free gingival margin (Fig. 9.4).
   (e) cross the maxillary midline at right angles, not diagonally.

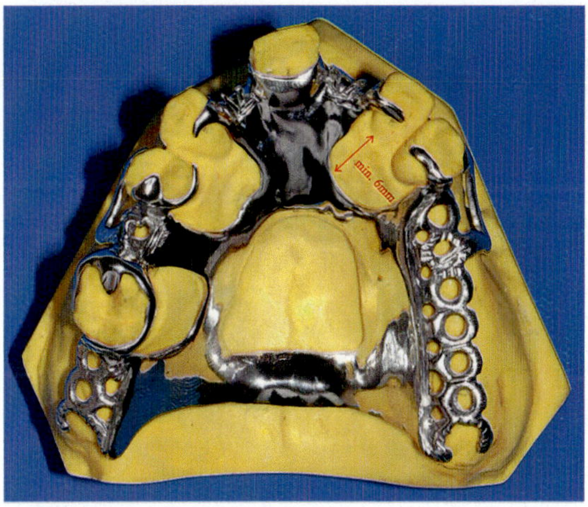

Fig. 9.3 Borders of a major connector should not be placed on the free gingival margin, instead of running away from the margins (at least 6 mm). Otherwise, it should be extended as a plate

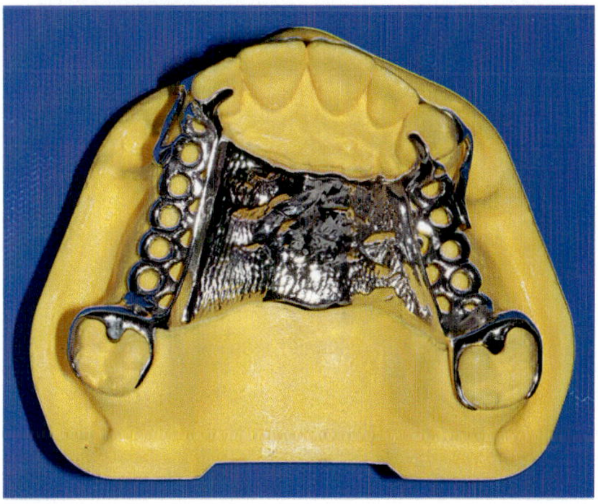

Fig. 9.4 The rugae should be replicated anatomically and borders of major connectors should not end on the crest of rugae

   (f) be beaded to increase the adaptation, to prevent debris from collecting beneath the major connector, and to minimize the casting shrinkage *in all maxillary major connectors* (0.5–1 mm wide and deep) (Fig. 9.5). Beading is not necessary in the mandibular major connector.

3. *Relief* is not required except for a palatal torus or prominent median palatal suture area in the *maxillary major connectors*, but it is often necessary between the rigid metal surfaces

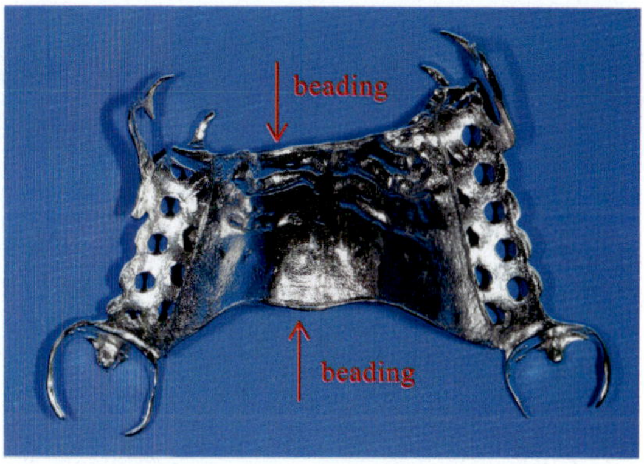

Fig. 9.5 Bead lines are used in all maxillary major connectors, not in mandibular major connectors

and the underlying soft tissues in the *mandibular major connectors.*

9.2.2 Maxillary Major Connectors

1. *Anteroposterior palatal strap.*
   (a) It can be used for Kennedy Class I, II, III, IV, and V partially edentulous arches (Fig. 9.6a–d).
   (b) It is structurally rigid with minimum bulk.
   (c) The anterior and lateral straps should be 6–8 mm wide. The posterior palatal strap can be 4 mm wide to increase patient comfort.
   (d) The palatal opening should be 15 mm or more in an anteroposterior dimension.
   (e) The anterior strap should not be placed beyond the most anterior rests.
   (f) The posterior strap should be placed as far back as possible but should not be in contact with the tissues of the movable soft palate.
   (g) When the presence of an inoperable torus that ends posteriorly 6–8 mm from the anterior of the junction of the hard and soft palates, an anteroposterior palatal strap can be used.
2. *Palatal strap.*
   (a) It is used in Kennedy Class III and VI partially edentulous arches if edentulous spaces are short (Fig. 9.7).

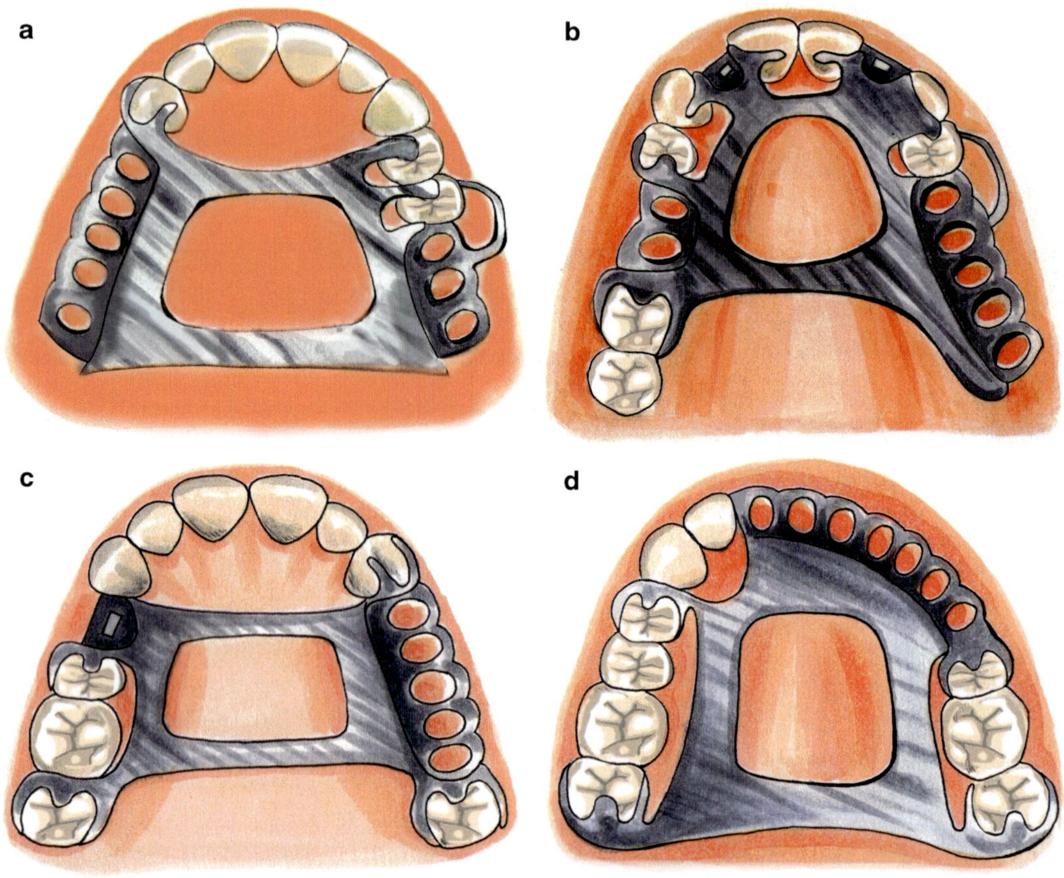

Fig. 9.6 (**a–d**) An anteroposterior palatal strap major connector can be a desirable choice for all maxillary arches except Kennedy-Applegate Class VI arches having short edentulous space. While anterior and lateral straps should be 6–8 mm wide, posterior strap should be 4 mm wide. The design example shown in (**d**) can also be used in Kennedy-Applegate Class V cases having weak anterior abutments. In distal extension bases, wrought wire retentive arms are indicated where clasp tips lie in front of the axis of rotation. For example, in the cases shown in (**a**), a wrought wire clasp can be used on the right canine abutment tooth

(b) The rigidity provided by a palatal strap is usually adequate if the anteroposterior dimension of a strap is a minimum of 8 mm.
(c) If there is a large torus, a palatal strap should not be used.

The anteroposterior palatal bar and the *palatal bar* mentioned in many textbooks are variations of the anteroposterior palatal strap and the palatal strap major connectors. They should be bulky in order to be rigid, and thus they are generally unacceptable for many patients and not recommended.

3. *Palatal plate.*
   (a) It is essentially used in Kennedy Class I partially edentulous arches where six or less anterior teeth remain, the abutments are periodontally weakened, and/or the support from the residual ridges is poor (Fig. 9.8a).
   (b) It is structurally rigid.
   (c) It covers one-half or more of the hard palate.
   (d) The posterior border extends to the junction of the hard and soft palates. The posterior palatal seal that is used with complete dentures should not be utilized

unless the posterior part is made of acrylic resin as seen in Fig. 9.8b; instead, a slight mechanical seal may be formed by ensuring the presence of a bead line along the posterior border of the major connector.

(e) If there is a large torus, a palatal plate should not be used.

(f) Three forms of the palatal plate can be used for different cases:
- It can cover two-thirds of the palate. The anterior border does not extend beyond the most anterior rests.
- The posterior part of the palatal plate can be formed as a gridwork design with the possibility of adding acrylic resin. This form allows for future relining (Fig.9.8b).
- Linguoplating can be used for indirect retention or subsequent replacement of natural teeth.

Modified palatal plate connector: It is used in Kennedy Class II partially edentulous arches. Anteroposterior dimension and form are done as palatal strap and continued backward, ending with a butt joint at the entrance to the hamular notch. The posterior border may not be extended to the junction of the hard and soft palates (Fig. 9.9).

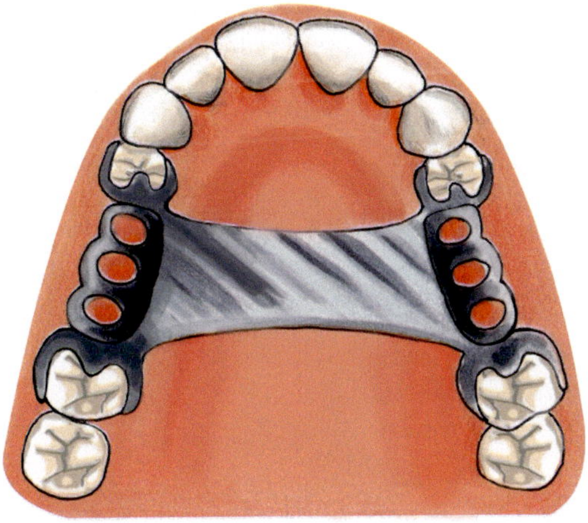

Fig. 9.7 A palatal strap major connector can be used in Kennedy Class III and Kennedy-Applegate Class VI arches having short edentulous spaces. Its anteroposterior dimension should be minimum 8 mm

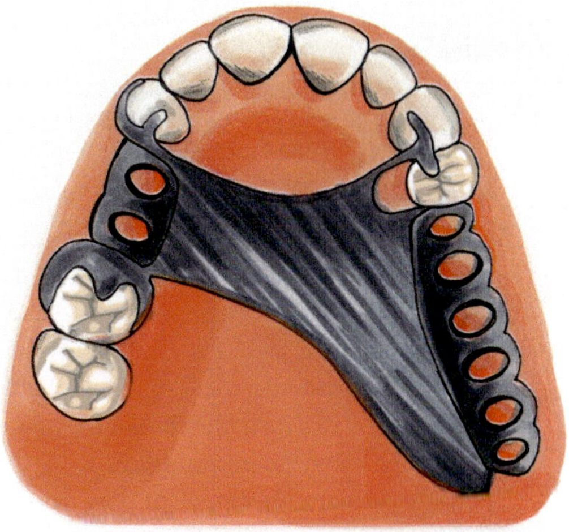

Fig. 9.9 A modified palatal plate major connector used in Kennedy Class II cases

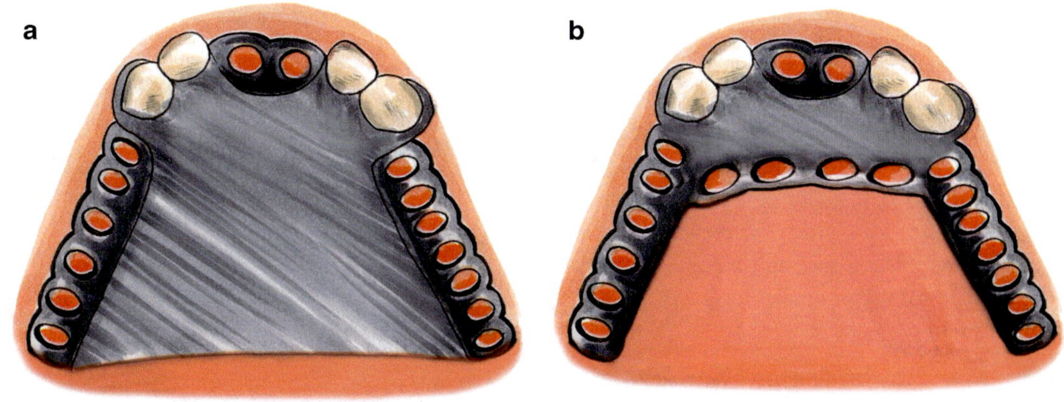

Fig. 9.8 (**a**, **b**) When maximum tissue support is necessary, a palatal plate major connector can be used. Posterior part of the major connector can be formed as a gridwork design. Wrought wire retentive arms can also be used on the canine abutments

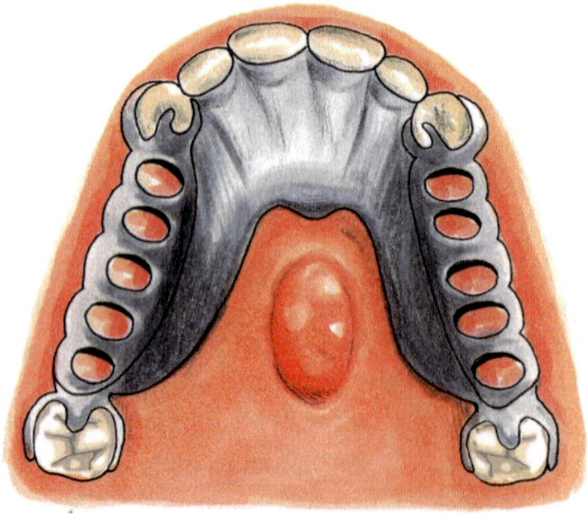

Fig. 9.10 A "U"-shaped or horse-shoe major connector. Its use is limited because the rigidity is not sufficient

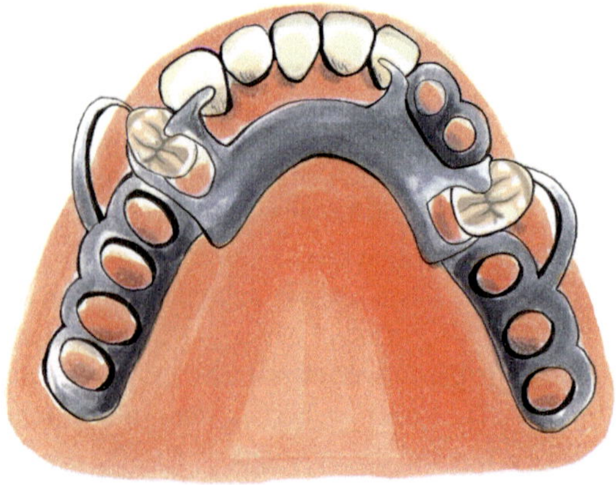

Fig. 9.11 If there is at least 7 mm vertical distance between the floor of the mouth and the gingival margins of the teeth when the tip of the patient's tongue is touching the anterior part of the palate, a lingual bar major connector can be used

4. *U-shaped or horseshoe.*
   (a) It is not structurally rigid, especially for the Kennedy Class I and II partially edentulous arches.
   (b) It is only used in cases with a prominent median suture line and if an inoperable torus extends to the posterior limit of the hard palate (Fig. 9.10). It can also be used when the patient insists on the use of her/his old denture's design, which is U-shaped or when she/he thinks they cannot tolerate the posterior portion of the major connector because of gag reflex. When it is used, the thickness of the framework should be increased if maximal rigidity is desired. This can be accomplished by use of two layers of pattern wax when the framework is made.

Rigidity is a very important factor that should be taken into consideration for major connectors because it has been shown that the rigid major connectors decrease both RPD and abutment tooth movement under loading. As described above, a major connector requires a minimum size for rigidity. Therefore, it is not recommended to reduce the metal framework for all types of major connectors.

9.2.3 Mandibular Major Connectors

1. *Lingual bar.*
   (a) It is structurally rigid if it is designed to a height of 4 mm and a thickness of 2 mm and is half pear-shaped in cross-section with the thin edge toward the teeth (Fig. 9.11).
   (b) The superior border of the bar should be 3 mm below the gingival margins. Therefore, it requires at least 7 mm of vertical space between the floor of the mouth and the gingival margins of the teeth when the tip of the patient's tongue is touching the anterior part of the palate.
   (c) It cannot be used when a large inoperable torus exists (Fig. 9.12).

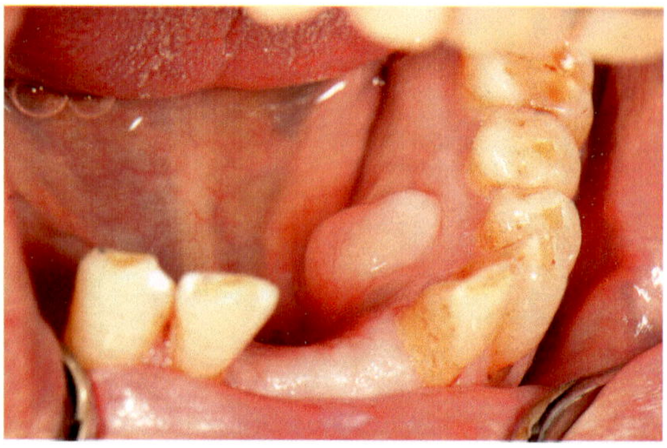

Fig. 9.12 In cases having large inoperable lingual torus, a lingual plate major connector should be used

2. *Lingual plate.*
   (a) It is structurally rigid.
   (b) It is an extended version of a lingual bar with a thin metal plate. The metal plate should cover the cingulum of the anterior

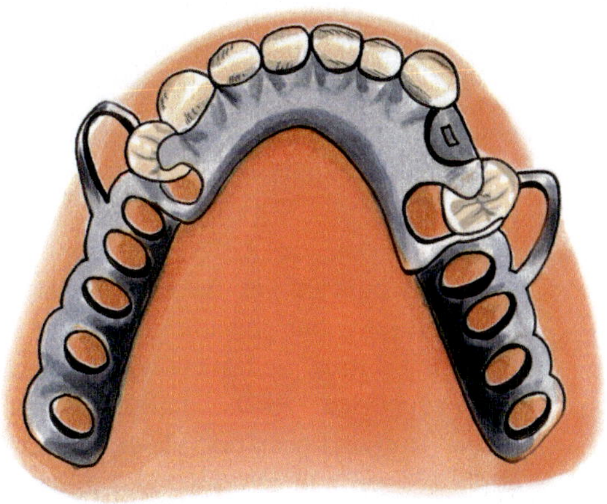

Fig. 9.13 The metal plate should cover the cingulum of the anterior teeth when a lingual plate major connector is used

teeth and the superior border must be scalloped (Fig. 9.13).

(c) When interproximal spaces exist between the anterior teeth, "stepbacks" can be designed to avoid a display of metal.

(d) It should have a terminal rest at each end regardless of the need for indirect retention.

(e) It can be used to stabilize mobile teeth, to facilitate repair in the presence of possible tooth loss, and in the presence of inoperable mandibular tori.

The Kennedy bar (double lingual bar/continuous bar), which is indicated when the axial alignment of the anterior teeth needs excessive blockout for the lingual plate and wide diastema exists, and the *labial bar,* which is indicated when excess lingually inclined anterior teeth exist, are mentioned in many textbooks. Both of them can create a food trap and can be disturbing to patients. Thus, they are not a practical solution, either esthetically or functionally, and are not mentioned in this chapter.

In case the inter occlusal distance is too limited to set up regular artificial teeth or due to existing deep-bite (severe vertical overlap), occlusal or palatal surfaces may be added to the framework design that can be engaged with veneering materials. This option allows easy handling of the posterior edentulous space and eliminates the risk of acrylic base fracture (Fig. 9.14).

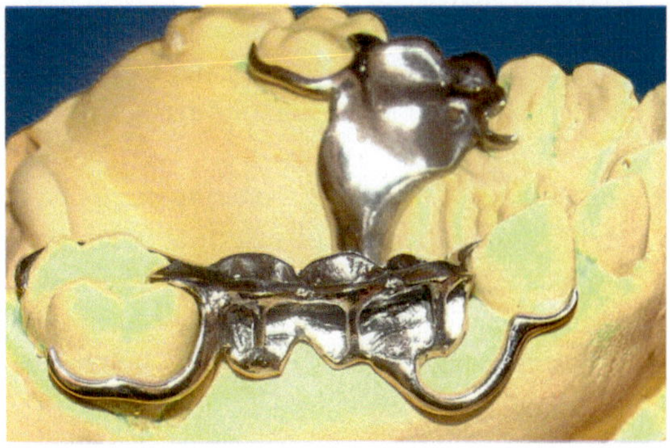

Fig. 9.14 An interim removable partial denture with metal occlusal surface. Metal occlusal or palatinal surfaces can be used in cases having insufficient interocclusal distance and severe vertical overlap

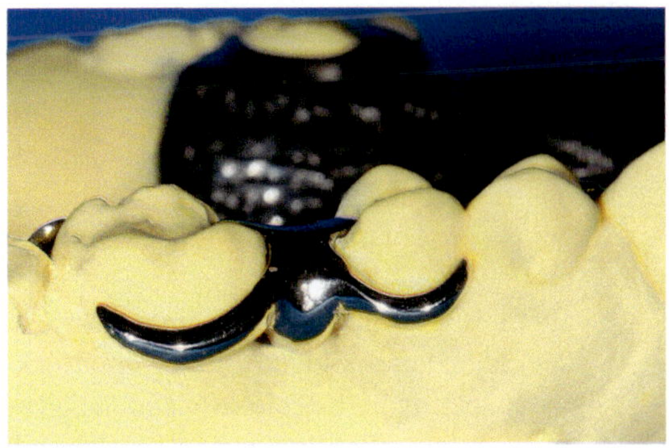

Fig. 9.15 If there is a short edentulous area that is not in the esthetic zone, it can be filled with just only metal to prevent food impaction and the migration of the teeth

In addition, in the presence of short spaces, insufficient room to set up artificial teeth can be closed only with metal if it does not cause esthetic problems. This will prevent food impaction and the migration of the teeth (Fig. 9.15).

Different study results showed that there was insufficient evidence to determine whether one design was better or worse than another regarding major/minor connectors and direct retainers in mandibular distal extension RPDs.

9.3 Minor Connectors

9.3.1 General Aspects of Minor Connectors

1. Minor connectors provide rigidity and unification by joining other components of a

framework to a major connector. Thus, the transmission of forces among the major connector, abutment teeth, and oral tissues can be achieved.
2. Minor connectors act as a bracing component and maintain the path of insertion when they are located on guiding planes.
3. Minor connectors should be rigid (except the fourth type) and placed so as not to irritate the surrounding tissues.

9.3.2 Types of Minor Connectors

1. Minor connectors that join clasp assemblies to major connectors. As they may be attached to the clasps, they can also be a separate entity.
   (a) Mostly, they are located on guiding planes or surfaces. Sometimes, it is necessary to put them on a tooth surface adjacent to another tooth. In this situation, it should be positioned in the associated lingual embrasure.
   (b) When it is formed as a separate entity, it should be approximately 1–1.5 mm thick with tapering both occlusally and facially. It is shifted slightly toward the lingual side to increase rigidity and enhance reciprocation (Fig. 9.16).
   (c) The guide (proximal) plate minor connector should cover about half the distance of the abutment tooth buccolingually (between the tips of the buccal and lingual cusps) and two-thirds the distance of the tooth occlusogingivally. It is effective to prepare a guide plane as close to the gingival margin as possible to reduce plaque accumulation (Figs. 9.16 and 9.17).
   (d) In distal extension RPDs, the proximal plate is in contact with the entire guiding plane initially, but physiological relief is necessary during the framework try-in. In tooth-supported RPDs, guiding plane preparation and proximal plates are generally longer, and physiological relief is not necessary. An elongated proximal plate that is parallel to the path of insertion may compensate for the loss of retention when an adequate guiding plane cannot be prepared.
   (e) If tooth surfaces are parallel to the path of placement, preparation of the guiding plane is not necessary (Preparation of the guiding planes on the abutment teeth is described in Chap. 7).
2. Minor connectors that join indirect retainers or auxiliary rests to major connectors.
   (a) They should be positioned in embrasures and should form right angles with the major connector, and junctions should be rounded. Although one study proposed to place a minor connector on the center of the lingual aspects of the maxillary abutment tooth to reduce the amount of gingival tissue coverage, more randomized

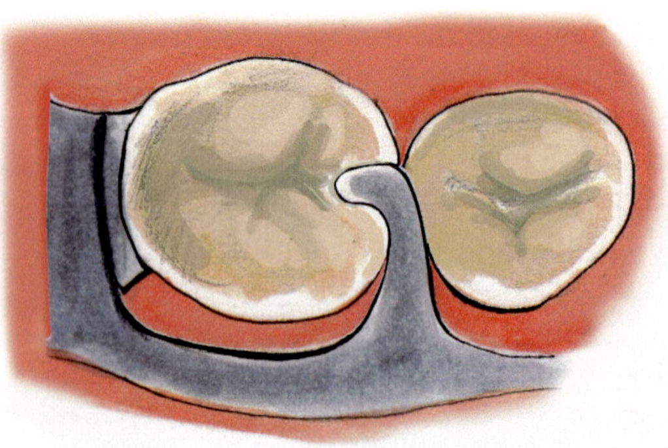

Fig. 9.16 If a proximal plate minor connector is formed as a separate entity, it is shifted slightly toward the lingual side

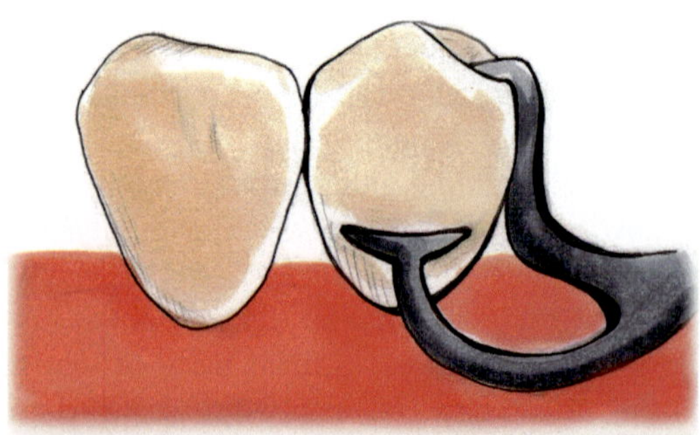

Fig. 9.17 A proximal plate minor connector should be placed on the guiding plane covering about two-thirds of the tooth occlusogingivally

clinical studies are needed to change the classical knowledge.

3. Minor connectors that join denture bases to major connectors.
   (a) They can be constructed in different designs such as mesh design, ladder-like design, loop design, or metal base with different retentive elements (such as bead, nailhead). Metal bases can be used instead of acrylic resin bases in tooth-borne RPDs where the short edentulous spaces exist (Fig. 9.18). Large openings in a retention design are generally more satisfactory than a mesh design which may result in further weakening of the resin (Fig. 9.19). In addition, it is recommended that the three structural designs that are superior to conventional design may also be considered along with the conventional designs.

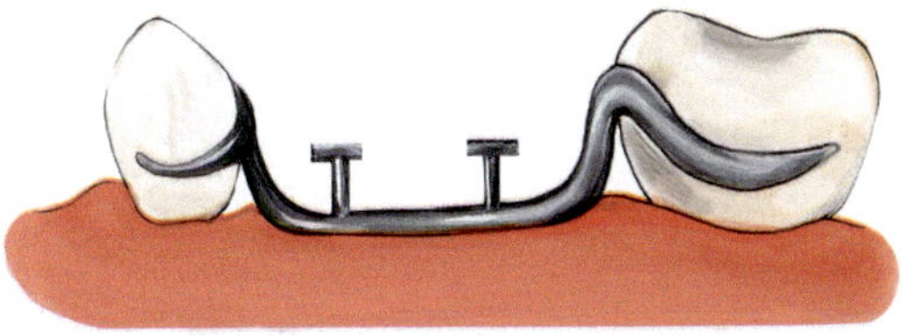

Fig. 9.18 Tissue surfaces can also be fabricated only metal in cases where tissue support and future relining are not necessary

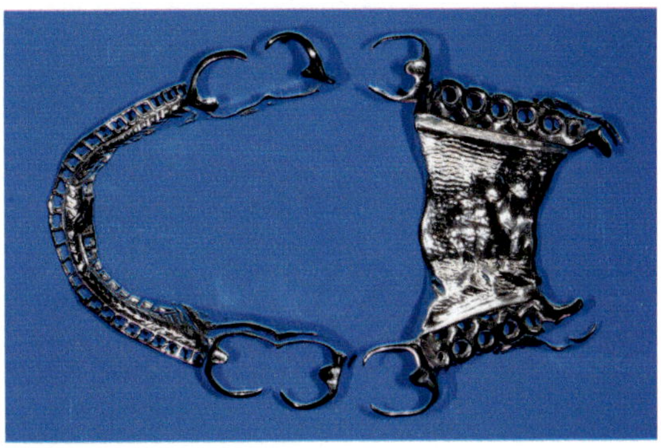

Fig. 9.19 Large opening gridwork designs such as ladder-like and loop designs (right) are more preferable than mesh design (left) considering the acrylic retention. But the thickness of these designs can complicate artificial tooth setting

   (b) In Kennedy Class I and II mandibular arches, the minor connector should extend about two-thirds the length of the edentulous ridge but should not be placed on the ascending portion of the ridge. It should be extended on both the buccal and lingual surfaces (Fig. 9.20).
   (c) In Kennedy Class I and II maxillary arches, they should be extended as far as possible posteriorly and the junction of the major and minor connectors should be located 2 mm medially from an imaginary line that would come into contact with the palatal surfaces of artificial teeth.
   (d) In free-end saddle partially edentulous cases, they must be finished with a "cast stop". Altered cast impression procedures result in an elevated cast stop from the residual ridge. The autopolymerizing acrylic resin can be added to compensate for this gap (Fig. 9.21a–c).
   (e) Relief under the minor connector should be started 1.5–2 mm away from the abutment tooth. Thus, metal/tissue contact can be created in this area.
   (f) A butt joint should be used to design the resin–metal interface (finishing line). The finishing line junction with the major connector should take the form of an angle not greater than 90°, therefore being somewhat undercut.

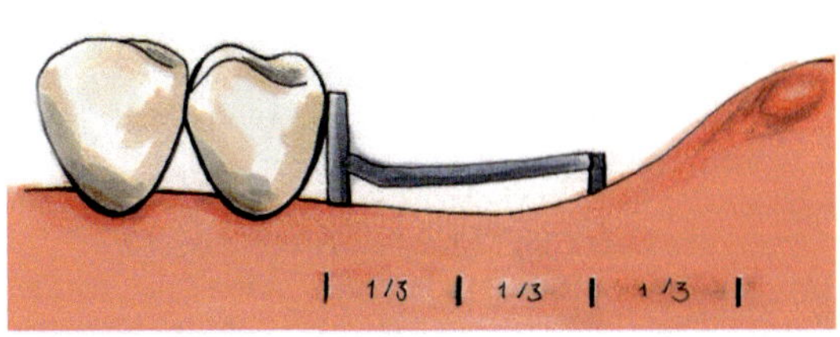

Fig. 9.20 In mandibular distal extension removable partial dentures, a gridwork minor connector should not be placed on the ascending portion of the ridge

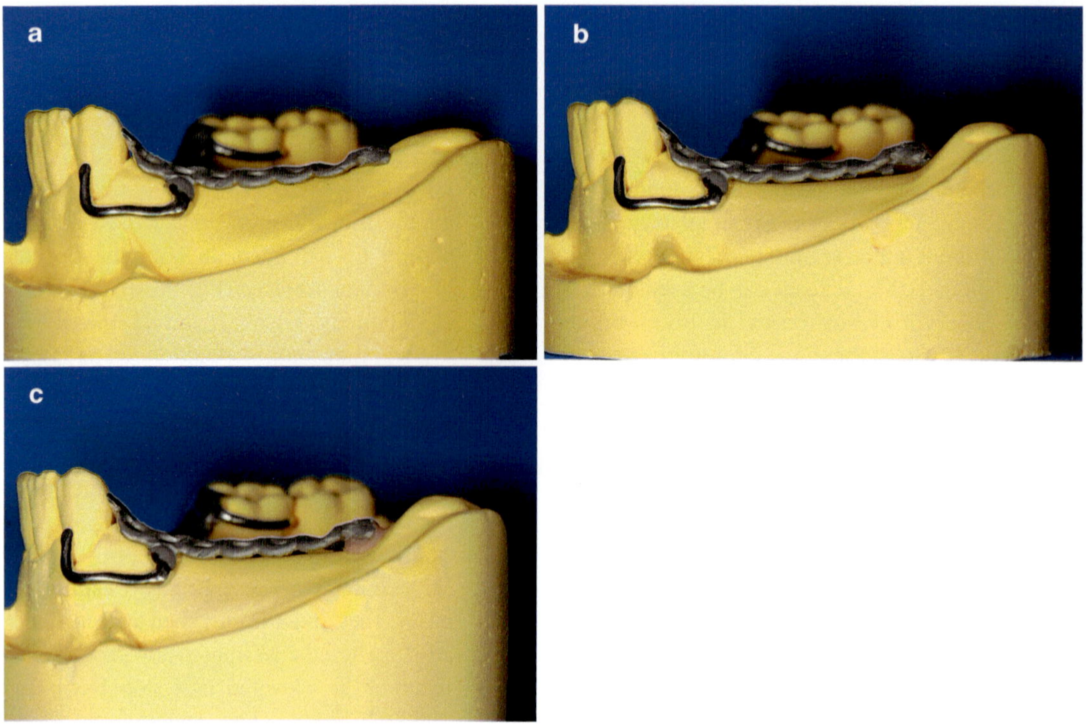

Fig. 9.21 (**a**–**c**) Metal cast stop can be modified with self-cure acrylic resin, if an altered cast impression has been performed

4. Minor connectors that serve as approach arms for vertical projection/bar-type clasps.

   These minor connectors support the clasps and do not need to be rigid (Fig. 9.1).

Further Reading

Akaltan F, Kaynak D. An evaluation of the effects of two distal extension removable partial denture designs on tooth stabilization and periodontal health. J Oral Rehabil. 2005;32:823–9.

Ben-Ur Z, Mijiritsky E, Gorfil C, Brosh T. Stiffness of different designs and cross-sections of maxillary and mandibular major connectors of removable partial dentures. J Prosthet Dent. 1999;81:526–32.

Bohnenkamp DM. Removable partial dentures: clinical concepts. Dent Clin North Am. 2014;58:69–89.

Carr AB, Brown DT. McCracken's removable partial prosthodontics. 13th ed. St. Louis, MO: Elsevier; 2016.

Chow TW, Clark RKF, Clarke DA. Improved designs for removable partial dentures in Kennedy class IV cases. Quintessence Int. 1988;19:797–800.

Dunny JA, King GE. Minor connector designs for anterior acrylic resin bases: a preliminary study. J Prosthet Dent. 1975;34:496–502.

Green LK, Hondrum SO. The effect of design modifications on the torsional and compressive rigidity of U-shaped palatal major connectors. J Prosthet Dent. 2003;89:400–7.

Hosman HJM. The influence of clasp design of distal extension removable partial dentures on the periodontium of the abutment teeth. Int J Prosthodont. 1990;3:256–65.

Itoh H, Baba K, Aridome K, Okada D, Tokuda A, Nishiyama A, Miura H, Igarashi Y. Effect of direct retainer and major connector designs on RPD and abutment tooth movement dynamics. J Oral Rehabil. 2008;35:810–5.

Jorge JH, Giampaolo ET, Vergani CE, Machado AL, Pavarina AC, Cardoso de Oliveira MR. Clinical evaluation of abutment teeth of removable partial denture by means of the periotest method. J Oral Rehabil. 2007;34:222–7.

Kapur KK, Deupree R, Dent RJ, Hasse AL. A randomized clinical trial of two basic removable partial denture designs. Part I: comparisons of five-year success rates and periodontal health. J Prosthet Dent. 1994;72:268–82.

Keyf F. Frequency of the various classes of removable partial dentures and selection of major connectors and direct/indirect retainers. Turk J Med Sci. 2001;31:445–9.

Kim JJ. Revisiting the removable partial denture. Dent Clin North Am. 2019;63:263–78.

LaVere AM, Krol AJ. Selection of a major connector for the extension-base removable partial denture. J Prosthet Dent. 1973;30:102–5.

Loney RW. Removable partial denture manual. Halifax, NS: Dalhousie University Faculty of Dentistry; 2011. http://removpros.dentistry.dal.ca/ewExternalFiles/RPD%20Manual%2011.pdf.

Nagayama T, Wada J, Watanabe C, Murakami N, Takakusaki K, Uchida H, Utsumi M, Wakabayashi N. Influence of retainer and major connector designs of removable partial dentures on the stabilization of mobile teeth: a preliminary study. Dent Mater J. 2020;39:89–100.

Ohkubo C, Abe M, Miyata T, Obana J. Comparative strengths of metal framework structures for removable partial dentures. J Prosthet Dent. 1997;78: 302–8.

Ohkubo C, Kurtz KS, Suzuki Y, Hanatani S, Abe M, Hosoi T. Comparative study of maxillary complete dentures constructed of metal base and metal structure framework. J Oral Rehabil. 2001;28:149–56.

Phoenix RD, Cagna DR, Defreest CF. Stewart's clinical removable partial prosthodontics. 4th ed. Chicago: Quintessence Publishing; 2008.

Pienkos TE, Morris WJ, Gronet PM, Cameron SM, Looney SW. The strength of multiple major connector designs under simulated functional loading. J Prosthet Dent. 2007;97:299–304.

Polychronakis N, Sotiriou M, Zissis A. A survey of removable partial denture casts and major connector designs found in commercial laboratories, Athens, Greece. J Prosthodont. 2013;22:245–9.

Pun DK, Waliszewski MP, Waliszewski KJ, Berzins D. Survey of partial removable dental prosthesis (partial RDP) types in a distinct patient population. J Prosthet Dent. 2011;106:48–56.

Radford DR, Walter JD. A variation in minor connector design for partial dentures. Int J Prosthodont. 1993;6:50–4.

Sato Y, Hosokawa R. Proximal plate in conventional circumferential cast clasp retention. J Prosthet Dent. 2000;83:319–22.

Shifman A, Ben-Ur Z. Prosthodontic treatment for the Applegate-Kennedy class V partially edentulous patient. J Prosthet Dent. 1996;76:212–8.

Shimura Y, Wadachi J, Nakamura T, Mizutani H, Igarashi Y. Influence of removable partial dentures on the formation of dental plaque on abutment teeth. J Prosthodont Res. 2010;54:29–35.

Stratton RJ, Wiebelt FJ. An atlas of removable partial denture design. Chicago: Quintessence Publishing Co.; 1988.

The glossary of prosthodontic terms: ninth edition. J Prosthet Dent. 2017;117(5S):e1–e105.

Rests and Rest Seats

10

Olcay Şakar

Abstract

Rests are vital for removable partial dentures (RPDs) to perform their optimal function. In addition to their several advantages described in this chapter, their most important benefits are preventing the RPD movement toward the tissue and transmitting the occlusal forces in a way that will not harm the abutment teeth. Their proper function can only be achieved if they seat on the well-prepared rest seats. Unfortunately, rest seat preparation is overlooked by many dentists and the size and shape of the preparations show variety even between prosthodontists. In this chapter, different forms of the rests, their appropriate rest seat preparations, and bonded rest seats are described along with the necessary equipment.

10.1 Definitions

Partial denture rest: A rigid extension of a fixed or removable dental prosthesis that prevents movement toward the mucosa and transmits functional forces to the teeth or dental implant.

Rest seat: The prepared recess in a tooth or restoration developed to receive the occlusal, incisal, cingulum, or lingual rest.

10.2 Functions of the Rests

Rests are used to:

1. Transmit the occlusal forces from the prosthesis to an abutment along the long axis of the tooth (Fig. 10.1).
2. Resist the denture base movement toward the soft tissue.
3. Prevent impingement on the gingival tissues.
4. Maintain clasps in the desired positions.
5. Prevent extrusion (displacement-migration) of the unopposed abutment teeth.

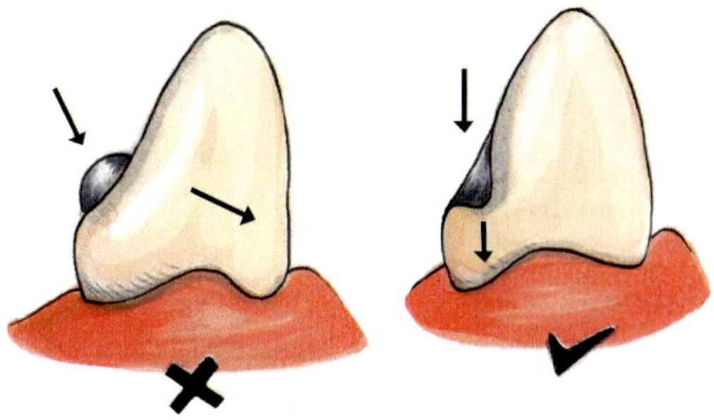

Fig. 10.1 A rest should be placed into a prepared rest seat. Otherwise occlusal forces cannot be transmitted from the denture to an abutment along the long axis of the tooth

O. Şakar (✉)
Faculty of Dentistry, Department of Prosthodontics, İstanbul University, İstanbul, Türkiye
e-mail: osakar@istanbul.edu.tr

O. Şakar (ed.), *Removable Partial Dentures*, https://doi.org/10.1007/978-3-031-47083-7_10

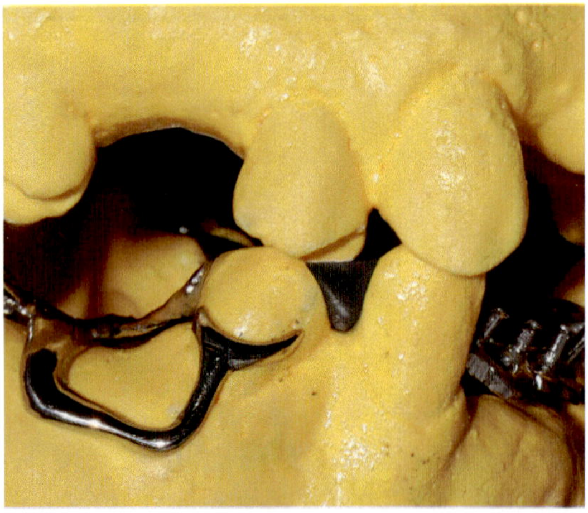

Fig. 10.2 Small spaces between teeth can be restored with back-to-back occlusal rests. Thus, reestablishing occlusion and preventing food impaction can be provided

6. Act as an indirect retainer in Kennedy Class I, II, and long-span IV partially edentulous arches (see Chap. 11).
7. Provide correct location of the denture in rebasing or altered cast impression procedures.
8. Reestablish occlusion (Fig. 10.2).
9. Prevent food impaction (Fig. 10.2).
10. Contribute to horizontal stabilization when placed on the anterior teeth.

10.3 Forms of Rest and Rest Seat Preparations

As a rule, a rest should be placed in the prepared rest seat and the preparation of a rest seat must be carried out after completing the guide surface preparation.

The rest seat preparation has to be performed in the manner described below to ensure the proper function of the rests. Preparations should be fabricated without undercut, sharp edges and angles, and should remain in enamel boundaries. When a metal-ceramic restoration with a rest seat has been fabricated, the rest seat should be on the metal surface and placed at least 1 mm away from the metal–ceramic junction. All-ceramic restorations have also been used in the abutment teeth of RPDs with a metal framework, as they are more esthetic and biocompatible. Although zirconia seems to be more durable in resisting posterior occlusal forces than resin composite and lithium disilicate, further studies investigating the veneering porcelain fracture frequency are required to draw more reliable conclusions. Also, when using digitally designed and manufactured restorations with the occlusal rest seat, it underlines the importance of checking the fit that should be the maximum contact area between the rest and the rest seat to prevent fracture. In addition, when placing a rest on a large amalgam restoration, possible complications should be considered, along with the patient's consent.

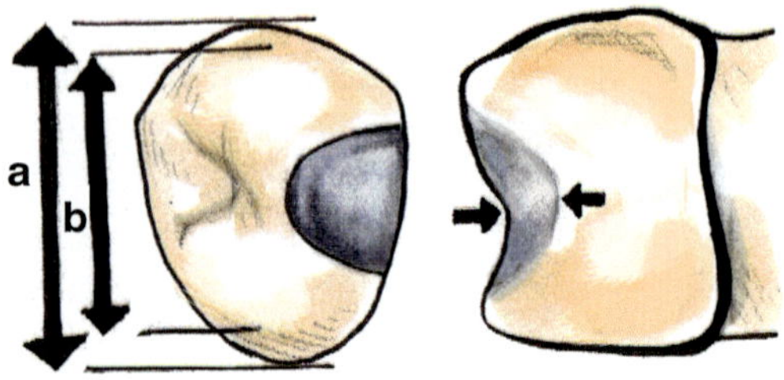

Fig. 10.3 Left: An occlusal rest size should be approximately A/3 or B/2. (a) Greatest buccolingual width. (b) The measurement between the cusp tips
Right: The depth of the occlusal rest should be 1–1.5 mm.

There are three major forms of the rests:

10.3.1 Occlusal Rests

The form of an occlusal rest should be a round, triangular shape from the occlusal view. Its base should be at the marginal ridge and its apex should extend toward the center of the tooth. The floor of the rest seat should be spoon-shaped from the sagittal view. The deepest part of an occlusal rest seat should be located near the center of the mesial or distal fossa. The depth of the rest should be 1.0–1.5 mm with the tapering center of the tooth measuring 0.5 mm in the sagittal plane (Fig. 10.3 Right). The recommended size of an occlusal rest is one-third to one-half the mesiodistal diameter of the abutment tooth and approximately one-half the buccolingual width of the abutment tooth measured between the cusp tips. This means that the width of the occlusal rest at the marginal ridge is approximately a minimum of 2.5 mm. (Figs. 10.3 and 10.4). In addition, if the rest does not have a sufficient bulk (approximately 1.5 mm.) over the marginal ridge, which is the most critical dimension, rest fractures may occur. Therefore, care should be taken to ensure adequate tooth reduction in this area.

The angle formed by the floor of the rest and the minor connector should be less than 90° so that the transmitted occlusal forces can be directed along the vertical axis of the tooth. If the angle is greater than 90°, the prosthesis can slip away from the abutment teeth. The appropriate angle can be achieved by preparing a spoon-shaped rest seat to avoid excess inclination, which is not recommended (Fig. 10.4).

Diamond burs with rounded ends and tapering sides can be used to prepare the rest seats

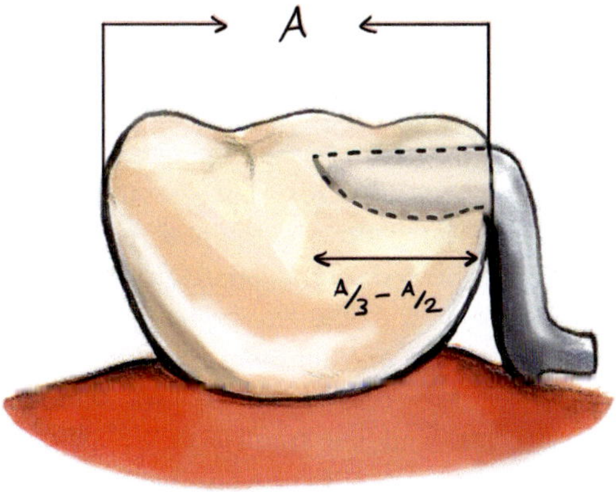

Fig. 10.4 A spoon-shaped occlusal rest should cover half or one-third of the mesiodistal length of the abutment tooth

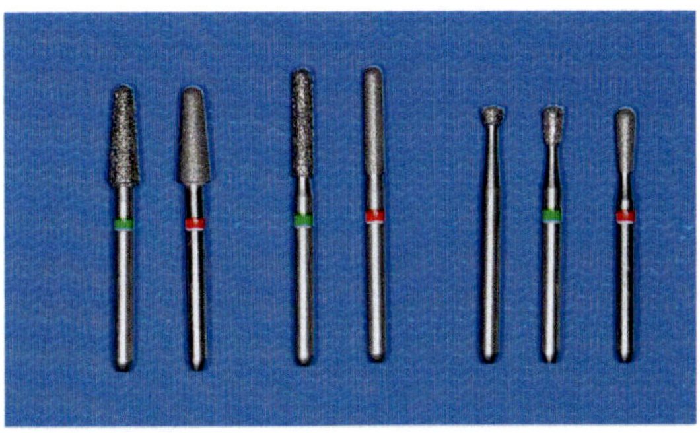

Fig. 10.5 The accessories for preparing rest seats

(Fig. 10.5). Using a round-shaped bur may cause a rest seat with a sharp edge or undercut.

Long box rests, which extend for more than half the mesiodistal width of a tooth, are used almost exclusively for the rotational path RPDs. This rest seat preparation is described in Chap. 12 (Fig. 12.14). If this rest is placed in a mesially inclined molar adjacent to the edentulous space, it can direct the forces along the long axis of the abutment tooth and thus the disto-occlusal rest may not be needed.

Onlay/overlay rests can be used on the tilted or infraoccluded teeth to restore occlusion or can be used for reestablishing occlusal vertical dimension and maximal intercuspal position in overlay RPDs. This process requires minimal preparation, including pits, fissures, and grooves, or no tooth preparation. Tooth preparation should include a guiding plane, especially when tilted teeth do not have enough guiding surface.

When *interproximal (embrasure) occlusal rests* are made, preparation of the rest seat extends over the occlusal embrasure of two approximating teeth. It is essential to remove sufficient tooth structure at the facial and lingual surfaces of the abutments and to permit the component to be shaped so that the occlusion will not be altered. Otherwise, fractures of the framework may occur. The contact between the teeth should be preserved to avoid tooth migration (Fig. 10.6). A diamond bur with a rounded end and tapering sides is also suitable for this preparation.

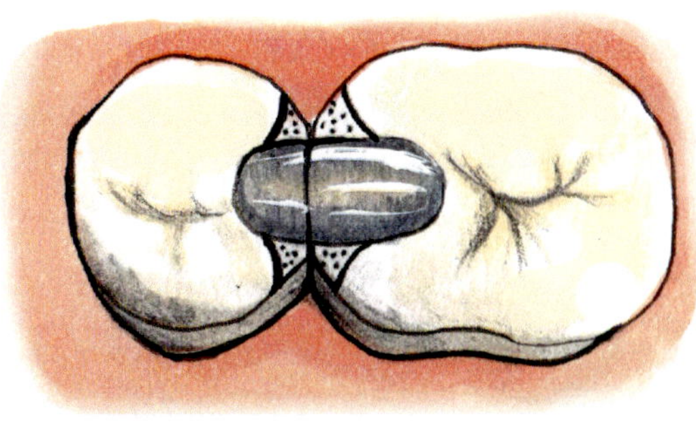

Fig. 10.6 An interproximal (embrasure) occlusal rest requires extra preparation of the dotted area. It is necessary to pay attention not to get lost of contact

10.3.2 Lingual (Cingulum) Rests

When posterior teeth are not present or available, *lingual rests* are utilized on anterior teeth, primarily on the canines. A satisfactory rest seat preparation can be made with minimal tooth reduction due to its well-developed cingulum (Fig. 10.7). If canines are missing, multiple incisors should receive rests to distribute the stress. It should be remembered that the preparation of lower anterior teeth may be risky because of the lack of thickness of their enamel.

A lingual rest seat preparation should be "V-shaped with a rounded base" when viewed in cross-section and "crescent-shaped" when viewed from the occluso-lingual aspect. An in-vitro study showed that among tooth-colored crown restorations with the same cingulum rest seat design, those which were zirconia-based had better fracture resistance than those with a lithium disilicate base. In addition, the rest seat design having a round shape floor with 0.5-mm radius curvature has shown better fracture resistance than the smaller radius design independent of crown material. The correct angulation of the floor of the rest seat should be less than 90° from the proximal view (Fig. 10.7). When a preparation has been made on a maxillary canine, the average dimensions should be 2.5–3 mm mesiodistally, 2 mm labiolingually, and 1.5 mm occlusogingivally. Preparation of a cingulum rest seat is accomplished using an inverted cone bur. Finishing touches should be performed with round-end burs (Fig. 10.5).

The incisor teeth, especially in the mandible, do not present suitable contours or depth of enamel for adequate preparation. In addition, it may create cleaning difficulties. When a cingulum is poorly developed, with insufficient bulk for the preparation of a cingulum rest seat, a rest seat can be made using composite resin (Fig. 10.8) and resin-bonded CoCr cast or laminates. Also, a new metal-ceramic restoration with lingual rest seat can be fabricated (see Chap. 7 and Fig. 7.10). Although more detailed studies are needed, long-term studies showed that the *bonded rest seats* can provide acceptable strength and longevity without damaging the periodontal tissues of the abutment teeth. While tooth preparation is needed for resin-bonded metal rest seats or laminates, composite resin rest seats can be fabricated by conserving the intact tooth and involving less cost. Rest seats are prepared at least 3 mm away from the cervical gingiva. The cervical portion of the composite resin should not be over-contoured, without sharp line angles, and should be well adapted and polished. It is also suggested to provide a composite resin rest seat after delivery of the RPD. The below-mentioned procedures should be followed: (1) A small groove is prepared as the floor of the rest on the lingual surface of the teeth. (2) After taking the impression, the rest seat is waxed above the groove on the working cast, and the framework is cast. (3) After finishing the RPD, the composite resin is filled in the gap and cured under the occlusal force. Thus, minimal preparation of the tooth and functional fitting can be provided.

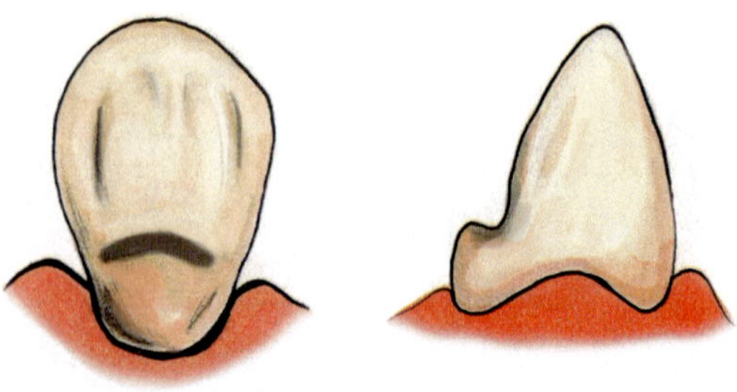

Fig. 10.7 A cingulum rest seat from lingual and sagittal view. The apex of the lingual rest preparation should be directed incisally

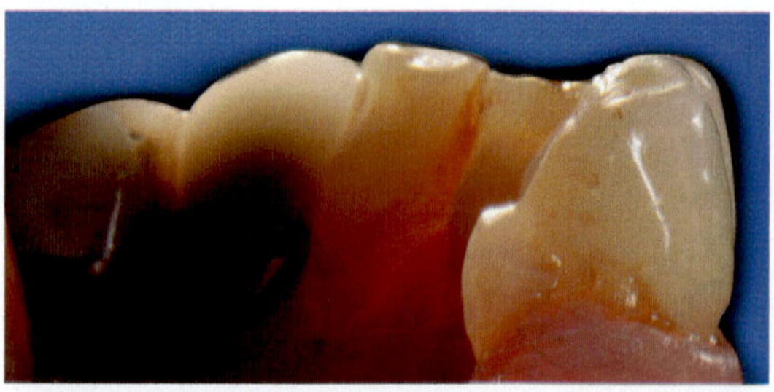

Fig. 10.8 A composite resin rest seat can be prepared when an anterior tooth have a cingulum with inadequate bulk for preparation

Ceramic orthodontic brackets have also been used as rest seats. It should be remembered that the removal of these brackets results in heat generation.

In some instances (such as poorly developed cingulum, lack of clearance in the opposing teeth), *round rest seats*, which are spoon-shaped like an occlusal rest seat, may be used. A reduction of the mesial marginal ridge is necessary to complete the preparation. Diamond burs with a rounded end and a tapering side, which match the tooth size, can be used to prepare the round lingual rest seats.

10.3.3 Incisal Rests

Incisal rests are less desirable than lingual rests, both esthetically and mechanically. Whenever possible, a lingual rest seat on the natural tooth or composite/cast/ laminate rest seats should be preferred instead of an incisal rest. A crown restoration with a lingual rest seat also can be used when it is indicated.

Incisal rest seat preparation should be "V-shaped with rounded base" placed on the mesial or distal incisal angle, and its deepest portion should be towards the center of the tooth. An incisal rest seat size should be approximately 2.5 mm mesiodistally and 1.5 mm occlusogingivally. The apex of the "V" should be rounded. An incisal rest seat has two parts slightly on the facial surface and a shallow one on the lingual surface (Fig. 10.9).

A silicone-based registration material or wax can be used to measure and verify the depth of the rest seat preparation (see Chap. 7, Fig.7.9). This procedure is also useful for detecting whether there is an undercut or not. After finishing the rest seat preparations, all sharp line angles and corners should be rounded and polished. Polishing is accomplished using a carborondum-impregnated rubber wheel or a low-speed handpiece. Fluoride should be applied after the alginate impression because some fluoride substitutes and irreversible hydrocolloids may be incompatible.

It has been shown that the pressure distribution under the distal extension base is affected by occlusal rest localization and the RPD design. *Rest localization* varies in different partially edentulous cases. In Kennedy I and II cases, mesial rest is preferred (Fig. 10.10). But in some cases (such as when abutment teeth are rotated and have a large restoration or a heavy centric contact on the mesial), a distal rest in a suitably prepared rest seat can be used. Long guiding planes with distal rests should not be used to

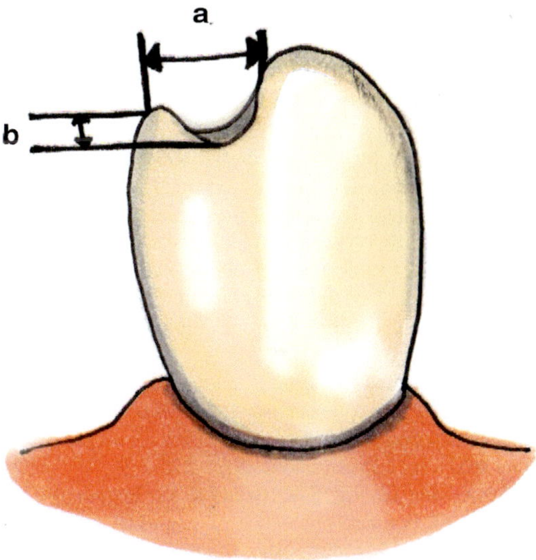

Fig. 10.9 "V"-shaped incisal rest seat dimensions should be approximately 2.5 mm mesiodistally (**a**) and 1.5 mm occlusogingivally (**b**)

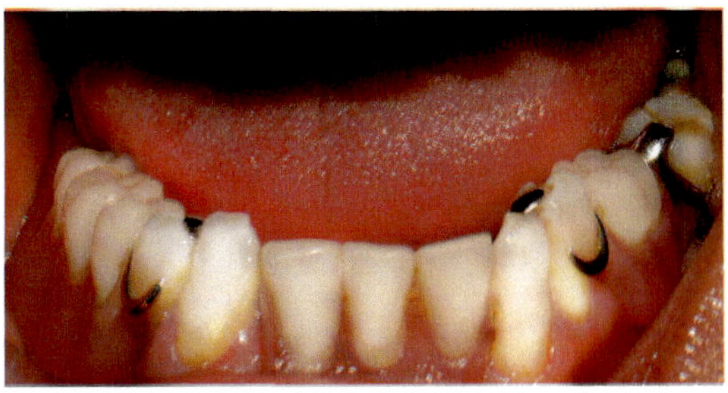

Fig. 10.10 In distal extension removable partial dentures, mesial rest is recommended. But a distal rest can be used in the presence of an abutment tooth being rotated or having large restoration and a heavy centric contact on the mesial

avoid potential torquing. In Kennedy III and IV cases, rests are placed adjacent to the edentulous space.

Further Reading

Carr AB, Brown DT. McCracken's removable partial prosthodontics. 13th ed. St. Louis, MO: Elsevier; 2016.

Carracho JF, Razzoog ME. Removable partial denture abutments restored with all-ceramic surveyed crowns. Quintessence Int. 2006;37:283–8.

Culwick PF, Howell PG, Faigenblum MJ. The size of occlusal rest seats prepared for removable partial dentures. Br Dent J. 2000;189:318–22.

Jones RM, Goodacre CJ, Brown DT, Munoz CA, Rake PC. Dentin exposure and decay incidence when removable partial denture rest seats are prepared in tooth structure. Int J Prosthodont. 1992;5:227–36.

Kancyper S, Sierraalta M, Razzoog ME. All-ceramic surveyed crowns for removable partial denture abutments. J Prosthet Dent. 2000;84:400–2.

Loney RW. Removable partial denture manual. Halifax, NS: Dalhousie University Faculty of Dentistry; 2011. http://removpros.dentistry.dal.ca/ewExternalFiles/RPD%20Manual%2011.pdf.

Maeda Y, Kinoshita Y, Satho H, Yang TC. Influence of bonded composite resin cingulum rest seats on abutment tooth periodontal tissues: a longitudinal prospective study. Int J Prosthodont. 2008;21:37–9.

Manchester JA, Chung KH, Brudvik JS, Ramos V Jr, Chen YW. Fracture resistance of cingulum rest seats in CAD-CAM tooth-colored crowns for removable partial denture abutments. J Prosthet Dent. 2019;121:828–35.

Miura S, Kasahara S, Yamauchi S, Katsuda Y, Harada A, Aida J, Egusa H. A possible risk of CAD/CAM-produced composite resin premolar crowns on a removable partial denture abutment tooth: a 3-year retrospective cohort study. J Prosthodont Res. 2019;63:78–84.

Ohkubo C, Shimizu S, Murata T, Miyama Y, Kurtz KS. Development of a lingual rest seat using adhesive composite resin after removable partial denture delivery. Eur J Prosthodont 2016;4:22–4.

Phoenix RD, Cagna DR, Defreest CF. Stewart's clinical removable partial prosthodontics. 4th ed. Chicago: Quintessence Publishing; 2008.

Pihlaja J, Näpänkangas R, Kuoppala R, Raustia A. Veneered zirconia crowns as abutment teeth for partial removable dental prostheses: a clinical 4-year retrospective study. J Prosthet Dent. 2015;114:633–6.

Rosenstiel SF, Land MF, Walter RD. Contemporary fixed prosthodontics. 6th ed. Philadelphia, PA: Elsevier; 2023.

Rudd RW, Bange AA, Rudd KD, Montalvo R. Preparing teeth to receive a removable partial denture. J Prosthet Dent. 1999;82:536–49.

Sato Y, Shindoi N, Koretake K, Hosokawa R. The effect of occlusal rest size and shape on yield strength. J Prosthet Dent. 2003;89:503–7.

Stratton RJ, Wiebelt FJ. An atlas of removable partial denture design. Chicago: Quintessence Publishing Co.; 1988.

Suenaga H, Kubo K, Hosokawa R, Kuriyagawa T, Sasaki K. Effects of occlusal rest design on pressure distribution beneath the denture base of a distal extension removable partial denture-an in vivo study. Int J Prosthodont. 2014;27:469–71.

The glossary of prosthodontic terms: ninth edition. J Prosthet Dent. 2017;117(5S):e1–e105.

Toth RW, Fiebiger GE, Mackert JR Jr, Goldman BM. Shear strength of lingual rest seats prepared in bonded composite. J Prosthet Dent. 1986;56:99–104.

Toth RW, Fiebiger GE, Mackert JR Jr, King GE, Goldman BM. Load cycling of lingual rest seats prepared in bonded composite. J Prosthet Dent. 1986;56:239–42.

Uchikura K, Murakami N, Yamazaki T, Lyu H, Nagata K, Ona M, Iwasaki N, Takahashi H, Wakabayashi N. Fracture resistance of CAD/CAM restorative materials in mismatched removable partial denture rests: an in vitro experimental and finite element analysis. Dent Mater J. 2022;41:466–72.

Direct and Indirect Retainers

11

Canan Bural Alan and Onur Geçkili

Abstract

The clasp assemblies act as the direct retainers of the removable partial dentures (RPDs) without precision attachments. In this chapter, infra- and supra-bulge clasp assemblies used in RPD design are described with their specific features. Components of the clasp assembly and factors that affect the retention of the clasp assembly are defined. In addition, the RPI clasp assembly that is used for the distal extension RPDs is explained in detail. Indirect retention (rests and minor connectors) and its principles to counteract the dislodgement of the RPD are also expressed.

11.1 Definitions

Circumferential clasp: A retainer that encircles a tooth by more than 180°, including opposite angles, and which generally contacts the tooth throughout the extent of the clasp, with at least one terminal located in an undercut area.

Clasp: The component of the clasp assembly that engages a portion of the tooth surface and either enters an undercut for retention or remains entirely above the height of contour to act as a reciprocating element; generally, it is used to stabilize and retain a removable partial denture.

Clasp assembly: The part of a removable dental prosthesis that acts as a direct retainer and/or stabilizer for a prosthesis by partially encompassing or contacting an abutment tooth— usage: components of the clasp assembly include the retentive clasp, the reciprocal clasp, the cingulum, incisal or occlusal rest, and the minor connector.

Convergence angle: The angle, measured in degrees as viewed in a given plane, formed by the axial walls when a tooth or machined surface on a metal or ceramic material is prepared for a fixed dental prosthesis.

Direct retainer: That component of a removable partial denture used to retain and prevent dislodgment, consisting of a clasp assembly or precision attachment.

Guiding planes: Two or more vertically parallel surfaces on abutment teeth and/or fixed dental prostheses oriented so as to contribute to the direction of the path of placement and removal of a removable partial denture, maxillofacial prosthesis, and overdenture.

Height of contour: A line encircling a tooth and designating its greatest circumference at a selected axial position determined by a dental surveyor; a line encircling a body designating its greatest circumference in a specified plane. **Synonym: survey line.**

C. Bural Alan (✉) · O. Geçkili
Faculty of Dentistry, Department of Prosthodontics, İstanbul University, İstanbul, Türkiye
e-mail: cbural@istanbul.edu.tr; geckili@istanbul.edu.tr

O. Şakar (ed.), *Removable Partial Dentures*, https://doi.org/10.1007/978-3-031-47083-7_11

I-bar clasp: An infrabulge retentive clasp that resembles an "I" as it approaches perpendicular to the facial height of contour.

Indirect retainer: The component of a removable partial denture that assists the direct retainer(s) in preventing displacement of the distal-extension denture base by functioning through lever action on the opposite side of the fulcrum line when the denture base attempts to move away from the tissues in pure rotation around the fulcrum line.

Indirect retention: The effect achieved by one or more indirect retainers of a partial removable denture that reduces the tendency for a denture base to move in an occlusal direction or rotate about the fulcrum line.

Infrabulge: That portion of the crown of a tooth apical to the survey line.

Infrabulge clasp: A removable partial denture retentive clasp that approaches the retentive undercut from a cervical or infrabulge direction.

Reciprocal clasp: A component of the clasp assembly specifically designed to provide reciprocation by engaging a reciprocal guiding plane; it counteracts the action of the clasp during removal and insertion of a removable partial denture. Synonym: bracing arm, reciprocal arm.

Reciprocation: The mechanism by which lateral forces generated by a retentive clasp passing over a height of contour are counterbalanced by a reciprocal clasp passing along a reciprocal guiding plane.

Retentive clasp: (1) a clasp specifically designed to provide retention by engaging an undercut; (2) a flexible segment of a removable partial denture that engages an undercut on an abutment and that is designed to retain the prosthesis.

RPI: Acronym for Rest, Proximal Plate, and I-BAR; the clasp components of one type of removable partial denture clasp assembly.

Suprabulge: That portion of a tooth or crown that converges toward the occlusal surface, i.e., above the height of contour.

Suprabulge clasp: Any removable partial denture retentive clasp that approaches the retentive undercut from an occlusal or suprabulge direction.

Survey line: A line produced on a cast by a surveyor marking the greatest prominence of contour in relation to the planned path of placement of a restoration.

11.2 Direct Retainers

The components of an RPD that resist forces to dislodge the prosthesis from the tissues or abutment teeth are called direct retainers. Direct retainers may be classified as follows:

1. Intracoronal:
   (a) Precision Attachments.
   (b) Semi-precision Attachments.
2. Extracoronal:
   (a) Retentive Clasp Assemblies.
      - Suprabulge.
      - Infrabulge.

   (b) Attachments.

11.2.1 Retentive Clasp Assemblies

The clasp assemblies act as the direct retainers of the RPDs without precision attachments. Retentive clasp assemblies denote the most usual method for extracoronal direct retention and are composed of the following parts:

1. *Rest:* The rigid extension of an RPD that contacts the occlusal surface, incisal edge, or cingulum of a tooth or restoration, the occlusal surface, incisal edge or cingulum of which may have been prepared to receive it.
2. *Retentive arm:* The portion of the clasp assembly that lies apical to the height of contour of the abutment tooth when the RPD is fully seated. Two types of retentive arms are present: suprabulge (Fig. 11.1) and infrabulge retentive arms (Fig. 11.2).
3. *Reciprocal element:* Every retentive clasp arm should be opposed by a reciprocal element capable of resisting pressures exerted by the retentive arm during insertion and removal of the RPD. When the retentive arm passes over

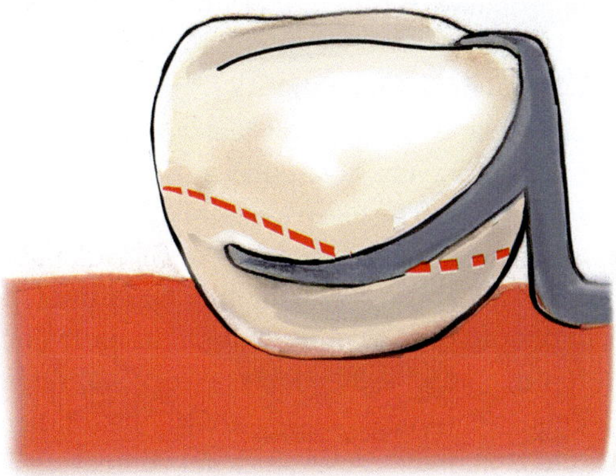

Fig. 11.1 Suprabulge retentive arm arising from the occlusal surface of the abutment tooth and reaching the undercut area

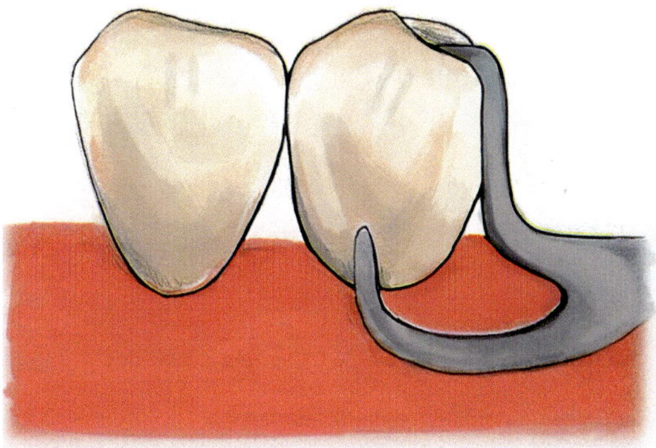

Fig. 11.2 Infrabulge retentive arm arising from the gingival surface of the abutment tooth and reaching the undercut area

the height of contour, the arm presents a small amount of flexure and this may cause lateral stress on the abutment tooth and should be neutralized by a rigid reciprocal element placed on the tooth surface opposite the retentive arm. Reciprocal elements may be a clasp, a combination of mesial and distal minor connectors, or a lingual plate. Reciprocal element should be located at the junction of the gingival and middle thirds of the abutment tooth (see Chap. 7).

4. *Body:* The rigid part of the clasp assembly that joins the rest and the shoulders of the clasp to the minor connector.

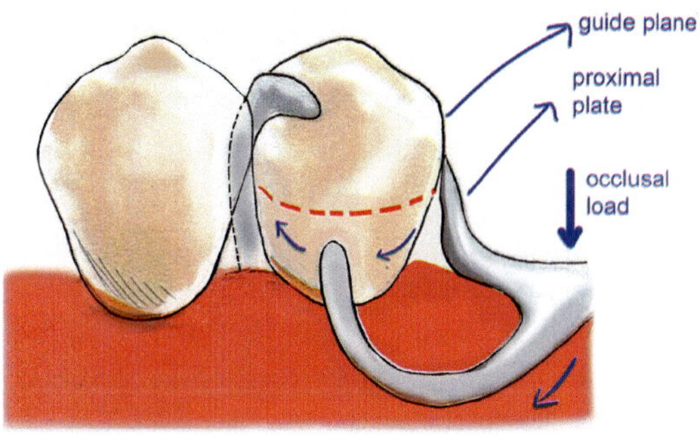

Fig. 11.3 The retentive arms that are located in undercuts on the abutments provide retention and this is called the primary retention. Secondary retention is delivered by the close relationship of the guiding planes, proximal plates and denture bases with minor connectors and of the major connectors with underlying tissues as the RPDs are subjected to occlusal loads

5. *Minor Connector:* This rigid component joins the body of the clasp assembly to the remainder of the framework (see Chap. 9).

A proper clasp assembly is required to provide the following:

1. Retention.
2. Support.
3. Stability.
4. Reciprocation.
5. Encirclement.
6. Passivity.

11.2.1.1 Retention

Retention is the capability of an RPD to resist vertical dislodging forces during function and probably the most important engagement of a clasp assembly. The dislodging forces may arise from the action of adherent foods or the gravity acting against a maxillary RPD. The retentive arms that are located in undercuts of the abutments provide retention, and this is called the primary retention (Fig. 11.3). Secondary retention is delivered by the close relationship of the guiding planes and denture bases with minor connectors and of the major connectors with underlying tissues (Fig. 11.3).

11.2.1.2 Support

Support is the ability of an RPD to resist vertical seating forces. Vertical seating forces are the forces acting on the RPDs toward the gingival direction during chewing or seating of the RPDs and are provided mainly by the rests.

11.2.1.3 Stability

Stability is the resistance of an RPD to horizontal forces and is maintained by reciprocal elements and minor connectors.

11.2.1.4 Reciprocation

When the retentive clasp passes over the height of contour of the abutment tooth, reciprocation of a clasp assembly prevents the lateral displacement of the abutment. This is probably one of the most important functions of a clasp assembly because it counteracts the periodontal harm and eventually the loss of the abutment teeth. Unlike the retentive arm, reciprocal elements touch the abutments at or above the height of contours to permit simultaneous contact of the retentive and the reciprocal elements during the insertion and removal of the RPDs (Fig. 11.4). The reciprocal arm should touch the tooth at the same time with the retentive arm to avoid the lateral displacements problems.

11.2.1.5 Encirclement

Encirclement is the specific feature of the clasp assembly to prevent horizontal movement of the abutment tooth. The clasp assembly must engage the tooth more than 180° with a direct contact (Fig. 11.5). This engagement may be in the type of continuous contact or discontinuous tooth contact in three areas as the occlusal rest, and retentive and reciprocal clasp areas. Insufficient encirclement may cause tooth movement away from the clasp assembly during functional movement of the RPD.

11.2.1.6 Passivity

When the RPD is completely seated, the clasp assembly should be passive and should not exert any force to the abutment tooth. This is called the passivity function of the clasp assembly and is very important for the periodontal health of the

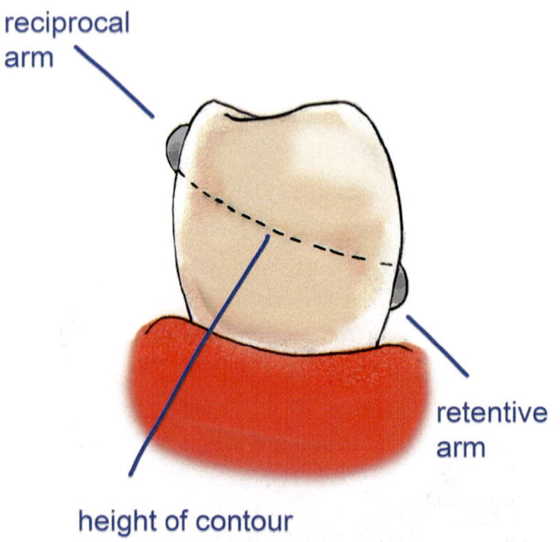

Fig. 11.4 Reciprocal elements touch the abutments at or above the height of contours to permit simultaneous contact of the retentive and the reciprocal elements during insertion and removal of the RPDs

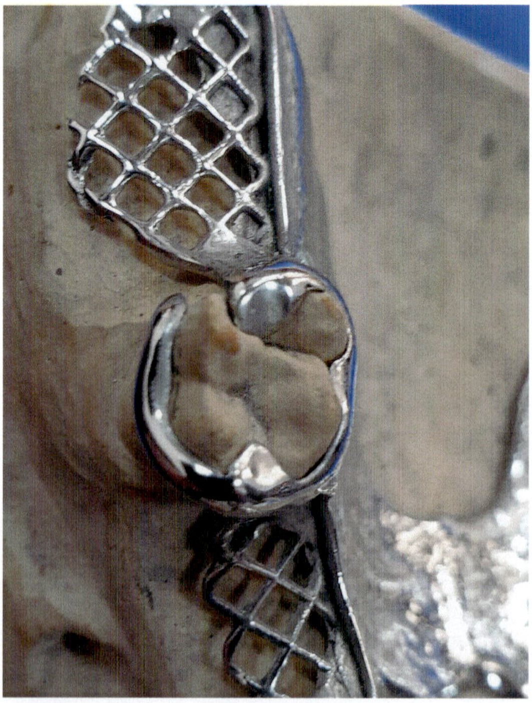

Fig. 11.5 The clasp assembly must engage the tooth more than 180° with a direct contact and this is called encirclement

abutment teeth. The retentive arm should be active only when the dislodging forces are applied to the RPDs. When no force is present, the retentive arm should be passive to prevent non-axial forces to the abutments.

11.2.2 Factors Affecting the Amount of Retention of a Clasp Assembly

The amount of retention provided by a clasp assembly is based on the following factors:

1. *Angle of convergence cervical to the height of contour*: The location of the retentive arm relative to the height of contour is very important for the retentive capabilities of the clasp assembly. The abutment tooth should have a convergence angle cervical to the height of contour to be retentive (Fig. 11.6). The angle of convergence in relation to the path of insertion when the cast is surveyed is vital for the appropriate position of the clasps (see Chap. 14). If the angle of convergence is not favorable for a particular path of placement under consideration, a different path of placement should be provided maintaining the suitable angle of convergence.
2. *Flexibility of the clasp arm*: The amount of retention depends on the flexibility of a clasp arm, and this is influenced by the following factors:
   (a) *Length*: Increasing the length of the clasp arm increases the flexibility. The flexibility of the clasp is directly proportional to the cube of its length if all other factors are equal. Clasp length is measured from the point where the taper begins. Using tapered retentive arms instead of straight ones increases the length.
   (b) *Diameter*: Cube of the thickness of the clasp arm is inversely proportional to its flexibility if all other factors are equal. The retentive clasp arm should have a uniform taper from the beginning of the body to its tip. So the average diameter will be between its origin and its terminal end. If the taper is not uniform, a point of flexure and consequently a point of weakness will happen at the narrowed part of the clasp. Therefore, the uniform taper of the retentive clasp is essential. To accomplish the ultimate uniform taper for a clasp arm to be flexible, its cross-sectional shoulder dimension should be twice the terminus.
   (c) *Cross-sectional form*: Clasps with round forms are more flexible than clasps with half-round forms. Round forms are flexible in any direction, whereas in half-round forms flexibility is limited to only one direction. But most cast clasps are

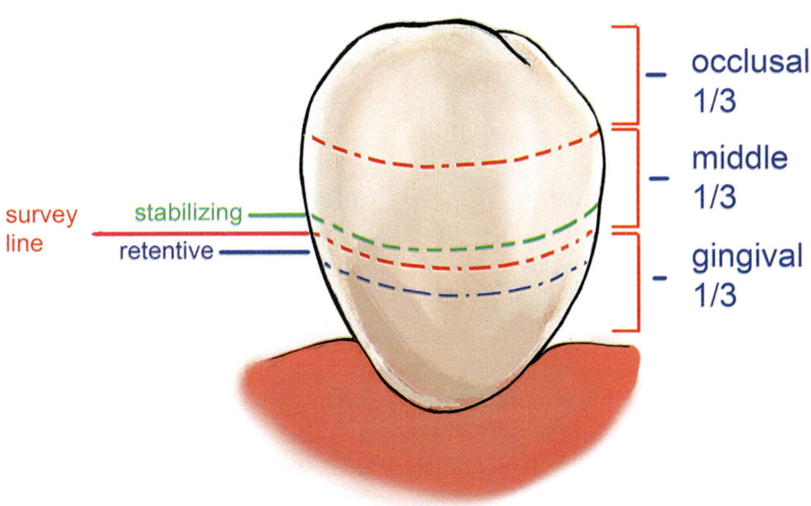

Fig. 11.6 The abutment tooth surface is divided into 3 according to the survey line as occlusal, middle and gingival 1/3. Location of the retentive arm relative to the height of contour is very important for the retentive capabilities of the clasp assembly. The abutment tooth should have an angle of convergence cervical to the height of contour to be retentive

half-round because it is very difficult to cast and polish a round form clasp. Therefore, it is more achievable to use half-round clasps with tooth-supported RPDs because, in distal extension RPDs, clasps should be flexible while insertion, removal, and function of the prosthesis.

(d) *Material:* Alloys with lower elastic moduli show more flexibility. Cast gold clasps are more flexible than the frequently used cast chromium-cobalt clasps but they are quite expensive. Therefore, it is much more reasonable for the practitioners to use wrought wire clasps when more flexibility is needed rather than gold clasps.

11.2.3 Types of Clasp Assemblies

According to the definition of DeVan, the portion of an abutment that converges toward the occlusal or incisal surface is called the suprabulge aspect, whereas the portion of the clinical crown that converges apically is called the infrabulge aspect of the abutment.

After the introduction of two terms infrabulge and suprabulge by DeVan, RPD clasps have been classified into two main categories:

1. Circumferential (suprabulge) clasps, and
2. Bar (infrabulge) clasps.

11.2.3.1 Circumferential (Suprabulge) Clasps

Circumferential clasps approach the desired undercut area from the occlusal direction. They may also be called as occlusally approaching clasps. Dr. Polk E. Akers has introduced and standardized the method of one-piece cast RPD with suprabulge clasps and therefore these clasps are often referred to as *Akers clasps*.

The cast circumferential clasp is the most commonly used clasp of all types. It is simple and easily constructed and repaired. Because of its retentive and stabilizing ability, it is commonly chosen for tooth-supported RPDs. For the tooth-supported RPDs, cast circumferential clasps may be replaced with bar clasps only if the esthetics is concerned or the undercut is approached better with an infrabulge system.

The following may be considered as the disadvantages of the cast circumferential clasps:

1. Not esthetic as compared with the bar clasps especially in the mandibular arch since more metal is displayed.
2. Covers a large amount of tooth surface that can cause caries or enamel decalcification if accurate oral hygiene is not maintained.
3. Its retention is not easily adjusted like the other cast clasp types because of the half-rounded form.

Design Principles: It has a supporting occlusal rest, a buccal retentive, and a lingual reciprocating arm encircling the abutment tooth by more than 180° (Fig. 11.7). The retentive arm approaches from the occlusal part, passes the height of contour, and enters the undercut area of the abutment tooth. Only the apical part of the retentive arm should engage the desired undercut, and the retentive arm should be long enough to ensure the desired flexibility. The retentive clasp arm should not be located too close to the gingival margin. The reciprocal arm may be located at or slightly above the height of contour on the lingual side of the tooth and should prevent lateral displacement of the abutment (Fig. 11.7).

A wide variety of circumferential clasp types are available but the less complex ones should be chosen for simplicity. Following are the cast circumferential clasp types:

1. *Simple circlet clasp*: It is a simple and widely used clasp and the clasp of choice for tooth-supported RPDs (Fig. 11.8a–c). Since the simple circlet clasp totally achieves the design requirements of support, stability, reciprocation, encirclement, and passivity; it is considered superior to the other designs of equal capabilities.
2. *Reverse circlet clasp*: The simple circlet design may also be used reversely and called as reverse circlet clasp. This design may be used when undercuts are present near the edentulous space (Fig. 11.9). Since the rest is located on

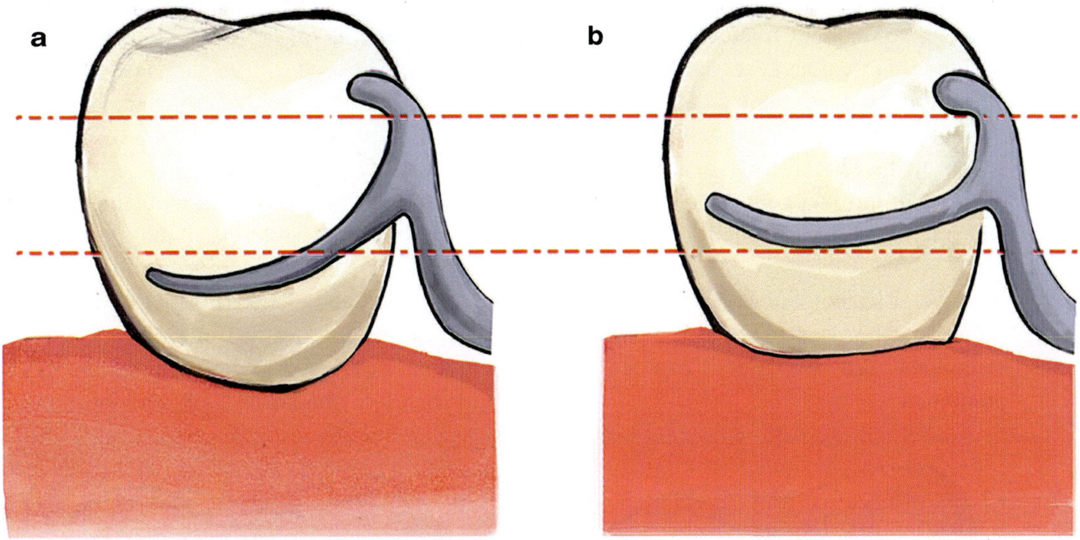

Fig. 11.7 The circumferential clasp has a supporting occlusal rest, a buccal retentive (**a**) and a lingual reciprocating arm (**b**) encircling the abutment tooth by more than 180°. The retentive arm approaches from the occlusal part, passes the height of contour and enters the undercut area of the abutment tooth (**a**). The reciprocal arm may be located at or slightly above the height of contour on the lingual side of the tooth and should prevent lateral displacement of the abutment (**b**)

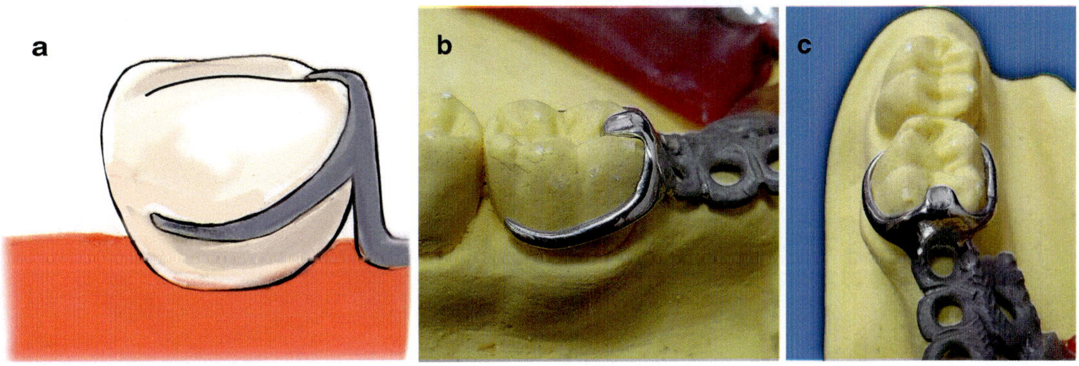

Fig. 11.8 (**a**) Simple circlet clasp is a simple and widely used clasp and the clasp of choice for tooth-supported removable partial dentures. (**b**) Cast simple circlet clasp (buccal view). (**c**) Cast simple circlet clasp (retentive arm on the buccal side, mesial rest on the occlusal surface, and reciprocating arm on the lingual side)

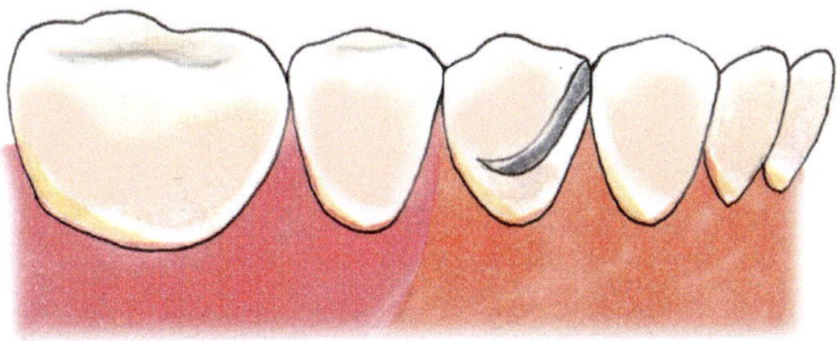

Fig. 11.9 The reverse circlet clasp is just the opposite of simple circlet clasp and may be used when undercuts are present near the edentulous space

the mesial side of the abutment and the clasp is projected from the mesial to the distal side, stresses are less transmitted to an abutment. This may be regarded as an advantage of the reverse circlet clasp and it may be used in Kennedy Class I and II situations. However, reverse circlet design has several disadvantages as listed below:

(a) The shoulder rests on the marginal ridges of the two adjacent teeth, and this may cause premature contact areas. These may result in consequent fractures when constructed thinner than necessary.

(b) Since no rest is present adjacent to the edentulous space to facilitate the releasing action of the retentive clasp, as the RPD moves during function, food impaction and trauma to the marginal gingiva may occur.

(c) The design is not esthetic and therefore should not be used especially when the abutments are maxillary canines or premolars.

Since the shortcomings are more than the benefits of the reverse circlet clasp, it should be used with caution, and infrabulge clasps should be preferred when the undercut is present, adjacent to the edentulous areas. If the anatomical contour apical to the abutment disallows the use of an infrabulge clasp, reverse circlet clasps may be selected.

3. *Ring clasp*: Ring clasps are usually used in tilted molar abutments (Fig. 11.10). A ring clasp originates mostly from the mesial rest, and it encircles nearly all of an abutment tooth and therefore should be used with caution in

a

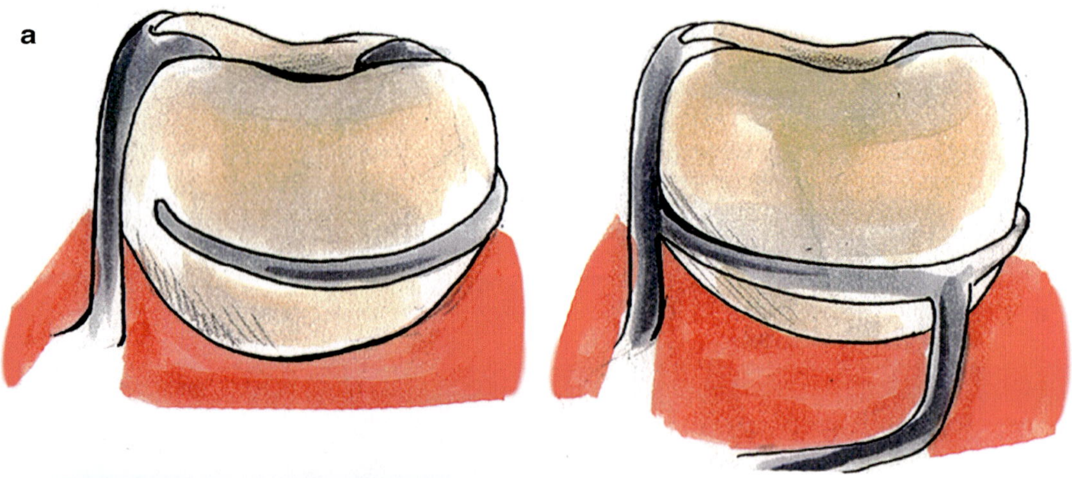

b

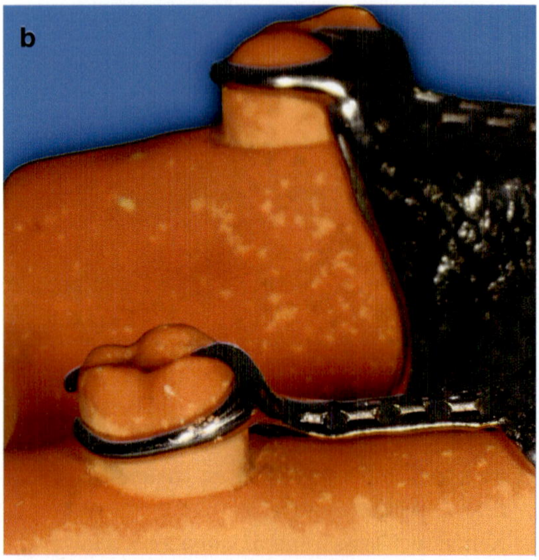

Fig. 11.10 (**a**) Ring clasp originates mostly from the mesial rest and it encircles nearly all of an abutment tooth. Although it is an effective clasp, it should not be considered when an alternative is present because it covers an extensive amount of abutment tooth structure. (**b**) Cast ring clasp (retentive arm on the buccal side and reciprocating arm on the lingual side)

order not to trigger caries and demineralization. In most of the cases, an additional rest is placed on the distal surface to provide extra support. A supporting structure on the nonretentive side will prevent the clasp arm from opening and closing with minimum or no reciprocation. Although it is an effective clasp, it should not be considered when an alternative is present because it covers an extensive amount of abutment tooth structure.

4. *Embrasure (double akers) clasps*: The embrasure clasp design is most frequently used in Kennedy Class II or Class III RPDs when no modification is present to service for additional clasp designs on the opposite side of the main edentulous areas (Fig. 11.11). It consists of two circumferential clasps heading to opposite sides joining in the body. It is a technique-sensitive clasp and both rest and interproximal embrasure preparation are essential when using this kind of clasp design in order not to cause fatigue failure and fracture which is a common complication (see Chap. 10). Therefore, too much tooth preparation is necessary before fabricating this clasp. Also when preparing the rest seats, it is very important not to lose the contact area of the abutments. Because of these technical hitches, this clasp should not be used if possible.
5. *Palatal clasp:* This unique clasp design may be used for esthetic reasons, especially when the abutments are maxillary premolars. It is well known that visible RPD components in these teeth are not well tolerated by the patients. Therefore, if precision attachments are not preferred by the patients because of financial reasons or mandatory tooth reduction, this design may be preferred. Palatal clasp design consists of a circumferential clasp engaging the mesio-palatal undercut of the premolar abutment and a small buccal plate to provide more than 180° encirclement of the abutment. In the design of this clasp, it is very important to analyze the study cast with a surveyor because mesio-palatal undercut is essential for the assembly to work properly. In case of prominent palatal undercut areas or small-sized premolars, in order not to cause a damaging effect on the abutments during insertion and removal of the RPDs, wrought gold wire clasps soldered or cast to the framework may be the solution (Fig. 11.12a–c).

Rarely used suprabulge clasps:

In this section, the suprabulge clasp types that are not common are explained briefly.

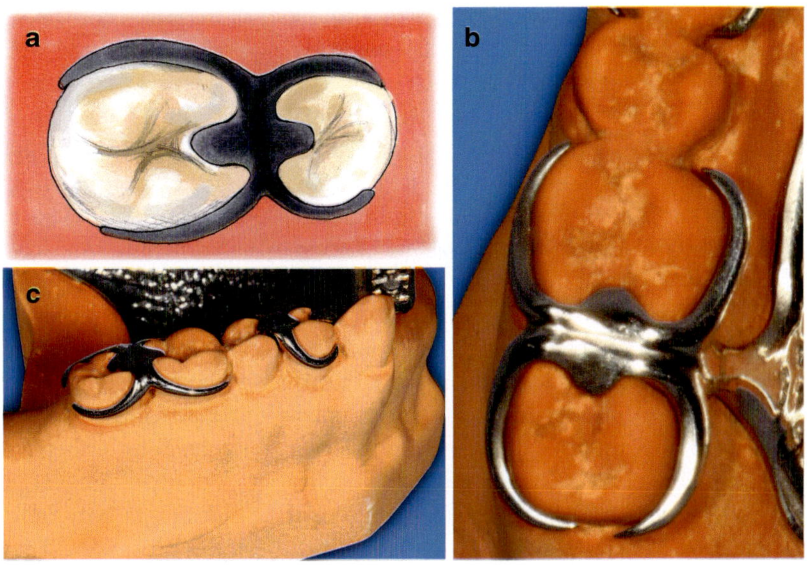

Fig. 11.11 (**a**) The embrasure clasp design consists of two circumferential clasps heading to opposite sides joining on the body. (**b**) Cast embrasure clasp (occlusal view). (**c**) Cast embrasure clasp designs with two retentive arms on the molar teeth and a single retentive arm on the premolar tooth

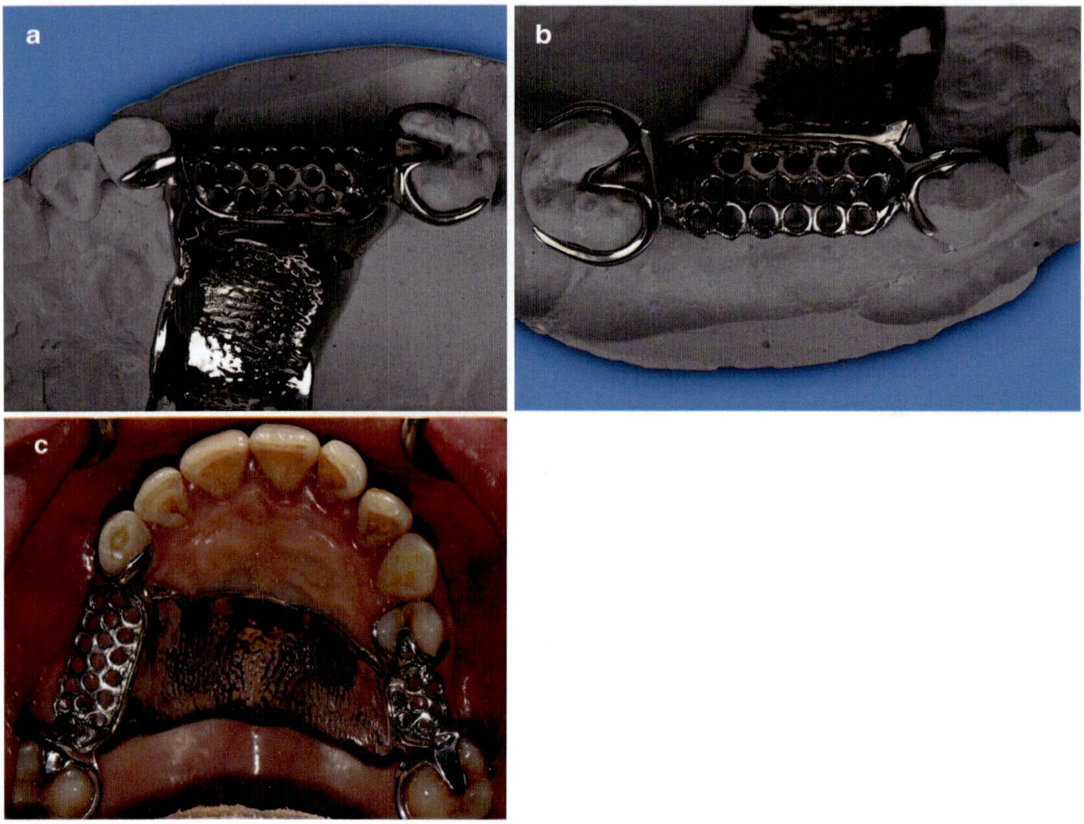

Fig. 11.12 (**a**) The retentive arm of the clasp was shortened on the canine to enhance esthetics (palatinal view). (**b**) The shortened retentive arm on the canine (buccal view). (**c**) Intra-oral view of the cast palatal clasp placed on the palatinal surface of the maxillary left first premolar

1. *Multiple clasps:* Multiple clasp is just a modification of the embrasure clasp to use for retaining the same kind of RPDs when the retentive areas are adjacent to each other. This design may also be used when the principal abutment tooth is periodontally compromised in tooth- or tissue-supported RPDs. The design consists of two opposing circumferential clasps joining at the terminal end of reciprocal arms (Fig. 11.13a).
2. *Half-and-half clasp*: A half-and-half clasp consists of a retentive arm on one tooth and a reciprocal arm on another (Fig. 11.14). Retentive arm arises from a minor connector and the reciprocal arm from another minor connector with or without an extra occlusal rest. It is designed to provide dual retention in unilateral RPDs.
3. *Reverse action (back action, reverse action, hairpin, fish hook) clasp*: Reverse action clasps are used when the undercut is present below the starting point of the clasp (Fig. 11.15a, b). It is not an esthetically acceptable clasp and therefore not preferred in the clinical practice.
4. *Onlay clasp*: This clasp type is used for both correcting the occlusion of infraoccluded abutments and maintaining retention (Fig. 11.16). It is hard to fabricate and complicated for the patients, and therefore an alternative design should be preferred if possible.
5. *Equipoise clasp*: Equipoise clasp is used for obtaining esthetic results and is a modified retentive lingual back-action clasp. This design is only indicated for the canines and the premolars. The retention of the clasp is

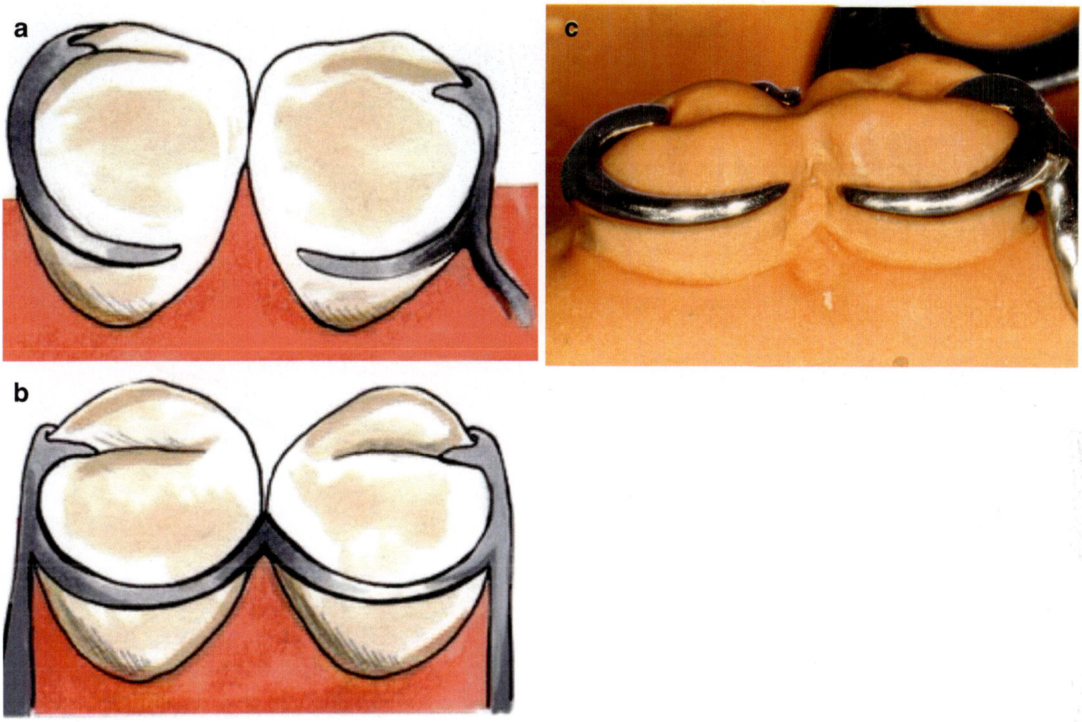

Fig. 11.13 Multiple clasp design consists of two opposing circumferential clasps. Retentive arms (**a**), joining at the terminal end of reciprocal arms (**b**), cast multiple clasp design (**c**)

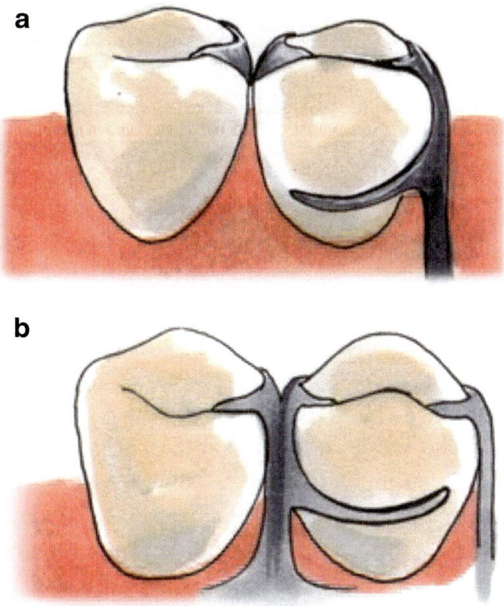

Fig. 11.14 Half-and-half clasp consists of a retentive (**a**) and a reciprocal arm (**b**) on different adjacent teeth. Retentive arm (**a**) arises from a minor connector and the reciprocal arm (**b**) from another minor connector with or without an extra occlusal rest

maintained by the friction of the clasp components on the surfaces of the abutments. The tip of the retentive clasp arm is at the junction of the vestibular and distal surfaces of the abutments (Fig. 11.17). Since the rests are placed away from edentulous areas, this clasp design can be used in Kennedy Class I and II situations and may be an alternative to RPI and RPA designs. The disadvantages of the equipoise clasp can be summarized as follows:

(a) 1.0 mm vertical interproximal reduction between abutment and the adjacent tooth should be employed for gaining space for the shoulder of the clasp assembly, and this reduction may cause sensitivity and increased proneness to caries. Therefore, it is much better to gain this space by making survey crown restorations and fabricating the RPD framework afterward.
(b) Poor reciprocation and lack of retention.
(c) The metal display of the shoulder between the abutment and the adjacent tooth.

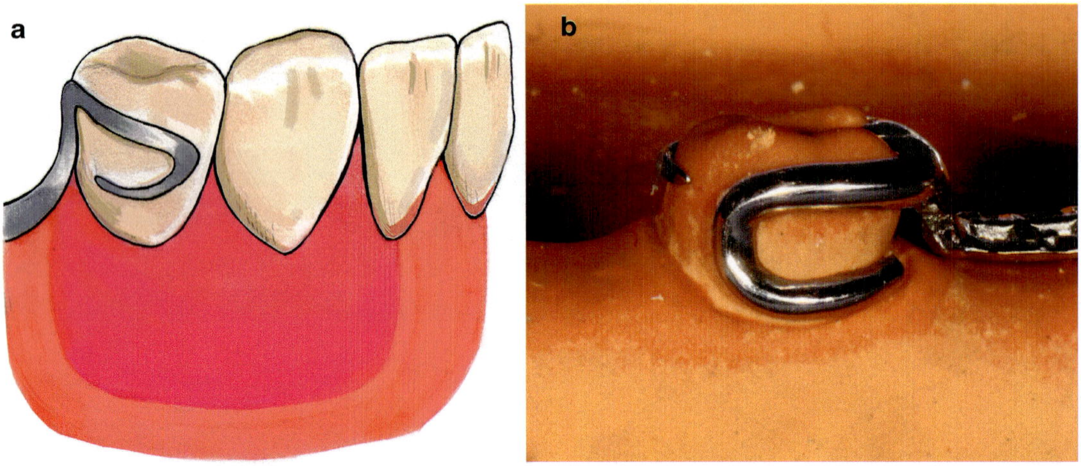

Fig. 11.15 (**a**) A reverse action clasp may be used when the undercut is present below the starting point of the clasp. (**b**) Cast reverse action clasp design

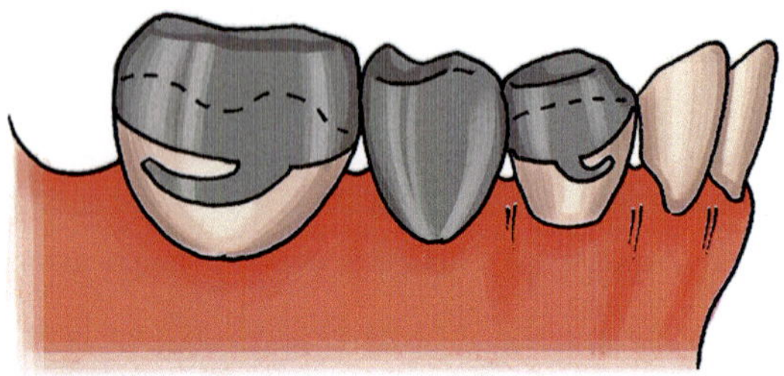

Fig. 11.16 Onlay clasp is used for both correcting the occlusion of infraoccluded abutment teeth and maintaining retention

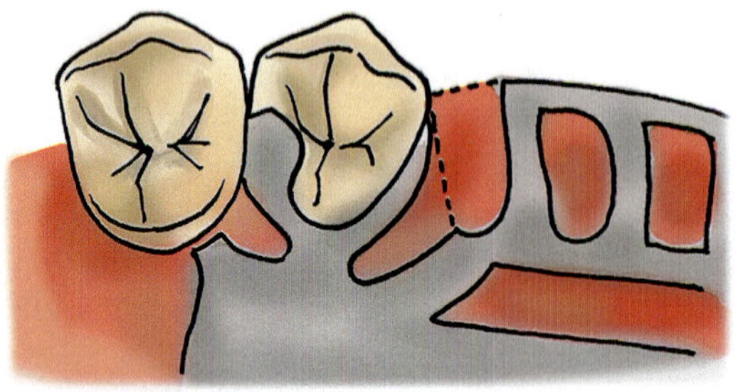

Fig. 11.17 The tip of the retentive arm of the equipoise clasp is at the junction of the vestibular and distal surfaces of the abutment

(d) Processing should be performed with caution. Excess acrylic resin may surround the equipoise clasp and the clasp may lose its retentive properties, and consequent unseating problems and damaging forces to the abutments may arise.

Because of the disadvantages, this clasp design has been modified over the years and named as *modified equipoise clasp*. In the most recent modified design, a surveyed metal-ceramic crown is fabricated on the abutment with a mesial reciprocating groove, a milled lingual ledge, and a 0.01″ distobuccal undercut to preserve the proximal contact between the adjacent tooth and the abutment and to overcome the inabilities of the former system.

Although this clasp design is not fully recognized by the dental literature, it has been shown that it is the most frequently used clasp system for the esthetic capabilities in some dental schools and has been in use for over 35 years.

6. *Saddle lock hidden clasp*

The saddle lock hidden clasp is generally not recommended for esthetic reasons. The mesial and distal proximal undercuts of natural abutments maintain retention of the design. Retentive clasp tips are located at each end of the saddle and locks the saddle to the ridge (Fig. 11.18). This hidden clasp has a very limited nature of usage because of a lack of reciprocation and retentive proper-

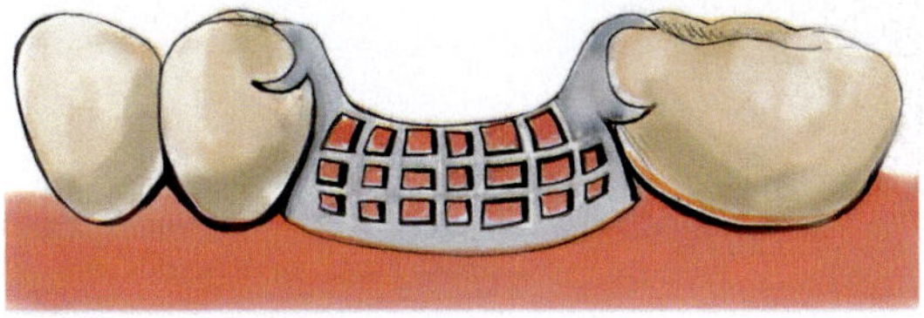

Fig. 11.18 Retentive tips of the saddle lock hidden clasp are located at each end of the saddle and locks the saddle to the ridge

ties. It can only be used in tooth-supported RPDs.

11.2.3.2 Bar (Infrabulge, Roach) Clasps

The infrabulge clasps have been given the names "bar" or "Roach" in 1930 by Dr. F. Ewing Roach. Just the opposite of circumferential clasp types, bar clasps originate from the RPD frameworks and engage the undercuts from gingival direction. Roach clasps are designed mainly for Kennedy Class I and Class II situations but they may also be used in tooth-supported RPDs. They are classified by the shape of retentive tips:

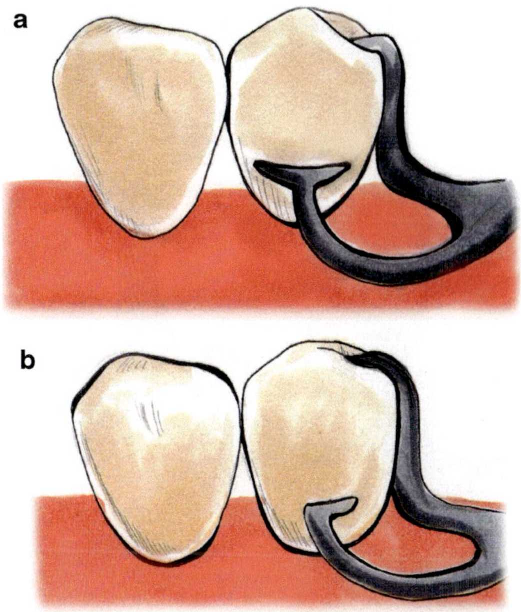

Fig. 11.19 T-clasp has an approach arm contacting the abutment at the height of contour and separating into two horizontal projections one of which extends towards the undercut area aimed at functioning for retention and the other over the undercut area to function for bracing and stabilization (**a**) whereas the modified T-clasp has only one projection, functioning for retention (**b**)

1. *T-clasp*: The T-clasp is a commonly used infrabulge clasp but is regarded as the most misused clasp type with the Y-clasp because the tooth coverage areas of these clasps are rarely necessary for providing retention. The approach arm contacts the abutment at the height of contour and separates into two horizontal projections, one of which extends toward the undercut area aimed at functioning for retention and the other over the undercut area to function for bracing and stabilization (Fig. 11.19). A T-clasp should not be used in a distal extension RPD if the only obtainable undercut is located on the mesiobuccal aspect of abutment.
2. *The modified T-clasp*: The difference between the modified T-clasp is the absence of one projection, which functions for bracing and stabilization (Fig. 11.19). The functioning properties are similar to the T-clasp. Since one of the projections is absent, this clasp type is more appropriate to use in abutment teeth with esthetic considerations such as canines and premolars.
3. *Y-clasp*: A Y-clasp is just an alteration of the T-clasp. The only difference is the mesial and distal projections are closer to the occlusal/incisal surface of the abutment (Fig. 11.20a, b). A Y-clasp encircles the abutment better than the T-clasp but it displays more metal and is more unesthetic.
4. *I-clasp*: An I-clasp is the bar-type clasp without any mesial and distal projections (Fig. 11.21a, b). The design is used with a mesial rest and a distal guide and will be discussed in detail below.

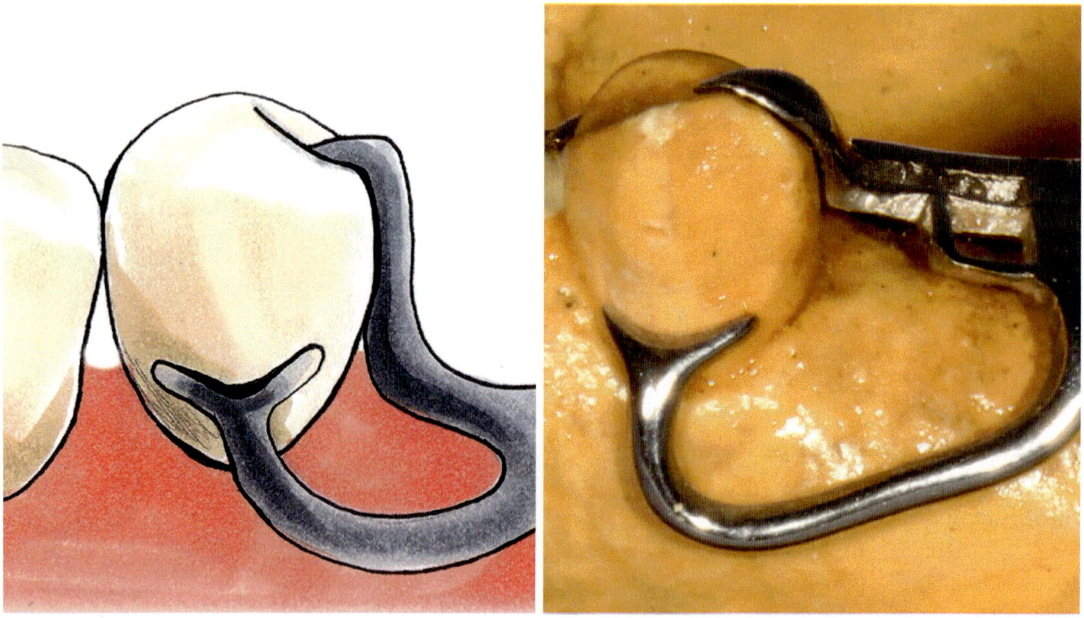

Fig. 11.20 Y clasp encircles the abutment better than the T-clasp but it displays more esthetic concerns

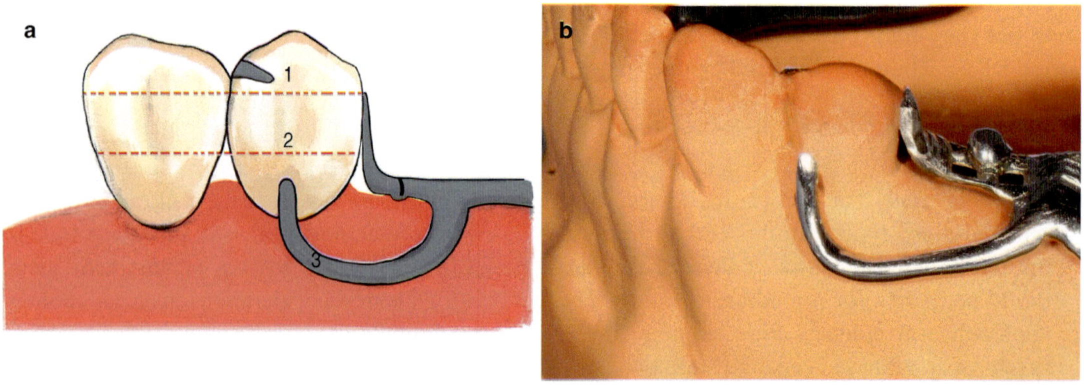

Fig. 11.21 (**a**) Three main components of RPI clasp assembly with specific features. (1) Mesially placed occlusal rest. (2) Proximal plate. (3) I-bar clasp. The proximal plate extends from the marginal ridge to the junction of the middle and gingival thirds of the proximal surface. (**b**) Cast RPI clasp design

11.2.4 Stress-Controlling Clasp Design for the Distal Extension Removable Partial Dentures

In distal extension RPDs, a Class I leverage system is formed by placing a distal rest on the abutment tooth as a fulcrum. In this type of leverage system, an effort arm is formed between the rest and the edentulous ridge whereas a resistance arm is formed between the rest and the retentive tip of the direct retainer. The effects of Class I leverage system are discussed in Chap. 4. To convert the Class I leverage system to a Class II leverage system is practically solved by placing a mesial rest on the abutment tooth to allow the rotational tissuewards movement of the RPD without excessive stress on the abutment teeth. This strategy has been generally called as a "mesial rest concept" in the dentistry for many years. This concept mainly includes the RPI (rest, proximal plate, and I-bar clasp) and RPA (rest, proximal plate, and Akers clasp) clasp designs.

11.2.4.1 RPI Clasp Design

In distal extension base RPD, the most accepted stress-releasing design described is the RPI system. RPI clasp design is a current concept of bar clasp system, which consists of three main components with specific features (Fig. 11.21a, b). All components must be properly designed and constructed to function effectively.

1. *Mesio-occlusal rest:* The rest is located on the mesio-occlusal surface of a premolar or mesio-lingual surface of a canine, with the minor connector placed into the mesiolingual embrasure. The minor connector should not be in contact with the adjacent tooth to prevent wedging. The rest acts as a fulcrum point for the rotational movement.
2. *Proximal plate:* A proximal plate is prepared on a distal guiding plane on the distal surface of the abutment tooth adjacent to the edentulous site. The bucco-lingual width of the plate is determined by the proximal contour of the abutment tooth. The plate is approximately 1–1.5 mm thick and extends from the marginal ridge to the junction of the middle and gingival thirds of the abutment tooth. The proximal plate should be designed as thinnest in the buccal and thickest at the lingual. The proximal plate extends lingually so that the distance between the minor connector and the proximal plate is less than the mesio-distal width of the tooth and joins the framework at a right angle (Fig. 11.22). The proximal plate in conjunction with the minor connector that supports the rest serves for stabilization and reciprocation against the force exerted by the retentive arm of the clasp during seating and removal of the RPD. The reciprocation is provided by the simultaneous contact of the proximal plate and the minor connector on the abutment tooth (Fig. 11.23). In cases where a simultaneous contact cannot be provided as may occur on the molar teeth, the retentive I-bar clasp should be positioned to engage the mesiobuccal undercut to receive reciprocation (Fig. 11.24). On narrow or tapered formed abutment tooth, such as mandibular premolars, the proximal plate should be designed narrow but it should be wide enough to prevent the lingual migration. The occlusal load on the extension base moves the proximal plate in a mesiogingival direction without torquing the tooth and

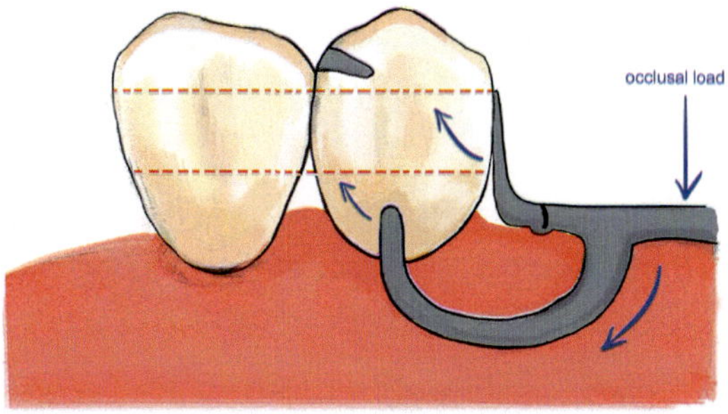

Fig. 11.23 The proximal plate serves for stabilization and reciprocation against the force exerted by the retentive arm of the clasp during seating and removal of the RPD. When an occlusal load is applied on the distal-extension base, rotation around the mesial rest causes the retentive tip of the I-bar clasp to move towards mesially. The reciprocation is provided by the simultaneous contact of the proximal plate and the minor connector on the abutment tooth

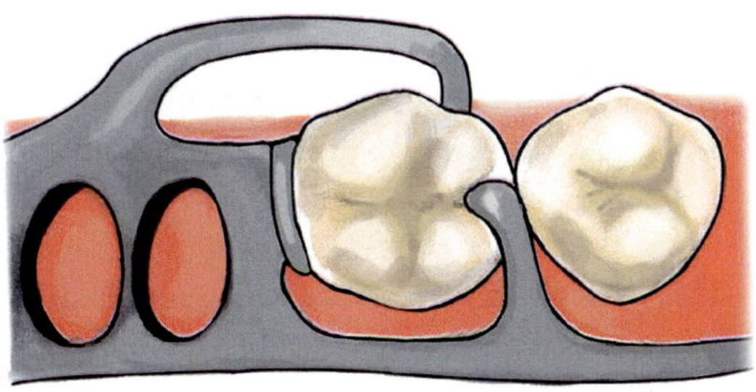

Fig. 11.22 The lingually extended proximal plate. The distance between the minor connector and the proximal plate should be designed less than the mesiodistal width of the tooth and the proximal plate should join the framework at a right angle

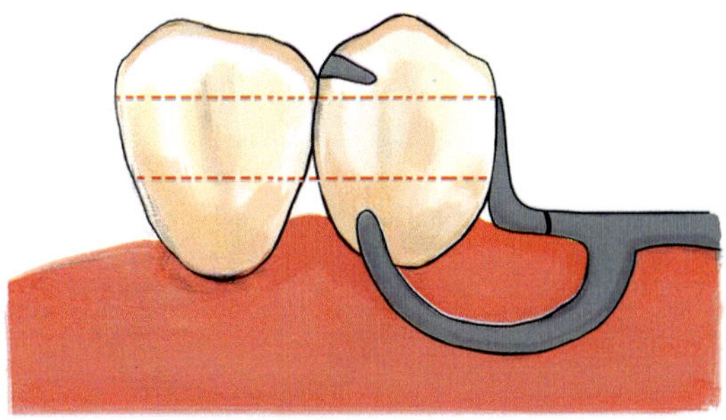

Fig. 11.24 When a simultaneous contact cannot be provided (e.g., on the molar teeth), the retentive I-bar clasp should be positioned to engage the mesiobuccal undercut to receive reciprocation

brings the plate into tight contact with the distal surface of the tooth.

There are three approaches for the proximal plate design in relation to the contact with the guiding plane

(a) The proximal plate extends to all entire length of the guiding plane (Fig. 11.25).
(b) The proximal plate extends from the marginal ridge to the junction of the middle and gingival thirds of the proximal surface (Fig. 11.21a).
(c) The proximal plate contacts approximately 1 mm of the apical portion of the guiding plane (Fig. 11.26).

The proximal plate should cervically extend and the distance to the mucosal contact point can be 2–3 mm. A physiological minimal relief is provided at the tooth–tissue junction to disengage under occlusal load (Fig. 11.27). Opening the embrasure spaces that might result in the food impaction prevents the impingement of the gingivae.

3. *I-bar clasp:* the clasp is located in the gingival third of the buccal surface of the premolar and on the mesiobuccal surface of the canine engaging 0.010 inch of buccal undercut. The I-bar originates from the grid work and approaches the tooth from the gingival direction and receives its reciprocation from the proximal plate. The clasp terminus disengages from the tooth when an occlusal load is applied to the adjacent distal extension base. No contact between the approaching arm and the tooth minimizes the lateral forces. The I-bar makes a 2 mm contact with the tooth and the bend in the I-bar should be located at least 3 mm. from the gingival margin to minimize the risk of the food accumulation and to increase the flexibility of the clasp arm (Fig. 11.28). The clasp is usually cast and is placed just below the height of contour line. The small terminus of the I-bar, minimal tooth contact, less retention, and less horizontal stability are the disadvantages of I-bar.

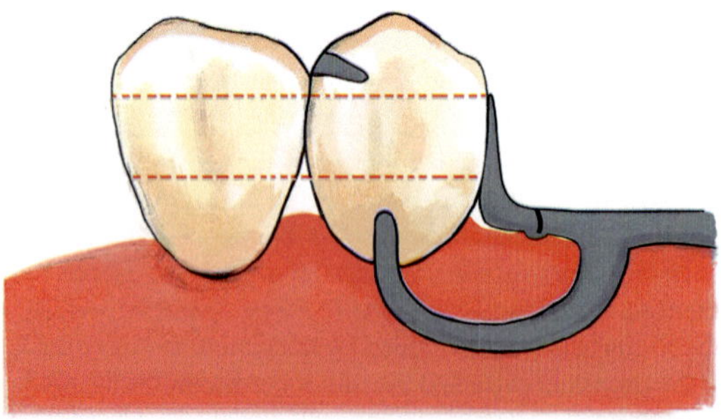

Fig. 11.25 The proximal plate extends to the entire length of the guiding plane

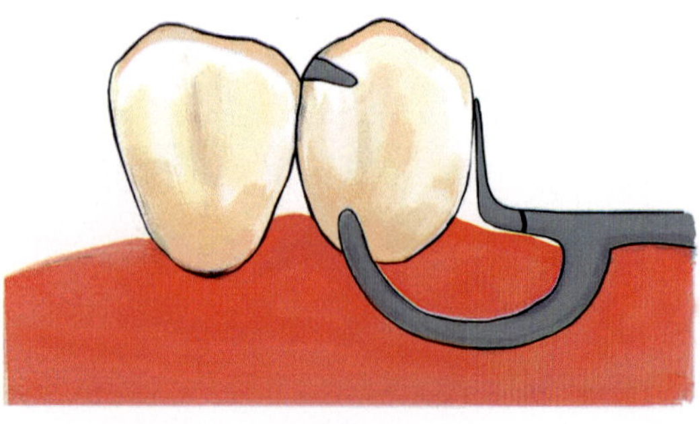

Fig. 11.26 The proximal plate contacts approximately 1 mm of apical portion of the guiding plane

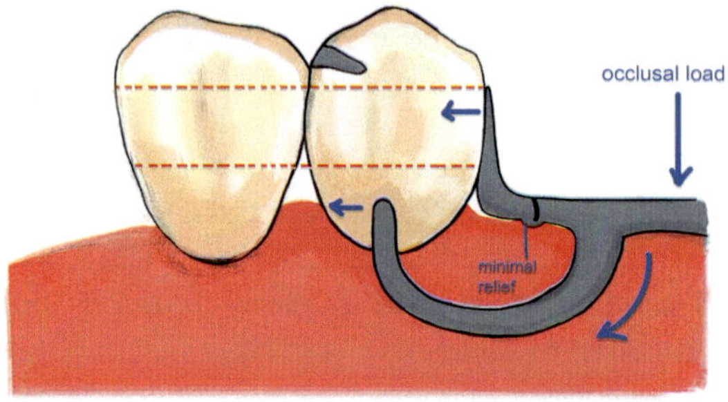

Fig. 11.27 A physiological minimal relief should be provided at the tooth-tissue junction to disengage under occlusal load. To prevent the gingival impingement, the embrasure spaces should be opened, but the space should not be too large to cause food accumulation

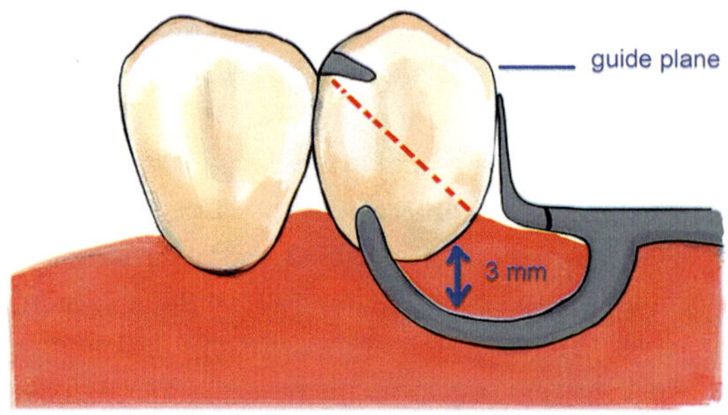

Fig. 11.28 The retentive tip makes a 2 mm contact with the tooth and the bend should be located at least 3 mm from the gingival margin to increase the flexibility of the clasp arm and to prevent the food accumulation

The location of the I-bar at the mesial is especially reasonable in symmetric distal extension base RPDs in which the axis of rotation around the most distal abutments with mesial rests is perpendicular to the longitudinal axis of the denture base and thus creating a Class II leverage system. However, in asymmetric distal extension base RPDs, the axis of rotation is shifted distally to the side of the short edentulous base. In this situation, the I-bar has a potential to move laterally with a Class I leverage effect. The solution may be the placement of the tip of the I-bar distal to the fulcrum line to minimize the potential torque. In clinical practice, when two teeth are splinted, the mesial rest is placed on the anterior tooth while the I-bar is placed on the posterior tooth. If a 3-unit fixed restoration is used, the same rule is to be followed.

The RPI design meets the need for vertical support, horizontal stabilization, retention, reciprocation, and passivity. In a finite element study, compared to Akers and embrasure clasp assemblies, it was shown that the RPI clasp assembly showed much lower stress concentration within the periodontal ligament and the buccal cortical bone supporting the abutment tooth, apical stress intensity distribution, distal displacement, and widest relative area of mucosal stress transfer suggesting a mechanical advantage. The RPI clasp contacts the tooth minimally and therefore is usually more esthetic than the other clasp arms. In addition, another important advantage of the RPI clasp is its avoidance of contact with the lingual surface of the abutment tooth. This design offers superior mechanical properties but manufacturing of this clasp design needs highly experimented technical skills.

However, in some cases, RPI clasp assembly cannot be applied due to some contraindications and limitations:

(a) Insufficient depth of vestibule: at least 3 mm distance for the vestibule depth is required for the clasp arm to approach the tooth.
(b) Tilting of the abutment tooth. Abutment tooth tilted too much in a lingual direction and therefore no buccal undercut area or tilted too much in a buccal direction.
(c) Buccal tissue undercut: a severe buccal tissue undercut causes the clasp arm to approach the tooth too far away from the gingiva. The need for extensive relief creates risk for the food accumulation under the clasp arm and the irritation of the mucosal tissue of the cheeks and the lips.
(d) Distobuccal undercut: if only a distobuccal undercut is available.
(e) Use of lingual plate as a major connector. If there is an elavated mouth floor, an appropriate proximal plate design can not be established.
(f) For some patients, the manipulation of the RPI might be difficult to grasp with finger or thumbnail for seating or removal of the RPD.
(g) Smile display: in patients where a great gingival tissue is displayed, use of I-bar might negatively affect the esthetics.

If RPI clasp design cannot be used due to above-mentioned clinical situations, then RPA clasp design may be the choice.

11.2.4.2 RPA Clasp Design

The RPA clasp design was developed to overcome the contraindications and limitations of the RPI design. In this design, the mesial rest and the proximal plate features are identically the same as those of RPI. The only difference is the use of an Akers clasp instead of the I-bar clasp (Fig. 11.29).

Akers clasp: The undercut will vary from 0.01 to 0.02 in. depending on the size of the abutment tooth. An Akers or a circumferential clasp

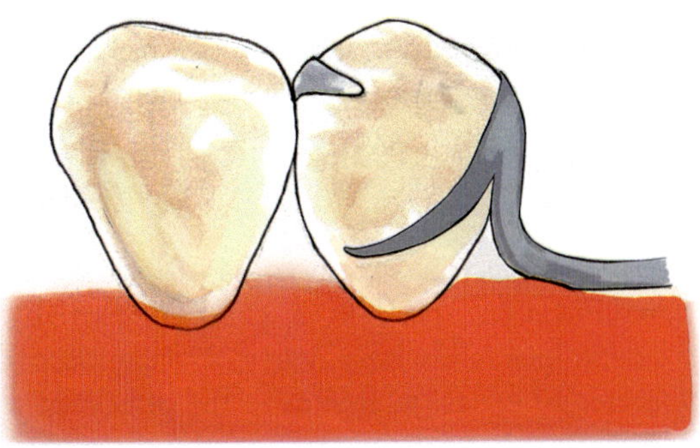

Fig. 11.29 The RPA clasp assembly. (1) Mesially placed occlusal rest, (2) the proximal plate, (3) Akers clasp instead of the I-bar clasp

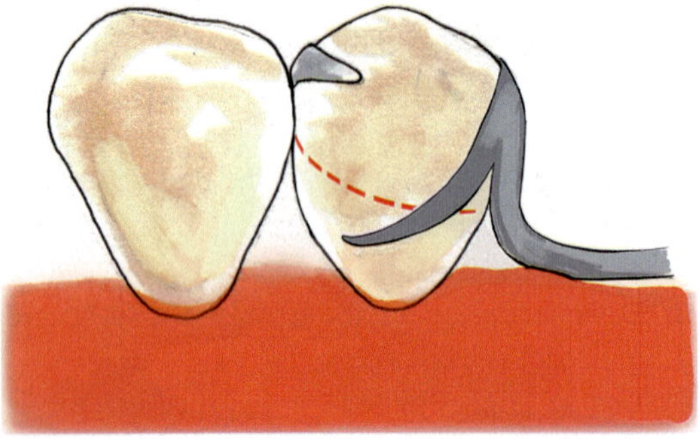

Fig. 11.30 The retentive arm of the Akers clasp in relation to the survey line should be correctly designed to ensure the success of the clasp assembly

arises from the superior portion of the proximal plate and extends around the tooth to engage in the mesiobuccal undercut. Under occlusal load during the rotational movement, the proximal plate will move gingivally and slightly mesially, the rigid portion of the clasp contacts the tooth along the survey line and moves gingivally and mesially while the retentive tip of the clasp also moves gingivally and mesially. The movement of the retentive tip of the clasp occurs due to the tissue relief for this design to be successfully functioning to avoid from torqueing of the abutment tooth. The success of the RPA clasp assembly is dependent on the proper positioning of the Akers clasp in relation to the survey line (Fig. 11.30).

11.2.4.3 Combination Clasp

To avoid the possible negative effects of the Class I leverage system, another clinical option is to use a combination clasp, which consists of an occlusal rest, cast reciprocal arm, and a tapered, round wrought-wire retentive clasp arm that is soldered to the cast framework (Fig. 11.31). The wrought wire retentive arm makes a line contact with the abutment tooth. This design is recommended:

1. For the anterior abutment of the posterior modification space in a Class II partially edentulous arch only when a mesiobuccal undercut exists, to minimize the effects of a first-class leverage system.
2. A severe buccal tissue undercut that does not permit the use of a bar clasp.

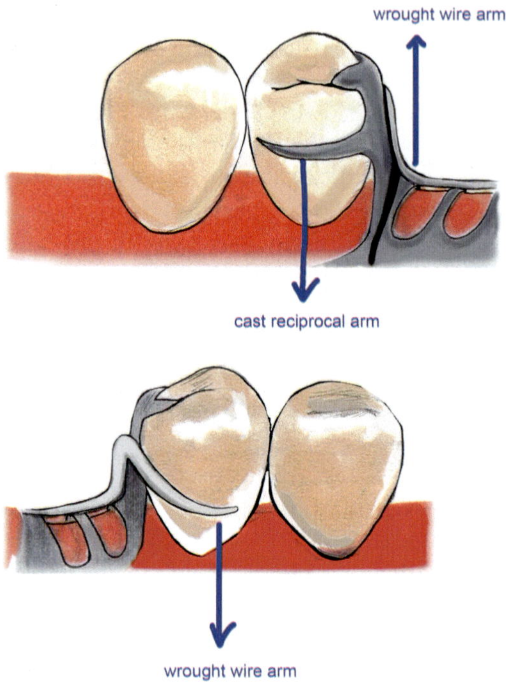

Fig. 11.31 Combination clasp: (1) Occlusal rest, (2) Cast reciprocal arm at the lingual side, (3) Tapered, round wrought-wire retentive clasp arm at the buccal side. The wrought wire is soldered to the cast metal framework

3. When flexibility is required on the abutment tooth adjacent to the distal extension base.
4. Rotation of abutment tooth.
5. Heavy centric contact or a large amalgam restoration on mesial half of the tooth.
6. On periodontally compromised abutment tooth when a cast bar-type clasp is not indicated.

The advantages of this clasp assembly are flexibility due to its circular cross-sectional form, adjustability when necessary, and appearance due to its round form and smaller diameter of 18 gauges. However, as disadvantages, it should be kept in mind that this clasp design needs extra steps in RPD fabrication, easily deformed, and less stabilization. This clasp system can be used even in 0.02 in. mesiobuccal undercuts due to its flexibility. These clasps may also be used in tooth-borne partial edentulous cases.

11.2.4.4 Rarely Used Infrabulge Clasps

1. *RLS system:* The RLS system uses the undercuts of the lingual surfaces of the abutment teeth. It involves a mesioocclusal rest, a distolingual L-bar direct retainer, and a distobuccal reciprocal element (Fig. 11.32). The clasp system uses the rationale for RPA and RPI systems. It can be used for the distal extension RPDs when there is no undercut present on the facial surface of the abutment teeth or when esthetics would be severely compromised with the use of RPI and RPA clasps.
2. *Twin-flex clasp (spring-clasp):* The twin-flex system uses a wrought wire soldered into a channel, which is cast into the major connector. It is claimed that the clasp is flexible and it does not produce torque to the abutment and can be used as an esthetic alternative for distal extension RPDs. The disadvantages include increased thickness of the major connector due to the channels, inability to be repaired and increased laboratory cost due to the complexity of the design. To overcome the toxicity associated with galvanic corrosion while soldering and the increased major connector thickness, the technique has been modified as twin-flex improved clasp. At this technique, the U-shaped wire is inserted from lingual to facial into the framework before tooth setup (Fig. 11.33). The RPD is flasked and finished afterward and the wire is adapted to the abutment by the clinician. This improved design can be adjusted or replaced easily.
3. *Round-rest, distal depression (RRDD) clasp:* The RRDD clasp has been designed for an esthetic alternative to conventional clasp types when the abutments are maxillary incisors or canines. It involves a round rest seat near the cingulum, a mesiolingual reciprocating plate, and a split minor connector engaging a distal depression for retention (Fig. 11.34). If the edentulous span is mesial to the abutment tooth, the system is called round-rest, mesial depression clasp. The RRDD clasp lacks the encirclement of a clasp assembly, therefore, it is not recommended for distal extension RPDs. The only indication is tooth-supported maxillary RPDs when the abutments are incisors or canines.
4. *The RPH Clasp:* The RPH clasp is the modification of the RPI system as: mesial rest (R), proximal plate (P), and horizontal retentive arm (H—RPH) (Fig. 11.35). The retentive arm is projected horizontally but since it touches the abutment only at its retentive tip, this clasp type is considered as an infrabulge clasp. The horizontal retentive arm may be cast half round, round, or maybe made-up from wrought wire according to the specific situation. This clasp may be an alternative to RPI clasp where there are soft tissue undercuts, high-frenal attachments, or shallow vestibular depth.

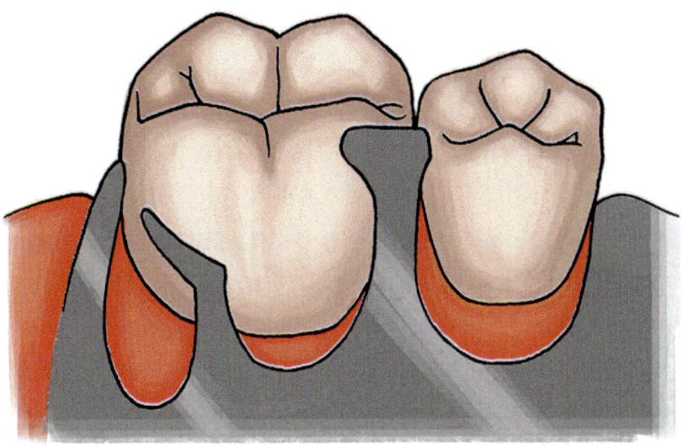

Fig. 11.32 The RLS system: (1) Mesioocclusal rest, (2) Distolingual L-bar direct retainer, (3) Distobuccal reciprocal element

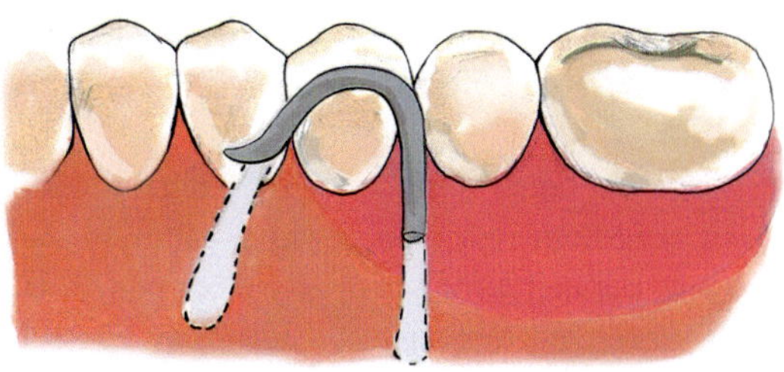

Fig. 11.33 The twin flex system uses a wrought wire soldered into a channel, which is cast into the major connector. The U-shaped wire is inserted from lingual to facial into the framework before tooth setup

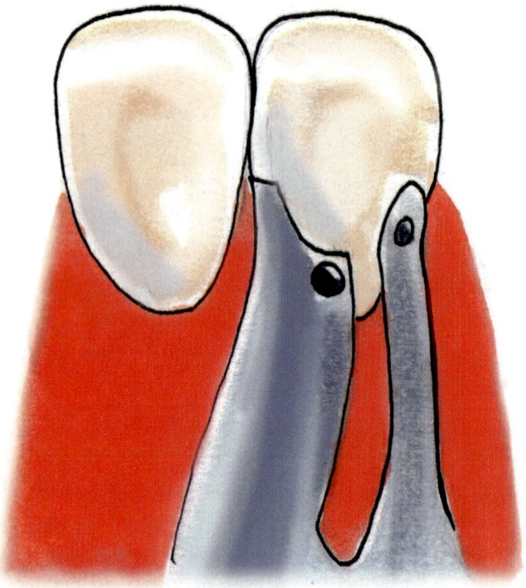

Fig. 11.34 Round-rest, distal depression clasp: (1) Round rest seat near the cingulum, (2) Mesiolingual reciprocating plate, (3) Split minor connector engaging a distal depression for retention

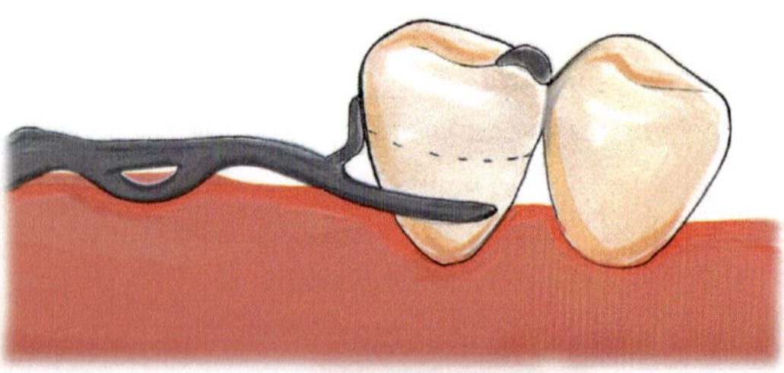

Fig. 11.35 The RPH clasp is the modification of the RPI system as mesial rest, proximal plate, and horizontal retentive arm

11.3 Indirect Retainers

An indirect retainer is an auxiliary occlusal, incisal, or cingulum rest that displays accurate and definitive contact with a properly designed, horizontally oriented rest seat. All Kennedy Class I, Class II, and Class IV RPDs require effective indirect retention. During mastication, the denture rotates around the fulcrum line (Fig. 11.36) that passes through the most posterior rests, causing the denture to move away from the tissues or move towards the tissue. This rotational movement is described in Chap. 4. When the denture base moves away from the supporting tissues, the anterior portion of the major connector impinges on the underlying supporting structures. This impingement may cause negative side effects such as trauma to the soft tissue or extensive destructive forces to the supporting teeth. The movement away from the tissues can be resisted by activation of the direct retainer, the stabilizing components of the clasp assembly, and the rigid indirect retainers.

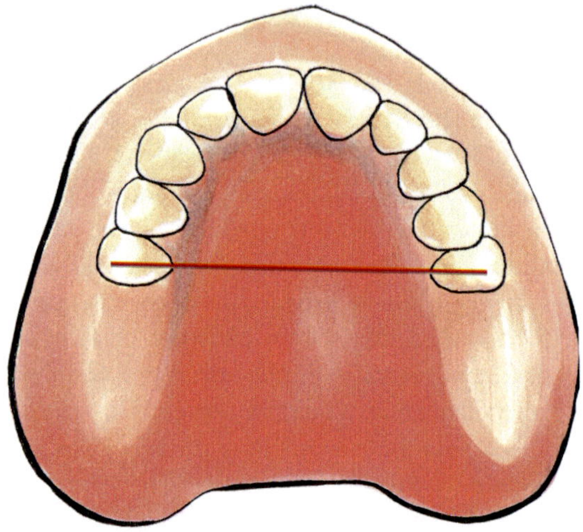

Fig. 11.36 Fulcrum line. The RPD rotates around the fulcrum line, which passes through the most posterior rests. This rotational movement causes the RPD to move away from the tissues or toward the tissue

The importance of the well-designed indirect retention (rests and minor connectors) counteracts these negative side effects. Indirect retention can only be achieved when one or more rigid indirect retainers are positioned in properly prepared rest seats. To prevent displacement of an extension base away from the tissues, practically one or more indirect retainers must be positioned perpendicular to the fulcrum line as far as possible to provide the best leverage system against dislodging forces (Fig. 11.37).

The effectiveness of the indirect retention will be increased as the distance to the fulcrum line increases. It is also important to choose the most suitable abutment tooth to place the rests for indirect retention. Although the most effective location

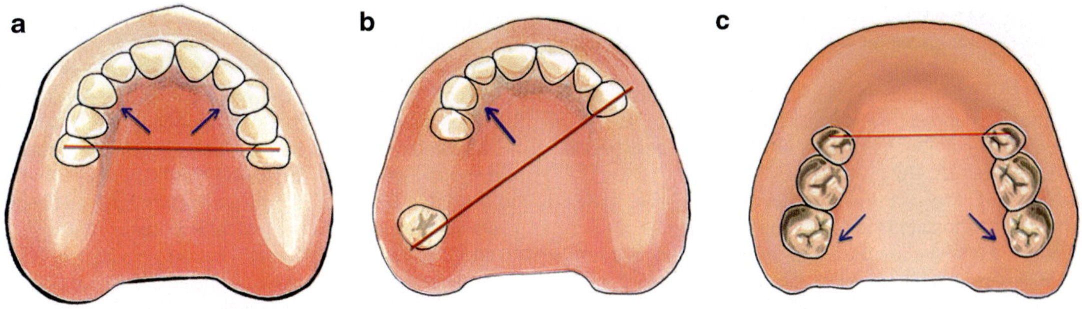

Fig. 11.37 One or more indirect retainers must be positioned perpendicular to the fulcrum line as far as possible to provide the best leverage system against dislodging forces. (**a**) In Kennedy Class I cases. (**b**) In Kennedy Class II cases, (**c**) In Kennedy Class IV cases

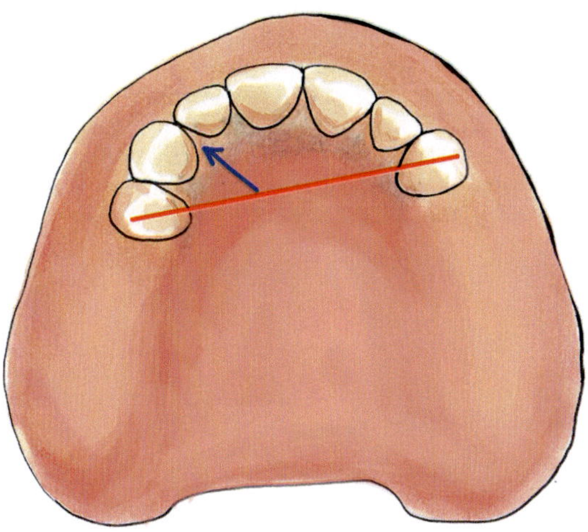

Fig. 11.38 Although it may not be as far from the fulcrum line, the most commonly used teeth are canines and premolars due to their increased periodontal support compared to incisal teeth

for indirect retention is the vicinity of an incisor tooth, rests for indirect retention are not preferred to be placed on the incisal teeth due to their lingual surface anatomy in clinical practice. For indirect retention, the most commonly used teeth are canines and premolars due to their increased periodontal support compared to incisal teeth even though they are not as far from the fulcrum line (Fig. 11.38). In these cases, choice of two locations for indirect retention might be clinically beneficial to compensate for the shorter distance to the fulcrum line. A cingulum rest is used for the purpose of indirect retention on a canine tooth and an occlusal rest for the premolar tooth to direct the forces axially. In cases of where only the use of indirect retention is available with the incisor teeth, an incisal rest seat should be prepared. In these situations, it may be more esthetically improved if crown restorations with the lingual rest seat are prepared. Lingual plating along with appropriate rest–rest seat combinations should be used to augment indirect retention. In Kennedy Class II cases, one indirect retainer on opposite side of distal extension base can be used.

Further Reading

Akers PE. Partial dentures. J Amer Dent Assoc. 1928;15:717–22.

Ancowitz S. Esthetic removable partial dentures. Gen Dent. 2004;52:453–9.

Aras M, Parab MM, Mascarenhas K. A stepwise approach towards planning of removable partial denture frameworks. EC Dent Sci. 2021;20:28–36.

Aviv I, Ben-Ur Z, Cardash HS, Fatael H. RLS—the lingually retained clasp assembly for distal extension removable partial dentures. Quintessence Int. 1990;21:221–3.

Balvinder SS, Mittal D. An overview of removable partial denture. Indian J Dent Sci. 2012;3:117–24.

Belles DM. The twin flex clasp: an esthetic alternative. J Prosthet Dent. 1997;77:450–2.

Ben-Ur Z, Gorfil C, Shifman A. Designing clasps for the asymmetric distal extension removable partial denture. Int J Prosthodont. 1996;9:374–8.

Brudvik JS, Palacios R. Lingual retention and the elimination of the visible clasp arm. J Esthet Restor Dent. 2007;19:247–54.

Carr AB, Brown DT. McCracken's removable partial prosthodontics. 13th ed. St. Louis, MO: Elsevier; 2016.

Cerkas L, Jaslow E. Saddle lock hidden clasp partial dentures. Compend Contin Educ Dent. 1991;12:746–52.

Chu CH, Chow TW. Esthetic design of removable partial dentures. Gen Dent. 2003;51:322–4.

DeVan MM. Preserving natural teeth through the use of clasps. J Prosthet Dent. 1955;5:208–14.

Eliason CM. RPA clasp design for distal-extension removable partial dentures. J Prosthet Dent. 1983;49:25–7.

Geckili O, Sulun T. Restoration of slightly infraoccluded premolars with ceramic onlays. Clin Dent Res. 2012;36:31–4.

Goodman JJ. The Equipoise removable rebturation. Trends Tech Contemp Dent Lab. 1991;8:45–52.

Hajjaj MS. Modified equipoise clasp: an esthetic option for removable dental prostheses. J Prosthodont. 2019;28:724–7.

Khan SB, Geerts GA. Aesthetic clasp design for removable partial dentures: a literature review. SADJ. 2005;60:190–4.

Krol AJ. RPI (rest, proximal plate, I bar) clasp retainer and its modifications. Dent Clin N Am. 1973;17:631–49.

Loney RW. Removable partial denture manual. Halifax, NS: Dalhousie University Faculty of Dentistry; 2011. http://removpros.dentistry.dal.ca/ewExternalFiles/RPD%20Manual%2011.pdf.

Nakamura Y, Kanbara R, Ochiai KT, Tanaka Y. A finite element evaluation of mechanical function for 3 distal extension partial dental prosthesis designs with a 3-dimensional nonlinear method for modeling soft tissue. J Prosthet Dent. 2014;112:972–80.

Nallaswamy. Textbook of prosthodontics. 2nd ed. New Delhi: Jaypee Brothers Medical Publishers; 2008.

Nazarova E, Taylor TD. The RPH clasp assembly: a simple alternative to traditional designs. J Prosthodont. 2012;21:331–3.

Nelson DR, von Gonten AS, Kelly TW Jr. The cast round RPA clasp. J Prosthet Dent. 1985;54:307–9.

Pardo-Mindan S, Ruiz-Villandiego JC. A flexible lingual clasp as an esthetic alternative: a clinical report. J Prosthet Dent. 1993;69:245–6.

Phoenix RD, Cagna DR, Defreest CF. Stewart's clinical removable partial prosthodontics. 4th ed. Chicago: Quintessence Publishing; 2008.

The glossary of prosthodontic terms: ninth edition. J Prosthet Dent. 2017;117(5S):e1–e105.

Yeung C, Yu OY, Lam WYH, Leung KCM, Wong AWY, Chu CH. Improving esthetics of removable partial dentures using palatal retentive arms. Clin Cosmet Investig Dent. 2020;12:391–7.

12 Esthetic Solutions for Removable Partial Dentures

Olcay Şakar

Abstract

Esthetic is a crucial factor in terms of patient acceptance and satisfaction with their dentures. The metal clasps located in the esthetic zone can be objectionable for many patients due to their appearance. Various solutions have been presented in the literature to address this esthetic issue.

The other chapters of the book present detailed information on the use of esthetic treatment alternatives in removable partial dentures (RPDs), such as precision attachments, double-crown systems, implants, and various metal clasp designs.

This chapter focuses on other widely accepted and used esthetic treatment alternatives which are non-metal clasp dentures with a metal framework produced from injection-molded thermoplastic resins and rotational path RPD design. The advantages, disadvantages, and the basic principles of clinical usage are presented.

Supplementary Information The online version contains supplementary material available at https://doi.org/10.1007/978-3-031-47083-7_12.

O. Şakar (✉)
Faculty of Dentistry, Department of Prosthodontics, İstanbul University, İstanbul, Türkiye
e-mail: osakar@istanbul.edu.tr

12.1 Definitions

Acrylic resin: (1) pertaining to polymers of acrylic acid, methacrylic acid, or acrylonitrile; (2) any of a group of thermoplastic resins made by polymerizing esters of acrylic or methylmethacrylate acids.

Injection molding: The adaptation of a plastic material to the negative form of a closed mold by forcing the material into the mold through appropriate gateways.

Non-metal clasp dentures: It is used to refer not only to dentures that do not contain any metal elements, but also to dentures that incorporate a metal rest or framework, and is defined as "the general name for removable partial dentures using denture base resins as the denture retentive parts".

Resin clasp: The resin retentive part of non-metal clasp dentures.

Rotational path removable partial denture: A removable partial denture that incorporates a curved, arcuate, or variable path of placement allowing one or more of the rigid components of the framework to gain access to and engage an undercut area.

Thermoplastic: A characteristic or property of a material that allows it to be softened by the application of heat and return to the hardened state on cooling.

O. Şakar (ed.), *Removable Partial Dentures*, https://doi.org/10.1007/978-3-031-47083-7_12

12.2 Non-metal Clasp Dentures

A conventional removable partial denture (RPD) generally consists of a CoCr (cobalt and chromium) alloy framework and heat-polymerized polymethyl methacrylate (PMMA)-based acrylic resin. Non-metal clasp dentures (NMCDs) described by Fueki et al. refer to RPDs with resin clasps that can be produced with or without a metal framework. Thermoplastic resin (TR) materials, such as polyoxymethylene, polyamide, polycarbonate, polyester, or acrylic resin constitute an alternative to the widely used conventional heat-polymerized PMMA denture base material. Injection molding is the most commonly used process for TR manufacturing. With the advent of digital technology, new materials known as high-performance polymers have emerged and, while there is a lack of long-term clinical studies, the use of metal-free polymer RPDs has also increased (see Part V). This section presents the advantages and disadvantages of *NMCDs produced with a metal framework and injection-molded TRs*, as well as fabrication techniques.

The basic requirement of a major connector is rigidity and occlusal rests are particularly critical in preventing movement of the denture base towards the soft tissue. A recent in-vitro study has shown that metal occlusal rests added to unilateral extension flexible resin framework RPDs are effective in reducing the vertical movement of the dentures. NMCDs that do not include a metal framework lead to traumatic damage to the periodontal tissue of the abutment teeth and impingement of the underlying tissue due to their flexibility.

In addition, it has been emphasized that a flexible denture base tends to undergo permanent deformation during chewing, and if vertical stress occurs later due to this deformation, the cancellous bone under the denture base may be resorbed. An in-vivo study supported the aforementioned result by indicating that heat-polymerized PMMA dentures without metal major connector/rest, similar to polyamide NMCDs, led to increased redness on the mucosa around the abutment tooth when compared to CoCr-RPDs. Despite their superior esthetics, polyamide dentures were found to have issues with surface roughness perceived by the tongue, difficulty in cleaning, and loss of retention. On the other hand, PMMA dentures were reported to cause speech difficulties and were described as cumbersome by the patients. Moreover, another study reported that RPDs made of PMMA and polyamide without a metal framework result in chewing deficiency compared to RPDs with a CoCr framework, which could potentially lead to an increase in body mass index. Consequently, NMCDs with a metal framework are rigid. Therefore, NMCDs including a metal structure with metal rest are recommended to avoid sinking and flexion of the denture base, and they can be used for all patients whose priority is esthetics.

However, NMCDs that do not include a metal structure can be treatment options for certain patients. For example, they can be used for patients with metal allergies or for those with only a few missing anterior teeth or a few missing teeth with occlusal support. They can also be used for maxillofacial defect patients for whom the dentures carry no functional load and for patients having diseases such as scleroderma that cause insufficient mouth opening, for patients who do not consent to the preparation of their abutment teeth even for rest seats and, for implant patients, as an interim denture.

Recently, there has been an increase in the use of injection-molded TR materials in dental practice and studies have been conducted to evaluate their physical properties and clinical outcomes. A 3-month randomized clinical trial reported that NMCDs made of a metal framework (CoCr) and TR denture base (polyester) including clasps, provided higher patient satisfaction and better oral health-related quality of life than the conventional RPDs. Although the results of TR studies are promising, the general consensus is that there is room for improvement in many of their properties to increase their clinical use. Therefore, their mechanical and physical properties, as well as their clinical usage, maintenance, and complications, will be described in the light of the studies undertaken hitherto. It should be kept in mind that the following advantages and disadvantages may vary depending on the specific material being used.

12.2.1 General Advantages of Non-metal Clasp Dentures and Thermoplastic Resin Materials

1. Esthetic appearance of NMCDs is more satisfactory than the conventional RPDs (Fig. 12.1a, b).
2. Wearing and fitting of NMCDs with thermoplastic resin base can be more suitable for patients due to the flexibility and softer surface of TRs compared to RPD with conventional heat-polymerized PMMA acrylic resin base.
3. TRs can be used in patients who have an allergy to metal.
4. TRs contain very little or no free monomer.
5. Creep resistance and fatigue strength of TRs are very high.
6. Although the flexural strength and modulus of elasticity (ME) of TRs are lower than conventional heat-polymerized PMMA resins, TRs demonstrate great toughness, impact strength, and strong resistance to fractures.
7. Flexibility of TRs can be enhanced by adding elastomeric resins.
8. TRs can be reinforced by adding glass filler or fibers.

12.2.2 General Disadvantages of Non-metal Clasp Dentures and Thermoplastic Resin Materials

1. The hardness and wear resistance of TRs are lower than those of conventional heat-polymerized PMMA resin, resulting in these resins being rougher than conventional PMMA resin.
2. TRs need special attention because they are affected by heat generation during polishing. If the glass transition temperature is exceeded, the structure may become rubbery.
3. The polished surface of the TRs may lose its brightness over time because they are softer than conventional heat-polymerized PMMA resin and more easily damaged by the scratch test. Therefore, NMCDs should be cleaned with a soft toothbrush without toothpaste and checked at short-term intervals. Discoloration and degradation of TRs may also be observed.
4. If the resin clasp is in the form of extending a part of the thermoplastic denture base resin, it covers the cervical area of the abutment teeth. This design may lead to periodontal problems. In addition, the thickness of the preformed clasps may cause the same problems. Therefore, careful cleaning and regular oral maintenance care are very important and poor oral hygiene can be considered as a contraindication factor.

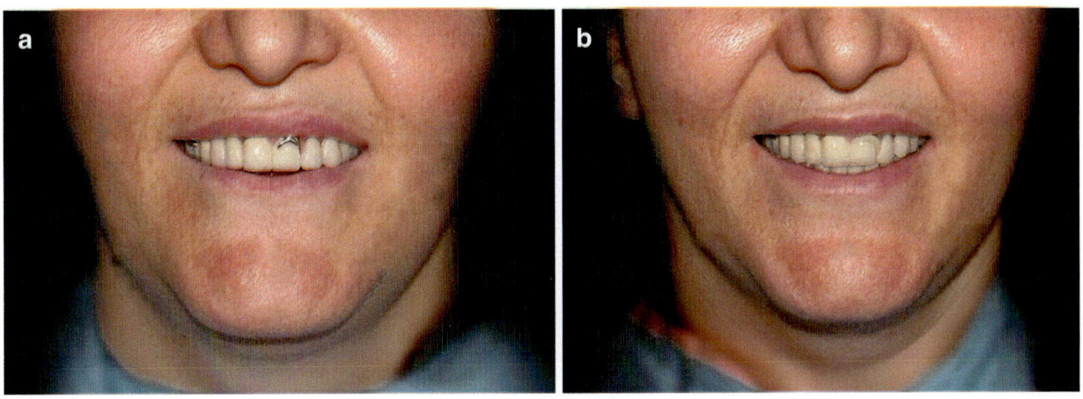

Fig. 12.1 (**a**, **b**) An acetal resin clasp in the anterior zone can be more satisfactory esthetically than a metal clasp

5. Adjusting and repairing NMCDs can be challenging because they generally do not chemically bond with the self-cure acrylic resin. It should be remembered that distal extension NMCDs should have maximum tissue support. An altered cast impression technique (see Chap. 8) can improve support in distal extension NMCDs and delay relining requirements.
6. Artificial tooth bonding with most thermoplastic materials is also non-chemical. Therefore, it is recommended to create a T-shaped tunnel in the artificial tooth for mechanical retention (Fig. 12.2).

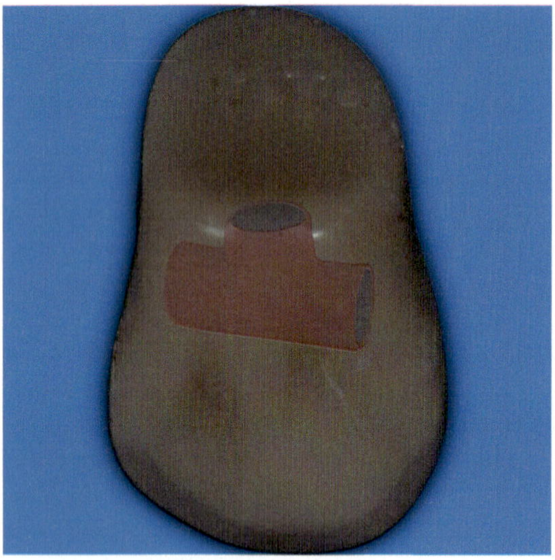

Fig. 12.2 Creating a T-shaped tunnel for mechanical retention between the thermoplastic resin material and the artificial tooth is recommended

7. NMCDs with TR base generally cost more than conventional RPDs.

12.2.3 The Basic Principles for Clinical Use of Non-metal Clasp Dentures with Different Thermoplastic Resin Materials

NMCDs should follow the same design principles as conventional RPDs with metal clasps except for the design of the resin clasp. TR clasps can be fabricated in two ways. In the first design, the resin clasp is in the form of extending a part of the thermoplastic denture base resin, and in the second design, a preformed resin clasp is used with a conventional heat-polymerized PMMA denture base material (Fig. 12.3a, b). As a general rule, the retentive force of a resin clasp is lower than a metal clasp. Therefore, to provide more retention and stability, while the resin clasps are used in the anterior teeth, metal clasps can be used in the posterior teeth. The design criteria of TR retainers depend on the ME of the resin. As the ME of the material increases, rigidity also increases. Hence, the material with the lower ME is more flexible and can be used in the deeper undercut (e.g., polyamides have lower ME than polyoxymethylenes).

The injection-molded TRs can be classified into various categories, but the physical properties of materials within the same category can vary even between different brands. Therefore,

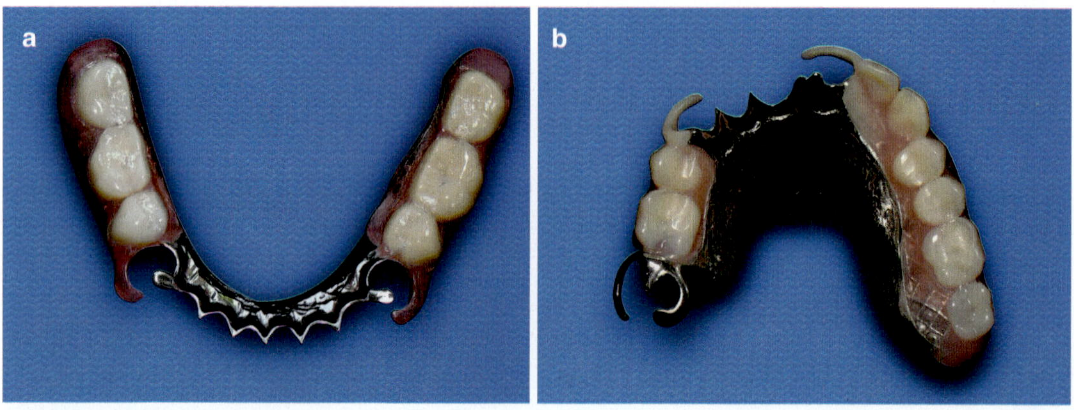

Fig. 12.3 (**a**, **b**) Non-metal clasp dentures should be fabricated with metal framework and its design should be same as conventional removable partial denture except the clasps

brand names are also mentioned while presenting the studies.

Polyoxymethylene (acetal resin) is a commonly used preformed clasp material in dentistry. It is also used as a base material for patients with an allergic reaction to metal framework because it is monomer-free. Although manufacturers suggest the use of this material without a metal framework, a metal framework offers better rigidity as is the case with other TRs.

It is suggested that this material is very strong, resists wear and fracture, and also exhibits high biocompatibility, creep resistance, fatigue endurance, dimensional stability, and chemical resistance. Although it is reported that the water sorption and the solubility of acetal resins were within ISO specification limits, an acetal resin (T.S.M. Acetal) showed clinically acceptable color changes with peroxide cleanser but unacceptable with hypochlorite cleanser. Recently a study result also revealed that acetal resin (T.S.M. Acetal) showed higher color changes caused by beverages than heat-polymerized PMMA (Paladon 65) and PEEK (BioHPP) and lower than polyamide (Valplast).

An acetal resin clasp is more flexible but has a lower retentive force than the CoCr clasp. Thus, it should be placed in deeper undercuts (approximately 0.5 mm) on abutments. It has been recommended that an acetal resin clasp should be fabricated shorter with a larger cross-sectional diameter to have a stiffness similar to a cast CoCr clasp (if all other variables are equal, an acetal resin clasp should be 5 mm long and 1.4 mm in diameter, instead of 15 mm long and 1 mm in diameter CoCr clasp-Dental D). A study result showed that a 1 kg force was required to dislodge Dental D clasp's tips by 0.5 mm, using its dimensions according to the manufacturer's recommendation (length 12 mm, thickness 1.9 mm tapering to 1.25 mm at the tip, width 2.8 mm tapering to 2.2 mm at the tip).

If plaque control is established, a thicker clasp will not be harmful to oral health. It is also recommended to benefit from guiding planes to provide more retention. Retention will also be affected by the number of clasps, the fit of the framework, and the depth of undercut (Fig. 12.4).

Acetal resin does not have natural translucency but is available in various color shades. It can be fabricated in the same shape as a metal clasp without covering the gingiva. A metal framework is fabricated in a conventional manner. After intraoral try-in of the framework, the jaw relations are recorded. In laboratory procedures, a wax pattern of an acetal resin clasp is manufactured and an injection is carried out and shaped in the metal framework's mesh. Thus, it is possible to check the retention and color harmony of acetal resin clasps during the esthetic try-in (Fig. 12.5).

Polyamides, commonly known as nylon/flexible dentures, have also become widely used in dentistry. Polyamides may be divided into two

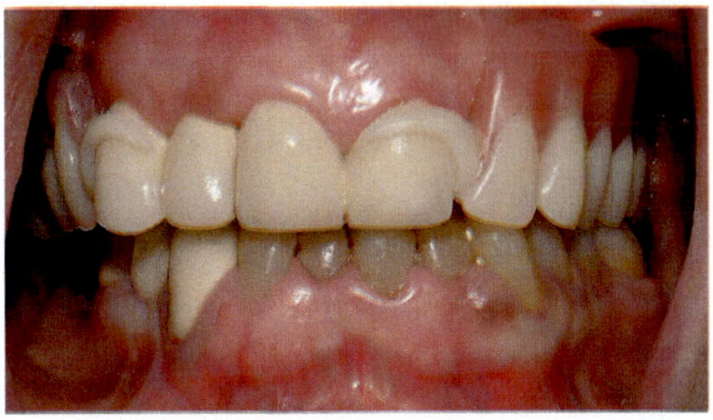

Fig. 12.4 The retention of an acetal resin clasp is less than a metal clasp. Therefore benefiting from the guiding planes and using sufficient undercut are necessary to obtain adequate retention

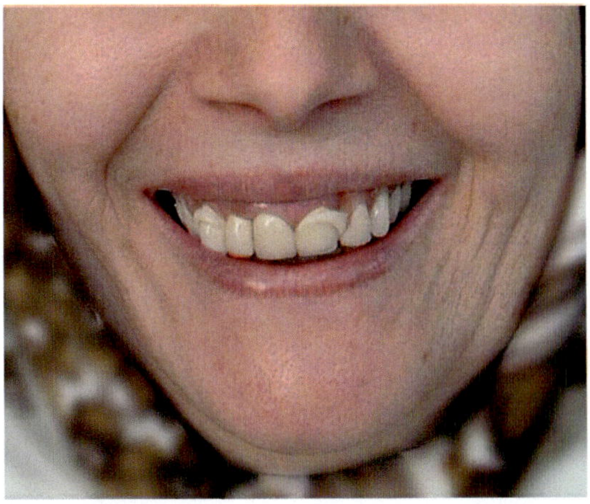

Fig. 12.5 Acetal resin clasp are fabricated before acrylic polymerization. Thus it is possible to check the retention and color harmony during the esthetic try-in

groups according to their flexural properties: soft-type (e.g., Valplast) and hard-type (e.g., Luciton FRS). Although the flexural properties of hard types are similar to those of polyester resins (e.g., EstheShot), soft types are similar to that of polypropylene resin (Unigum). The most noteworthy and clinically important additional differences from the above-mentioned advantages and disadvantages are as follows for commonly used materials:

Valplast's and Deflex's colors harmonize well with the color shades of the gums (Fig. 12.6a–c). Valplast can be disinfected with glutaraldehyde or sodium hypochlorite without changing its surface roughness. But a study showed that the all three denture cleansers (Corega, Protefix, Val-Clean) increased surface roughness of the polyamide materials (Valplast, Deflex). Sunflex has higher flexural and impact strength than Valplast. After immersion disinfection (Val-Clean), it has been shown that while the impact strength, namely rigidity, increased in Valplast, there were no significant changes in Sunflex.

Color changes (Valplast) can occur with some foods and beverages such as coffee, tea, wine, and curry. A study result showed that Deflex also displayed more color changes when compared to PMMA. The results of another study showed that although all the TRs examined showed clinically significant color change, polyamides (Valplast, Lucitone, Smiletone) had the lowest color stability among Polyester (Estheshot-Bright), Acrylic resin (Acrytone) and, Polypropylene (Weldenz). Polishing and grinding are easier for Lucitone FRS because it is harder than Valplast and highly resistant to abrasion. However, the risk of fracture, color instability, and the difficulty of relining and repairing are considered disadvantages.

As Valplast and Lucitone FRS do not bond to acrylic resins, treating the surface with 4-Acryloyloxyethyl trimellitate anhydride/methyl methacrylate-tri-n-butylborane (4-META/MMA-TBB) resin after sandblasting/tribochemical silica coating has been recommended. Ultimate is a relatively new material about which there is little information. Relining and repairing

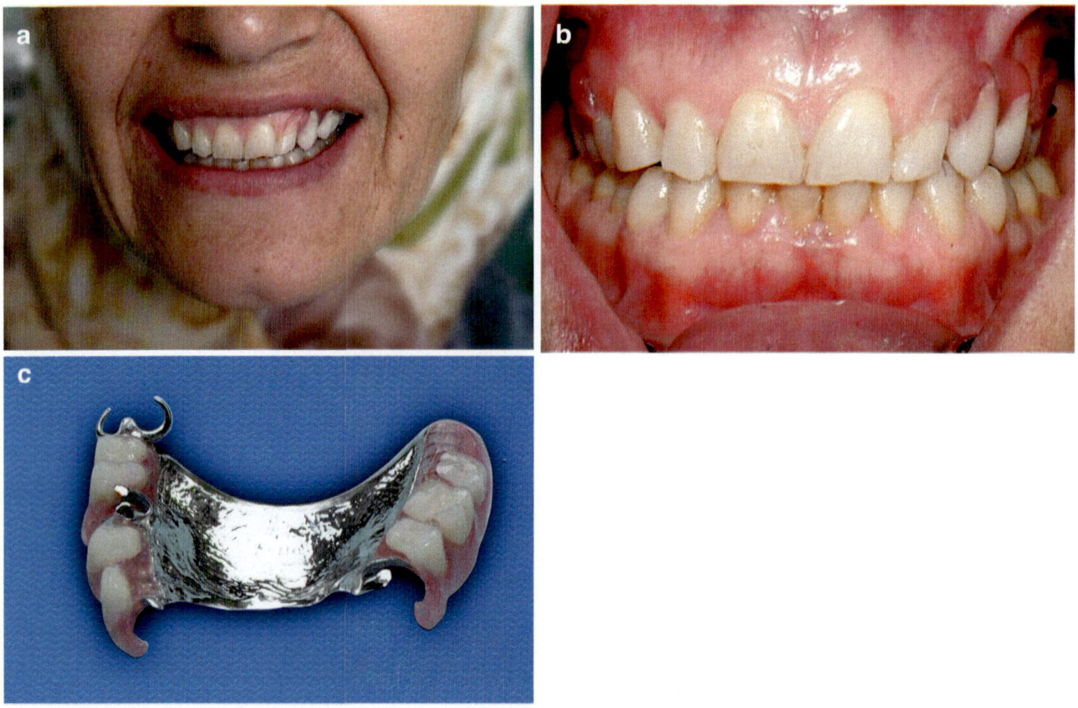

Fig. 12.6 (**a–c**) Polyamide base removable partial denture's color harmonizes well with the color of the gums

can be fabricated by reinjection of the material, and it can also be used for the relining and repairing of the Lucitone FRS.

It was shown that a polyamide denture base (Flexiplast) becomes more than 7 times smoother and a processed polymethylmethacrylate becomes more than 20 times smoother when they are polished with the same conventional polishing technique. However, it was emphasized that the polished polyamide was within clinically acceptable norms.

Polyesters (EstheShot, EstheShot Bright) TR materials have lower resilience and better fitting than polyamides and polycarbonates, but they have a greater risk of fracture. The fitting accuracy of polyester is superior to heat-cured PMMA resin. Surface roughness and the water sorption of polyesters are also lower than that of polyamides. Unlike polyamides, repairing and relining are possible with self-curing resin. However, tribochemical silica coating and 4-META/MMA-TBB resin are suggested to provide more secure bonding. Alkaline denture cleaners may lead to degradation on the surface of the polyesters.

Polycarbonates generally have higher flexural strength, elastic modulus, and proportional limit than those of polyesters and polyamides. Reigning which is a *polycarbonate* has similar physical properties to polyesters but lower water absorbency. It can be reinjected to repair the broken clasp. Another polycarbonate material Reigning N's surface is harder than polyamides and polyesters. Consequently, it is found that the wear depth of polycarbonate (Reigning N) was lower than that of polyamide (Lucitone FRS, Valplast), PMMA (Acrytone), and polyester (EstheShot, EstheShot Bright). Discoloration is less than in other resins. Similar to Estheshot, it bonds to self-cure resin more securely with tribochemical silica coating and 4-META/MMA-TBB resin. Artificial teeth exist of the same material which therefore do not need special retention for both materials. Denture cleaners do not affect the material.

Polyetheretherketone (PEEK) and *polyetherketoneketone (PEKK) aryl ketone polymer (AKP)* are called new-generation high-performance polymers. They are produced in enamel colors in different shades, including gingival color. Similar to other TR materials, high-performance polymer resin clasps also show less retention than CoCr clasps. Therefore, they should be prepared more thickly and placed in a deeper undercut than metal clasps. Although various in-vitro studies use different dimensions for optimum clasp design, the issue of minimum 0.5 mm undercut requirement is clear. These materials are generally produced with digital production techniques, including major connectors and clasps. Detailed information is presented in Chap. 19.

There are also *acrylic resin* (e.g., Acrytone, Acryshot) and lately *polypropylene* (e.g. Weldenz, Unigum) TR materials used in dentistry. A recent study revealed that polypropylene (Weldenz) showed the lowest flexural strength/hardness value among polyester (Estheshot-Bright), acrylic resin (Acrytone), and polyamides (Valplast, Lucitone, Smiletone). And also Weldenz showed less water sorption than Acrytone and Lucitone. However, flexural strength of Unigum was found to be similar to that of Valplast in another study but as with Weldenz it also exhibited the lower water sorption than acrylic resins, polyamides, polycarbonate, and polyesters.

The retentive forces of all TR clasps depend on different factors such as ME, thickness and width of the resin, and the amount of the undercut. If a TR clasp is fabricated as an extending part of the denture base, depending on the properties of the TR material and the depth of the sulcus the recommended width of the retentive arm is approximately 5.0–8.0 mm and the thickness of the clasp arm is 1.0–1.5 mm (Fig. 12.7a, b). Thus, in clinically short crowns with inadequate sulcus depth and/or an excessive undercut in the tissue part, the width of the retentive arm may not be properly designed. In the case of missing molars, a study indicated that if there is a presence of 0.75 mm undercut on the second premolar, a polyamide resin clasp covering only the buccal surface is desirable, but in the presence of a 0.50 mm undercut, a resin clasp should also be extended to the buccal surface of the first premo-

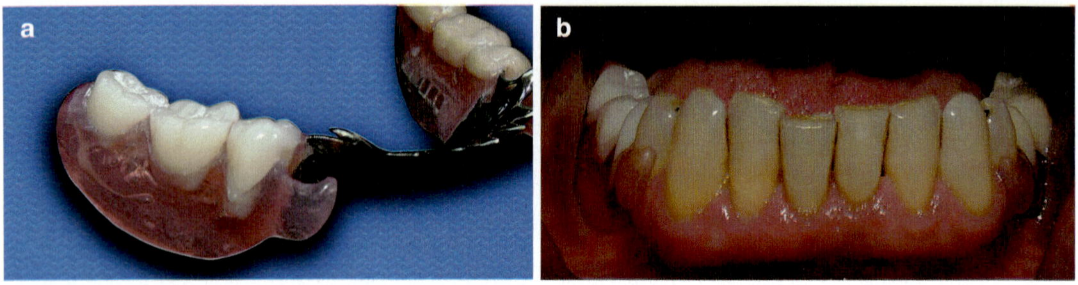

Fig. 12.7 (**a**, **b**) If a thermoplastic resin clasp is fabricated as an extending part of the denture base, the recommended width of the retentive arm is approximately 5.0–8.0 mm and the thickness of the clasp arm is 1.0–1.5 mm

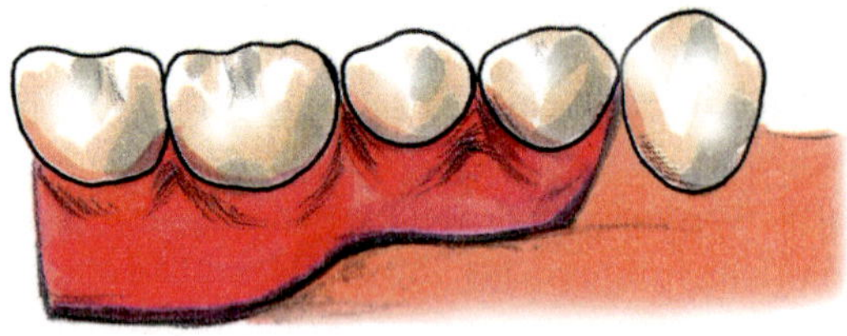

Fig. 12.8 In cases having no molars, in the presence of 0.5 mm undercut on the second premolar, a thermoplastic resin clasp may be extended to buccal surface of the first premolar to obtain adequate retention

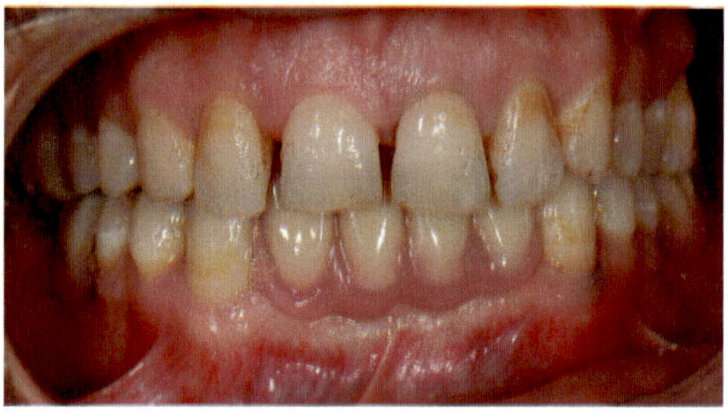

Fig. 12.9 If appropriate cases are chosen, a correctly designed rotational path RPD will be very satisfactory esthetic solution for patients

lar (Fig. 12.8). If a deeper undercut was found to be more effective than that of a design covering the anterior abutment tooth, it is also necessary to use lingual and proximal undercuts to increase retention. However, it should be kept in mind that further studies on the design of the resin clasps are still needed.

In clinical steps, the metal framework is fabricated. Jaw relations are recorded. Artificial teeth are arranged. After completing the esthetic try-in, the denture is forwarded to the laboratory. The metal clasps are removed at this stage. The denture base, including the clasps, is manufactured from TR.

Valplast's manufacturer suggests that after immersing the finished denture in hot tap water for approximately 60 s, insertion into the patient's mouth can aid adaptation or the same method can be applied to tighten and loosen the clasps. In addition, it is necessary to use the trimming and polishing equipment the manufacturer recommends.

In light of the above data, it is clear that more in-vitro and long-term in-vivo studies should be performed on TRs and the dentist should have detailed information about the material before its clinical application.

12.3 Rotational Path Removable Partial Dentures

It is possible to eliminate the clasps in the esthetic zone by using the rotational path of placement (Fig. 12.9). In addition, in the presence of severely tilted teeth, the placement of the RPD is possible by using the rotational path design. A straight path of placement is used in the conventional design. But, in the rotational path design, one portion of the framework is seated first, and later the other portion of the framework is seated (Fig 12.10). Retention is obtained from the proximal undercuts adjacent to the edentulous spaces. Rigid retentive units consist of a rest and a minor connector. The retentive minor connector is frequently formed with a gingival extension on the teeth.

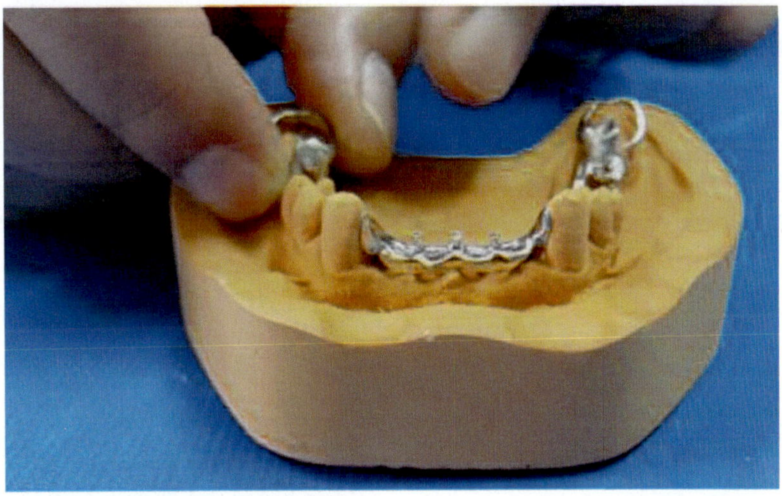

Fig. 12.10 Placement of a rotational path RPD is different from a conventional RPD. While straight path of placement is used in conventional RPDs, rotational path RPD's one portion is placed first, and later the other portion is placed. Path of placement shows differences according to the rotational centers (Video 12.1)

The primary indication of the rotational path design is for tooth-bounded partially edentulous arches. Namely, applying this design is more suitable for Kennedy Class III and IV cases. One clinical study that evaluated Kennedy Class III and II (without anterior modification) case results revealed that the rigid retainers demonstrated support, stability, retention, adequate encirclement, and passivity at the end of 10 years or more follow-up. Further clinical studies are still needed to expand the indications for this design.

12.3.1 Advantages of the Rotational Path Removable Partial Denture Design

1. The clasps can be eliminated in the esthetic zone.
2. Plaque accumulation may be decreased by reducing tooth coverage.
3. Preparation on the abutment teeth is minimally invasive.
4. Facial or lingual undercuts are not necessary for retention.
5. Further tipping of the abutment tooth can be prevented by a rigid retainer.

12.3.2 Disadvantages of the Rotational Path Removable Partial Denture Design

1. Fabrication and adjustment may be more difficult when compared to conventional design because dental technicians are less familiar with this design and processing errors are less tolerable.
2. The well-prepared rest seat preparation is vital.

There are two categories of rotational path designs. In *Category I design*, the rotational centers of the framework are located at the ends of the rests of the rigid retainers. The rotational centers are seated first, and then the entire prosthesis is placed in its final position. Depending on esthetic and periodontal considerations, the anterior or posterior portion of the RPD is placed first. Elimination of either anterior or posterior clasps with this design is possible. If the anterior portion of the prosthesis is placed first, the path of placement is termed *anteroposterior*, and generally, it is used to eliminate the anterior clasp (Fig. 12.11a, b). If the posterior portion is placed

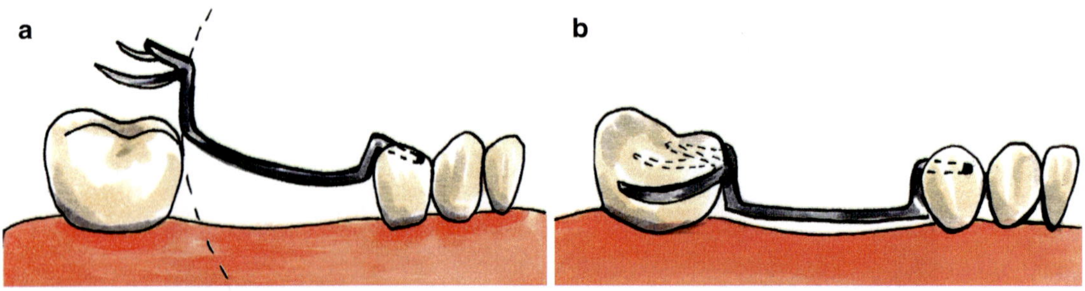

Fig. 12.11 (**a**, **b**) Anteroposterior Category I rotational path design

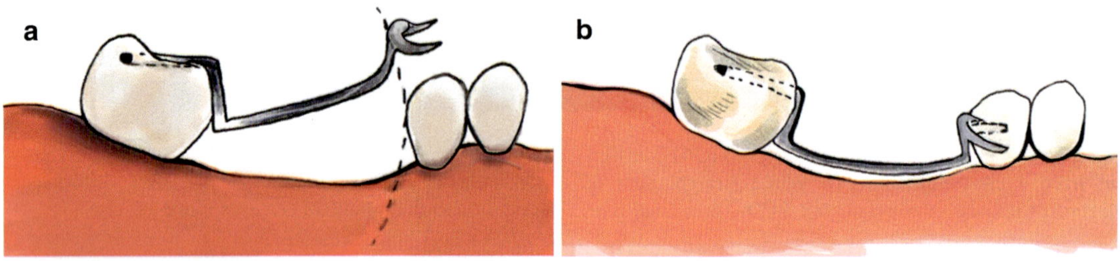

Fig. 12.12 (**a**, **b**) Posteroanterior Category I rotational path design

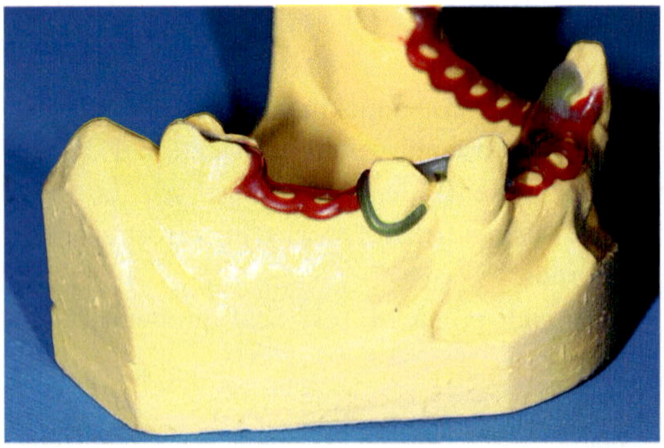

Fig. 12.13 In cases having mesially tilted molars, posteroanterior category I rotational path design can be used and minor connector on the mesial guiding plane of the molar abutment serve as retentive unit

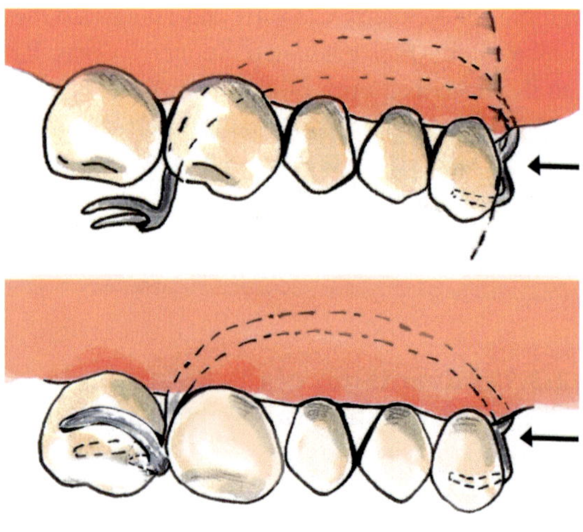

Fig. 12.14 Category II rotational path design

first, the path is termed *posteroanterior*, and generally, it is used to eliminate the posterior clasp (Fig. 12.12a, b). When molar abutments are tipped mesially, this design offers a great advantage (Fig. 12.13).

In *Category II designs*, rotational centers are placed gingivally as rigid extensions of the minor connectors and are primarily used to replace anterior teeth with the elimination of anterior clasps (Fig. 12.14). This category includes all lateral paths. Rests in the rotational path design show small differences from conventional design. In posteroanterior category I design rest seats should be prepared 1.5 to 2 mm deep occlusogingivally with nearly parallel buccal and lingual walls on the molar abutments. Rest seat preparation should be extended to more than half the mesiodistal width of the occlusal surface to provide bracing and vertical distribution of the forces to the abutment teeth and to prevent tooth migration. If the center of rotation is positioned at the distal third to half of the occlusal surface interference will not appear, regardless of the extent of inclination of the molars and interference testing will not be required. The preparation of the irregular outline form also prevents migration (Fig. 12.15). If molars are also tipped lingually, their rest seat walls should be prepared parallel to each other.

A cingulum rest seat on the anterior teeth should be prepared. When a suitable cingulum does not exist, it can be provided by acid-etched composite resin or fabricating a crown restoration. The outline form of the preparation should be an inverted "U" or "V" and extend to more than one-half the mesiodistal width of the anterior tooth.

Conventional clasping and rest can be used wherever necessary in all designs. Regardless of the design category, rigid retainers should be passive during and after seating of the framework, and therefore they do not require reciprocation.

It is important to remember that the lingual bar design causes fewer problems when establishing a rotational path of insertion in the mandible. The lingual plate is more likely to cause interference as the surface covered is much greater. So, if possible, a lingual bar should be preferred to a lingual plate.

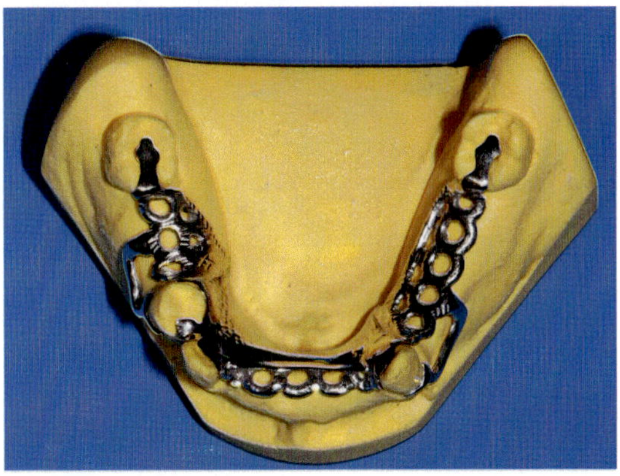

Fig. 12.15 On the molars that the clasps are eliminated, rest seat preparations are extended to more than half the mesiodistal width with an irregular outline form

12.3.3 Steps of Clinical and Surveying Procedures

1. The patient's acceptance and coordination are assessed. Intraoral evaluation is performed to determine whether a rotational path design is possible or not. Moreover, the presence of proximal undercuts, the location and number of edentulous areas, and the arch form are evaluated. Occlusal relationships are assessed both clinically and on the mounted casts. Then the study casts are investigated in terms of adequate undercuts when the cast is surveyed with a zero-degree tilt. Rest and retentive areas are also investigated. The amount of undercut should be approximately 0.5 mm in the retentive area. Although guiding plates are not usually recommended for this design, recontouring in the required areas is performed to minimize the amount of relief.
2. Rest seat preparation is performed. If there is no proper cingulum to prepare the rest seat and/or adequate undercut, crown or bonded composite resin restorations can be provided. Composite restorations are generally recommended in completing rest seats to improve contours and to alleviate the patient's financial constraints.

   After the final impression, the cast is surveyed again. The height of contours are drawn at two different positions (at the zero-degree and tilted positions) (Fig. 12.16a–c). Retentive areas and undercuts are indicated on the cast. The analyzing rod is utilized to assess whether access exists for the rests to be seated. If not, extra preparation is required which eventually needs a new impression.
3. An acrylic prototype resembling the metal framework may be helpful to check the rotational path of insertion. Thus, any obstacles detected during try-in can be handled before casting.
4. During the adjustment of the metal framework, care should be given to preserve the surface of minor connectors that are facing abutment teeth and act as rigid retainers. If necessary, these surfaces should be adjusted

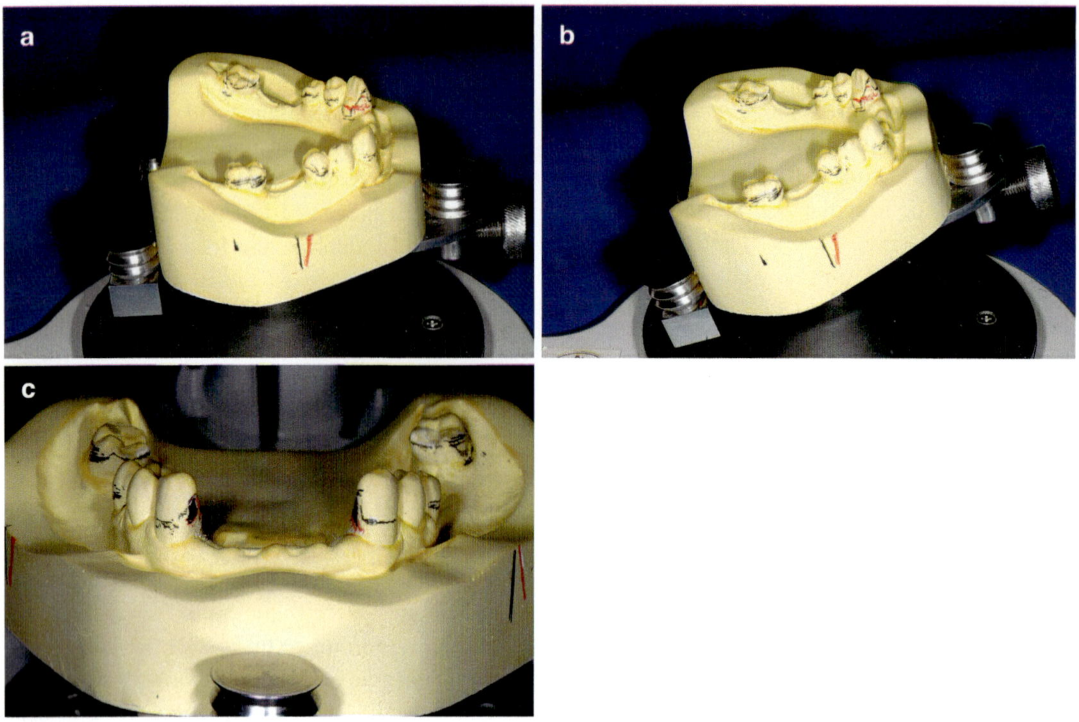

Fig. 12.16 (**a**–**c**) Rotational path RPD's retentive areas are determined on the surveyor. The height of contours are drawn first at zero-degree (**a**) and later at tilted positions (**b**). Retentive minor connector will be placed between the two lines (**c**)

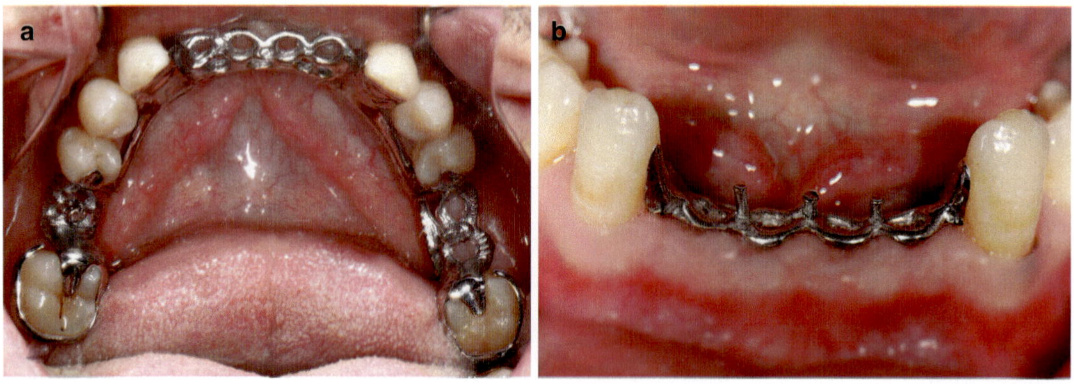

Fig. 12.17 (**a**, **b**) Retentive minor connector should be adjusted chairside by the dentist and technician should be warned not to grind these areas

chairside by the dentist (Fig. 12.17a, b). However, any interference with the framework regarding the rotational path of insertion has to be eliminated during laboratory finishing.

5. To determine the shape and amount of blockout under the minor connector and whether there is adequate undercut for the rigid retentive component, a pair of compasses can be used (Fig. 12.18). The free arm tip of the compass is used to evaluate the undercut area during motion around the other arm tip which is fixed at the rotation axis. If multiple edentulous areas exist, a sufficient blockout of undesirable undercuts should be planned for all minor connectors.

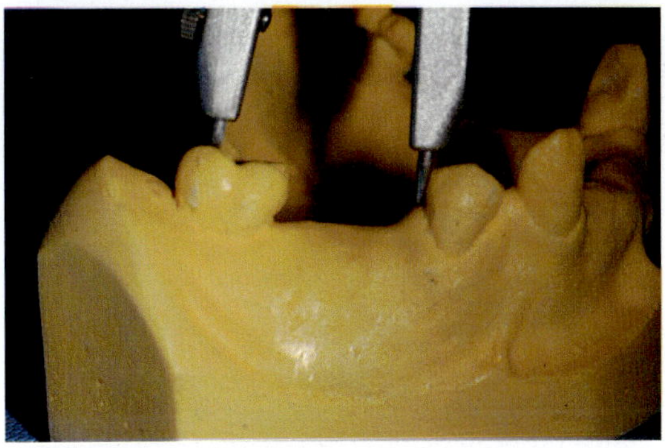

Fig. 12.18 A pair of compasses can be used to assess undercut areas in terms of both amount of adequate undercut and block-out on abutment teeth

Further Reading

Abuzar MA, Bellur S, Duong N, Kim BB, Lu P, Palfreyman N, Surendran D, Tran VT. Evaluating surface roughness of a polyamide denture base material in comparison with poly (methyl methacrylate). J Oral Sci. 2010;52:577–81.

Arda T, Arıkan A. An in vitro comparison of retentive force and deformation of acetal resin and cobalt-chromium clasps. J Prosthet Dent. 2005;94:267–74.

Arikan A, Ozkan YK, Arda T, Akalın B. An in vitro investigation of water sorption and solubility of two acetal denture base materials. Eur J Prosthodont Restor Dent. 2005;13:119–22.

Arikan A, Ozkan YK, Arda T, Akalin B. Effect of 180 days of water storage on the transverse strength of acetal resin denture base material. J Prosthodont. 2010;19:47–51.

Aysan I, Uçar Y, Üşümez A. A comparison of the color stability of three different base materials in the different solutions. J Dent Fac Atatürk Uni. 2011;21:219–25.

Baharav H, Ben-Ur Z, Laufer BZ, Cardash HS. Removable partial denture with a lateral rotational path of insertion. Quintessence Int. 1995;26:531–3.

Barraclough O, Gray D, Ali Z, Nattress B. Modern partial dentures-part 1: novel manufacturing techniques. Br Dent J. 2021;230:651–7.

Campbell SD, Cooper L, Craddock H, Hyde TP, Nattress B, Pavitt SH, Seymour DW. Removable partial dentures: the clinical need for innovation. J Prosthet Dent. 2017;118:273–80.

Carreiro Ada F, Machado AL, Giampaolo ET, Santana IL, Vergani CE. Dual path: a concept to improve the esthetic replacement of missing anterior teeth with a removable partial denture. J Prosthodont. 2008;17:586–90.

Chow TW, Clark RK, Clarke DA. Improved designs for removable partial dentures in Kennedy class IV cases. Quintessence Int. 1988;19:797–800.

Donovan T. Use of the rotational path removable partial denture concept in a Kennedy Class II patient: a case report. J Esthet Restor Dent. 2008;20:294–9.

Durkan R, Ayaz EA, Bagis B, Gurbuz A, Ozturk N, Korkmaz FM. Comparative effects of denture cleansers on physical properties of polyamide and polymethyl methacrylate base polymers. Dent Mater J. 2013;32:367–75.

Firtell DN, Jacobson TE. Removable partial dentures with rotational paths of insertion: problem analysis. J Prosthet Dent. 1983;50:8–15.

Fitton JS, Davies EH, Howlett JA, Pearson GJ. The physical properties of a polyacetal denture resin. Clin Mater. 1994;17:125–9.

Fueki K, Ohkubo C, Yatabe M, Arakawa I, Arita M, Ino S, Kanamori T, Kawai Y, Kawara M, Komiyama O, Suzuki T, Nagata K, Hosoki M, Masumi S, Yamauchi M, Aita H, Ono T, Kondo H, Tamaki K, Matsuka Y, Tsukasaki H, Fujisawa M, Baba K, Koyano K, Yatani H. Clinical application of removable partial dentures using thermoplastic resin-part I: definition and indication of non-metal clasp dentures. J Prosthodont Res. 2014a;58:3–10.

Fueki K, Ohkubo C, Yatabe M, Arakawa I, Arita M, Ino S, Kanamori T, Kawai Y, Kawara M, Komiyama O, Suzuki T, Nagata K, Hosoki M, Masumi S, Yamauchi M, Aita H, Ono T, Kondo H, Tamaki K, Matsuka Y, Tsukasaki H, Fujisawa M, Baba K, Koyano K, Yatani H. Clinical application of removable partial dentures using thermoplastic resin. Part II: material properties and clinical features of non-metal clasp dentures. J Prosthodont Res. 2014b;58:71–84.

Fueki K, Yoshida-Kohno E, Wakabayashi N. Oral health-related quality of life in patients with non-metal clasp dentures: a randomised cross-over trial. J Oral Rehabil. 2017;44:405–13.

Fueki K, Yoshida-Kohno E, Inamochi Y, Wakabayashi N. Patient satisfaction and preference with thermoplastic resin removable partial dentures: a randomised cross-over trial. J Prosthodont Res. 2020;64:20–5.

Fueki K, Inamochi Y, Yoshida-Kohno E, Wakabayashi N. Cost-effectiveness analysis of prosthetic treatment with thermoplastic resin removable partial dentures. J Prosthodont Res. 2021;65:52–5.

Fueki K, Inamochi Y, Yoshida-Kohno E, Wakabayashi N. Short-term effect of thermoplastic resin removable partial dentures on periodontal health: a randomized cross-over trial. J Prosthodont Res. 2022;66:167–75.

Gray D, Barraclough O, Ali Z, Nattress B. Modern partial dentures-part 2: a review of novel metal-free materials and innovations in polymers. Br Dent J. 2021;230:813–8.

Hamanaka I, Shimizu H, Takahashi Y. Shear bond strength of an autopolymerizing repair resin to injection-molded thermoplastic denture base resins. Acta Odontol Scand. 2013;71:1250–4.

Hamanaka I, Iwamoto M, Lassila LVJ, Vallittu PK, Takahashi Y. Wear resistance of injection-molded thermoplastic denture base resins. Acta Biomater Odontol Scand. 2016;2:31–7.

Hamanaka I, Shimizu H, Takahashi Y. Bond strength of a chairside autopolymerizing reline resin to injection-molded thermoplastic denture base resins. J Prosthodont Res. 2017;61:67–72.

Horie N, Ouchi T, Nishiyama R, Usuda S, Morikawa S, Asoda S, Nakagawa T. Vertical displacement in unilat-

eral extension base flexible removable dentures. Bull Tokyo Dent Coll. 2019;60:233–9.
Huang CT, Liu FC, Luk KC. Interference factors regarding the path of insertion of rotational-path removable partial dentures. Biom J. 2017;40:69–75.
Ito M, Wee AG, Miyamoto T, Kawai Y. The combination of a nylon and traditional partial removable dental prosthesis for improved esthetics: a clinical report. J Prosthet Dent. 2013;109:5–8.
Jacobson TE. Rotational path partial denture design: a 10-year clinical follow-up-part I. J Prosthet Dent. 1994;71:271–7.
Jacobson TE. Rotational path partial denture design: a 10-year clinical follow-up-part II. J Prosthet Dent. 1994;71:278–82.
Kawara M, Iwata Y, Iwasaki M, Komoda Y, Iida T, Asano T, Komiyama O. Scratch test of thermoplastic denture base resins for non-metal clasp dentures. J Prosthodont Res. 2014;58:35–40.
Kim MH, Heo SJ, Kim SK, Koak JY. Full mouth rehabilitation of destroyed dentition with rotational path removable partial denture: a case report. J Adv Prosthodont. 2010;2:46–9.
Krol AJ, Finzen FC. Rotational path removable partial dentures: Part 1. Replacement of posterior teeth. In J Prosthodont. 1988;1:17–27.
Krol AJ, Finzen FC. Rotational path removable partial dentures: Part 2. Replacement of anterior teeth. Int J Prosthodont. 1988;1:135–42.
Kurtulmus H, Kumbuloglu O, Aktas RT, Kurtulmus A, Boyacioglu H, Oral O, User A. Effects of saliva and nasal secretion on some physical properties of four different resin materials. Med Oral Patol Oral Cir Bucal. 2010;15:e969–75.
Lee HH, Lee JH, Yang TH, Kim YJ, Kim SC, Kim GR, Kim HR, Lee CJ, Okubo C. Evaluation of the flexural mechanical properties of various thermoplastic denture base polymers. Dent Mater J. 2018;37:950–6.
Lekha K, Savitha NP, Roseline M, Nadiger RK. Acetal resin as an esthetic clasp material. J Interdiscip Dent. 2012;2:11–4.
Manzon L, Fratto G, Poli O, Infusino E. Patient and clinical evaluation of traditional metal and polyamide removable partial dentures in an elderly cohort. J Prosthodont. 2019;28:868–75.
Negrutiu M, Sinescu C, Romanu M, Pop D, Lakatos S. Thermoplastic resins for flexible framework removable partial dentures. TMJ. 2005;55:295–9.
Osada H, Shimpo H, Hayakawa T, Ohkubo C. Influence of thickness and undercut of thermoplastic resin clasps on retentive force. Dent Mater J. 2013;32:381–9.
Ozkan Y, Arikan A, Akalin B, Arda T. A study to assess the colour stability of acetal resins subjected to thermocycling. Eur J Prosthodont Restor Dent. 2005;13:10–4.
Papathanasiou I, Papavasiliou G, Kamposiora P, Zoidis P. Effect of staining solutions on color stability, gloss and surface roughness of removable partial dental prosthetic polymers. J Prosthodont. 2022;31:65–71.
Polyzois G, Niarchou A, Ntala P, Pantopoulos A, Frangou M. The effect of immersion cleansers on gloss, colour and sorption of acetal denture base material. Gerodontology. 2013;30:150–6.
Sasaki H, Hamanaka I, Takahashi Y, Kawaguchi T. Effect of reinforcement on the flexural properties of injection-molded thermoplastic denture base resins. J Prosthodont. 2017;26:302–8.
Schierz O, Schmohl L, Hahnel S, Rauch A. Polyoxymethylene as material for removable partial dentures-a literature review and illustrating case report. J Clin Med. 2021;10:1458.
Sequeira AL, Narayan AI, George VT. Effects of nonaldehyde immersion disinfection on the mechanical properties of flexible denture materials. J Prosthet Dent. 2019;121:843–7.
Song SY, Kim KS, Lee JY, Shin SW. Physical properties and color stability of injection-molded thermoplastic denture base resins. J Adv Prosthodont. 2019;11:32–40.
Suh JS, Billy EJ. Rotational path removable partial denture (RPD): conservative esthetic treatment option for the edentulous mandibular anterior region: a case report. J Esthet Restor Dent. 2008;20:98–105.
Taguchi Y, Shimamura I, Sakurai K. Effect of buccal part designs of polyamide resin partial removable dental prosthesis on retentive force. J Prosthodont Res. 2011;55:44–7.
Takabayashi Y. Characteristics of denture thermoplastic resins for non-metal clasp dentures. Dent Mater J. 2010;29:353–61.
Tannous F, Steiner M, Shahin R, Kern M. Retentive forces and fatigue resistance of thermoplastic resin clasps. Dent Mater. 2012;28:273–8.
Tashiro S, Kawaguchi T, Hamanaka I, Takahashi Y. Bond strength of artificial teeth to thermoplastic denture base resin for injection molding. Dent Mater J. 2021;40:657–63.
The glossary of prosthodontic terms: ninth edition. J Prosthet Dent. 2017;117(5S):e1–e105.
Turner JW, Radford DR, Sherriff M. Flexural properties and surface finishing of acetal resin denture clasps. J Prosthodont. 1999;8:188–95.
Ucar Y, Akova T, Aysan I. Mechanical properties of polyamide versus different PMMA denture base materials. J Prosthodont. 2012;21:173–6.
Vozza I, Manzon L, Passarelli PC, Pranno N, Poli O, Grippaudo C. The effects of wearing a removable-partial-denture on the bite forces: a cross-sectional study. Int J Environ Res Public Health. 2021;18:11401.
Wada J, Fueki K, Yatabe M, Takahashi H, Wakabayashi N. A comparison of the fitting accuracy of thermoplastic denture base resins used in non-metal clasp dentures to a conventional heat-cured acrylic resin. Acta Odontol Scand. 2015;73:33–7.
Wieckiewicz M, Opitz V, Richter G, Boening KW. Physical properties of polyamide-12 versus PMMA denture base material. Biomed Res Int. 2014;2014:150298.
Zheng J, Aarts JM, Ma S, Waddell JN, Choi JJE. Different undercut depths influence on fatigue behavior and retentive force of removable partial denture clasp materials: a systematic review. J Prosthodont. 2023;32:108–15.

Establishing Occlusal Relationships

13

Tonguç Sülün

Abstract

Establishing occlusal relationships for partial edentulous patients is a critical step in ensuring proper function and long-term success of dental restorations. The process involves a comprehensive evaluation of the patient's occlusion, including tooth position, occlusal plane, and interocclusal distance. This evaluation helps the dentist determine the most appropriate occlusal scheme for the restoration, which may include bilateral balanced occlusion, group function, or canine guidance. Proper occlusal relationships can also help prevent occlusal trauma, tooth wear, and temporomandibular joint (TMJ) dysfunction. With careful consideration and planning, establishing occlusal relationships for partial edentulous patients can lead to successful, functional, and aesthetically pleasing restorations.

13.1 Definitions

Anterior guide pin: That component of an articulator, generally a rigid rod attached to one member, contacting the anterior guide table on the opposing member. It is used for the purpose of maintaining the established vertical separation. The anterior guide pin and table, together with the condylar elements, direct the movements of the articulators' separate members.

Arcon: A contraction of the words "articulator" and "condyle" used to describe an articulator containing the condylar path elements within its upper member and the condylar elements within the lower member.

Arcon articulator: An articulator that applies the arcon design; this instrument maintains anatomic guidelines by the use of condylar analogs in the mandibular element and fossae assemblies within the maxillary element.

Bennett angle: The angle formed between the sagittal plane and the average path of the advancing condyle as viewed in the horizontal plane during lateral mandibular movements.

Centric relation : A maxillomandibular relationship, independent of tooth contact, in which the condyles articulate in the anterior-superior position against the posterior slopes of the articular eminences; in this position, the mandible is restricted to a purely rotary movement; from this unstrained, physiologic, maxillomandibular relationship, the patient can make vertical, lateral or protrusive movements; it is a clinically useful, repeatable reference position.

Centric relation record: A registration of the relationship of the maxillae to the mandible when the mandible is in centric relation. The registra-

Supplementary Information The online version contains supplementary material available at https://doi.org/10.1007/978-3-031-47083-7_13.

T. Sülün (✉)
Faculty of Dentistry, Department of Prosthodontics, İstanbul University, İstanbul, Türkiye
e-mail: tsulun@istanbul.edu.tr

O. Şakar (ed.), *Removable Partial Dentures*, https://doi.org/10.1007/978-3-031-47083-7_13

tion may be obtained either intraorally or extraorally (synoym, ***checkbite***).

Curvilinear: Consisting of or bounded by curved lines; represented by a curved line.

Deprogrammer: Various types of devices or materials used to alter the proprioceptive mechanism during mandibular closure.

Gothic arch tracer: The device that produces a tracing that resembles an arrowhead or a gothic arch. The device is attached to the opposing arches. The shape of the tracing depends on the relative location of the marking point and the tracing table. The apex of a properly made tracing is considered to indicate centric relation.

Maximal intercuspal position: The complete intercuspation of the opposing teeth independent of condylar position, sometimes referred to as the best fit of the teeth regardless of the condylar position.

Split-cast mounting: 1. a procedure for placing indexed casts on an articulator to facilitate their removal and replacement on the instrument; 2. the procedure for verifying the accuracy of the maxillomandibular relation record (synoym, **split cast method**).

There are multiple ways to achieve a proper occlusion in a partially edentulous patient. It is important to know that every patient has individual functional and aesthetical needs and expectations. The clinician has to decide first if the existing natural or artificial occlusion of the patient is acceptable or if there is anything to change in intercuspal position and/or occlusal vertical dimension. In cases that require a reestablishment of the existing occlusion, a functional pretreatment is generally necessary.

When there is an extremely worn dentition, it may cause a decrease in the occlusal vertical dimension of the patient (Fig. 13.1a, b). So we have to reestablish a new one. However there are many cases with severely worn dentition where occlusal vertical dimension is not decreased. Up to date, there is no explanation in the literature that explains why the occlusal vertical dimension is somethimes preserved by the remodelling process in the alveolar bone and sometimes not. Nevertheless, the rehabilitation of these cases is the most challenging part of the prosthetic dentistry. Reestablishing the occlusal vertical dimension of these patients to achieve a sufficient interocclusal space will be explained in Chap. 21. However, it is important to point out here that this process may take 4–10 weeks. Only after a sufficient pretreatment procedure the final denture should be prepared.

In cases with decreased occlusal vertical dimension due to worn dentition or where the residual dentition has no occluding contacts, the recording of vertical jaw relations is nearly the same as in complete denture patients. This procedure will also be explained in Chap. 21.

First of all, it is important to decide whether there is an acceptable intercuspal position, if not, the centric relation (CR) of the patient should be recorded.

13.2 Deciding the Type of Horizontal Relation

13.2.1 Using the Maximal Intercuspal Position as a Reference

- Where the patient has no temporomandibular disorder (TMD) or functional problems in the stomatognathic system.

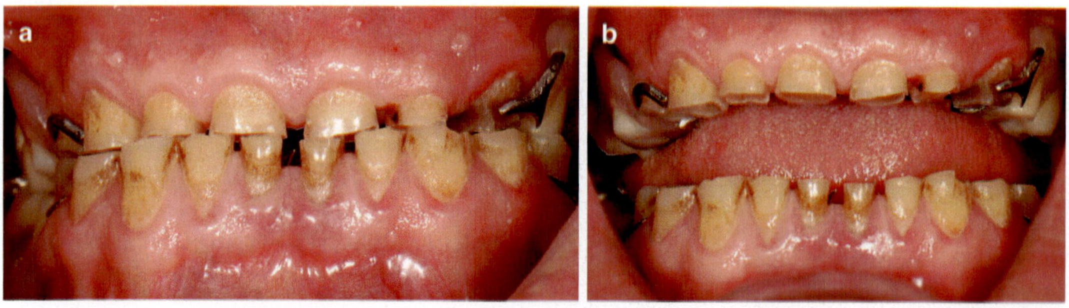

Fig. 13.1 (**a**) A patient with severely worn dentition with the removable partial denture in maximal intercuspal position. (**b**) Intraoral view of the existing removable partial dentures

- Where there is no need to change the occlusal vertical dimension.
- Where there are sufficient occluding posterior teeth.
- In patients with small gaps in dentition.

13.2.2 Using the Centric Relation as a Reference

- Where the patient has TMD or functional problems in the stomatognathic system.
- Where the occlusal vertical dimension needs to be increased.
- Where there are no occluding teeth or only the anteriors are in contact.
- Where complex treatment modalities, full mouth rehabilitation, etc. are needed.

13.2.3 Exceptional Cases in Using Maximal Intercuspal position/ Centric Relation as a Reference

- Geriatric patients with pseudo-prognathism. Because of the lack of the neuromuscular adaptation of these patients, it's logical to prefer the habitual intercuspal position as a reference.
- Patients with extreme Angle Class II Div 1 jaw relations (Fig. 13.2a, b).

These patients have an extreme dual bite which is present when the antero-posterior difference between the CR and maximal intercuspal position (MIP) exceeds 2 mm, and if two occlusal positions can easily be repeated. If the CR is recorded as a reference in these patients, a considerable overjet occurs in between the anterior teeth (Fig. 13.3). So the patient will never be able to close her/his jaw in a more anterior position. And if the maximum intercuspation is created in CR, a freedom-in-centric concept will not help. Obviously, because of the proprioceptive receptors in the periodontium, patients tend to close their mandible in a position with maximum tooth contact. Thus, the restorative occlusion and maximum intercuspation should be created in MIP and only then the occlusal equilibration should be prepared from MIP to CR, for both groups of patients. Finding and recording the MIP when there are no occluding teeth anymore is a challenging procedure. Owing to this difficulty, the best way is using an intra-oral gothic arch-tracing device. After the patient traces the gothic arch, the tip of the arrow will mark the surrounding counters of the metal plate. Then the surface is repainted and the patient is asked to tap her/his mandible several times. After a while, there is a gathering of points in the painted surface which is called the "adduction point." This point or area can now be used for recording the MIP (Figs. 13.4a, b and 13.5a–e).

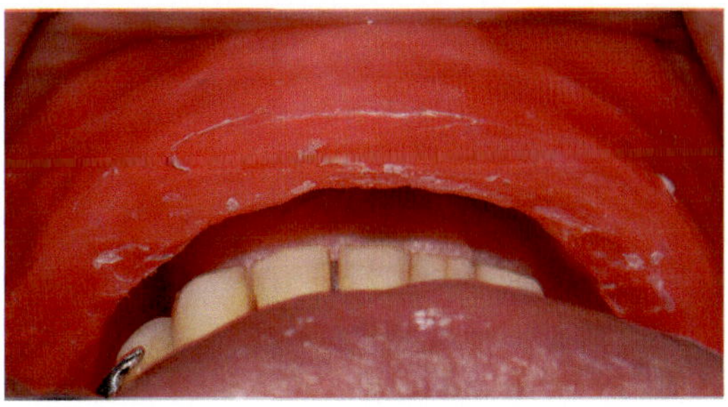

Fig. 13.3 A case with maxillary complete and mandibular Kennedy Class I edentulism. The occlusion in CR. Please notice the extreme overjet

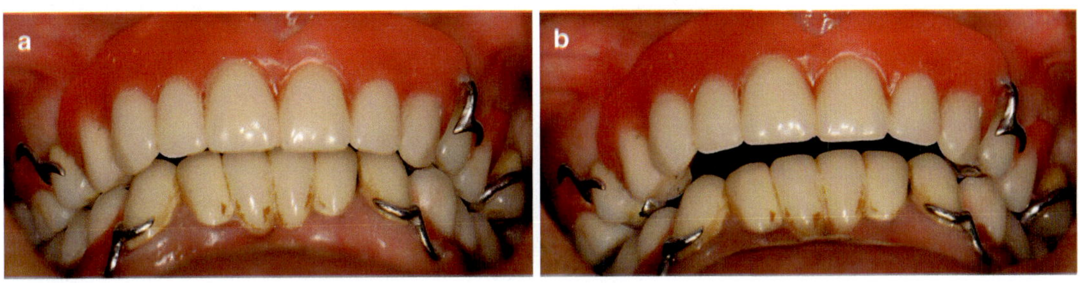

Fig. 13.2 (**a**) Intraoral view of the wax try-in of a removable partial denture in maximum intercuspal position. (**b**) Intraoral view of the wax try-in of a removable partial denture in CR

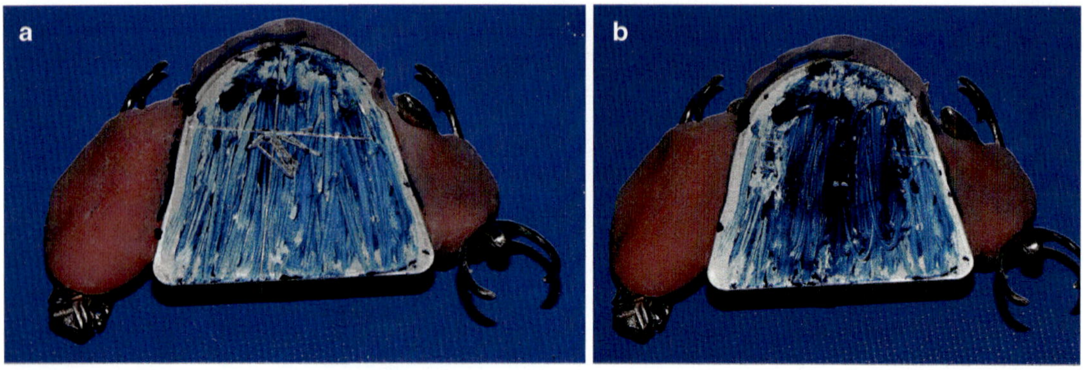

Fig. 13.4 (**a**) The gothic arch tracing of the case in Fig. 13.3. (**b**) The tapping point. Notice the difference between the tapping point and the apex of the gothic arch

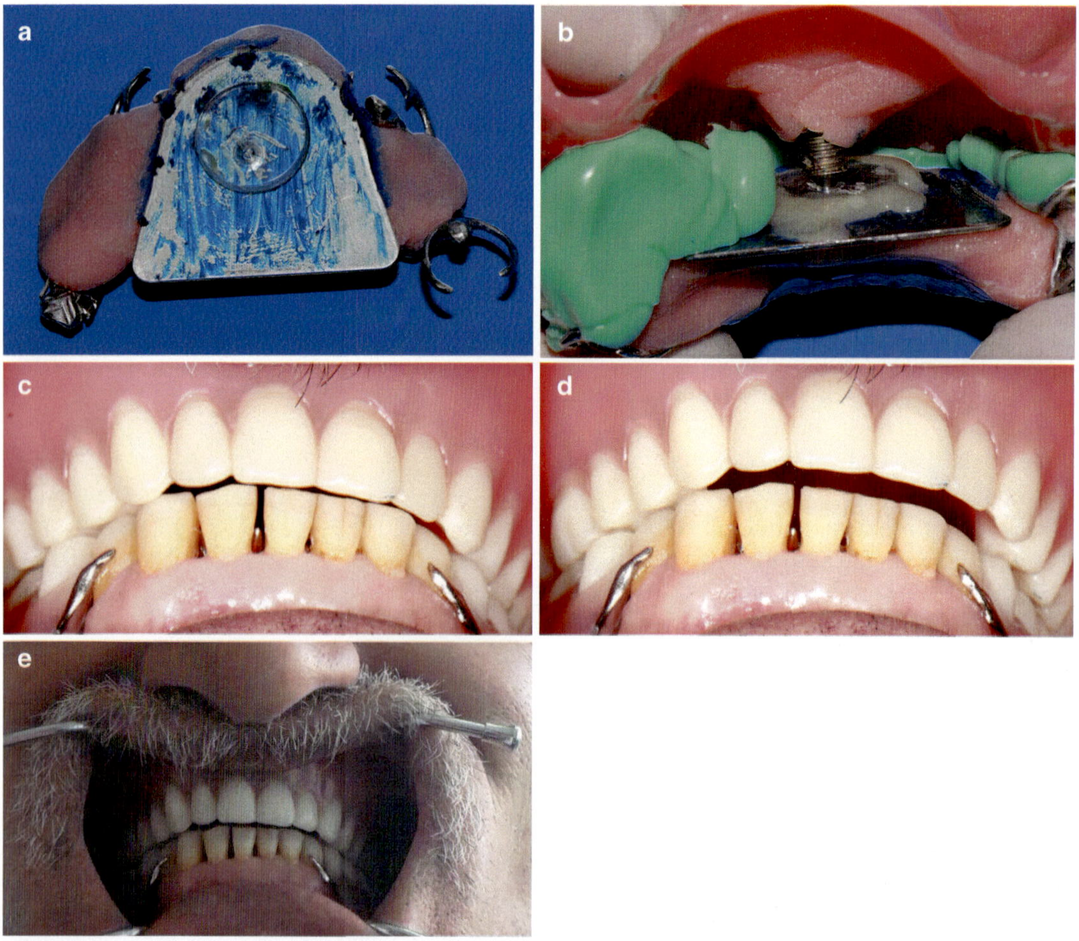

Fig. 13.5 (**a**) In this case the tapping point is chosen as a reference for centric record instead of the apex of the gothic arch. (**b**) The centric record. Lingual view. (**c**) The intraoral view of the prosthesis in MIP. (**d**) The intraoral view of the prosthesis in CR (**e**) The slide between MIP and CR (Video 13.1)

After deciding between MIP or CR as a reference, the next logical step is to choose the method for recording the horizontal jaw relations. According to the type of partial edentulism, we can use a base plate and occlusion rims or opt for the check-bite method.

13.3 Deciding the Type of Base Plate

13.3.1 Using a Base Plate (or Metal Framework) and Occlusion Rims to Record Horizontal Jaw Relations

- Where no teeth are in contact with the antagonist.
- Where the teeth are severely worn and the occlusal vertical dimension is decreased.
- Where just the anterior teeth are in contact.

13.3.2 Using Check-Bite Method to Record Horizontal Jaw Relations

- Where sufficient teeth are in contact with an acceptable occlusal relationship.
- Where sufficient teeth are in contact and there are some premature occlusal contacts with or without a major discrepancy between MIP and CR.

Using the check-bite method for recording the horizontal relationship is only preferred when mounting the master casts to the articulator. If the patient has an acceptable occlusion and no TMD or functional disorders of the masticatory system, the softened wax blocks or other materials like bite registration silicones can be used directly as recording materials. However in cases with occlusal discrepancies or disharmonies, we should use an anterior bite-plane (so-called deprogrammer): In some cases, a premature occlusal contact can be the reason of the destruction of the periodontal ligaments along with bacterial insertion and that may cause the mobility of the tooth. If the clinician does not use a deprogrammer between the anterior teeth, the patient will bite on the tooth and it will move to a wrong position resulting in failure of transferring the mandibular position with premature occlusal contact to the articulator.

In cases with discrepancies between MIP and CR and/or functional disorders of masticatory system, it is a challenging act to bring the mandible to the desired position. The deprogrammer behaves like a short-term occlusal splint to stabilize the muscles and temporomandibular joints (TMJ) of the patients.

An anterior bite plane which produces a gap of 1.5–2 mm between premolar teeth is an ideal construction. It is important to know that in patients with an uncontrolled and extreme bite force, it is preferable to use a deprogrammer made of an impression compound instead of acrylic resin. Because excessive biting on the anterior bite plane may cause a retrusive movement of the mandible especially if the surface inclination of the deprogrammer is not correctly perpendicular against the axis of mandibular anterior teeth. The anterior bite plane made of an impression compound will immediately crack if the patient bites intensely. Thus, this material plays a safety mechanism role for the gentle bite of the patient.

13.4 Articulators

First of all, to analyze the occlusion and to fabricate a potential interim prosthesis or an occlusal device, the above-mentioned records should be transferred to the articulator. There are basically two ways for this procedure:

- Positioning both maxillary and mandibular master casts with the bite registration according the instructions of the articulator company. As landmarks, the incisal pin and the two notches besides the articulator's frames are used. If these landmarks are used to correct the occlusion plane of the master casts, the positions will be usually in the center of the articulator and parallel to the floor.
- Using a face-bow to transfer the maxillary (usually) cast to the articulator. In current dental literature, there is a discussion about the necessity of face-bow usage.

13.4.1 Using Face-Bow

According to the *Glossary of Prosthetic Terms*, face-bow is an instrument used to record the spatial relationship of the maxillary arch to some anatomic reference point or points and then transfer this relationship to an articulator. So, by using a face-bow the distance between each tooth and center of condyles will be transferred just as it is in the skull. For a compass, if the distance between needle and printer differs, printer draws circles with a different radius. Just as here, teeth which have different distances from the center of rotation (condyle's or rather centers of articulators' condylar spheres) draw different circles during the opening and closing movement of mandible. This means, when changes are made in the occlusal vertical dimension or during adapting the casts with a recorded check-bite (without a contact of opposite dentitions), different ways of opening and closing occur. If a face-bow is used in the transfer, the opening and closing ways will be the same as it is in the patient's mouth. Therefore, changes that are made with the articulator will also be the same as in the mouth.

The theoretical situation described above is well known since the first face-bow was introduced by Snow in 1907. However, in recent years, prosthetic literature shows that benefits of face-bows do not affect the clinical success as previously expected. Scientific studies claim that the clinical success of the prosthesis tend not to change with or without using the face-bow. However, little information has been given about types of occlusion or morphological characteristics of patients included in these scientific studies. For an individual who has a normal-sized cranium and Angle Class I occlusal relation, the location of the casts which are transferred using a face-bow to the articulator is nearly the same as the location of the casts which are transferred arbitrarily (without using a face-bow). This occurs because articulators are fabricated in compliance with average characteristics of morphometric cranial properties and Class I occlusal relations. Thus, using a face-bow on normal individuals does not have a significant impact on the direction of opening and closing or functional pathways occurring during eccentric movements. Once this is acknowledged, the absence of a significant difference between treatment success and patient satisfaction should be regarded as normal.

Situations requiring face-bow usage can be outlined as following:

In cases with prognathia inferior or retrognati inferior, extremely small or gigantic skeletal structure and laterognathia.

In cases with normal occlusion and morphometric characteristics, a face-bow transfer should only be applied if a full-mouth fixed prosthetic rehabilitation especially with gnathological problems is indicated.

In all other cases, like fixed partial dentures with a few units and removable partial dentures, the use of a face-bow is up to the practitioner's preference.

13.4.2 Important Aspects of Articulator Selection

Articulators are devices used by dentists and dental technicians. But prosthetic procedures can be easier and faster only if these two professions work harmoniously together. During intensive clinical work, it is difficult for a dentist to spare time for laboratory procedures such as mounting casts and adjusting articulators. These procedures are mainly applied by the dental technician alone. However, in order to provide the necessary guidance, the dentist should know about articulators as much as the dental technician. By the same token, although face-bow applications are only performed by a dentist, a technician should have the practical and theoretical knowledge about face-bow as he/she is the one transferring face-bow records to the articulator. Therefore, the dentists and technicians should encourage each other to work with the same articulator system to eliminate any deficiency.

The following titles describe the properties of a suitable articulator. In the market, there is an abundance of articulators possessing these properties. Be it as it may, the dentist should go for the same articulator used by his technician. In such cases, the dentist no longer has to send the face-bow to the technician, but only the appropriate part, the biting fork with the wax record will prove sufficient. The technician can readily transfer the face-bow recording to an articulator produced by the same company. Needless to say, in order to perform all these procedures correctly, the articulators have to be calibrated by the company beforehand.

13.4.3 Properties of a Suitable Articulator

1. Has to be Rigid

It is an indispensable point for an articulator to be made of a rigid material. It is impossible to maintain centric relation correctly for an articulator which is made of a flexible and deformable material.

2. Should Maintain the Centric Relation

The most important property of an articulator is maintaining the CR, so the articulator should be rigid and should have an efficient centric lock mechanism. This is especially crucial for arcon articulators. Non-arcon articulators however can maintain CR very easily due to their typical structure.

3. Should Receive Face-Bow Recording

The classification of modern articulators was altered due to their ability of face-bow transfer. Face-bows are indispensable elements for an articulator to mimic real jaw movements. If casts are mounted without face-bow records, the articulator will not be able to imitate mandibular movements even if it has been adjusted precisely.

4. Should Have a Vertical Pin and Incisive Table

Articulators should maintain intermaxillary relations accurately. Also occlusal vertical dimension should be determined carefully for the prosthetic procedures. This can be preserved only if the device has a vertical pin. Within the determined vertical relation, changes during the prosthesis construction can be monitored by the dental technician and clinician. In addition, the numerical values of occlusal vertical dimension changes can also be recorded.

Almost all of the articulators have an incisive table. Not only the condylar path inclination but also the incisive path inclination should be individually adjustable. Incisive table can be adjusted in three different ways:

- It can be adjusted in lateral and protrusive ways with the screws (e.g., Dentatus).
- It can be adjusted by choosing the appropriate angled table (e.g., Gerber Condylator).
- Cold-curing acrylic resin is put on the the incisive table and the incisive path inclination can be adjusted by moving the vertical pin with the guidance of casts (e.g., SAM). After polymerization of the resin, an individually adjusted incisive table is ready to use. This procedure is used especially in cases which have anterior fixed hybrid rehabilitation. Primary casts which are made from unprepared tooth impressions are mounted to the articulator. Then the acrylic table is formed by using casts' incisive path inclination. After the preparation of the teeth, casts for the fixed restorations can be constructed by using this acrylic incisive table.

5. Protrusive Condylar Path Should Be Adjustable and Curvilinear

The condylar pathways of the average value articulators are not adjustable. There is no objection to use these articulators with simple restorations stated above. However, an articulator should lend itself for all kind of prosthetic works. At the end of the day, the choice of utilizing various abilities should be left to the dentist's preference depending on the type of the prosthetic procedure. One should also be reminded that the individually adjusted protrusive condylar path provides a customized occlusal morphology of the posterior teeth and a palatal concavity of the upper incisors as well.

In this method, protrusive records are completed following the centric record at the same appointment. Later upper and lower casts are mounted to the articulator using centric records. The centric locks are loosened in order to allow eccentric movements. Protrusive records are placed on the lower teeth and the upper casts are seated on it while the condylar path inclination of the device is fixed to 30°. If both of the patient's condyle protrusive condylar path inclinations are not 30°, the upper casts can't match with the record. For both sides, the protrusive condylar path inclination is moved above and below 30°, until the upper casts are properly seated; thus, this will be the patient's individual protrusive condylar path inclination. Doing this method with an upper cast which is mounted with the split-cast method is a more reliable way in avoiding the deformation of the bite registration material.

An appropriate articulator should have not only an adjustable condylar mechanism, but also this mechanism should have a correct curvilinear design. For an articulator with a linear condylar path, it is simply impossible to mimic natural mandibular movements.

6. Should Simulate the Bennett Movement (Figs. 13.6, 13.7, 13.8, 13.9, 13.10 and 13.11)

Bennett movement is known as 1 mm entire shifting of the mandible during lateral movement. Timing of this lateral shifting can be different. Immediate side shift is defined as shifting of the mandible at the beginning of the mandibular movement followed by the rotation of the working side condyle and moving of the non-working side condyle in an anterior, medial and caudal direction. This movement is observed in 80% of the population, yet it is hard to record. Because this movement occurs at the beginning of chewing hard food, as the food softens, the range of the movement decreases. This motion has an impact on the occlusal morphology. In a person

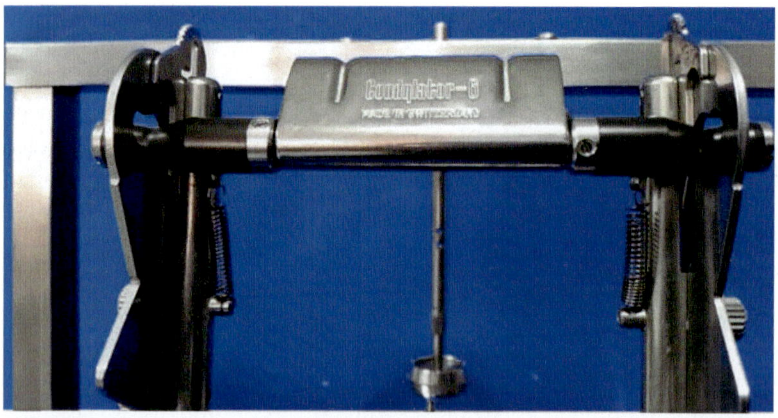

Fig. 13.6 The articular mechanism of the Gerber Condylator. The latero-protrusive movement (Video 13.2)

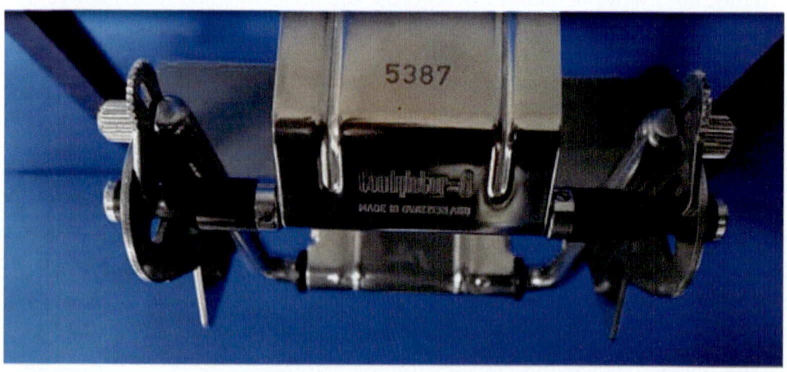

Fig. 13.7 The articular mechanism of the Gerber Condylator. The pure lateral movement (Bennett movement). Upper view (Video 13.3)

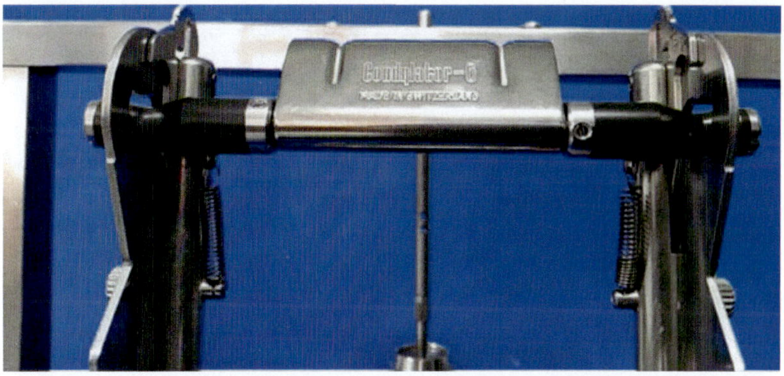

Fig. 13.8 The articular mechanism of the Gerber Condylator. The pure lateral movement (Bennett movement). Back view (Video 13.4)

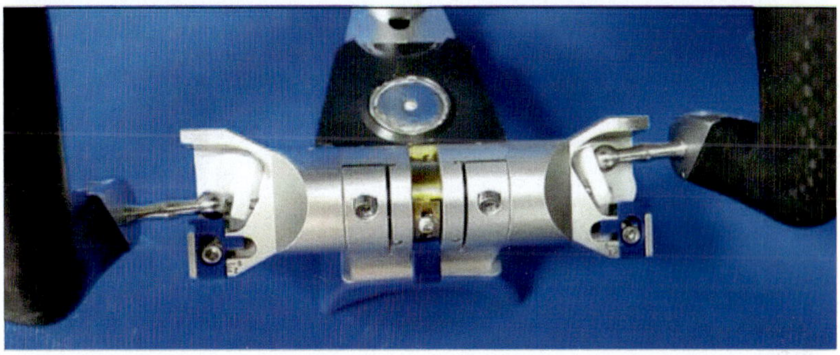

Fig. 13.9 The articular mechanism of the Girbach Artex articulator. The latero-protrusive movement (Video 13.5)

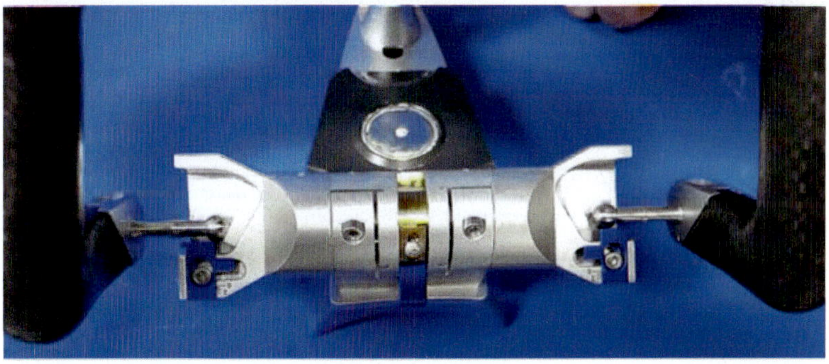

Fig. 13.10 The articular mechanism of the Girbach Artex articulator. The pure lateral movement (Bennett movement) (Video 13.6)

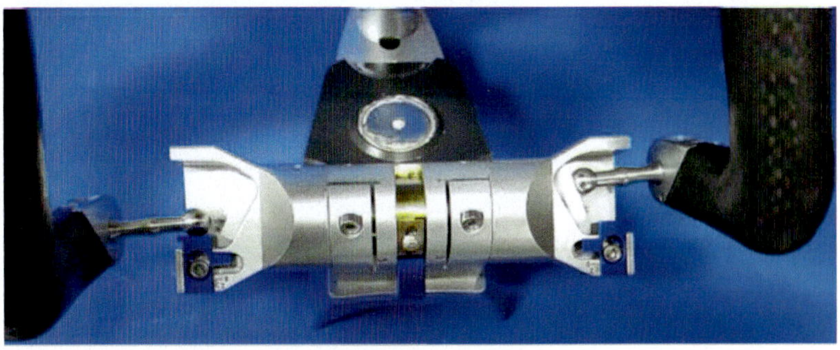

Fig. 13.11 The articular mechanism of the Girbach Artex articulator. The latero-protrusive movement with immediate side shift (Video 13.7)

who has immediate side-shift movement, the angle between latero-mediotrusive functional ways is larger on the occlusal surfaces of the molars. If a person can do this movement where the articulator cannot, the functional ways of prosthesis are going to be formed with steeper angles. And when this prosthesis is used by the patient, there will certainly be occlusal interferences between cusps while chewing hard food. This happens especially on nonworking side. It is nearly impossible to determine this interference in the mouth. In patients with complete dentures, this interferences cause destabilization of lower denture and sore points at mandible. Also with fixed prosthesis, repeated fractures on occlusal surfaces of second molars, periodontal problems of the same tooth, and also myofascial pain at masseter muscle should be expected. Therefore, a patient will be more satisfied with his/her prosthesis that is produced using an articulator that contains an immediate-side-shift mechanism.

7. Should Simulate the Retrusive Movement (Figs. 13.12 and 13.13)

Most of the articulators are capable of making lateral and protrusive movements and some of them are even individually adjustable. Nevertheless, most of them cannot mimic the retrusive movement, which has an importance in chewing as shown by Gerber and Pretti for many years. In some cases horizontal jaw relations have to be recorded in MIP and then the occlusion has to be adjusted in direction to CR. Thus, an articulator with a retrusion mechanism is necessary. Otherwise, the clinician should adjust the occlusion by grinding the restoration to create the retrusive facets which will damage the occlusal morphology and cause waste of time at the chair site.

Commercially available articulators may differ from each other in retrusive mechanisms. For example, while the direction of the retral movement of Artex (Girbach) articulator is backward and upward, this direction in Gerber Condylator

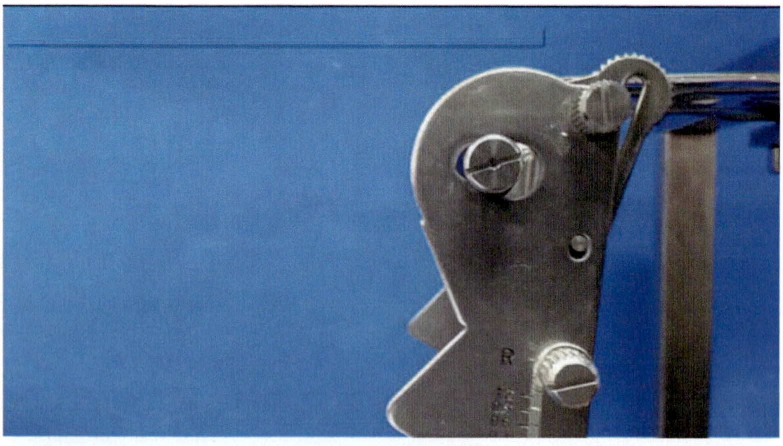

Fig. 13.12 The articular mechanism of the Gerber Condylator. The protrusive and retrusive movement (Video 13.8)

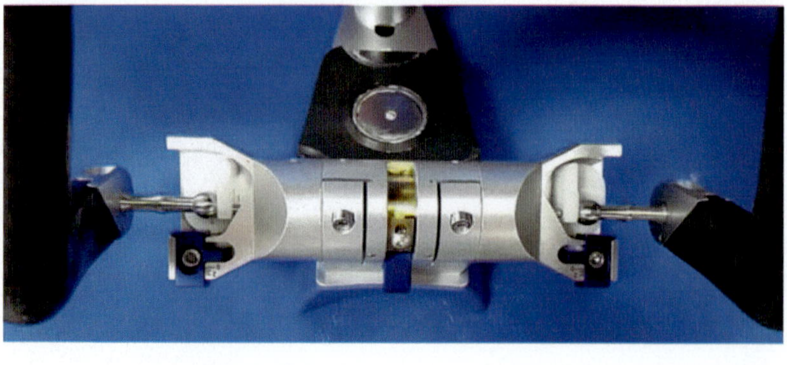

Fig. 13.13 The articular mechanism of the Girbach Artex articulator. The retrusive movement (Video 13.9)

is backward and downward. A study in recent years encouraged that both movement patterns may occur in natural dentition.

13.5 Clinical Procedure

After checking the fit and occlusal relation to the antagonist teeth of the metal framework it can be used as a base plate (Fig. 13.14). The denture base retentive mesh of the framework has a distal tissue stop in free-ending cases. However, this stop is mostly not sufficient because of the varied mucosa flexibility. Therefore, prior to the occlusion rims the clinician should create a wax stop between the retentive mesh and the tissue surface of the cast. First a softened wax is placed on the cast and the heated metal framework is then placed on the cast. It is dangerous to heat the metal casting on the flame because of the overheating risk. Therefore, heating the framework in boiled water is safer. The dentist should concentrate on visualizing the fit of all component of the framework on the cast. After placing the cast into cold water, the metal framework is removed from the cast and the excess wax under the major and minor connectors and guiding surfaces is scraped apart (Fig. 13.15). The framework is then rechecked for the perfect fit in the mouth and the occlusion rims are formed on the casts (Fig. 13.16). First the maxillary framework with occlusion rims is placed in the mouth and the occlusal plane is adjusted parallel to the Camper's plane and the straight line between the pupils (Fig. 13.17). In cases with infra- or supra-erupted existing teeth or in cases where the occlusal plane is not parallel to these planes and the patient is reluctant to the preparation of the teeth, the occlusion rims are formed accordingly. After the occlusal plane is formed on the occlusion rims, the buccal contact of the occlusion rim is created. The occlusion rims should have a

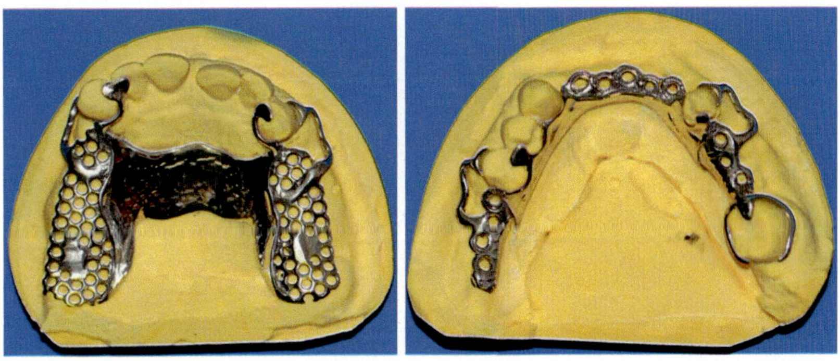

Fig. 13.14 The metal frameworks that will be used as base plates

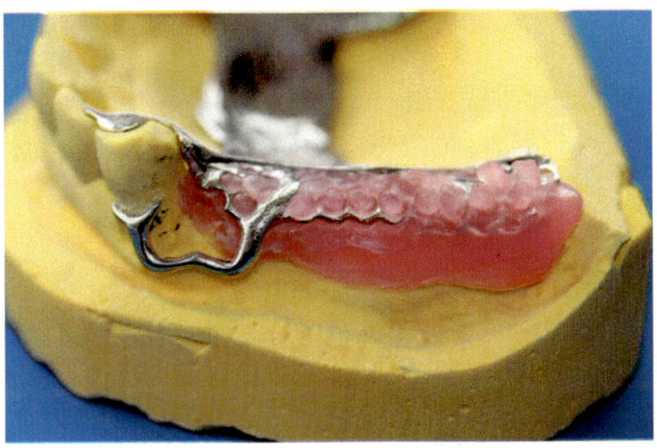

Fig. 13.15 The retentive mesh of the metal framework is supported with wax

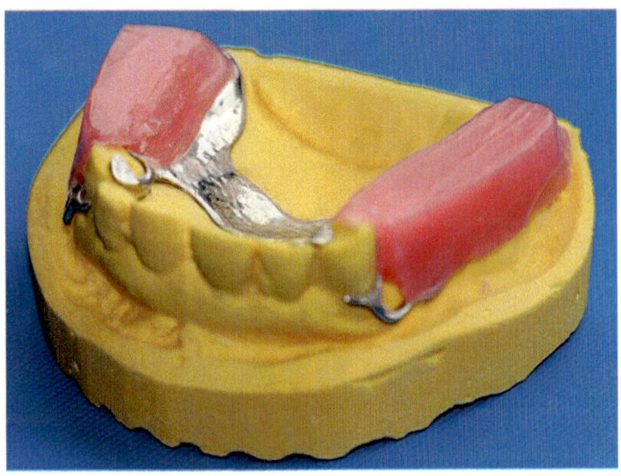

Fig. 13.16 The occlusion rim is finished for the record of vertical and horizontal intermaxillary relations

gentle contact with the buccal mucosa (Fig. 13.18). Only now, the mandibular metal framework with occlusion rims can be placed in the mouth to decide on the vertical and horizontal intermaxillary relationship (Fig. 13.19). If there is no antagonist of occluding teeth the occlusal vertical dimension is determined same as in complete denture fabrication. If there are occluding teeth the occlusal vertical dimension should mostly not be altered. However in cases with decreased occlusal vertical dimension, the cast analysis should be carried out before the metal frameworks are fabricated. As mentioned before, the CR is determined and recorded in most of the cases in CR. However in Angle Class II Div 1 patients and pseudoprognathic cases, the MIP should be preferred. Prior to the fixation of the centric relation record, a face-bow record can be done if deemed necessary (Fig. 13.20a, b). After that, the centric relation record is made using a bite silicone material (Fig. 13.21). The frameworks are placed to the casts and the record is checked accordingly (Fig. 13.22). As a final step, casts are transferred to the articulator and the arrangement of the artificial teeth is now finished (Chap. 14) (Fig. 13.23a, c).

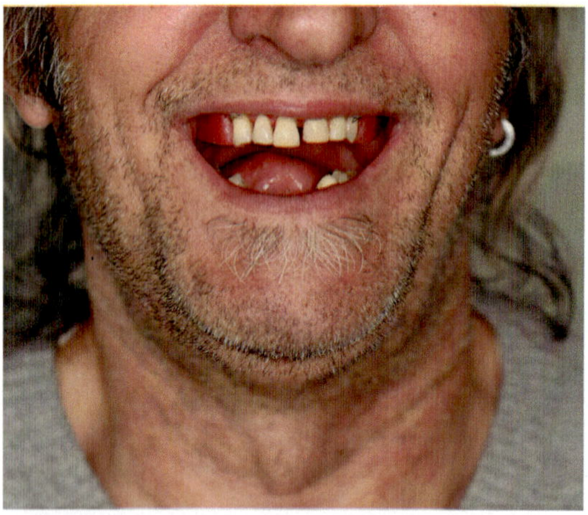

Fig. 13.17 The upper occlusion rim in the mouth of the patient. The occlusal plane is adjusted first

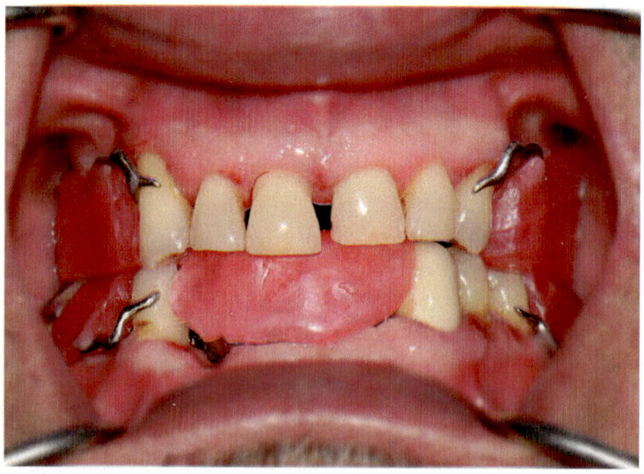

Fig. 13.19 The vertical and horizontal intermaxillary relations are adjusted

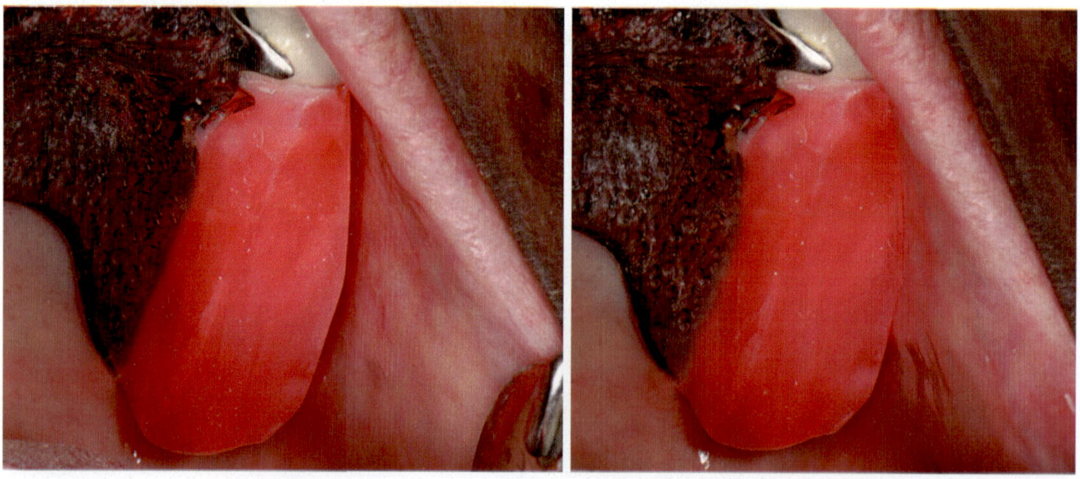

Fig. 13.18 The upper occlusion rim in the mouth of the patient. Please notice the contact between buccal mucosa and occlusion rim

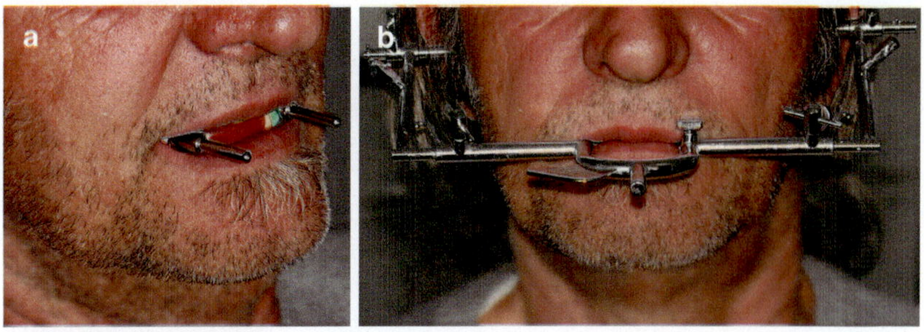

Fig. 13.20 (**a**) The intra-oral metal frame of the face-bow is adapted on the mandibular arch. (**b**) The face-bow transfer

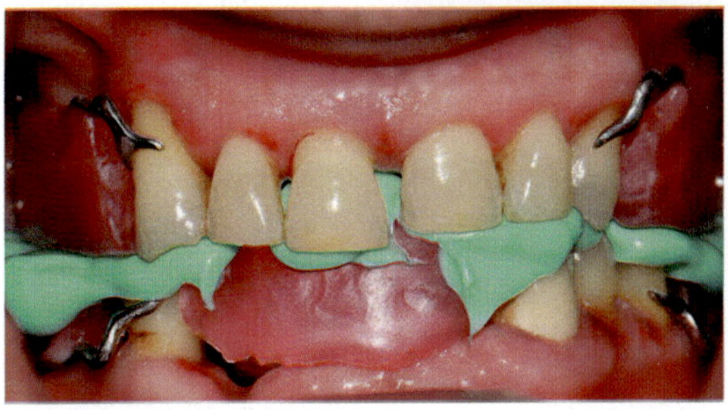

Fig. 13.21 After the face-bow transfer the centric relation record is made

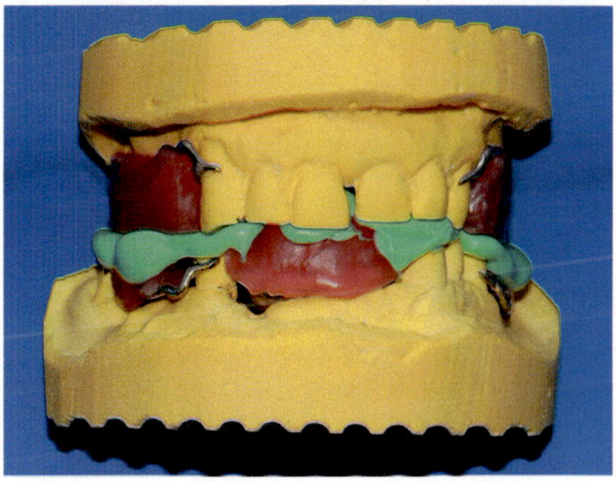

Fig. 13.22 The centric relation record is checked with the casts

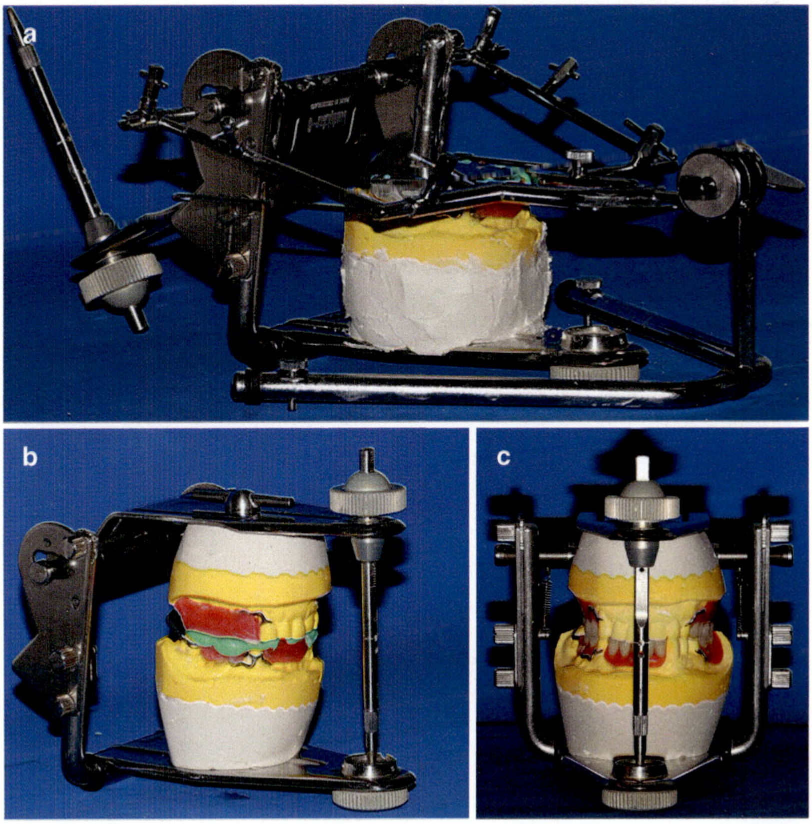

Fig. 13.23 (**a**) First the mandibular cast is transferred to the articulator using face-bow record. (**b**) Afterward the maxillary cast is transferred to the articulator using centric relation record. (**c**) The teeth arrangement is finished

Further Reading

Al-Fahd AA. Facebow transfer does not achieve better clinical results than simpler approaches in complete denture prosthodontics. J Evid Based Dent Pract. 2016;16:182–3.

Amorim VC, Laganá DC, de Paula Eduardo JV, Zanetti AL. Analysis of the condyle/fossa relationship before and after prosthetic rehabilitation with maxillary complete denture and mandibular removable partial denture. J Prosthet Dent. 2003;89:508–14.

Beck HO. Choosing the articulator. J Am Dent Assoc. 1962;64:468–74.

Carlsson GE. Some dogmas related to prosthodontics, temporomandibular disorders and occlusion. Acta Odontol Scand. 2010;68:313–22.

Carr A, Brown D, McCracken W. McCracken's removable partial prosthodontics.13th ed. St. Louis, MO: Elsevier Mosby; 2015.

Collet HA. The movements of temporomandibular joints and their relation to the problems of occlusion. J Prosthet Dent. 1955;5:486–96.

Davies SJ, Gray RM, McCord JF. Good occlusal practice in removable prosthodontics. Br Dent J. 2001;191:670.

Egermark-Eriksson I, Carlsson GE, Ingervall B. Function and dysfunction of the masticatory system in individuals with dual bite. Eur J Orthod. 1979;1:107–17.

Eliss E 3rd, Tharanon W, Gabgrell K. Accuracy of face bow transfer: effect on surgical prediction and post surgical result. J Oral Maxillo Fac Surg. 1992;50:562–7.

Ellinger CW, Wesley RC, Abadi BJ, Armentrout TM. Patient response to variations in denture technique. Part VII: twenty-year patient status. J Prosthet Dent. 1989;62:45–8.

Ferrario VF, Forza C, Mianni A Jr, Serrao G, Tartaklia G. Open-close movements in the human temporomandibular joint: does a pure rotation around the intercondylar hinge exist? J Oral Rehabil. 1996;23:401–8.

Gerber A. Kiefergelenk und Zahnokklusion DZZ 1971; 26:119–141.

Gerber A. Okkusiondiagnostik bei defektem und prosthetisch versogtem Gebbiss. Zahnaerztliche Welt. 1978;87:436–47.

Gernet W, Beuer F. Zahnärztliche Prothetik. Stuttgart: Thieme; 2007.

Goska JR, Christensen LV. Comparison of cast positions by using four face bows. J Prosthet Dent. 1988;59:42–4.

Graber G, Besimo C, Wiehl P, Rateitschak K. Farbatlanten der Zahnmedizin. Stuttgart: Thieme; 1992.

Grossmann Y, Sadan A. The prosthodontic concept of crown-to-root ratio: a review of the literature. J Prosthet Dent. 2005;93:559–62.

Kinderdnecht KE, Vonk GK, Billy EJ, Li SH. The effect of deprogrammer on the position of the terminal transverse horizontal axis of the mandible. J Prosthet Dent. 1992;68:123–31.

Kotwall KR. The need to use arbitrary face-bow when remonuting complete dentures with inter occlusal records. J Prosthet Dent. 1979;42:224–7.

Loney RW. Removable partial denture manual. Halifax, NS: Dalhousie University Faculty of Dentistry; 2011. http://removpros.dentistry.dal.ca/ewExternalFiles/RPD%20Manual%2011.pdf.

Miller E, Grasso J. Removable partial prosthodontics. Baltimore, MA: Williams & Wilkins; 1981.

Mohl ND, Zarb GA, Carlsson GE. Lehrbuch der Okklusion. Berlin: Quintessenz Verlags-GmbH; 1990.

Morneburg T, Pröshcel HA. Differences between traces adjacent condlylar points and their impact on clinical evaluation of condyle motion. Int J Prosthodont. 1998;11:317–24.

Öwall B, Kaeyser AF, Carlsson GE. Prosthodontics. Principles and management strategies. Mosby-Wolfe Pub; 1996.

Palla S. Dr. A. Gerber, a European pioneer in the craniomandibular field. Cranio. 1988;6:1; Guest Editorial.

Piehslinger E, Celar A, Celar R, Jager W, Slavicek R. Reproducibility of the condylar reference position. J Orofac Pain. 1993;7:68–75.

Preti G. Prosthetic rehabilitation. London: Quintessence Pub; 2008

Rues S, Lenz J, Türp JC, Schweizerhof K, Schindler HJ. Muscle and joint forces under variable equilibrium states of the mandible. Clin Oral Investig. 2011;15:737–47.

Santos JJ. Occlusion. Chicago, IL: Quintessence Pub. Co.; 2007.

Simpson JW, Hesby RA, Pfeifer DL, Pelleu GB Jr. Arbitrary mandibular hinge axis locations. J Prosthet Dent. 1984;51:819–22.

Strub JR, Türp JC, Witkowski S, Hürzeler MB, Kern M. Curriculum Prothetik. Band 3. Qintessenz Verlag; 2005. p. 467–75.

The glossary of prosthodontic terms: ninth edition. J Prosthet Dent. 2017;117(5S):e1–e105.

Thorp ER, Smith DE, Nicholls JI. Evaluation of the use of a face bow in complete denture occlusion. J Prosthet Dent. 1978;39:5–15.

von Stein-Lausnitz M, Schmid S, Blankenstein FH, Peroz I, Beuer F, Sterzenbach G. Influence of a face-bow on oral health-related quality of life after changing the vertical dimension in the articulator: a randomized controlled trial. Part II. Clin Oral Investig. 2018;22:433–42.

von Stein-Lausnitz M, Sterzenbach G, Helm I, Zorn A, Blankenstein FH, Ruge S, Kordaß B, Beuer F, Peroz

I. Does a face-bow lead to better occlusion in complete dentures? A randomized controlled trial: part I. Clin Oral Investig. 2018;22:773–82.
Yamashita S, Ai M, Hashii K, Akiyama S, Koike H, Numao H. Relationship between tooth contacts in the retruded contact position and mandibular positioning during retrusion. J Oral Rehabil. 2006;33:800–6.
Yuan JC, Sukotjo C. Occlusion for implant-supported fixed dental prostheses in partially edentulous patients: a literature review and current concepts. J Periodont Implant Sci. 2013;43:51–7.

Surveying and Laboratory Procedures

14

Burç Gençel and Max Bosshart

Abstract

The quality of prosthetic rehabilitation highly depends on the level of collaboration between the dentist and the dental technician. The technician provides material for clinical procedures by processing the material delivered from the clinic. The quantity and the quality of material delivered to the dental laboratory draw the borders to the dental technician. For example, the fit of a custom impression tray to the impression area can at most be as good as its fit to the cast that it is constructed on which is bound to the quality of the preliminary impression. Written and verbal communication is another key factor to achieve better results from physical materials exchanged after each phase of the overall treatment. Throughout this reciprocal workflow, the responsibility of the outcome is on the clinician. Therefore, in addition to performing proper clinical work, the dentist must be equipped with not necessarily the ability but the knowledge of laboratory procedures to be able to manage the overall process accordingly. Clinicians' use of a dental surveyor in planning and designing removable partial dentures (RPDs) improves the quality of preprosthetic preparations and the resultant prosthesis. The basic principles of surveying and steps of laboratory procedures are summarized in this chapter.

B. Gençel (✉)
Dental Laboratory Technology Program, İstanbul University-Cerrahpaşa, İstanbul, Türkiye
e-mail: bgencel@iuc.edu.tr

M. Bosshart
Dental Technology Center Zurich, Zurich, Switzerland

14.1 Definitions

Angle of gingival convergence: The angle of gingival convergence is located apical to the height of contour on the abutment tooth; it can be identified by viewing the angle formed by the tooth surface gingival to the survey line and the analyzing rod or undercut gauge of a surveyor as it contacts the height of contour.

CAD-CAM: Acronym for Computer-Aided Design-Computer-Aided Manufacturing (or Computer-Assisted Machining): the Computer Numerical Control (CNC) subtractive fabrication of a 3D object; in dentistry, it is a CAD-CAM technology used to produce different types of prostheses, including crowns, veneers, inlays, onlays, fixed dental prostheses, removable dental prostheses, dental implant prostheses, and orthodontic and other devices.

Clasp assembly: The part of a removable partial denture that acts as a direct retainer and/or stabilizer for a prosthesis by partially encompassing or contacting an abutment tooth. Components of the clasp assembly include the retentive clasp,

O. Şakar (ed.), *Removable Partial Dentures*, https://doi.org/10.1007/978-3-031-47083-7_14

reciprocal clasp, cingulum/incisal or occlusal rest, and minor connector.

Dental plaster: The beta-form of calcium sulfate hemihydrate; a fibrous aggregate of fine crystals with capillary pores that are irregular in shape and porous in character.

Dental stone: The alpha-form of calcium sulfate hemihydrate with physical properties superior to the beta-form (dental plaster); the alpha-form, a-calcium sulfate hemihydrate, is created when the dihydrate of gypsum is heated under steam pressure resulting in the formation of dense rods or prisms, and is, therefore, more dense than the b-calcium sulfate hemihydrate (dental plaster). Synonym, **Gypsum**.

Direct metal laser sintering: Acronym is DMLS. An additive CAM technique which uses a sintering of metal alloy powder to develop 3D objects.

Guiding planes: Two or more vertically parallel surfaces on abutment teeth and/or fixed dental prostheses oriented so as to contribute to the direction of the path of placement and removal of a removable partial denture, maxillofacial prosthesis, and overdenture. Synonym, **Guiding planes**.

Infrabulge clasp: A removable partial denture retentive clasp that approaches the retentive undercut from a cervical or infrabulge direction.

Lingualized occlusion: This form of denture occlusion articulates the maxillary lingual cusps with the mandibular occlusal surfaces in centric occlusion, working and nonworking mandibular positions.

Occlusion rim: Occluding surfaces fabricated on interim or final denture bases for the purpose of making maxillomandibular relation records and arranging teeth. Synonym, **Record rim**.

Parallelometer: (1) An instrument used for determining the exact parallel relationships of lines, structures, and surfaces in dental casts and prostheses; (2) an apparatus used for making one object parallel with another object, as in paralleling attachments and abutments for fixed dental prostheses or precision attachments for removable dental prostheses. Synonym, **Surveyor**.

Path of insertion: The specific direction in which a prosthesis is placed on the residual alveolar ridge, abutment teeth, dental implant abutment(s), or attachments. Synonym, **Path of placement**.

Reciprocal clasp: A component of the clasp assembly specifically designed to provide reciprocation by engaging a reciprocal guiding plane; it counteracts the action of the clasp during removal and insertion of a removable partial denture. Synonyms, **Bracing arm and Reciprocal arm**.

Reciprocation: (1) The mechanism by which lateral forces generated by a retentive clasp passing over a height of contour are counterbalanced by a reciprocal clasp passing along a reciprocal guiding plane.

Retentive clasp: (1) A clasp specifically designed to provide retention by engaging an undercut; (2) a flexible segment of a removable partial denture that engages an undercut on an abutment and that is designed to retain the prosthesis. Synonym, **Retention arm**.

RPD: Acronym for Removable Partial Denture. A removable denture that replaces some teeth in a partially edentulous arch; the removable partial denture can be readily inserted and removed from the mouth by the patient.

Stabilizing circumferential clasp: A circumferential clasp that is relatively rigid and contacts the height of contour of the tooth without retentive force.

Stereolithography: Acronym is SLA; a computer numerical control (CNC) additive fabrication of an object; in dentistry, it relates to the laser initiation of light-reactive resin layering to make replicas of casts and devices; alternative to processes of casting, injection molding and vacuum thermoforming.

Suprabulge: That portion of a tooth or crown that converges toward the occlusal surface above the height of contour.

Suprabulge clasp: Any removable partial denture retentive clasp that approaches the retentive undercut from an occlusal or suprabulge direction.

Survey: (1) To examine as to condition, value, or situation; to appraise; (2) to determine the form and position of a given entity by means of taking linear and angular measurements; (3) to inspect or scrutinize; (4) the procedure of locating and delineating the contour and position of the abutment teeth and associated structures before designing a removable partial denture.

Survey line: A line produced on a cast by a surveyor marking the greatest prominence of contour in relation to the planned path of placement of a restoration. Synonym, **Height of contour**.

Surveyed diagnostic cast for removable partial denture: A diagnostic cast before tooth preparations with essential survey for diagnosis and treatment planning for a removable partial denture; the cast is used to determine an acceptable path of placement, guiding planes, location and measurement of retentive undercuts indicative with clasp flexibility, location of tooth and bony interferences, a favorable design relative to aesthetics, charting of existing foundation restorations relative to design, location of occlusal contacts relative to design, location of horizontal height of contours, and placement of tripodal marks.

Surveyed definitive cast for removable partial denture: A master cast after tooth preparations with survey for blockout and duplication or optical scan for a removable partial denture; this cast is used to determine an acceptable path of placement, guiding planes, location and measurement of retentive undercuts indicative with clasp flexibility, location of tooth and bony undercuts, location of occlusal contacts relative to design, location of horizontal height of contours, and placement of tripodal marks.

Surveying: An analysis and comparison of the prominence of intraoral contours associated with the fabrication of a dental prosthesis.

Surveyor: A paralleling instrument used in making a dental prosthesis to locate and delineate the contours and relative positions of abutment teeth and associated structures. Synonym, **Parallelometer**.

Undercut: (1) The portion of the surface of an object that is below the height of contour in relationship to the path of placement; (2) the contour of a cross-sectional portion of a residual ridge or dental arch that prevents the insertion of a dental prosthesis; (3) any irregularity in the wall of a prepared tooth that prevents the withdrawal or seating of a wax pattern or indirect restoration.

14.2 Surveying

14.2.1 Structural Units of a Surveyor

Basically a surveyor is used to analyze the axial surfaces of teeth and other areas of a cast in relation to vertical plane. There are almost a dozen different designs of surveyors; however, all of them function according to the simple principle of the first parallelometer that Fortunati used in 1918.

Main structural components of a surveyor are a horizontal bench with a cast holder which is capable of tilting and a vertical arm hanging at a right angle to the bench which works with the surveying tools. The tilting table of the cast holder allows the individual horizontal plane for each cast to be adjusted, so that the vertical arm functions perpendicularly to this acquired horizontal plane. The vertical arm can move up and down and its position can be fixed at any point. The functions of the surveying tools around the axial surfaces of the cast can be provided by the sliding ability of the cast holder over the bench top or the roaming ability of the vertical arm over the horizontal plane, which depends on the design of the surveyor; however most available models are decorated with both functions which provide easy and smooth operation. Main tools of surveying are the analyzing rod, carbon marker, and undercut gauges. The analyzing rod visuals the surfaces in relation to vertical plane, the carbon marker basically draws the survey line, and undercut gauges measure the depth of undercuts. Carving knife is also a useful tool especially during the evaluation of abutment teeth (Fig. 14.1).

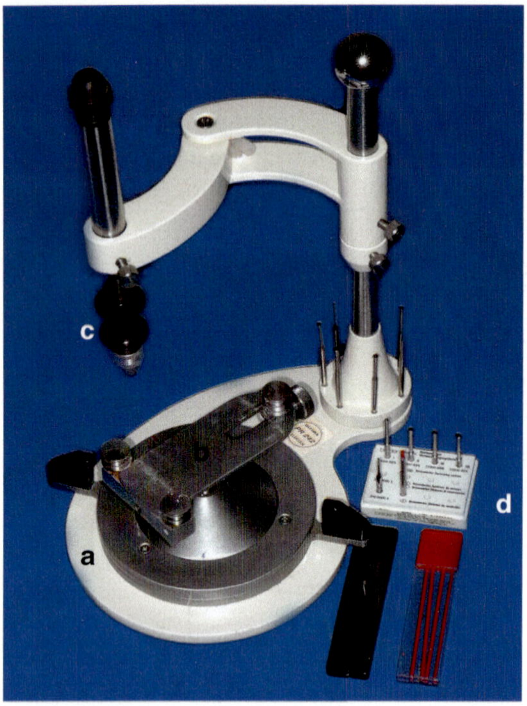

Fig. 14.1 Structural units and accessories of a surveyor. (**a**) Horizontal bench (**b**) Cast holder (**c**) Vertical arm (**d**) Analyzing tools (analyzing rod, carbon marker, undercut gauges and spare marker tips)

14.2.2 Objective of Surveying

Partial edentulism is usually associated with edentulous areas of alveolar ridge accompanied by single or groups of teeth lacking relative parallelism and proper contours, which turn the design process into a biomechanical challenge. The biologic and mechanical principles are integrated to planning, design, and construction phases by means of the surveyor.

The surveying procedure reveals the designer the physical characteristics of the denture-related tissues that will simplify or complicate the design of a successful prosthesis like

- the amount and locations of undercuts on abutment teeth;
- soft and hard tissue interferences;
- guiding plane surfaces.

The acquired data, along with esthetic considerations, will help to determine a path of insertion and to establish the design of the prosthesis. With the benefits of surveying, an RPD with satisfactory aesthetics and calculated retention which allows easy insertion and removal by the patient can be constructed. Furthermore, the reduced gaps between the guiding surfaces not only improve aesthetics but also minimize food retention as well.

In case a surveyor is not used, the independently designed components of an RPD cannot be correlated to each other. Each one bearing a different path of placement, they cannot align to a single path of insertion, at least, without exerting uncontrolled, probably harming, forces to the remaining structures or they cannot be inserted as a single unit at all.

14.2.3 Surveying: The Procedure

There are two stages of surveying. A preparatory analysis of the diagnostic cast is made to determine the favorable path of insertion and related necessary preparations before the final impression is made. Once the mouth preparation is complete, the definitive surveying is made on the master cast.

14.2.3.1 Systematic Steps of Surveying

1. Mount the cast on the surveyor, adjust the plane of occlusion as parallel as possible to the horizontal plane, and lock the tilting mechanism.
   (a) It is very important to safely fix the cast on the cast holder. During surveying a number of precise measurements will be marked on the plaster surface. If the position of the cast is somewhat lost on the holder before tripoding, exact repositioning of the cast on the holder may not be possible. This may result in confusing marks on measured surfaces.
   (b) Fixing the vertical arm close to the occlusal plane and checking the distance to each tooth while roaming may help to adjust the plane of occlusion (Fig. 14.2).
2. The analyzing rod fundamentally is the tool for determining the path of insertion. Attach the analyzing rod and make sure its range of vertical motion covers the area between the

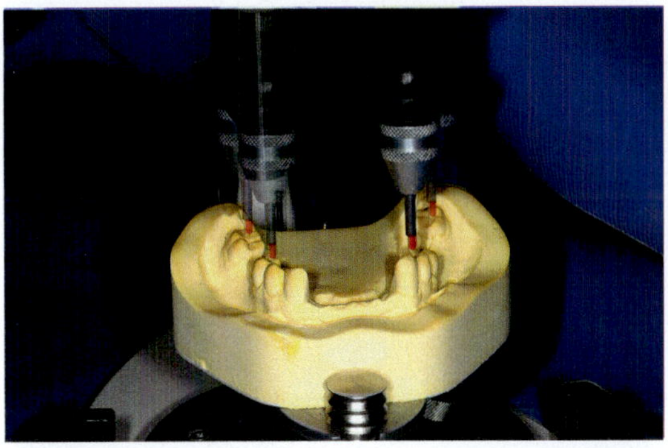

Fig. 14.2 Orientation of occlusal plane. Fix the cast holder when the distances between the occlusal surfaces and the vertical arm are equal

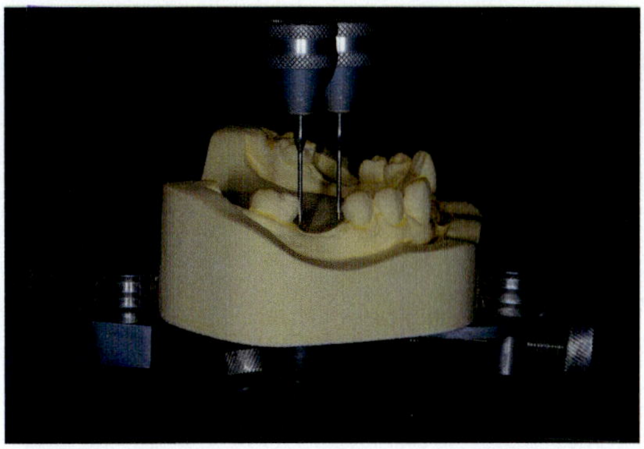

Fig. 14.3 The evaluation of axial surfaces in relation to path of placement

average occlusal plane and the bottom of vestibular pouch. The rod provides visual help to allocate undercut areas. Roaming in contact with the abutment teeth, it reveals the location and relative amounts of undercuts. After initial observation tilting mechanism of the cast holder is released to distribute the undercut areas for adjustment of retention, minimizing food traps, and enhancing aesthetics. The procedure is repeated on the cast until optimum distribution of undercuts is achieved. Once the final tilt is decided, the vertical arm indicates the direction of the path of insertion.

Regarding the path of insertion, it is primarily dependent on the non-retentive undercut areas on the lateral surfaces of abutment teeth facing edentulous spaces.

In most cases, dead zones, dark triangles between the guiding plates and the gingival borders are present. To avoid large food traps and improper guiding surfaces tilt the cast to set the vertical rod as the angle-bisector between the long axes of relevant abutment teeth. Practically, the dark zones are thus evenly shared (Fig. 14.3).

Some cases require esthetic priorities due to missing anterior teeth. To eliminate the dark gaps on axial undercuts and avoid visible clasp arms these undercuts must be engaged to provide retention to the RPD. This is possible by employing a rotational path of insertion. Establishment of the rotational path of insertion provides retention from anterior teeth by engaging the guiding plates as retentive components (Fig. 14.4a and b) (See Chap. 12).

The retentive undercuts of possible abutment teeth should also be evaluated in this step. Inspect the buccal surfaces of teeth to determine the locations of retention arms. The cast may have to be tilted, usually slightly, to adjust retentive areas. Once the final tilt of the cast is decided the vertical arm indicates the path of insertion.

(a) Tilting the cast changes the height of contour for all teeth simultaneously.

3. After determining the path of insertion, the analyzing rod is replaced with the carbon marker tool. The tool consists of a carbon marker placed in a pipe like protective casing. It is applied on the relevant teeth like the analyzing rod (Fig. 14.5).
   (a) The lateral side of the marker must be in contact with the most prominent circumference of teeth, not the tip. If the tip is marking the surface, it is probably working within the suprabulge area and not drawing the actual survey line.
   (b) In case a second survey line with an altered inclination of the cast need to be drawn, different colored markers prevent confusion between different survey lines.
4. The carbon marker is replaced with an undercut gauge after survey lines are drawn.

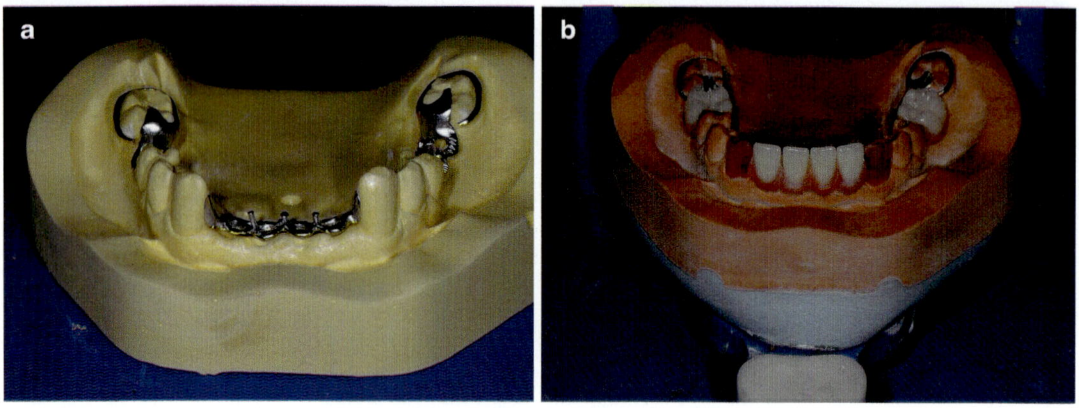

Fig. 14.4 (**a** and **b**) Using axial surfaces of abutment teeth for retention. Rotational path of insertion allows a clasp-free design at the aesthetic region

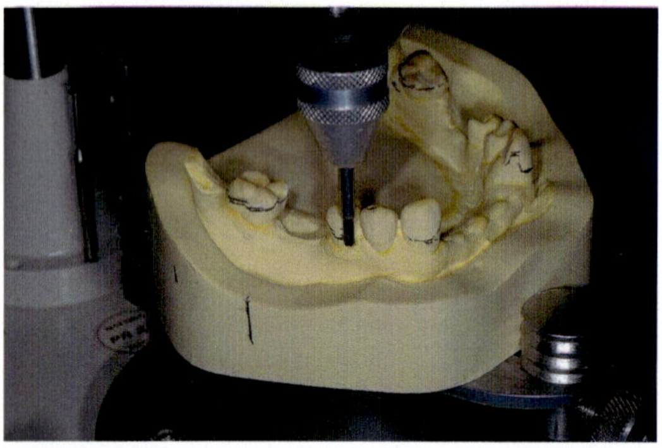

Fig. 14.5 Drawing the survey line. The carbon marker should travel on most prominent circumference of teeth. If the tip of the marker is drawing then it is operating in the suprabulge area. If it is in contact with the gingiva and no survey line is drawn then there is no retentive undercut on that particular tooth

The shape of an undercut gauge is like a regular nail, only the tip is not pointed and the head projection from the shaft is scaled. They are conventionally available in three sizes as 0.25, 0.50, and 0.75 mm. The retentive tip of a cast clasp arm should be located in a 0.25 mm undercut; if the clasp arm will be of wrought wire, then it may occupy a 0.50 mm depth. To use a 0.75 mm undercut, which is very rarely needed, the retention arm should be made from wrought wire and be at least 8 mm long, otherwise it may apply excessive forces on abutment teeth during insertion and removal of the denture. Deeper undercuts can only be used with resin clasp arms (see Chap. 12).

Select the appropriate gauge according to your choice of retention arm. Locate the proper spot for the clasp tip on the abutment tooth and mark it as a point with a pencil. This is where your retention arm will end (Fig. 14.6a, b).

14.2.3.2 Tripoding

Before removing the cast from the cast holder its position should be recorded, so that it can be remounted on another surveyor with the same path of insertion by the dental technician. This is referred to as "tripoding." Tripoding also allows the dentist to check the laboratory work.

Making three lines as lateral projections of the analyzing rod on three different lateral walls of the cast is one of three options for tripoding. Re-attach the analyzing rod, thrust its lateral side on one of the lateral walls of the cast, and use it as a ruler while drawing a straight line parallel to the path of insertion. Repeat the procedure on two other side walls of the cast. For finding the same path of insertion the cast is mounted on a surveyor and the tilt of the cast is adjusted until the three lines become parallel with the analyzing rod (Fig. 14.7).

Another technique is to fix the vertical movement of the carbon marker at an appropriate height where it can make contact with three distant points on the cast without interfering with the present drawings. Each of these points is marked with two short lines perpendicular to each other with the dot being at the junction and

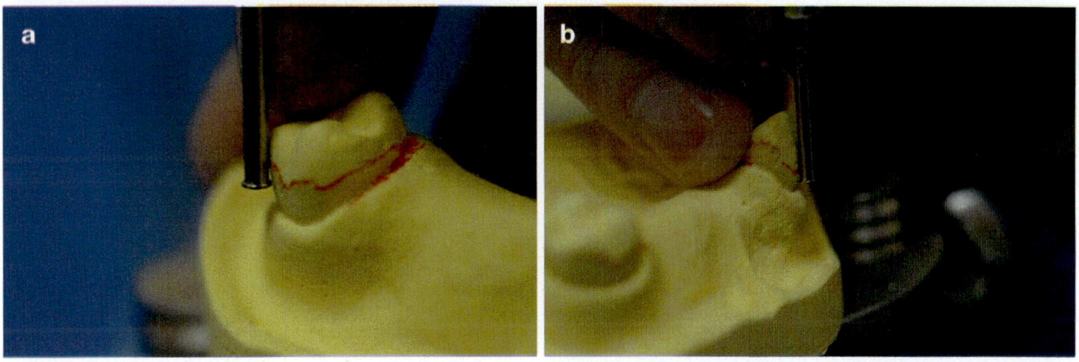

Fig. 14.6 (**a**, **b**) Determining the suitable spot for the retention arm on the abutment tooth. The undercut gauge contacts both the height of contour and point of desired amount of retentive undercut. (**a**) Location of the retentive arm tip for a circumferential clasp. (**b**) Location of the retentive arm for a bar clasp

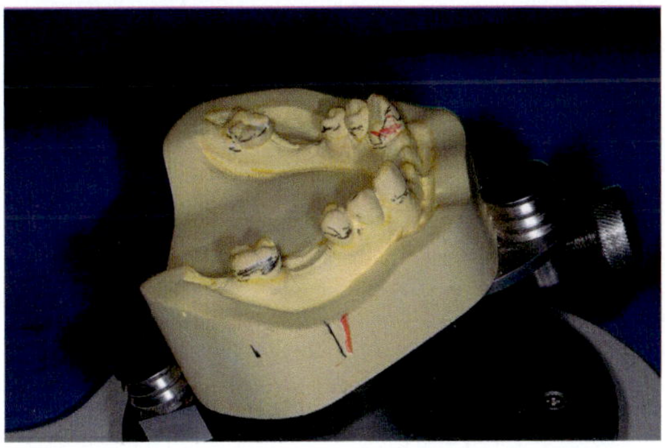

Fig. 14.7 Tripoding by drawing parallel projections on the axial surfaces of the cast. These lines should be parallel to the path of insertion and should be drawn on three sides of the cast. In case two different paths are determined they should be marked with different colored markers. The analyzing rod can be used as a ruler while drawing

the formed plus sign is encircled. The color of the pencil should be in contrast with the color of the plaster. When transferred to another surveyor, the height of the analyzing rod and the inclination of the cast are adjusted to provide the same contacts between the three points and the tip of the rod. Like the three-line method, the adjustments may take some time to achieve accurate alignment (Fig. 14.8).

Embedding a flat metal shaft, like an analyzing rod, or a simple hand-piece bur can also be used to tripod the cast. A small cavity, a little larger than a bur shaft and about 5 to 10 mm in depth is drilled on an available location on the cast. The flat shaft or the bur is mounted on the vertical arm, naturally in exact alignment with the path of placement. The drilled cavity is filled with either a few drops of plaster or acrylic resin and the mounted shaft is placed and fixed in contact with the bottom of the cavity. After the filling material is set the vertical arm is detached and the rod is left on the cast which can now be mounted on any surveyor without error very easily (Fig. 14.9a–c). There are even commercially available pins to apply with this technique.

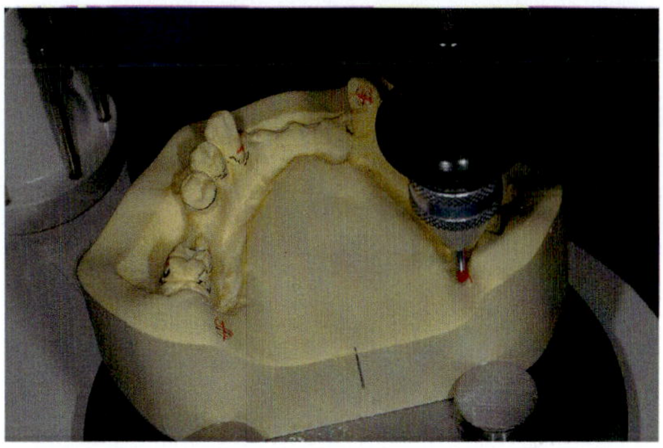

Fig. 14.8 Tripoding by marking three distant points on the cast. The vertical arm draws horizontal lines. Make vertical lines with a red pencil, intersect the two lines in their middle, and circle the + sign to locate the markings

14.2.3.3 Evaluation of Potential Abutment Teeth

Surveying reveals the options for defeating any obstacles to benefit from abutment teeth for

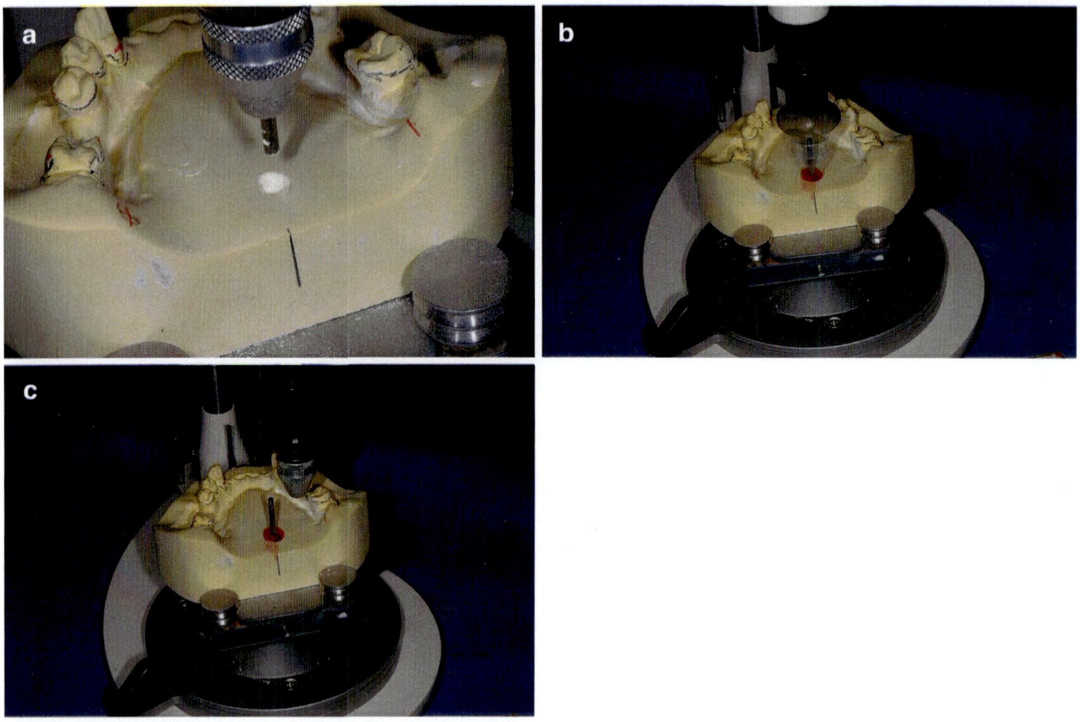

Fig. 14.9 (**a–c**) Tripoding by embedding a straight rod in the surveyed cast. (**a**) A hole is drilled on the cast and the rod is attached to the vertical arm. (**b**) The cavity is filled with acrylic resin and the rod is fixed in contact with the bottom of the cavity. (**c**) Vertical arm is detached, and the rod is aligned with the path of placement

retention, reciprocation, stabilization, and path of placement. These options include the following:

- Minor grinding of teeth
- Adhesive restorations
- Fixed prosthesis

  to integrate the tooth into the definitive design
- Extraction
- Ignoring

  to create a design without involving a particular tooth

Guiding Planes/Guiding Plates

Axial walls of abutment teeth, sometimes along with reciprocating surfaces, guide the prosthesis from the initial contact with teeth to the final seating through the defined path of placement. The potential guiding surfaces are evaluated with the surveyor and adjusted if necessary.

Once the path of insertion is decided, if the height of contour on a desired guiding surface appears to be narrow and too close to the plane of occlusion (within the occlusal 1/3 of abutment teeth), the surface can be altered with a simple grinding. A proper guiding plane is prepared that is covering nearly 1/3 of tooth height and bearing a smaller dead zone close to the gingiva. Grinding of the diagnostic cast on the surveyor will be the reference to the preparative clinical procedure (see Chap. 7).

Retention

In case, when the amount of retentive undercut is not sufficient or there is no undercut at all on a particular tooth which otherwise is a potential abutment, the ability to provide retention should be added. It is possible to correct the position of tipped or rotated teeth with orthodontics; however, it mostly is not practical due to added cost and time to finish the overall treatment. Common solutions are re-contouring of teeth to create an angle of gingival convergence either by grinding the enamel surface or with an adhesive restoration. If one of these options is not capable of handling the situation then we are left with the choice of a full crown restoration. Occasionally, extraction of a severely malpositioned tooth may be necessary when its existence interferes with any proper design alternatives for the framework.

Conversely, when the survey line is too high and/or the retentive undercut is sharply too deep to allow a proper clasp design, the tooth can be altered to serve efficiently with one of the options above.

Reciprocation

One of the overlooked issues regarding clasp design is the establishment of reciprocation. A reciprocal component can only reciprocate the action of the retention arm during insertion and removal only if it contacts the abutment tooth simultaneously with the retention arm if not before. Furthermore, it should continuously keep its contact while the retentive arm slides over the survey line until the framework is fully seated. This requires a flat surface for the reciprocating unit that is parallel to the path of insertion and as wide as the vertical travel of the clasp tip from its initial contact to final seating. This flat surface almost never exists on natural teeth. The reciprocating surfaces of teeth should be integrated to the path of insertion either by grinding or by a restorative alternative (see Chap. 7).

14.2.3.4 Grinding the Diagnostic Cast

The controlled grinding of tooth surfaces on the surveyor can be done with the help of undercut gauges.

When the analyzing rod slides almost in contact with the potential retentive surface but reveals no suitable undercut area, grinding within the enamel layer may be a solution. After surveying with the analyzing rod, the possible location of the clasp tip is marked with a pencil on the abutment tooth. The manual grinding of the plaster surface can be done with a round-tipped modeling knife until the 0.25 mm gauge fits the undercut that is carved. This provides sufficient retention for a cast metal clasp arm without removing excessive amounts of tooth structure.

The guiding planes can also be arranged with the help of undercut gauges. The marking rod is replaced with a 0.25 mm undercut gauge and the point where the gauge contacts the plaster on the axial surface is marked with a pencil. The grinding of the surface, parallel to the path of insertion, can be done with the carving knife of the surveyor. The procedure can be repeated if sufficient width of plane is not achieved. Even if a third carving is needed the amount of lost enamel thickness will correspond to 0.75 mm which is often possible without exposing any dentin tissue.

With the path of insertion decided and possible preparations carried out, the design of the framework should be studied on the diagnostic cast.

The final shape of the diagnostic cast is the reference to alterations that must be made in the mouth. There are several methods to guide clinical procedures to imitate the changes on the study cast but usually the simple marks drawn on the cast are sufficient. Having worked on the study cast the dentist can easily repeat similar preparations in the mouth before making the final impression.

The final analysis is made on the master cast with the same order. After the survey line is drawn the design of the metal framework can be transferred to the master cast.

14.3 Laboratory Procedures

14.3.1 Final Casts, Mounting in the Articulator and Diagnostic Wax-up

The master cast is preferably prepared with Type IV dental stone if the finishing of the acrylic will be made with an autopolymerizing polymethyl methacrylate denture base material (Fig. 14.10).

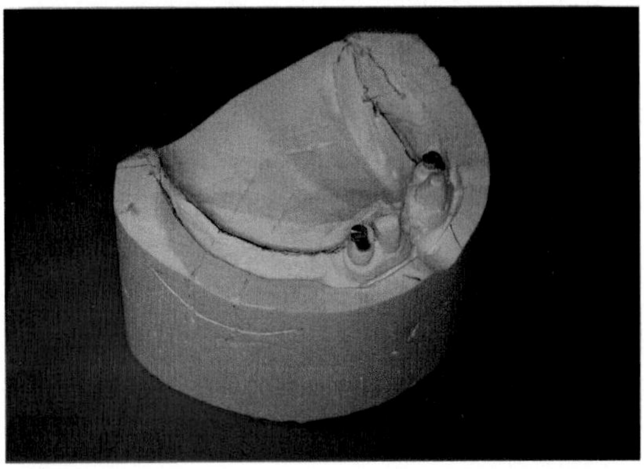

Fig. 14.10 Master cast prepared with Type IV dental stone

However, Type III dental stone is commonly the regular material to prepare diagnostic or master casts for all kinds of removable appliances including RPDs. The occlusal surface of the opposing impression can be constructed with polyurethane as an alternative to dental stones (Fig. 14.11). This material is more resistant to abrasions than plaster but less precise and is more heat sensitive.

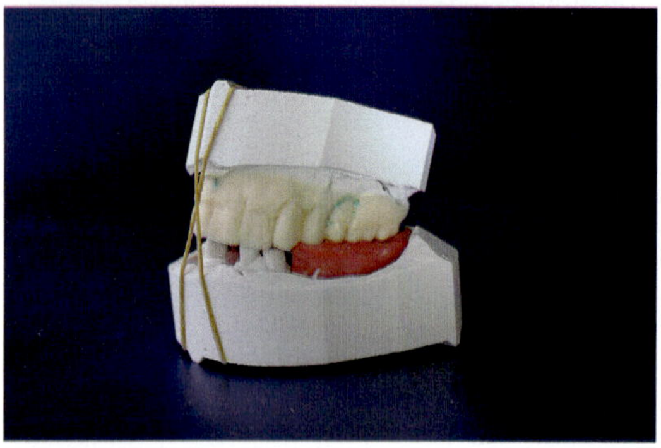

Fig. 14.11 Centric record: The wax occlusion rim should provide sufficient contacts with the corresponding surfeces of the opposing model

A mounting table helps in mounting the models on the articulator. For the Gerber articulator it is attached to the upper side of the articulator for transferring the mandibular cast along with the average occlusal plane according to its design. The more common designs of articulators accept the transfer of the average occlusal plane through the transfer of the maxillary cast or occlusion rims (Fig. 14.12a and b). Individual transfer of the occlusal plane requires the articulator-specific facebow transfer for each patient.

As it is not always easy to establish vertical dimensions once the models are in the articulator, a diagnostic wax-up may be helpful to readjust the vertical dimension (Fig. 14.13).

14.3.2 Model Analysis: Mounting of Posterior Teeth

Functional analysis of the crestline is an invaluable guide for the arrangement of posterior teeth.

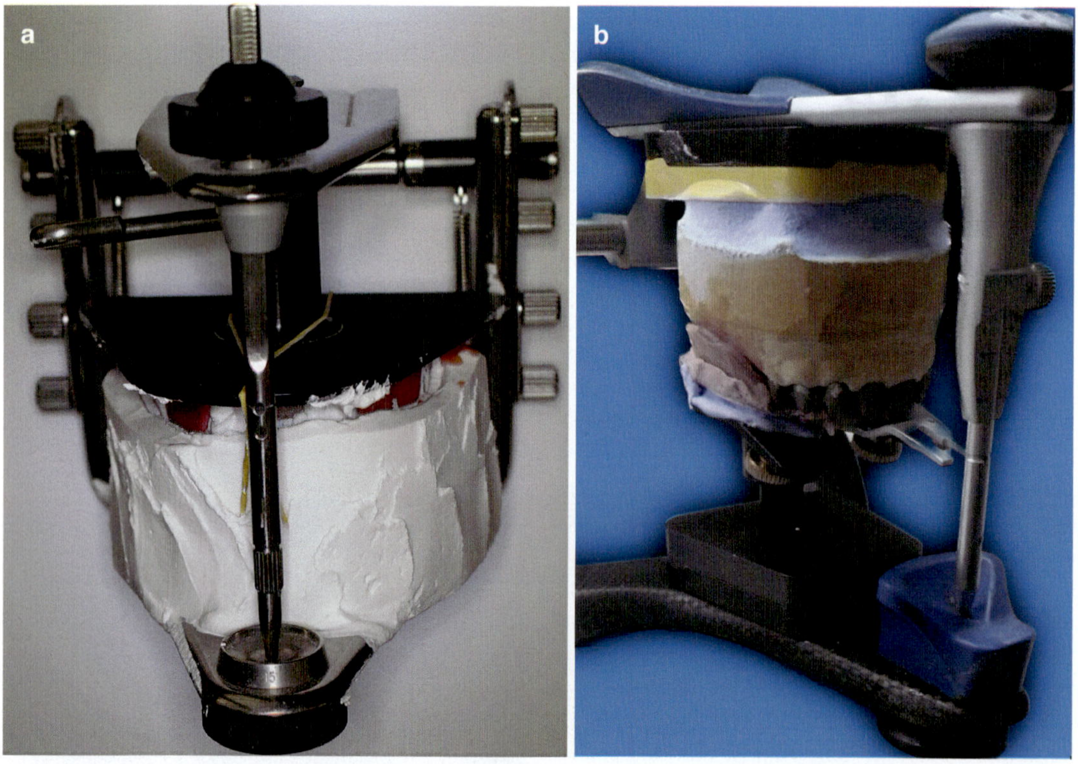

Fig. 14.12 (**a**) Mandibular cast is mounted on the Gerber articulator. (**b**) Transfer of the plane of occlusion by mounting the maxillary cast is a more common design for other articulators

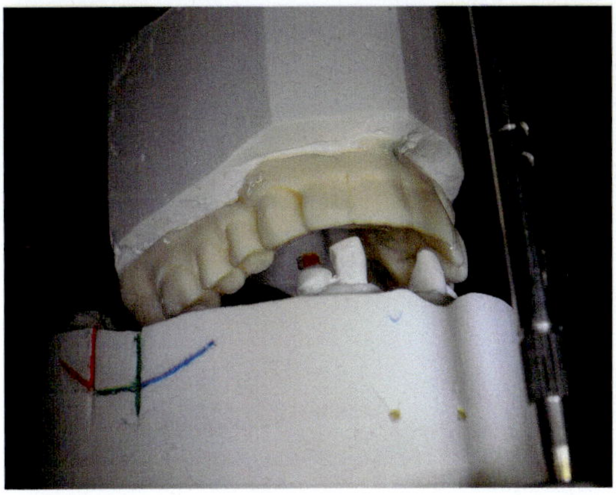

Fig. 14.13 Vertical dimension for occlusion and centric relation according to the record by the clinician

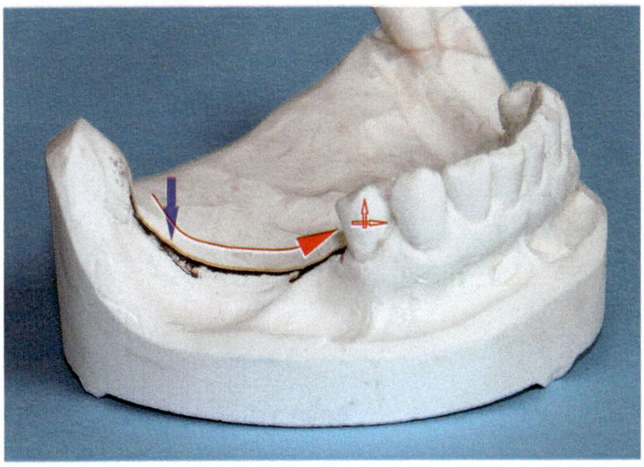

Fig. 14.14 The blue arrow represents the chewing pressure in the area of the last molar. If chewing force occurs on this tooth, the resulting force produces pressure in the direction of the red arrow

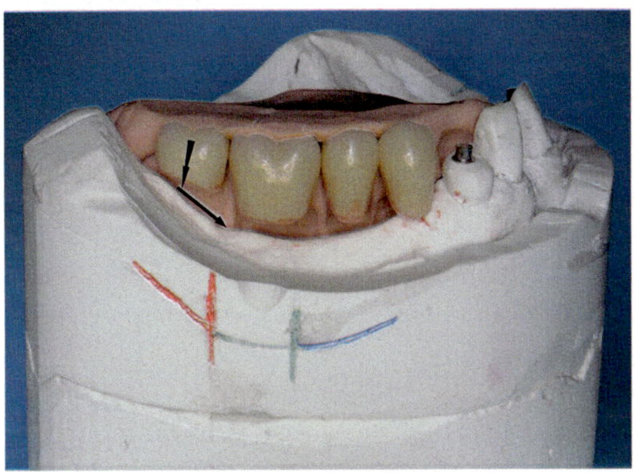

Fig. 14.15 The last molar is placed over a steep surface. The resulting chewing force (black arrows) can damage the ball attachment on the root of the canine

It is simply done by tracing the lateral crest profile on the side of the model by the help of a compass. The analysis provides information to achieve superior function from posterior teeth (Figs. 14.14 and 14.15).

14.3.2.1 Occlusion: Sagittal Stability

An inadequate occlusion may produce horizontal forces (Figs. 14.14, 14.15 and 14.16) which could cause periodontal problems and ultimately the loss of the abutment tooth.

To prevent undesired horizontal forces on mandibular cases, examine the alveolar ridge and mark a red vertical line indicating the anterior border of the steep slope starting from the retromolar pad area. No tooth should be in occlusal contact beyond this line. The deepest area on the alveolar crest is for the first molar. This specific location is marked with a green line (Fig. 14.16).

Tooth arrangement should be made before the fabrication of the metal framework and follow the model analysis described above (Figs. 14.16, 14.17, 14.18 and 14.19).

14.3.2.2 Occlusion –Transversal Stability

With free-end saddles, the antero-posterior line of the occlusal contact originates on the last tooth or root with an attachment and its posterior support is the alveolar ridge (Figs. 14.20 and 14.21). Forces occurring outside the center of the alveolar ridge produce torsion on the free-end saddle

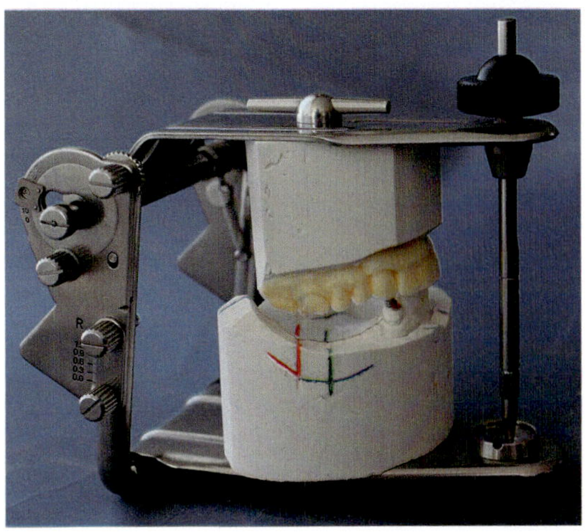

Fig. 14.16 The model analysis is executed with the cast mounted on the Gerber Condylator

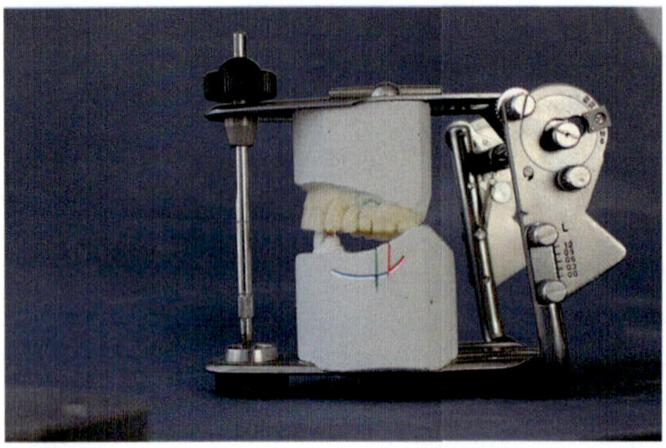

Fig. 14.17 The model analysis on the left side can be different from the right side

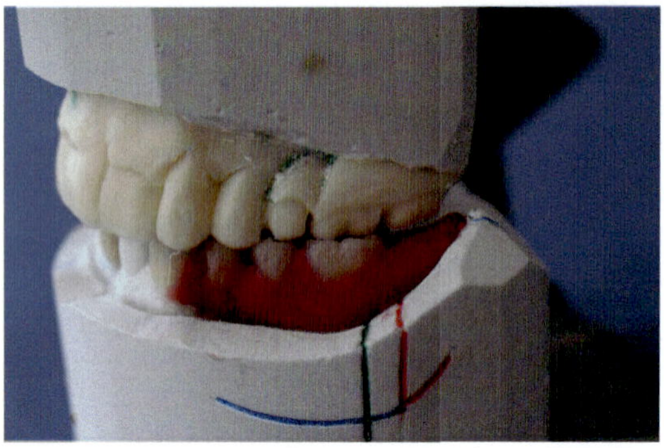

Fig. 14.18 Posterior tooth arrangement according to the model analysis

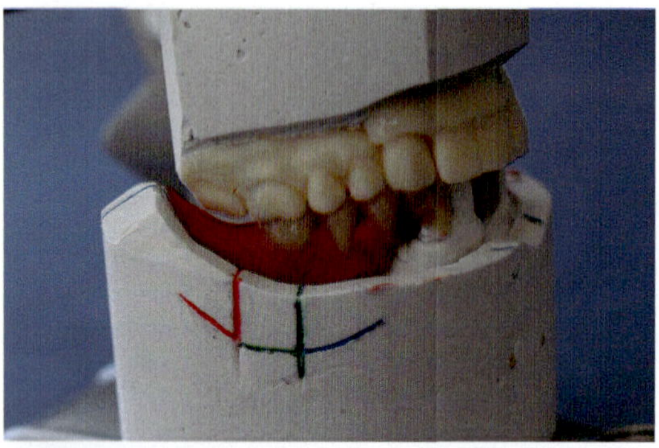

Fig. 14.19 Posterior tooth arrangement according to the model analysis

and can overload the abutment tooth. The use of the lingualized occlusal concept offers a good

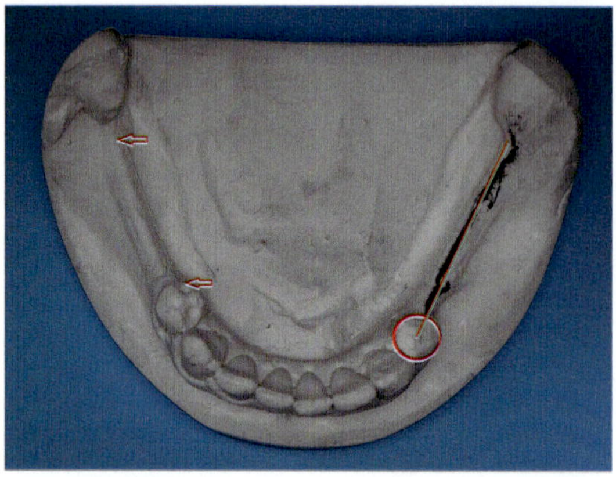

Fig. 14.20 On the left side of the case, the center of the alveolar ridge is marked with a lead pencil leading to the abutment tooth (red circle)

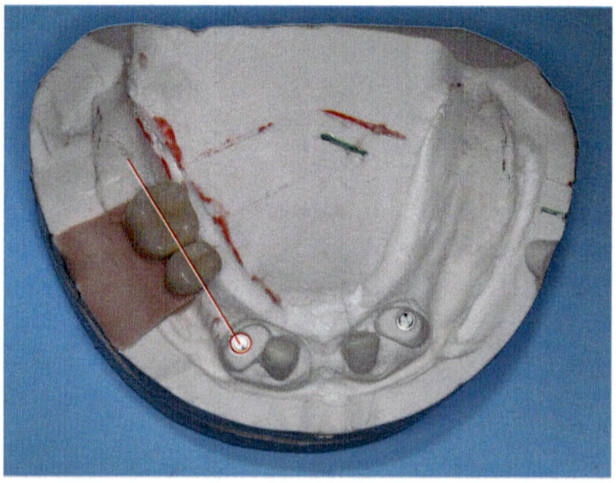

Fig. 14.21 In a case with attachments and free-end saddles, the center of the supporting alveolar ridge crosses over the center of the lower teeth

solution for keeping the occlusal forces as close as possible to the antero-posterior line (Figs. 14.22 and 14.23a). The lingualized occlusion is also recommended for maxillary RPDs with free-end saddles, based on the same principle as shown in the Figs. 14.19, 14.20, 14.21 and 14.22 for mandibular RPDs.

Different cases require different types of occlusal relations (Fig. 14.23a–d). These are explained in Chap. 13 "Establishing occlusal relationships."

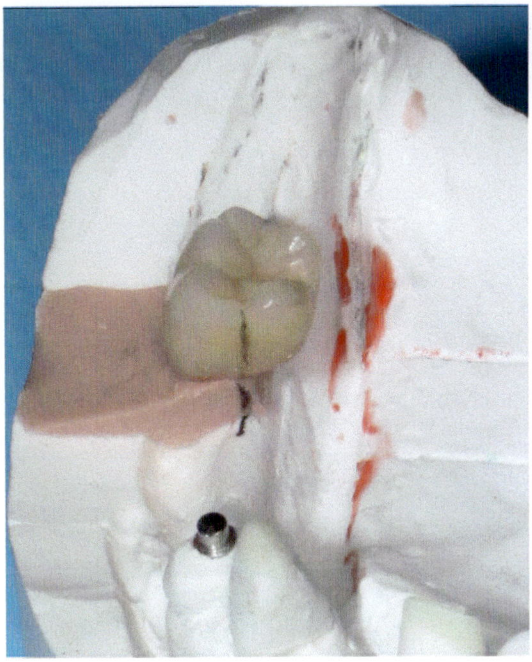

Fig. 14.22 Control of the position of the molar in relation to the alveolar ridge. The tooth is not obstructing the space for the tongue and will get a tight contact to the buccinator muscle

14.3.3 Try-in and Preparation for the Cast Metal Frame

Aesthetics and occlusion must be established first and tried-in before constructing the metal framework (Fig. 14.24). This way, the metal framework can be precisely designed according to the arrangement of teeth without disturbing the esthetics of the case (Figs. 14.25 and 14.26). Overly constructed frameworks are still common and it is preferable to work with a minimum adequate size and number of clasps for hygienic reasons. There is always a risk of secondary caries and periodontal involvement underneath the clasps.

If artificial anterior teeth are part of the case, a new try-in is recommended once the metal framework has been completed.

After final try-in the work is sent to the dental laboratory for finishing procedures.

14.3.3.1 Planning

Well thought-out plans avoid complication. This involves a collaborative effort between clinician and laboratory technician. The technician should be informed of which teeth are solid and able to

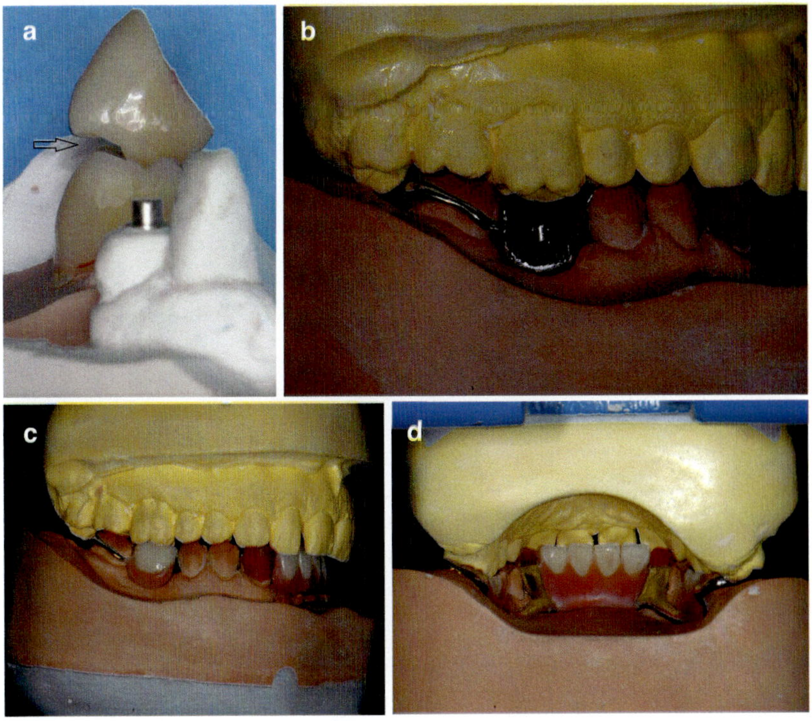

Fig. 14.23 (**a**) Placement of the upper molar according to lingualized occlusion. The buccal cusp is out of contact by 2 mm. (**b**, **c**, and **d**) However, opposing dentition may not allow that amount of buccal clearance. The type of occlusion for posterior teeth arrangement is therefore a case-specific choice

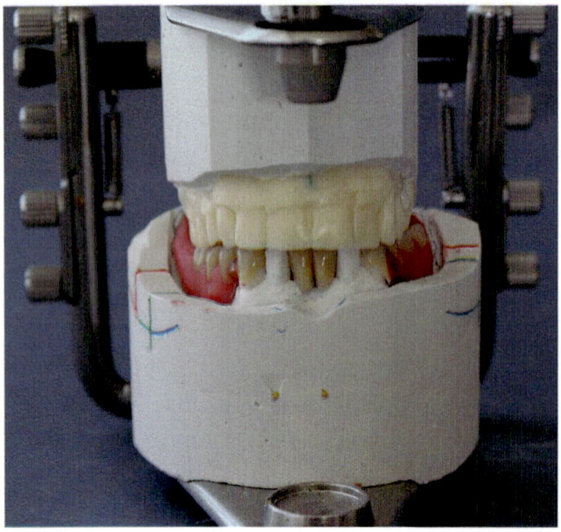

Fig. 14.24 Once aesthetics and occlusion are satisfactory, plaster or silicon keys are made over the teeth

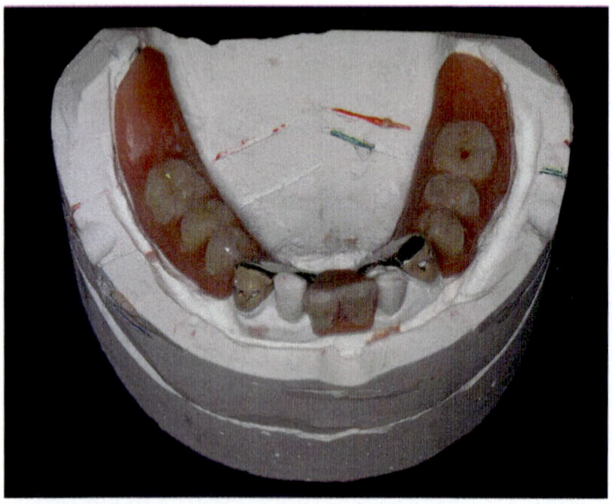

Fig. 14.25 Grooves are cut outside the casting

support the load of the partial denture and which teeth must be avoided or only stabilized by including them in the metal frame.

The planning begins with surveying and making a simple drawing on the diagnostic model (Fig. 14.27). After mouth preparation the master cast is surveyed, tripoded, and delivered to the lab with the desired design transferred to the definitive cast. Important information can be drawn on the work authorization form as seen in Fig. 14.28.

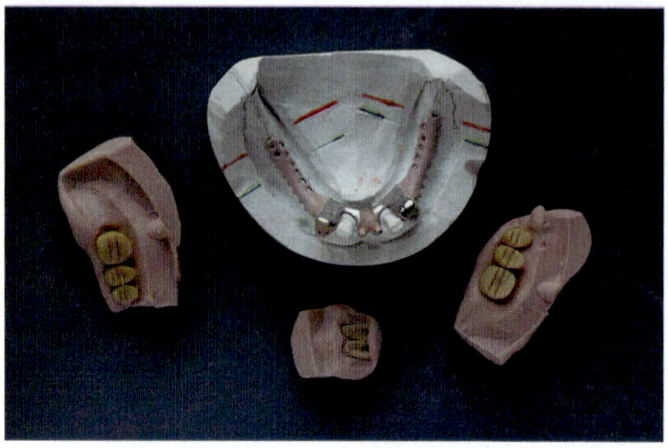

Fig. 14.26 The grooves assist in repositioning the keys when remounting the teeth once the metal frame has been completed. Especially for aesthetics, it is recommended to repeat the try-in when anterior teeth are arranged

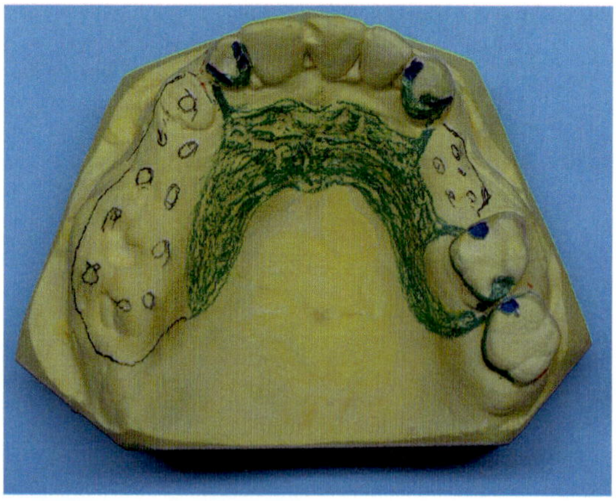

Fig. 14.27 Initial design of the framework on the diagnostic cast

14.3.3.2 The Bios and the Ney Clasp Systems

The form of the Bios clasp is different and offers better precision to determine the force of retention. Because the clasp arm of the Bios system is symmetrical and progressively conic (Fig. 14.29), its sectional form is like a wire cut in half (Fig. 14.30). The cross-section of clasps for the Ney system is ovoid with a flat surface. In the oral cavity, the Bios clasp is less visible (Fig. 14.31a, b) and reduces the risk of secondary caries. However, the Ney system is the commonly preferred clasp system for RPDs.

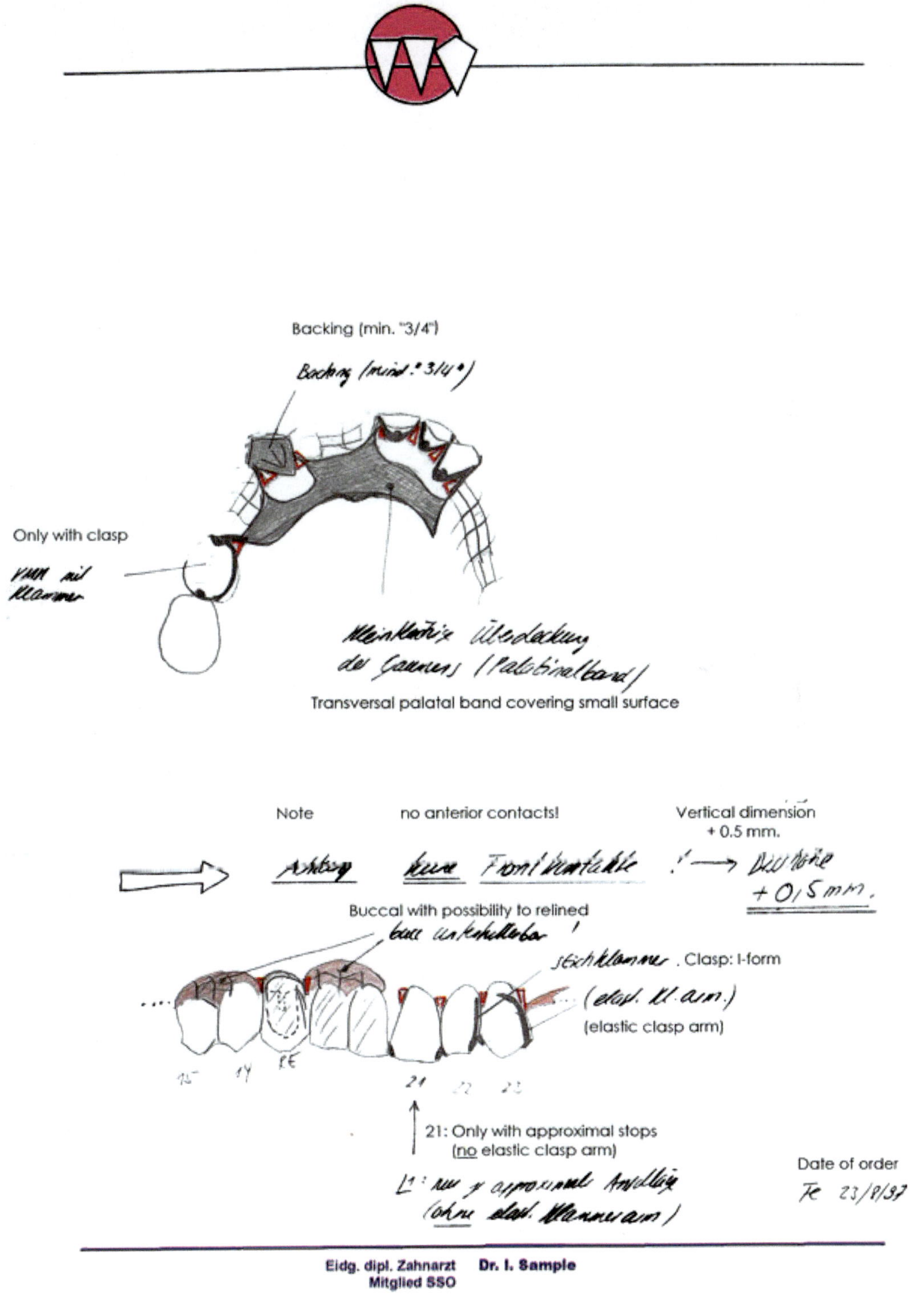

Fig. 14.28 A typical example of a hand-written "work authorization form" including the details of the framework as the dentist designed it and all complementary information that the clinician sends to the laboratory. It is more descriptive when the written instructions are associated with a detailed drawing of the case and the design

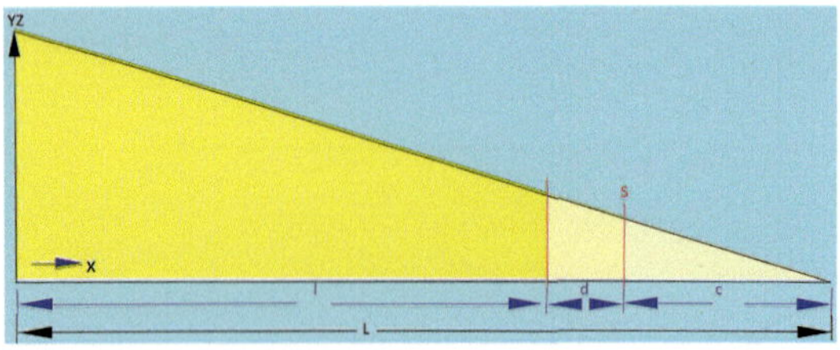

Fig. 14.29 If the retention of the clasp arm must be less flexible, the tip can be shortened. That symmetrically increases the force of retention

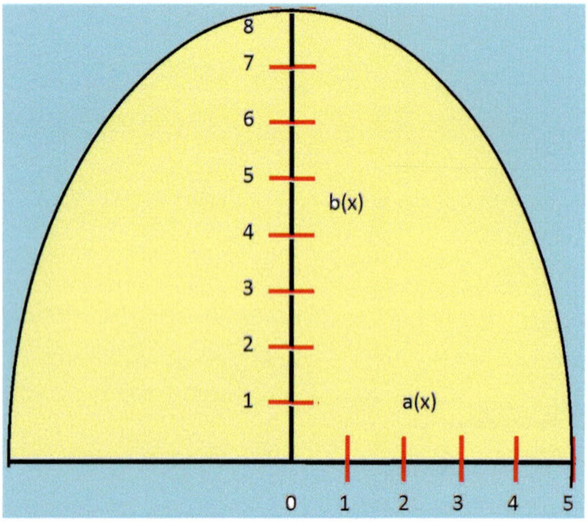

Fig. 14.30 Diametric form of a Bios clasp. The contact surface to the natural tooth is small

14.3.3.3 Construction of the Metal Framework

Construction of the framework is conventionally done by casting (Fig. 14.32). CoCr alloys are regularly used for the purpose. Titanium is an alternative which is lighter and more flexible than CoCr and reveals better results with CAD-CAM manufacturing. Due to material properties, titanium frameworks are less prone to show plastic deformation and assumed to be more bio-friendly; however their flexibility threatens the acrylic-metal base connection. Breaking of the

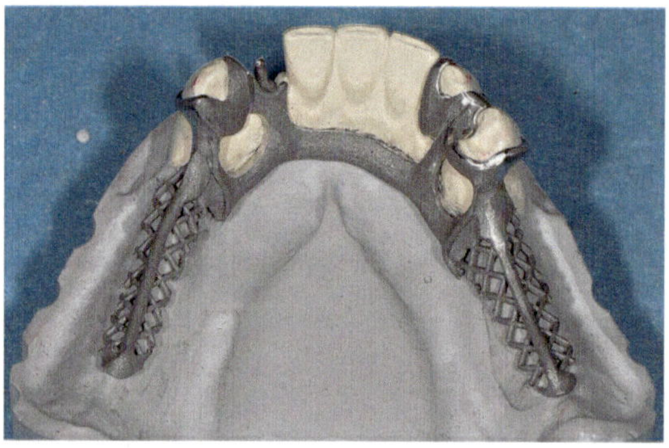

Fig. 14.32 CoCr framework constructed by conventional casting

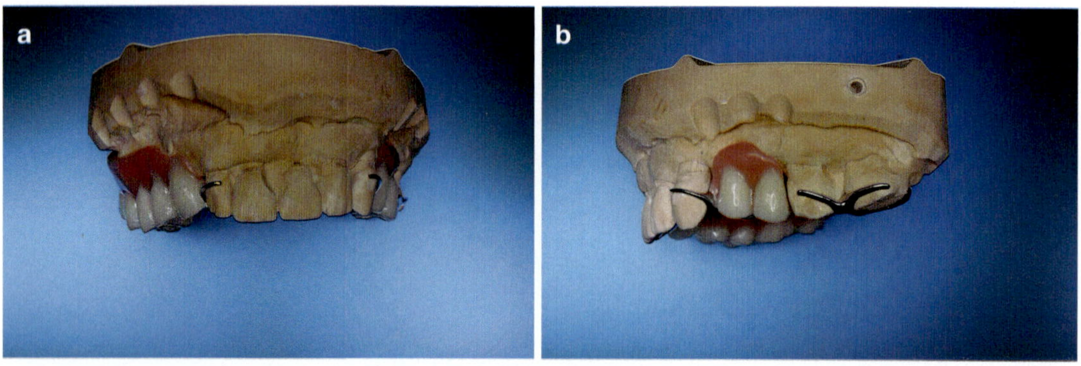

Fig. 14.31 (**a**, **b**) Notice the location of retention arms on the abutment teeth. Without surveying, most technicians would locate them closer to gingival border which would result in excessive forces acting on the abutment teeth during placement and removal of the prosthesis

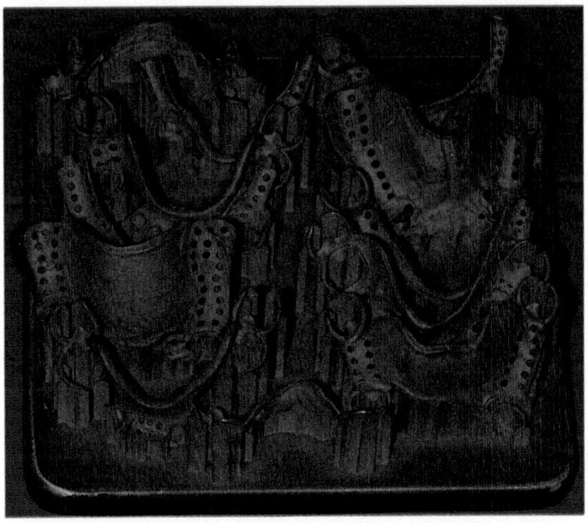

Fig. 14.33 Metal frameworks produced by direct metal laser sintering

acrylic saddles may be expected. However, a two-year clinical study showed no significant difference between the clinical successes of the two materials.

Additive and subtractive CAD-CAM techniques like direct metal laser sintering and CAD-CAM milling are modern production techniques for the production of metal frameworks. The digital production of the framework requires a digital design or the transfer of the framework design to the computer media. Digital systems show better dimensional stability and require less complicated laboratory work when compared to casting. The nature of direct metal laser sintering is more suitable to the complex design of frameworks (Fig. 14.33). Current techniques and procedures of digital manufacturing of RPDs are explained in Part V: "Digital Workflow of Removable Partial Dentures."

Further Reading

Ahmad I, Waters NE. Accuracy of dental surveyors. J Dent. 1991;19:181–5.

Ansari IH. A procedure for reorienting a cast on a surveyor. J Prosthet Dent. 1994;72:104–7.

Au AR, Lechner SK, Thomas CJ, Mori T, Chung P. Titanium for removable partial dentures (III): 2-year clinical follow-up in an undergraduate programme. J Oral Rehabil. 2000;27:979–85.

Bezzon OL, Mattos MG, Ribeiro RF. Surveying removable partial dentures: the importance of guiding planes and path of insertion for stability. J Prosthet Dent. 1997;78:412–8.

Bezzon OL, Ribeiro RF, Pagnano VO. Device for recording the path of insertion for removable partial dentures. J Prosthet Dent. 2000;84:136–8.

Bhola S, Hellyer PH, Radford DR. The importance of communication in the construction of partial dentures. Br Dent J. 2018;224:853–6.

Bohnenkamp DM. Removable partial dentures: clinical concepts. Dent Clin North Am. 2014;58:69–89.

Bowley JF, Cipra DL, Herman PF. Evaluation of the accuracy of cast reorientation to a surveyor by prosthodontic residents. J Prosthet Dent. 1992;68:294–8.

Carr AB, Brown DT. McCracken's removable partial prosthodontics. 13th ed. St. Louis, MO: Elsevier; 2016.

Carreiro Ada F, Machado AL, Giampaolo ET, Santana IL, Vergani CE. Dual path: a concept to improve the esthetic replacement of missing anterior teeth with a removable partial denture. J Prosthodont. 2008;17:586–90.

Chen YC, Chang MC, Hsiao WY, Chen YC. Castability of a Ti-7.5Mo alloy for fabricating frameworks for removable partial dentures. J Prosthet Dent. 2023;130:646–53.

Dikbas I, Ozkurt Z, Kazazoglu E. Predoctoral prosthodontic curricula on removable partial dentures: survey of Turkish dental schools. J Dent Educ. 2013;77:85–92.

Engelmeier RL. The history and development of the dental surveyor: part I. J Prosthodont. 2002a;11:11–8.

Engelmeier RL. The history and development of the dental surveyor: part II. J Prosthodont. 2002b;11:122–30.

Engelmeier RL. The history and development of the dental surveyor: part III. J Prosthodont. 2004;13:195–202.

Han J, Wang Y, Lü P. A preliminary report of designing removable partial denture frameworks using a specifically developed software package. Int J Prosthodont. 2010;23:370–5.

Jayachandran S, Ramachandran CR, Varghese R. Occlusal plane orientation: a statistical and clinical analysis in different clinical situations. J Prosthodont. 2008;17:572–5.

Johnson A, Wildgoose DG. Partial denture design comparisons between inexperienced and experienced undergraduate students and the teaching staff of a UK dental school. Br Dent J. 2010;209:287–92.

Krikos AA. Preparing guide planes for removable partial dentures. J Prosthet Dent. 1975;34:152–5.

Lang LA, Tulunoğlu I. A critically appraised topic review of computer-aided design/computer-aided machining of removable partial denture frameworks. Dent Clin North Am. 2014;58:247–55.

Loney RW. Removable partial denture manual. Halifax, NS: Dalhousie University Faculty of Dentistry; 2011. http://removpros.dentistry.dal.ca/ewExternalFiles/RPD%20Manual%2011.pdf.

Nokubi T, Ono T, Morimitsu T, Ikebe K, Yasui S, Kita S, Okuno Y. Clinical application of a newly devel-

oped surveying system for designing and fabricating removable partial dentures. J Osaka Univ Dent Sch. 1992;32:104–17.
Ohkubo C, Hanatani S, Hosoi T. Present status of titanium removable dentures-a review of the literature. J Oral Rehabil. 2008;35:706–14.
Ohkubo C, Sato Y, Nishiyama Y, Suzuki Y. Titanium removable denture based on a one-metal rehabilitation concept. Dent Mater J. 2017;36:517–23.
Pavarina AC, Machado AL, Vergani CE, Giampaolo ET. Preparation of composite retentive areas for removable partial denture retainers. J Prosthet Dent. 2002;88:218–20.
Phoenix RD, Cagna DR, Defreest CF. Stewart's clinical removable partial prosthodontics. 4th ed. Chicago: Quintessence Publishing; 2008.
Rashedi B, Petropoulos VC. Preclinical removable partial dentures curriculum survey. J Prosthodont. 2003;12:116–23.
Rudd RW, Bange AA, Rudd KD, Montalvo R. Preparing teeth to receive a removable partial denture. J Prosthet Dent. 1999;82:536–49.
Shifman A, Ben-Ur Z. Prosthodontic treatment for the Applegate-Kennedy class V partially edentulous patient. J Prosthet Dent. 1996;76:212–8.
Steas AD. Recording and reproducing the tilt of a cast on a surveyor. J Prosthet Dent. 1987;57:121–5.
Suh JS, Billy EJ. Rotational path removable partial denture (RPD): conservative esthetic treatment option for the edentulous mandibular anterior region: a case report. J Esthet Restor Dent. 2008;20:98–105.
The glossary of prosthodontic terms: ninth edition. J Prosthet Dent. 2017;117(5S):e1–e105.
Varjão FM. Use of transparent vinyl polysiloxane in a minimally invasive approach for creating composite resin undercuts for partial removable dental prostheses. J Prosthet Dent. 2012;107:55–8.
Waghorn S, Kuzmanovic DV. Technique for preparation of parallel guiding planes for removable partial dentures. J Prosthet Dent. 2004;92:200–1.
Williams RJ, Bibb R, Eggbeer D, Collis J. Use of CAD/CAM technology to fabricate a removable partial denture framework. J Prosthet Dent. 2006;96:96–9.
Wu J, Wang X, Zhao X, Zhang C, Gao B. A study on the fabrication method of removable partial denture framework by computer-aided design and rapid prototyping. Rapid Prototyp J. 2012;18:318–23.

Initial Placement and Adjustments 15

Tonguç Sülün

Abstract

Initial placement and adjustments of removable partial dentures (RPDs) are crucial steps in ensuring optimal function and patient comfort. The process involves a series of appointments during which the dentist evaluates the fit, stability, and retention of the RPD, as well as the occlusion and esthetics. Adjustments may be needed to improve the fit, reduce pressure points, and ensure proper occlusion. The dentist may also need to make adjustments to the clasps and framework to improve retention and stability. With careful planning and adjustments, RPDs can restore patients' ability to speak, chew, and smile with confidence, improving their overall quality of life. The clinicians mostly underestimate the appointment for the delivery of RPD. However, this appointment is as significant as other procedures. Thus, it is important to offer sufficient time and effort for this appointment.

T. Sülün (✉)
Faculty of Dentistry, Department of Prosthodontics, İstanbul University, İstanbul, Türkiye
e-mail: tsulun@istanbul.edu.tr

15.1 Definitions

Bruxism: (1) The parafunctional grinding of teeth; (2) an oral habit consisting of involuntary rhythmic or spasmodic nonfunctional gnashing, grinding, or clenching of teeth, in other than chewing movements of the mandible, which may lead to occlusal trauma.

Centric stop: Opposing cuspal/fossae contacts that maintain the occlusal vertical dimension between the opposing arches.

Denture border: (1) The margin of the denture base at the junction of the cameo surface and the intaglio surface; (2) the peripheral border of a denture base at the facial, lingual, and posterior limits.

Disclusion: The separation of opposing teeth during eccentric movements of the mandible.

Pressure indicating paste: Any substance applied to a dental prosthesis, that, when seated on a structure, demonstrates the adaptation of the prosthesis to the structure it opposes.

15.2 The Timing of Delivery Appointment

Clinicians mostly underestimate the appointment for the delivery of RPD. However this appointment is as significant as other procedures. Thus it is important to offer sufficient time and effort for this appointment.

O. Şakar (ed.), *Removable Partial Dentures*, https://doi.org/10.1007/978-3-031-47083-7_15

1. The delivery of the prosthesis should be early in the morning to have time for a double check after the patient used the RPD for several hours.
2. This appointment should not be placed in the last day of the week. It is important to give the patient the chance for a second appointment the day after. Although the patient has no complaints with the denture or can remove the prosthesis for one day if any, patients mostly favor to see the dentist immediately.

15.3 The Goals of Delivery Appointment

15.3.1 Making the Insertion of the Removable Partial Denture Comfortable By Adjusting the Clasp Arms, Overpressure Points on the Impression Surface and Overextended Borders

Normally checking and adjusting the framework should have been done at the previous appointment. Therefore, this procedure takes a short time. The fit of the RPD will not be proper if the undercut areas in soft tissue weren't correctly blocked out by the dental technician or if too much polymerization shrinkage had occurred. In these cases, the metal framework cannot be seated exactly on the abutment teeth. Thus, not the framework but the intaglio acrylic surfaces should be analyzed. Also, the retention of the RPD can be too strong or too weak due to the messy job of the dental technician. The clasp arms should be adjusted accordingly using a proper clasp bending pliers.

After this procedure if the RPD still doesn't fit properly, the guiding surfaces of the framework should be checked. In most cases, an excessive acrylic on this surface is responsible for the lack of the fit of the RPD. Indicator material, articulating paper, or occlusion sprays can be used to detect the place which blocks the path of insertion (Fig. 15.1a–c).

The fit of the RPD will not be correct if any overpressure points on the impression surface or overextended borders are present. To detect the pressure points, the best method is using pressure indicating paste (PIP). To apply the paste on the impression surfaces correctly, the base should be dried before. A stiff-bristled brush is used to coat the surface with a thin layer of PIP. The brush marks should be visible (Fig. 15.2). Before applying in the mouth of the patient, the prosthesis is best sprayed with silicone oil to avoid from the paste sticking to the oral mucosa. The RPD is then placed in the mouth carefully and the patient is asked to bite on a cotton roll gently for few seconds. If the paste has lost the brush marks and a tissue pattern is visible, the fit of the base with the mucosa is correct. If the brush marks are still there in some places, there is no contact in these parts of the base (Fig. 15.3). And if there is no paste anymore on some areas, these are the overpressure points and should be adjusted before the delivery of the prosthesis to the patient.

The overextended borders of the prosthesis should also be adjusted before the delivery. This can worsen the retention of the RPD or can cause ulceration in the soft tissue. A visual examination during functional movements of the patient is mostly enough to detect the overextended border. However sometimes it is very difficult to identify the exact place. Thus, using a light-body silicone impression material will be helpful to detect the part needs to be shortened. A thin coat of silicone material is placed on the tissue surface of the RPD. After that the patient makes functional movements. The impression material is easily wriggled out from the extended border. This part is then shortened accordingly.

15.3.2 Checking the Esthetics of the Prosthesis and Making Individualization By Cosmetic Grinding

The esthetical try-in procedures are not so difficult in RPD treatment compared with complete dentures or fixed partial dentures. Most RPDs are prepared to replace the posterior teeth. However, in cases with the lack of anterior teeth, individualization of the artificial teeth is mostly necessary. Nowadays there are plenty of individualization composite sets in dental market. If porcelain teeth were used, a conventional technique can be used. It is also important to note that if a

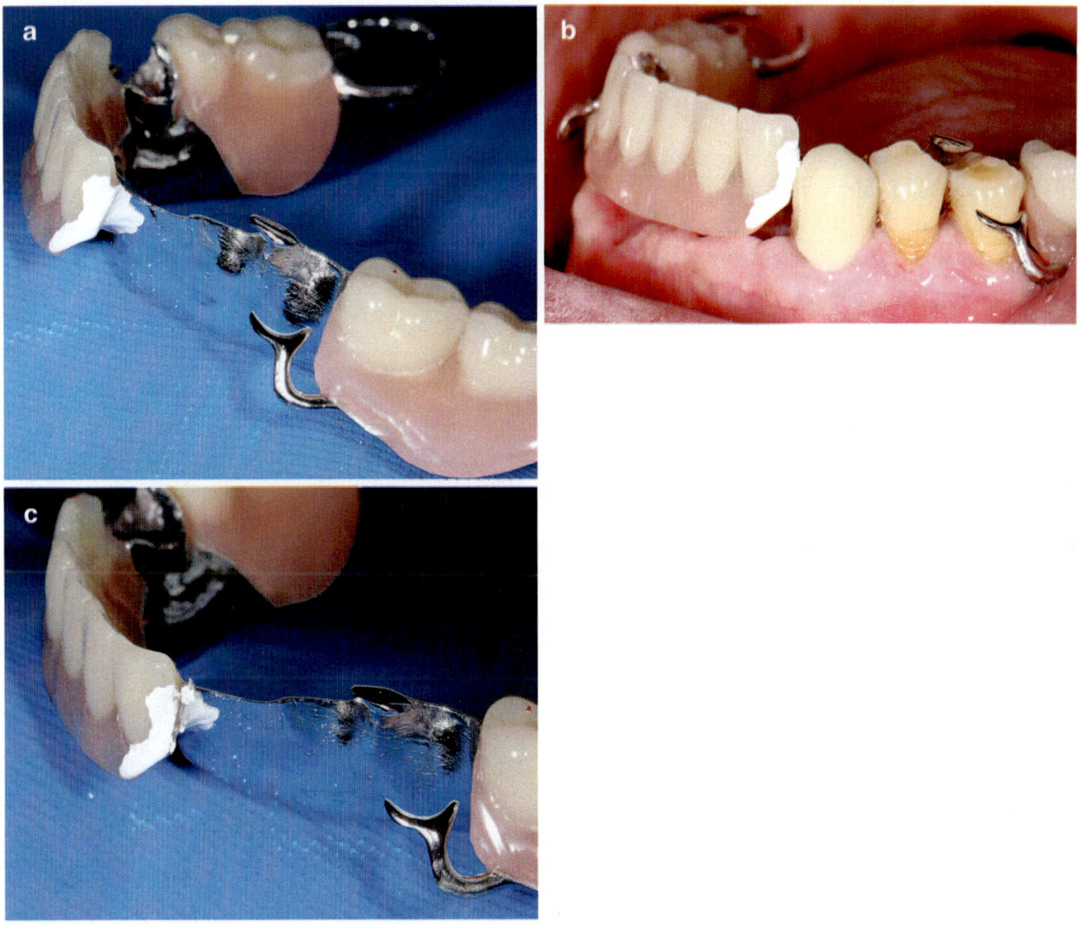

Fig. 15.1 Mandibular prosthesis is not seated correctly to the place. (**a**) The guided surface is painted with a thin layer of indicator material. (**b**) The prosthesis is forced to be placed in the mouth of the patient. (**c**) The indicator material is scratched over the acrylic surface. The part is then grinded carefully

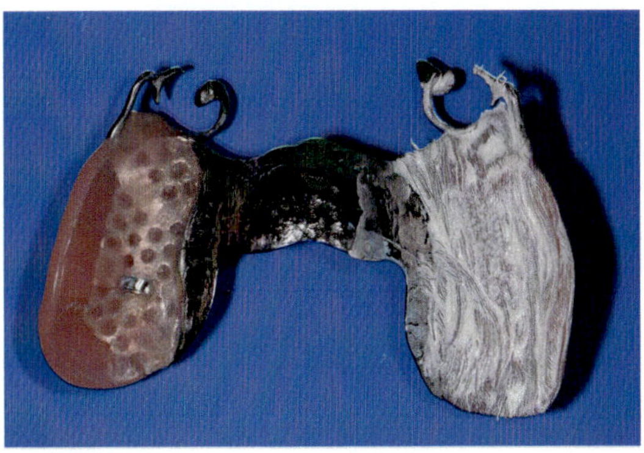

Fig. 15.2 The impression surface of the prosthesis is painted with PIP

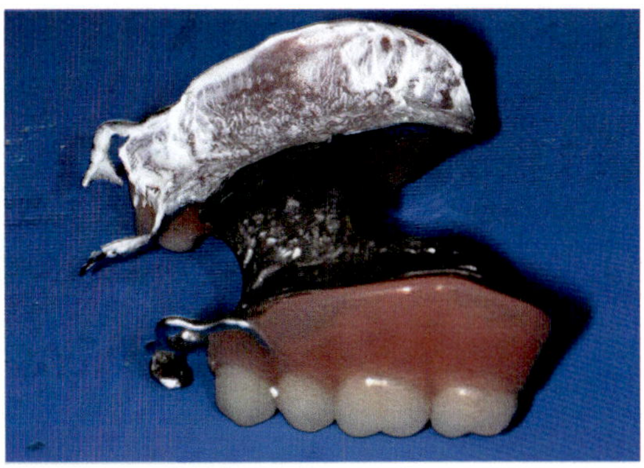

Fig. 15.3 Notice the overpressure point in PIP

crown restoration for the abutment tooth was planned, the selection and arrangement of the artificial teeth should be prepared before the esthetic work of the crown was finished. It is the easiest way to achieve the best esthetic harmony between artificial teeth and crown restoration. The dental technician makes the esthetic labial surface of the crown according to the artificial teeth. Otherwise, it will be quite difficult to achieve an esthetic result in a combined prosthesis.

15.3.3 Adjusting Centric and Eccentric Occlusion

Prior to the delivery of the prosthesis to the patient, the clinician must be sure that the occlusion is perfect. It is unexpected that the metal framework disturbs the occlusal balance. The contacts of the occlusal rests with the antagonist teeth have to be checked before. However, if the fit of the RPD is not ideal, a gap between the occlusal rest and seat may be seen easily. Thus, in such a case, the fit of the RPD should be checked again.

The most expected problem with the occlusion is the premature occlusal contacts of the artificial teeth on RPD. This problem can be solved easily by systematic occlusal grinding in the mouth. However, in cases with a huge occlusal first contacts or disclusion of the posterior artificial teeth the best way is to remount the prosthesis to the articulator and to make the corrections in dental laboratory. The best method is to take a new centric relation record using a silicone bite registration material and impression compound. The impression compound is softened first and applied on the maxillary incisors to create a deprogrammer. After the deprogrammer is hardened, the contact of the mandibular incisors with the flat surface of the impression compound is checked. This surface should be prepared perpendicular to the long axis of the lower incisors. A disclusion of 2–3 mm between the posterior teeth in centric and eccentric occlusion is ideal to make a centric relation record. After that silicone bite registration material is applied between the posterior teeth (Fig. 15.4). Following alginate impressions of both jaws are taken (Fig. 15.5). The RPD should stay within the impression. A remount cast is formed after all undercut places, clasps, and proximal plates are blocked out with wax. These remount casts are then transferred to

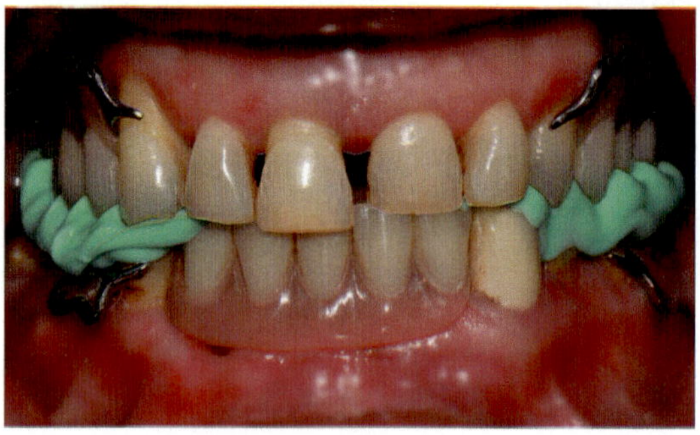

Fig. 15.4 The occlusion of the prosthesis is not sufficient. Thus, a centric relation record is made

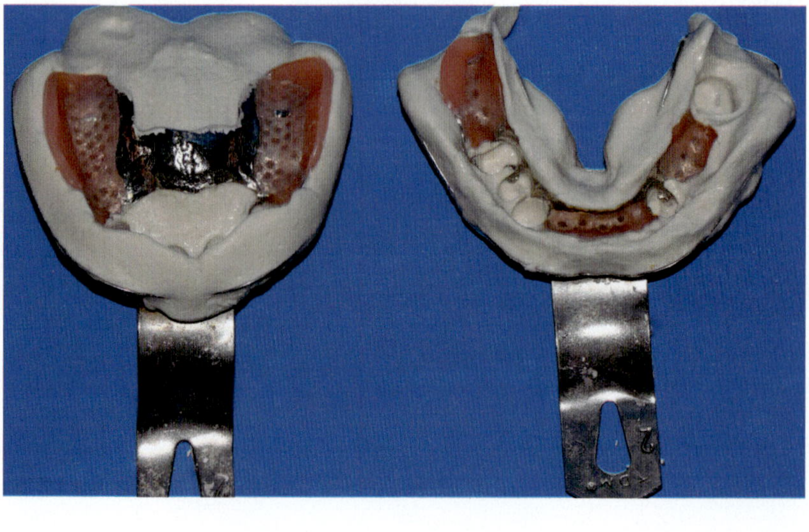

Fig. 15.5 Alginate impressions are made for lower and upper jaws

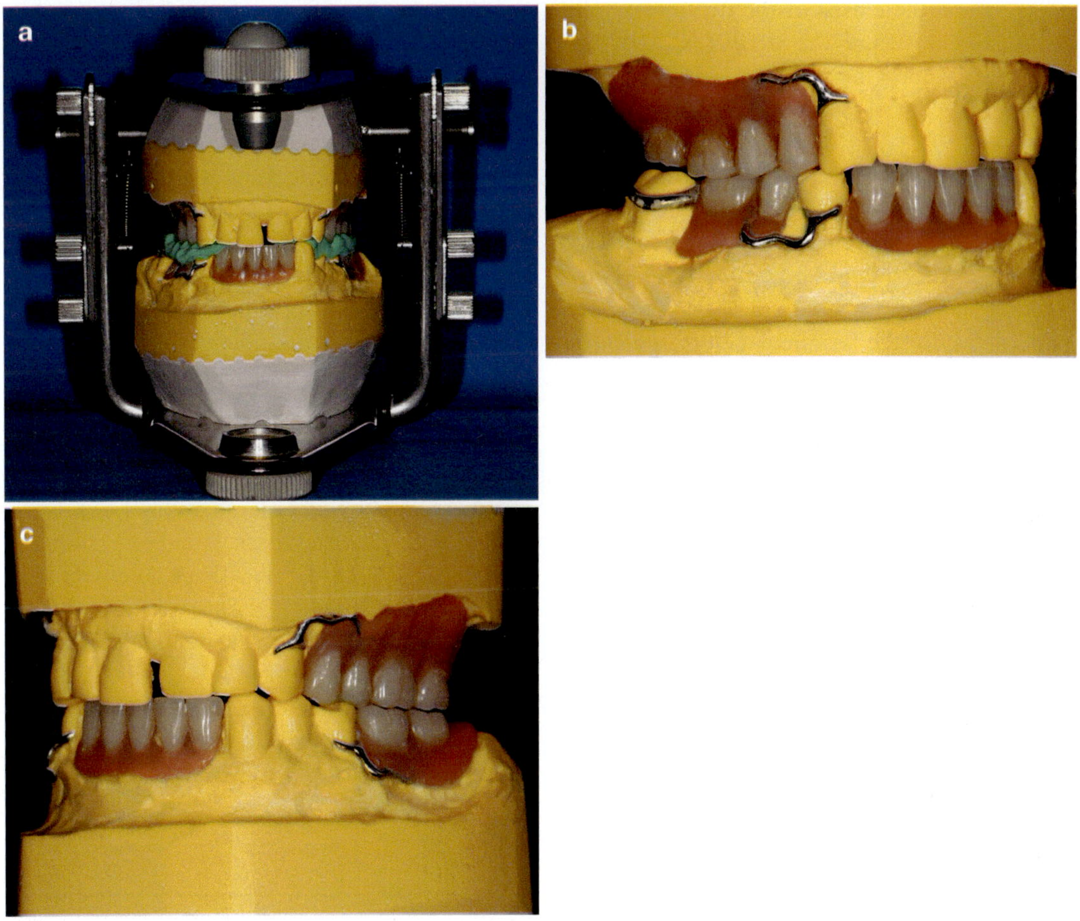

Fig. 15.6 (**a**) The remount casts are mounted to the articulator. (**b**) There are no occluding contacts (right side view). (**c**) There are no occluding contacts (left side view)

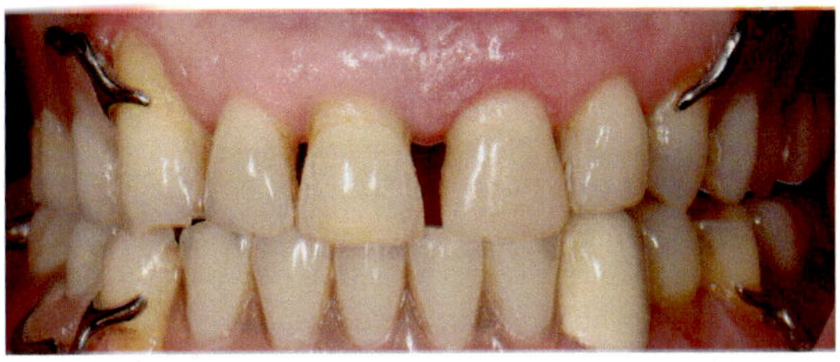

Fig. 15.7 The adjusted prosthesis in the mouth of the patient. Notice the restored left central tooth, too

an articulator using the interocclusal record (Fig. 15.6a–c). The occlusion is corrected and the RPDs are placed to the mouth of the patient (Fig. 15.7).

Occlusal grinding of the artificial teeth in RPD is a very easy process and similar to the method used for complete dentures.

15.3.4 Instructing the Patient How to Maintain the Prosthesis, the Mouth, and the Remaining Teeth

First of all, the patient should be informed about the importance of path of insertion. The patient should understand that his/her prosthesis can be inserted and removed in only one direction. Therefore, the first insertion and removal of the RPD should be performed by the clinician while the patient observes the process. After that, the mirror is held by the doctor and the patient tries carefully to insert and remove the RPD into the mouth. The patient should be warned not to place the prosthesis by biting on it but instead to guide into the seated position when the tips of fingers are on the clasps of the prosthesis. The patient should secure the perfect seat of the prosthesis by applying pressure along the incisal and/or occlusal surfaces of the artificial teeth.

For the removal of the prosthesis, the patient should use the thumbnails for the mandibular RPD and the index fingers for the maxillary RPD. The force should be applied to the clasp shoulders equally for both sides. Applying the force directly to the terminals can result in the distortion of the clasp arms. Trying to remove the prosthesis from the acrylic is not recommended because of the risk of the mucosal irritation. There is, however, no other way to remove the precision attachment RPDs. As a solution a metal pin is constructed in the framework which is then covered with acrylic resin and only the tip stays on the polished surface of the RPD. This is a good retentive part to apply force with the finger nails. However, patients find these parts mostly irritating. Another way to remove the precision attachment RPDs is holding the prosthesis using thumb and index fingers of the same hand.

It is crucial to inform the patient that the prosthesis and the teeth should be kept clean. The patient must understand that, lack of hygiene is more hazardous for the development of caries when using an RPD. Especially the areas between minor connectors and oral tissues are prone to food accumulation. A normal stimulation of tongue and food contact is lacking in these areas. Therefore, the patient should give extra effort to massage these parts using a toothbrush to simulate the normal function. The patient should be informed not to use toothpaste for cleaning the RPD. Toothpastes contain mostly abrasive particles which can easily damage the acrylic surfaces of the denture. A denture-cleaning solution can be used for extra cleaning especially for older and handicapped patients (see Chaps. 24 and 25).

Despite every effort of the dentist, the character, age, neuromuscular adaptation capability, and expectations of the patient make it sometimes very difficult to adapt to the new denture. Thus, the patient should be informed of the possible discomfort in the first days, e.g., soreness, difficulty with phonetics, discomfort, gagging. Patients mostly like to know that these difficulties can be solved easily in the control appointments. It is vital to inform the patients about the importance of the periodic recalls.

Night wear of the prosthesis is a controversial issue in current dental literature. Because of hygienic reasons and from a physiologic point of view, it is better to take the prosthesis out at night. However, in cases with severe bruxism, it is better to advise the patient to keep the prosthesis in mouth while sleeping because of the better distribution of the occlusal loads. Another example is the typical patient with maxillary complete denture and mandibular RPD. These patients mostly like to wear his/her complete denture at night. If the patient is insistent about this routine, it is better to advise the patient to wear also the mandibular prosthesis. Otherwise, the risk of the resorption of the anterior part of the maxillary crest will be higher.

Further Reading

Carr AB, Brown DT. McCracken's removable partial prosthodontics. 13th ed. St. Louis, MO: Elsevier; 2016.

Gernet W, Beuer F. Zahnärztliche Prothetik. Stuttgart: Thieme; 2007.

Graber G, Besimo C, Wiehl P, Rateitschak K. Farbatlanten der Zahnmedizin. Stuttgart: Thieme; 1992.

Loney RW. Removable partial denture manual. Halifax, NS: Dalhousie University Faculty of Dentistry; 2011. http://removpros.dentistry.dal.ca/ewExternalFiles/RPD%20Manual%2011.pdf.

Miller E, Grasso J. Removable partial prosthodontics. Baltimore, MA: Williams & Wilkins; 1981.

Preti G. Prosthetic rehabilitation. London: Quintessence Pub; 2008.

Santos JJ. Occlusion. Chicago, IL: Quintessence Pub. Co.; 2007.

The glossary of prosthodontic terms: ninth edition. J Prosthet Dent. 2017;117(5S):e1–e105.

Part IV

Advanced Retention and Support Auxiliaries for Removable Partial Dentures

16 Attachments and Double Crown Systems for Removable Partial Dentures

Ahmet Altuğ Çilingir

Abstract

There is a lack of evidence-based knowledge to dominate clinical decision-making about attachments in removable partial dentures. Even though the use of attachments in clinical dentistry is very regular, selecting the appropriate attachment for a particular case can sometimes be challenging. This chapter explains a brief classification of attachments, attachments' resilience capacities, step-by-step detailed clinical cases, and clinical hints in decision-making.

16.1 Definitions

Attachment: (1) A mechanical device for the fixation, retention, and stabilization of a prosthesis; (2) a retainer consisting of a metal receptacle and a closely fitting part; the former (the female {matrix} component) is usually contained within the normal or expanded contours of the crown of the abutment tooth, and the latter (the male {patrix} component) is attached to a pontic or the denture framework.

A. A. Çilingir (✉)
Faculty of Dentistry, Department of Prosthodontics, Trakya University, Edirne, Türkiye
e-mail: aaltugcilingir@trakya.edu.tr

Extracoronal attachment: Any prefabricated attachment for support and retention of a removable dental prosthesis; the retentive components (the matrix and patrix components or clasp) are positioned outside the normal contour of the abutment tooth.

Frictional attachment: A precision or semiprecision attachment that achieves retention by metal-to-metal contact without springs, clips, or other mechanical means of retention.

Intracoronal attachment: Any prefabricated or custom-made attachment for support and retention of a fixed or removable dental prosthesis; the patrix and matrix components are positioned within the normal contours of the abutment tooth.

Overdenture: Any removable dental prosthesis that covers and rests on one or more remaining natural teeth, the roots of natural teeth, and/or dental implants; a dental prosthesis that covers and is partially supported by natural teeth, natural tooth roots, and/or dental implants.

Precision attachment: (1) A retainer consisting of a metal receptacle (matrix) and a closely fitting part (patrix); the matrix is usually contained within the normal or expanded contours of the crown on the abutment tooth/dental implant, and the patrix is attached to a pontic or the removable dental prosthesis framework; (2) an interlocking device, one component of which is fixed to an abutment or abutments, and the other is integrated into a removable dental prosthesis to stabilize and/or retain it.

O. Şakar (ed.), *Removable Partial Dentures*, https://doi.org/10.1007/978-3-031-47083-7_16

Precision rest: A prefabricated, rigid metallic patrix in a fixed or removable partial denture that fits intimately into the matrix portion of a precision attachment in a restoration.

Resilient attachment (1998): An attachment designed to give a tooth-, soft tissue-, or implant-borne removable dental prosthesis sufficient mechanical flexion to withstand the variations in seating of the prosthesis as a result of deformations of the mucosa and underlying tissues to avoid placing excessive stress on the abutments.

Semiprecision attachment: A laboratory-fabricated rigid metallic patrix of a fixed or removable partial denture that fits into a matrix in a cast restoration, allowing some movement between the components; attachments with plastic components are often called semiprecision attachments even if prefabricated (not laboratory fabricated).

Telescopic crown: An artificial crown (framework) constructed to fit over a coping, another crown, a bar connector, or any other suitable rigid support for the dental prosthesis.

Precision attachments offer aesthetic solutions to patients unsatisfied with the appearance of their conventional removable partial denture (RPD). An attachment should replace the functions of a direct retainer. Basically, it should provide support, stabilization, and retention; therefore, it should be designed to have specific parts acting instead of an occlusal rest (1), a reciprocal arm (2), and a retentive arm (3) (Fig. 16.1).

Attachments are divided into two main categories as precision and semi-precision attachments. Precision attachments are manufactured precisely from a special metal alloy at a level of 0.01 mm tolerance. Matrix and patrix are both prefabricated and have advantages, such as ease of changing the parts when necessary and exhibition of less wear compared to semi-precision attachments. On the other hand, the main disadvantage of using precision attachments is the high cost. Semi-precision attachments are fabricated using wax, plastic, or refractory patterns. These patterns are attached to wax patterns of crowns or removable partial denture frameworks and are cast together with various metal alloys. Conventional casting procedures may negatively affect precision; therefore, these attachments are called "semi-precision" attachments. Easier fabrication, lower cost, and absence of welding are the main advantages of semi-precision attachments.

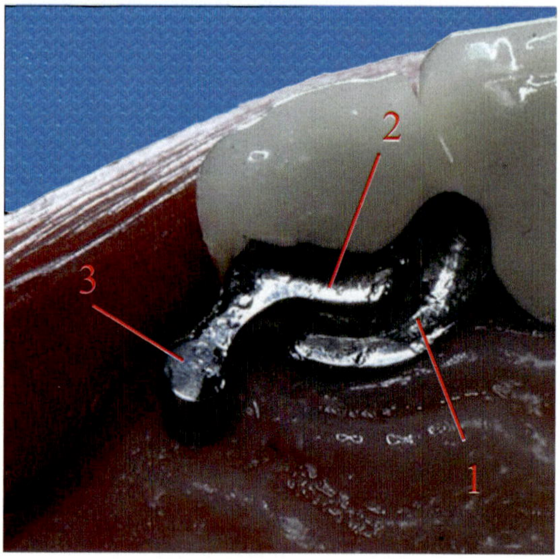

Fig. 16.1 An attachment should have parts of a direct retainer assembly: (1) an occlusal rest, (2) a reciprocal arm, and (3) a retentive arm

16.2 Classification of Attachments

There are two different main classifications according to the function and location of the attachments. RPDs transfer occlusal forces to supporting tissues like teeth and alveolar bone by their structural components. Resilient attachments transfer occlusal loads to alveolar tissues better than non-resilient attachments.

Non-resilient attachments, theoretically, do not allow any movement between their parts. However, a slight amount of movement will occur after the wear of the components.

16.2.1 Classification of Attachments According to Their Function

Deciding the attachment type is one of the most critical issues in planning an attachment-retained RPD. The length of the edentulous space, Kennedy's classification of partial edentulism, periodontal health of abutment teeth, and the patient's oral hygiene status should be considered while deciding the type of attachment.

Solid Attachments

Class 1a Solid, rigid, non-resilient (Fig. 16.2)
Class 1b Solid, rigid, non-resilient, lockable with an extra part (Fig. 16.2)

Resilient Attachments

Class 2 Vertical resilient (Fig. 16.3)
Class 3 Hinge resilient (Fig. 16.4)
Class 4 Vertical and hinge resilient (Fig. 16.5)
Class 5 Rotational and vertical resilient (Fig. 16.6);
Class 6 Universal, omni-planar (Fig. 16.7)

Class 1a

These attachments do not allow any movement between abutment teeth and RPD. Most of the intracoronal attachments are in this group. Solid, rigid, non-resilient characteristics of these attachments give them a very limited range of indica-

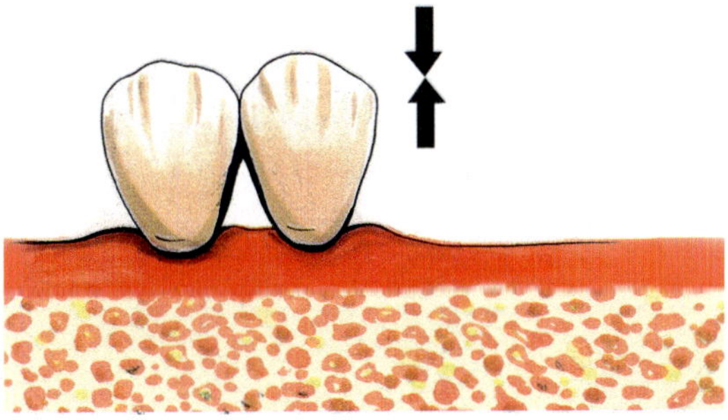

Fig. 16.2 Attachment classification: Class 1a or Class 1b rigid attachment

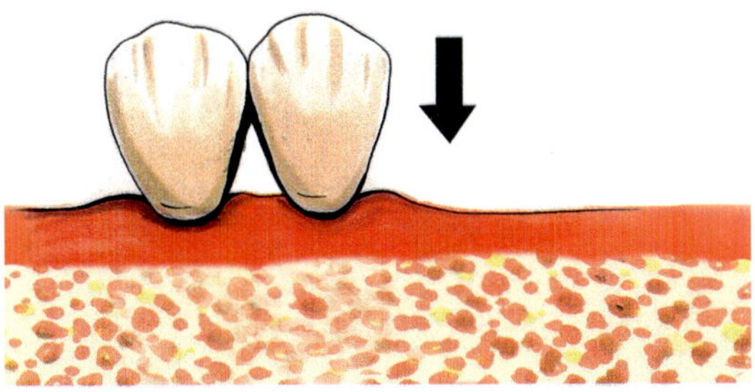

Fig. 16.3 Attachment classification: Class 2 vertical resilient

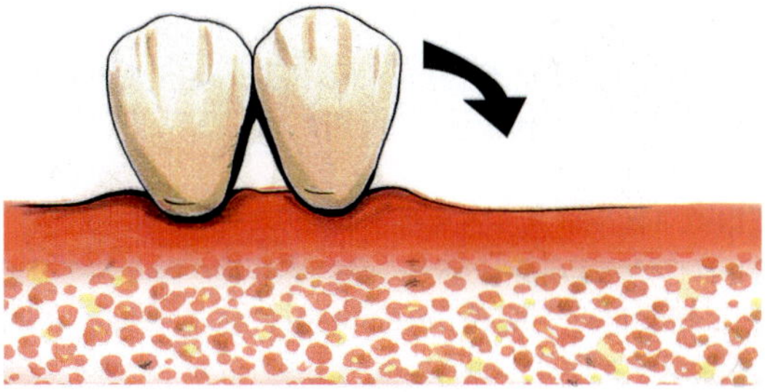

Fig. 16.4 Attachment classification: Class 3 hinge resilient

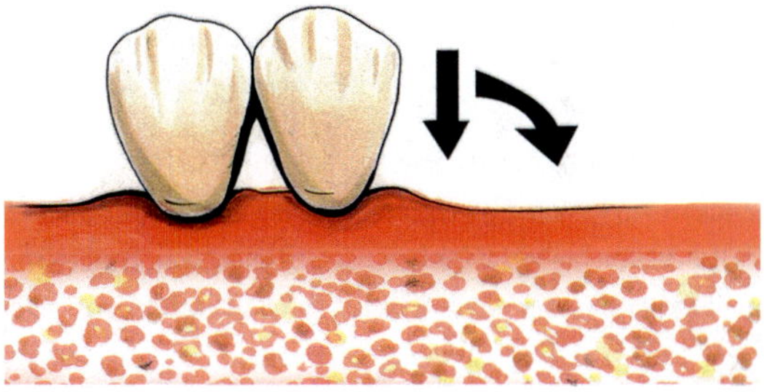

Fig. 16.5 Attachment classification: Class 4 vertical and hinge resilient

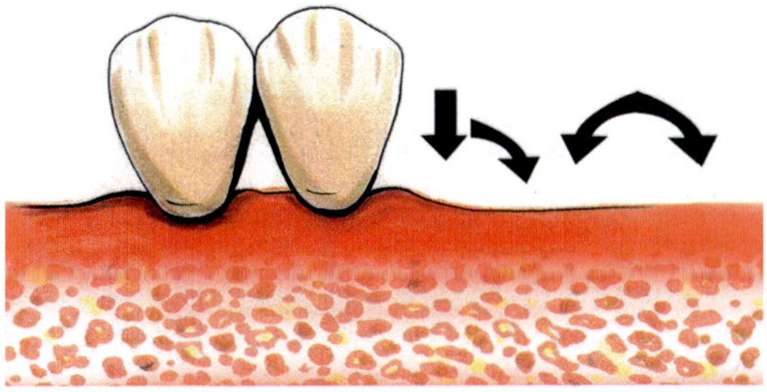

Fig. 16.6 Attachment classification: Class 5 rotational and vertical resilient

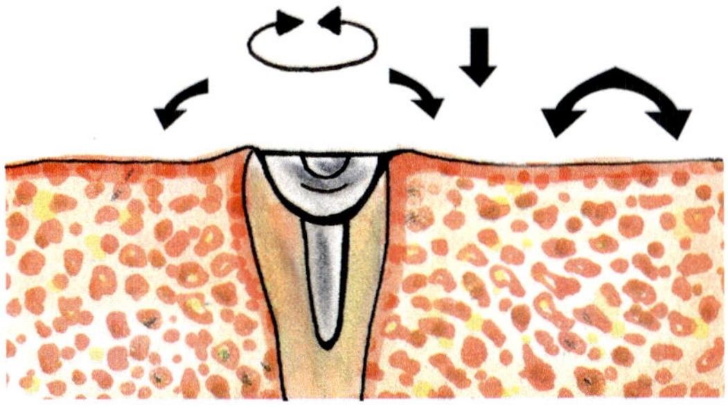

Fig. 16.7 Attachment classification: Class 6 universal, omni-planar

tions like tooth-supported RPDs. Chayes, Crismani, and McCollum are the commonly used attachments in this group (Fig. 16.2).

Class 1b

These attachments are very similar to class 1a attachments. The difference in this group is the presence of an additional part that locks the attachment components. They are also solid, rigid, and non-resilient and are only used in tooth-supported RPDs. Schatzmann and Stern Latch may be regarded as the most preferred class 1b attachments (Fig. 16.2).

Class 2

Class 2-type attachments have only vertical resilience. Only vertical occlusal loads are transferred to the alveolar ridge while the RPD is in function. Resilient Dolder and Hader bar attachments are cited in this group when two or more bar units with resilience parts and metal riders are used (Fig. 16.3).

Class 3

These attachments have hinge resilience and are mostly extracoronal. They allow RPDs to make rotational movements around the fulcrum line. Dalbo, Preci-Vertix, and Variosoft are the most favored class 3 attachments (Fig. 16.4).

Class 4

This group of attachments combines the features of class 2 and class 3 attachments. Under functional loads, they show both hinge movements and vertical resilience. Dalbo S is an example of a class 4 attachment (Fig. 16.5).

Class 5

These attachments have a motion capacity in all directions and therefore show all the resilience mechanisms. ASC 52 and Ceka may be presented as examples for this attachment group (Fig. 16.6).

Class 6

Most stud attachments belong to this group. Universal and omni-planar attachments have a motion capacity in all directions; they even allow rotation around their long axis if a single abutment is used to retain an overdenture (Fig. 16.7).

16.2.2 Classification of Attachments According to Their Location on Abutment Teeth

A wide variety of shapes and sizes of precision attachments have been offered for the use of prosthetic dentistry over the years. Information on the clinical use and technical features of some of these attachments on cases will be given below.

1. Intracoronal attachments (Fig. 16.8)
2. Extracoronal attachments (Fig. 16.9)
3. Stud-type attachments (radicular/intraradicular) (Fig. 16.10)
4. Bar-type attachments (Fig. 16.11)

Intracoronal Attachments

Generally, intracoronal attachments are non-resilient and provide all functions of direct retainers. The main advantage of intracoronal attachments is the direction of occlusal forces parallel to the long axis of abutment teeth. On the other hand, the necessity of box preparation leads to more reduction of abutment teeth, and their non-resilient nature makes them unfavorable for distal extension RPDs (Fig. 16.8).

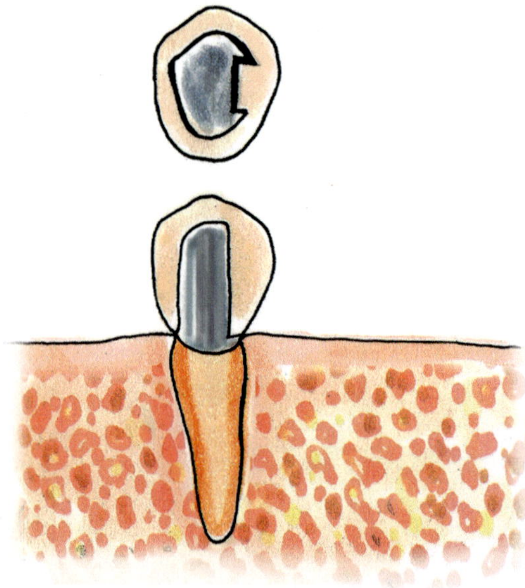

Fig. 16.8 Box-type tooth preparation of abutment teeth for intracoronal attachments

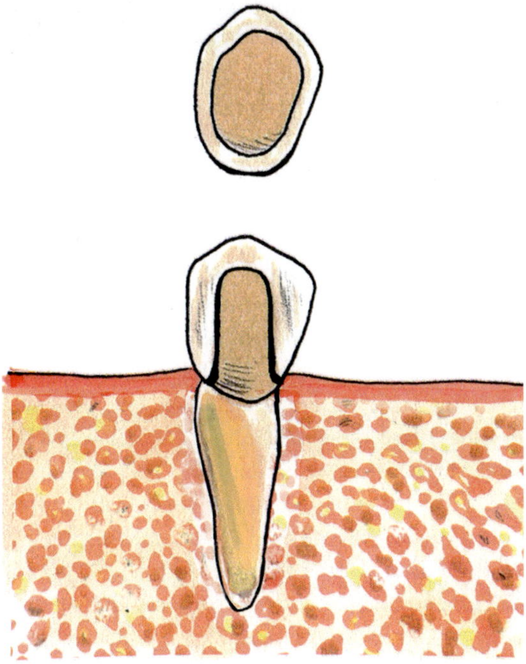

Fig. 16.9 Regular tooth preparation of abutment teeth for extracoronal attachments

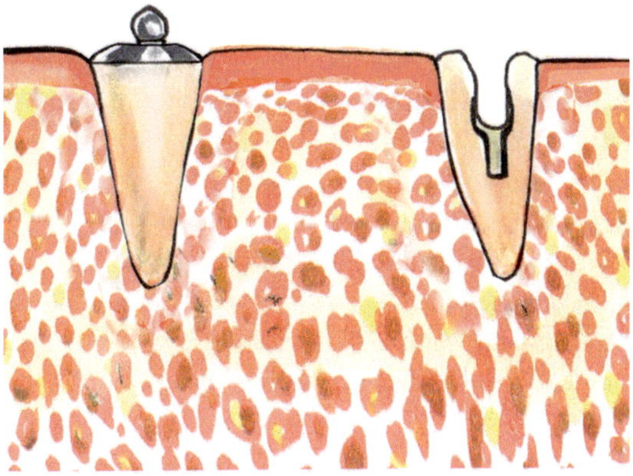

Fig. 16.10 Stud type attachments (radicular/intraradicular)

Intracoronal attachments consist of two parts: a groove and a flange. Groove is embedded into the crown, and the flange is merged into the RPD. Herman Chayes designed a T-shaped attachment in 1906 which was the first commercially available intracoronal attachment and is still in the market with a few modifications. His design has particular functions of a clasp, like retention and support. The retention mechanism

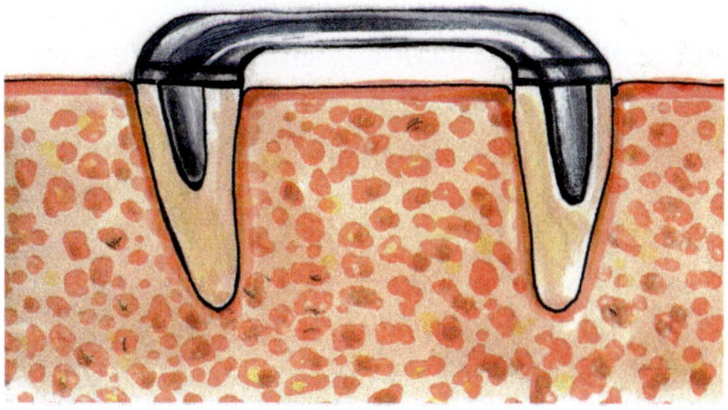

Fig. 16.11 Bar-type attachments

is maintained by the surface contact area between the attachment parts. Later, Chayes designed another H-shaped intracoronal attachment in 1912 with significant advantages over earlier T-shaped ones. The external flange of an H-shaped attachment increases the surface area twice and provides extra strength. Chayes attachment is a class 1a rigid attachment and should only be used with tooth-supported RPDs. Continuous insertion and removal of the RPDs may decrease the friction-dependent retention of these attachments. A razor blade or a scalpel may adjust the retention by opening the two parts of the attachments. Manufacturers fabricate numerous attachments, and the correct attachment type selection depends on the shape and size. The Crismani, McCollum, and Stern Latch are the commonly used examples of intracoronal rigid attachments. The Crismani intracoronal attachments are available in two different dimensions. The unit is regularly 7 mm long but can be shortened to 2 mm. The Crismani attachment is a class 1a rigid attachment having a dovetail design with a central groove for adjustment and should only be used with tooth-supported RPDs. The McCollum attachment is also a class 1a rigid attachment and should only be used with tooth-supported RPDs. Stern Latch is an intracoronal rigid precision attachment for non-resilient RPDs. The Stern Latch intracoronal attachments are precisely manufactured to "0.0001" tolerances which correspond to the interchangeability of parts. The female part of Stern Latch may either be soldered to crowns or cast with precious and non-precious alloys. The male part of Stern Latch may be soldered or laser welded to the

RPD framework or cast with gold alloys. For the abutment tooth selection, a minimum of 4 mm vertical and buccolingual length is required. It should be underlined that the patients who will use the RPDs with these attachments should be capable of using this mechanism, and the patients should be warned about this situation before starting the treatment.

The clinician adjusts the attachment chairside to provide the minimum retention necessary to hold the denture in place. Too much retention will cause excessive attachment wear, making the denture challenging to insert and remove. The clinician should try the denture in the mouth, enlarge the retention split slightly, and reseat the RPD. If the RPD retention is insufficient, the procedure should be repeated.

Extracoronal Attachments

Resilient and non-resilient types of extracoronal attachments are available in the market. The abutment teeth are prepared with less reduction, and the need for endodontic treatment is reduced with extracoronal attachments compared to intracoronal alternatives (Fig. 16.9). They also provide an easy path of insertion. Most extracoronal attachments have variable resilience mechanisms. Hygiene management may be compromised as the extracoronal parts cover extra surfaces for plaque accumulation. Cleaning the attachment parts with a toothbrush is difficult, and regular flossing is required. Mouthwash and rinse may also help oral hygiene management. Long extracoronal attachments have mechanical advantages like altered stability and increased retention area. However, plaque accumulation and space requirement for the attachments within the denture base may be regarded as disadvantages. Extracoronal attachments should be placed on the midline of the residual alveolar ridge. However, if this placement provokes aesthetic considerations, they may be positioned slightly lingually. Too lingually set attachments may cause problems like undesirable artificial tooth placement and over-contoured denture bases. The lingual or palatal bracing arm should be prepared for most extracoronal attachments in the form of a reciprocal arm and an occlusal rest. If the bracing arm ends with an interlock, attachments become more rigid. Distal extension RPDs require a minimum of two splinted abutment teeth on either side. Still, if six or fewer anterior teeth remain, splinting them together is necessary to form one rigid abutment. If less than four mandibular anterior teeth remain, fabricating an overdenture is much better.

Dalbo S

Dalbo S may be regarded as one of the most prevalent class 4 precision extracoronal attachments. The male part is soldered to the abutment crowns, and it comprises an L-shaped bar with a resilient ball joint with vertical translation and rotation. There are two types of Dalbo S attachment systems, bilateral and unilateral. The unilateral model has an enlarged lateral surface area, providing more resistance to lateral displacing forces. Using a bracing arm with the Dalbo S attachment is unnecessary because the attachment design has a reciprocation system embedded in its body. The precise contact between the vertical surface of the male unit and the female part prevents the distal denture base from dislodging through the mucosa, providing a perfect indirect retainer mechanism. The female part has an inside spring that provides a 0.4 mm vertical resilience to the prosthesis and a lamellar design, which makes it achievable to adjust the retention force. The buccal/lingual flanges of the lamellar design are slightly bent to adjust the retention. The main disadvantages of the Dalbo S attachment are the space requirement of the female in the RPD and vertical load transfer away from the long axis of the abutment tooth.

Dalbo Mini

Dalbo mini is a class 3 extracoronal attachment with a simplified female compared to Dalbo S. The female part of the Dalbo mini does not have a spring, which allows vertical resilience. Dalbo mini has all the advantages of Dalbo S with less space requirement for the female having a lamellar design in the RPD.

Preci-Vertix

Preci-Vertix is a class 3 semi-precision extracoronal attachment. Easy fabrication procedures and servicing, aesthetics, compatibility with any dental alloy, cost-effectiveness, and excellent patient comfort may be regarded as the advantages of this attachment. The vertical height of the male is 5.9 mm but can be reduced to 3 mm when necessary. In case of buccolingual space restrictions, Preci-Vertix is one of the best attachment solutions. A shoulder for a lingual bracing arm is recommended, and this shoulder may be finished with an interlock which gives more rigidity to the RPD. There are different female elastic clips with three friction levels (yellow standard friction, white reduced friction, and red increased friction levels). The castable plastic patterns are placed on the abutment crowns with the aid of a surveyor. The wax pattern is cast with a proper alloy and finished. Yellow female is inserted on the male part, a refractory model is fabricated, and the framework is waxed. After the framework is cast and finished, yellow elastic clips are inserted into the places prepared. The elastic clips are subjected to wear over time, but it is very easy to replace them (Figs. 16.12, 16.13, 16.14, 16.15, 16.16, 16.17, 16.18, 16.19, 16.20, 16.21, 16.22, and 16.23).

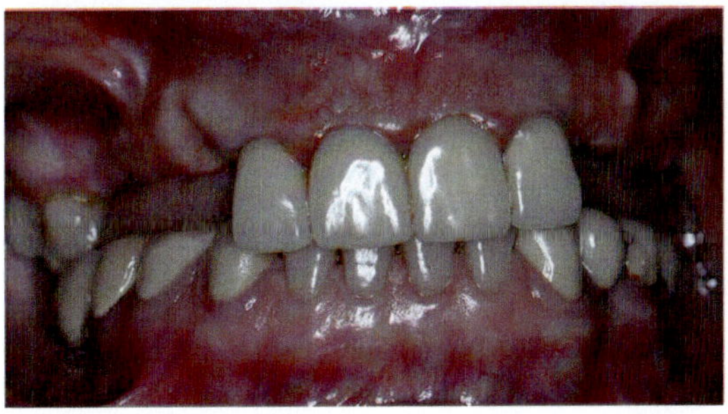

Fig. 16.12 Patient demands for attachment retained removable partial denture

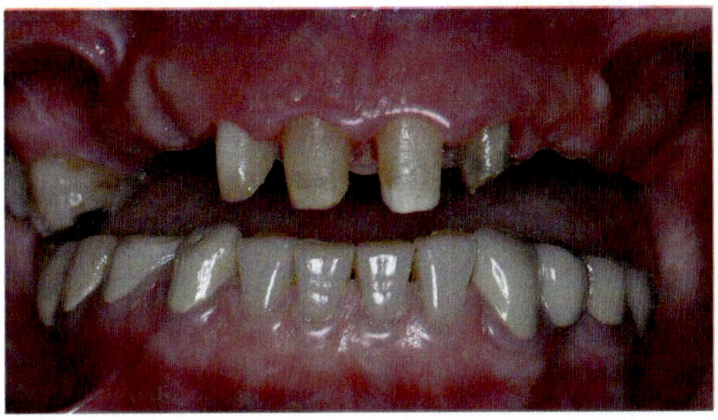

Fig. 16.13 Tooth preparation for extracoronal attachments

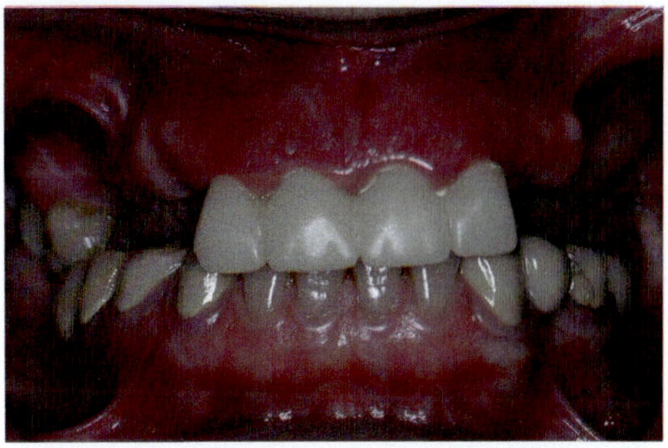

Fig. 16.14 Provisional crowns are cemented

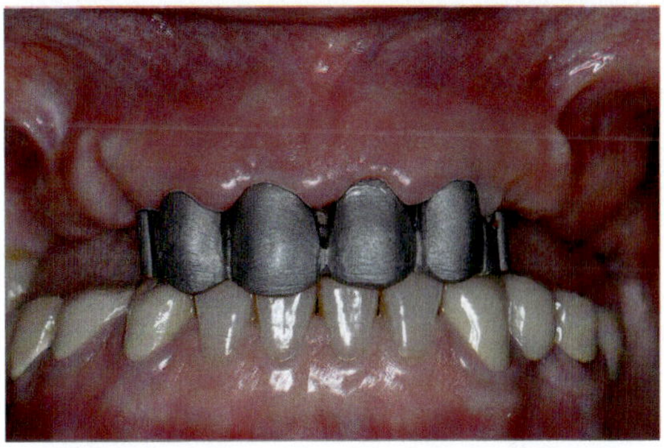

Fig. 16.15 Metal try-in for metal ceramic crowns with Preci-Vertix extracoronal attachments

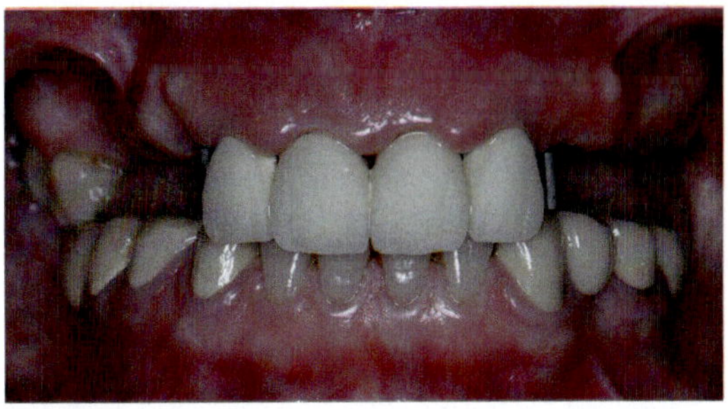

Fig. 16.16 Esthetic try-in for metal ceramic crowns with Preci-Vertix extracoronal attachments

MK1

MK1 is a solid (rigid) semi-precision class 1b attachment. It is indicated mainly for unilateral distal extension RPDs. It is a frictionless attachment; no wear is expected on the moving parts in time. The modular and simple design of MK1 permits the easy exchange of the parts of the attachment. MK1 has an aperture at the buccal

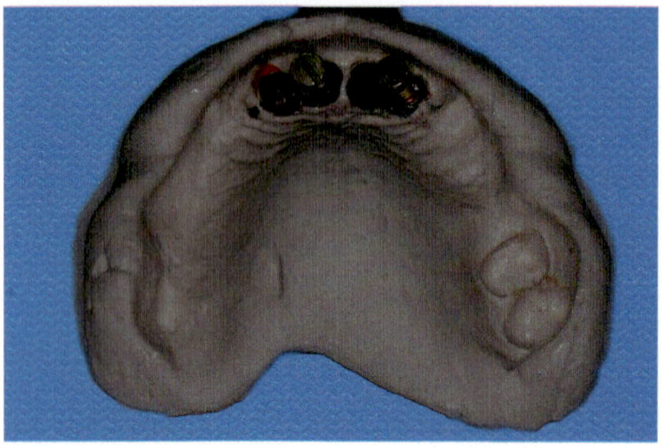

Fig. 16.17 An impression is made using a reversible hydrocolloid impression material with the crowns in place for the RPD framework

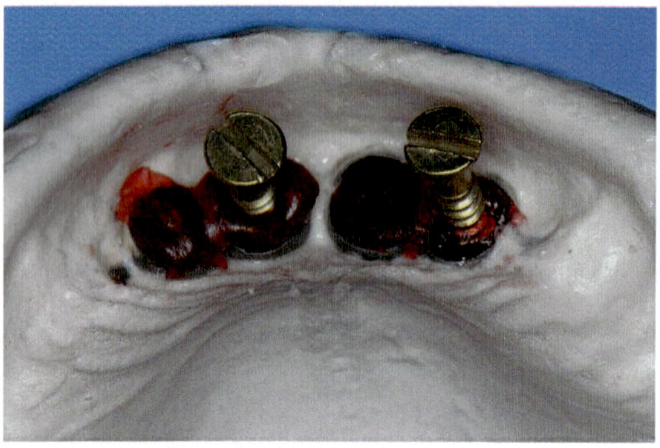

Fig. 16.18 The intaglio surfaces of the crowns are poured using autopolymerizing acrylic resin (pattern resin) using retentive dies

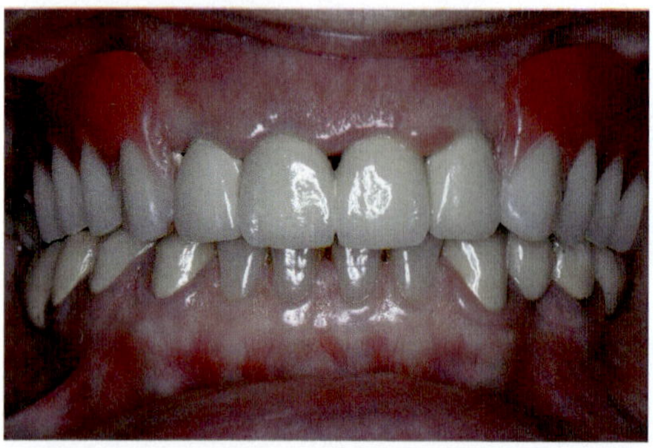

Fig. 16.19 Esthetic try-in is performed taking into consideration the occlusal contacts, centric relation, and occlusal vertical dimension

side of the RPD acting as a locking mechanism and a small key to open this lock which is provided by the manufacturer. Splinting the abutment crowns as much as possible is recommended in order to avoid decementation. Regular controls for the need for relining/rebasing of the RPDs should be checked in order to avoid the possible destructive occlusal forces generated by the rigid behavior of the attachment. After relining/rebasing, if the RPD does not fit its place easily, the interface between the interproximal area of the denture and the abutment crowns should be

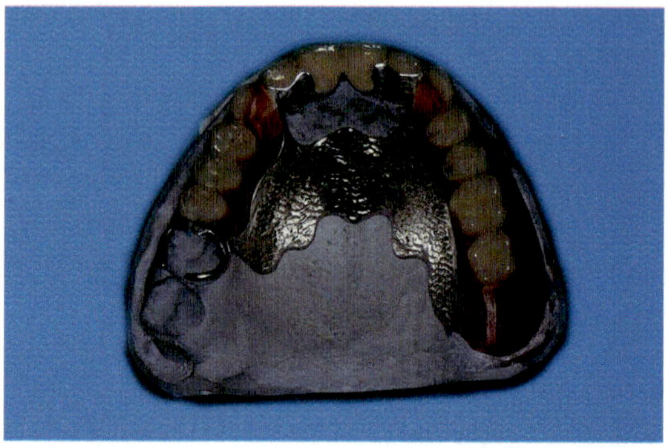

Fig. 16.20 Occlusal view of esthetic try-in on plaster model

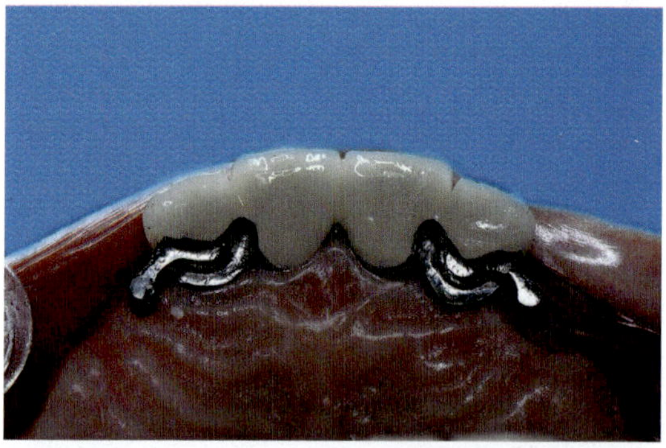

Fig. 16.21 Occlusal view of cemented metal ceramic crowns with attachments and precisely milled shoulders

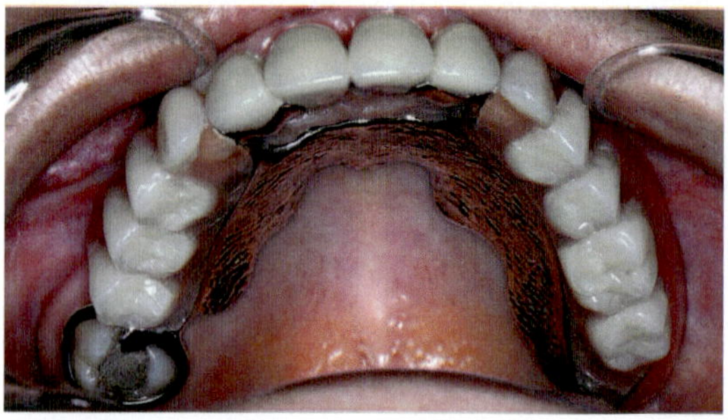

Fig. 16.22 Occlusal view of entire maxillary arch with attachment-retained RPD

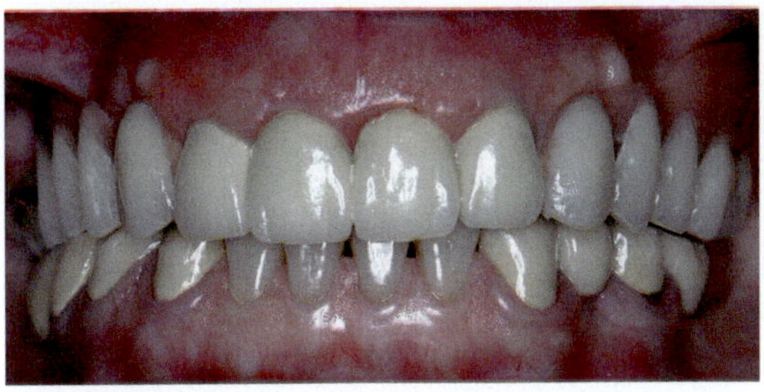

Fig. 16.23 Intra-oral view of attachment-retained RPD

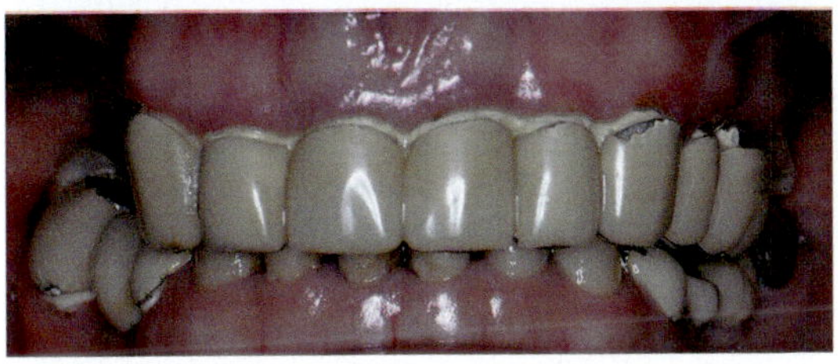

Fig. 16.24 A pure Kennedy Class II patient with metal plastic old crowns

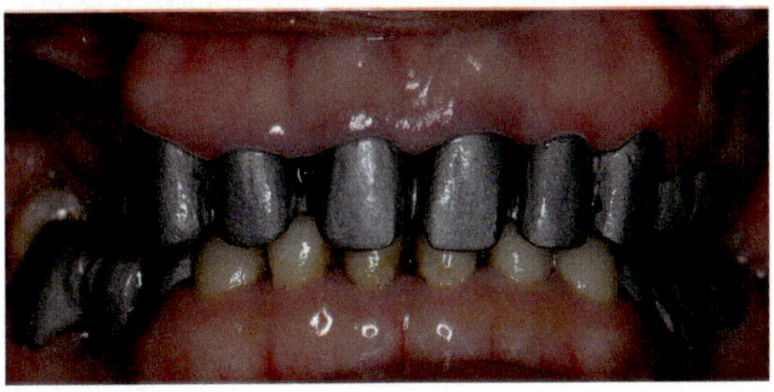

Fig. 16.25 Try-in of metal framework with a unilateral MK 1 attachment

checked. If there is excess acrylic resin, it should be ground carefully until the RPD fits the crowns submissively. A bracing arm is also recommended for stability. The difficulties in learning and using the locking mechanism by the patients may be considered as the main disadvantage of the MK1 attachment system. A clinical case of MK 1 is shown in figures (Figs. 16.24, 16.25, 16.26, 16.27, 16.28, 16.29, 16.30, and 16.31).

Ceka

Ceka attachment is a class 5 attachment allowing movement in rotational and vertical resilient all directions under functional occlusal loads. Ceka attachment has a male pin attached to the RPD

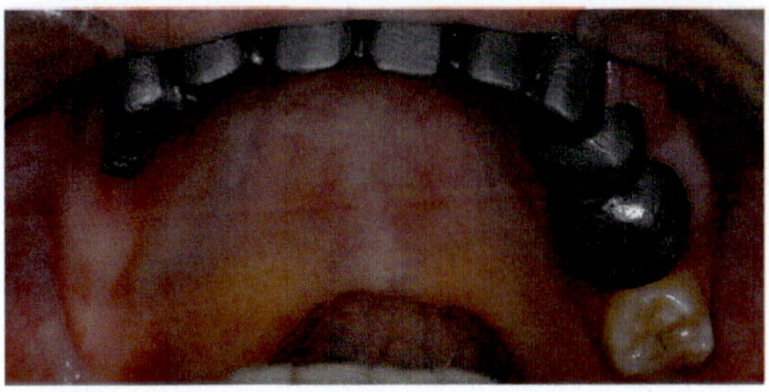

Fig. 16.26 Occlusal view of entire arch with metal framework

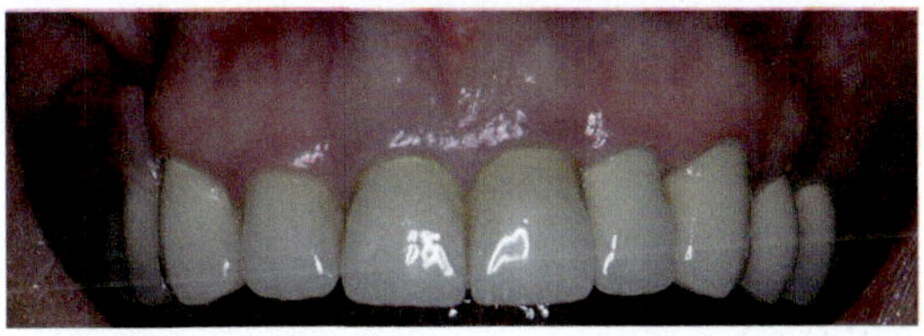

Fig. 16.27 Intra-oral view of metal porcelain crowns with unilateral MK 1 attachment-retained RPD

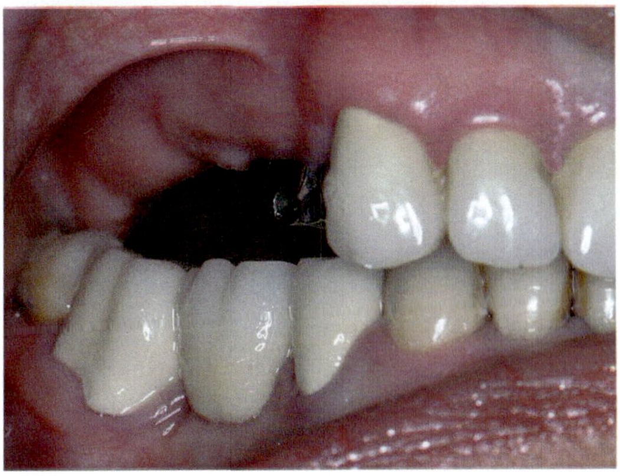

Fig. 16.28 Lateral view of unilateral MK 1 attachment

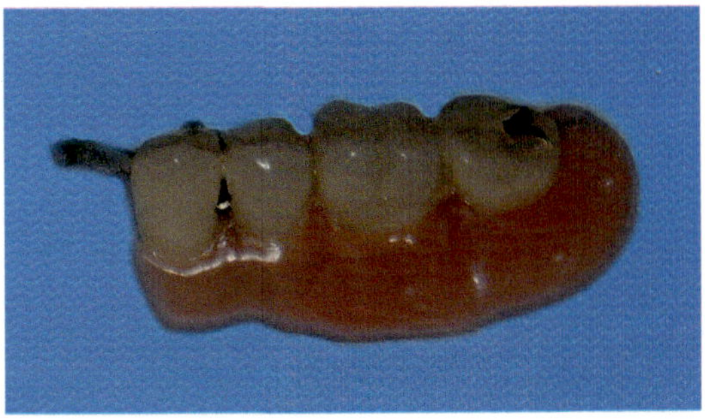

Fig. 16.29 Unilateral RPD with MK 1 attachment

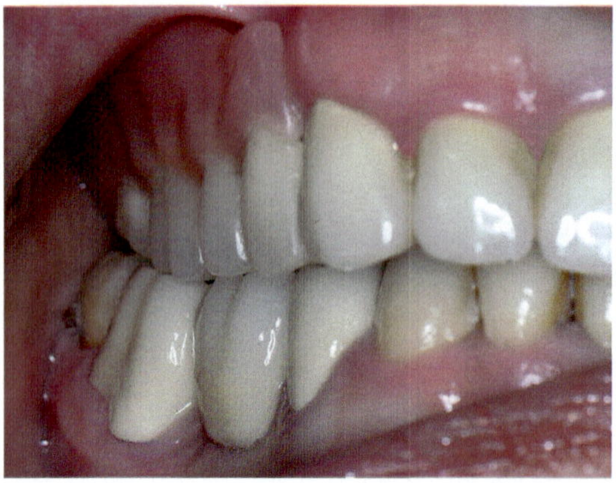

Fig. 16.30 Lateral view of fixed partial denture (FPD) and RPD with MK 1 attachment in situ

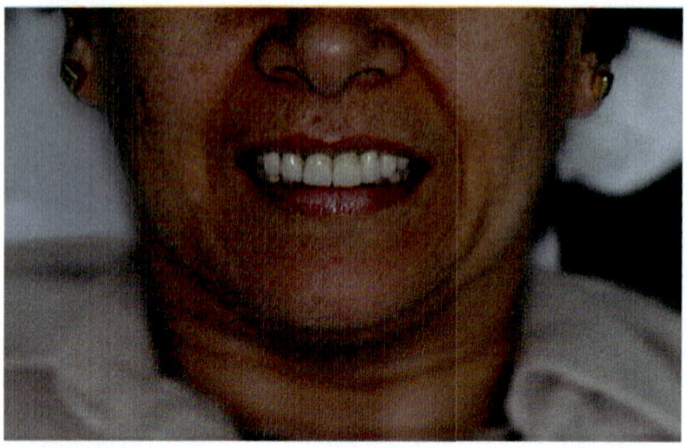

Fig. 16.31 The smile of the patient

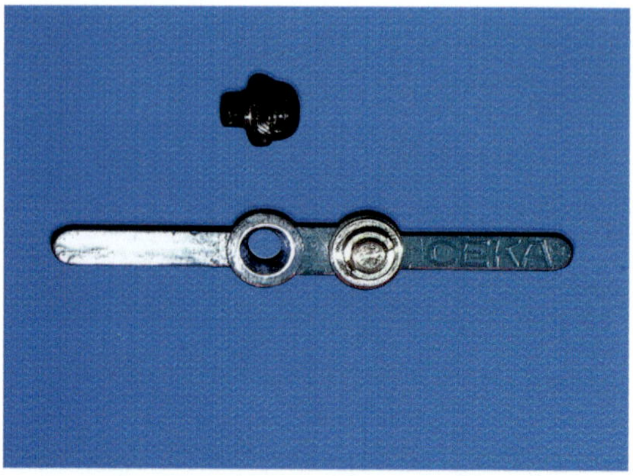

Fig. 16.32 The female part of the attachment has different castable forms with precious or non-precious alloys and a prefabricated form made-up with high fusing alloys. The prefabric model for casting with a non-precious metal is shown

and a female part joined to the abutment crowns. As with the other attachments, Ceka needs at least a 5 mm abutment length. Additionally, sufficient buccolingual space to cover the 4 mm diameter of the ring and allowing an adequate denture base thickness are required. Ceka attachment acts like a direct retainer so it should be combined with an occlusal rest and a lingual bracing arm with a shoulder. This arm prevents lateral movements of the RPD and guides it while seating in place. Ceka system includes both resilient and rigid attachment types. Resilient Ceka has a spacer between the male and female parts while processing the RPD. The manufacturer produces special equipment for activating and deactivating the male part to adjust the retention force. Additionally, the precision and semi-precision form of the Ceka attachment is available in the market. The female part of the attachment has different castable forms with precious or non-precious alloys and a prefabricated form made up of high-fusing alloys (Fig. 16.32). The female ring should be placed as close as possible to the mucosa in order to overcome the vertical space requirement, gingival hyperplasia, and torque forces acting on the abutments. The retention force should be adjusted with the aid of proper adjustment tools supplied by the manufacturer; otherwise, male-retaining pins may be easily damaged. The retention force of the male pins should be reduced when the denture is delivered for the first time. Relining/rebasing the RPDs requires care and precision. A specific spacer should be inserted between the male and female parts before making the impression. The pressure for seating the denture while making the impression for relining/rebasing should be applied from bracing arms, occlusal rest, and over the attachments. An overall impression with an irreversible hydrocolloid should be made for removing the RPD from the mouth. The spacer must be used while processing the relining procedures in the laboratory. The spacer will be removed when the denture is seated in place after relining/rebasing.

ASC 52

ASC 52 is also a class 5 attachment allowing movement in all directions under functional occlusal loads. Precision and semi-precision types of ASC 52 are available for different applications. The main advantage of ASC 52 is the stress-breaking feature that is designed from the cardan joint according to the requirements of dentistry, and therefore it is indicated for bilateral distal extension cases with elastic mucosa. ASC 52 has two different male parts with protection and without protection (Fig. 16.33). The RPD is easily inserted and removed without any risk to the abutment teeth. The removable part of the RPD is attached securely to the abutment tooth without applying any destructive loads. The retention mechanism is based on the special adaptation principle of the ball/socket joint. The female part of the attachment may either be cast or welded to the abutment crowns. The prefabricated male part is embedded in the RPD. The retention force and movement capacity of the RPD is adjusted from the spring located in the male part with a specific screwdriver. The retention spring and the ball can be easily changed if they are worn. A clinical case of ASC 52 is shown in figures (Figs. 16.34, 16.35, 16.36, 16.37, 16.38, 16.39, 16.40, 16.41, and 16.42).

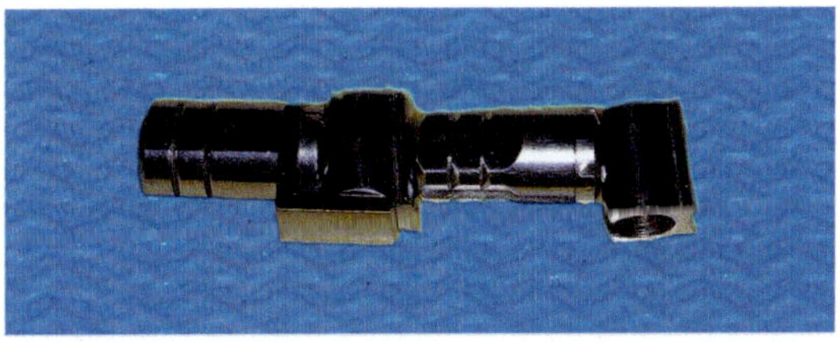

Fig. 16.33 The ASC 52 has two different male parts with protection and without protection

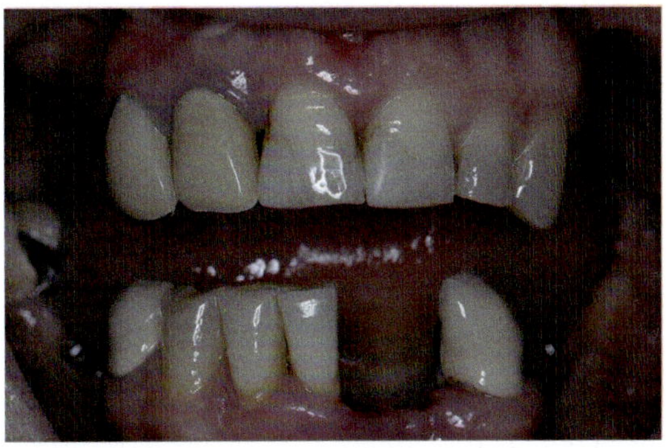

Fig. 16.34 Initial intraoral status

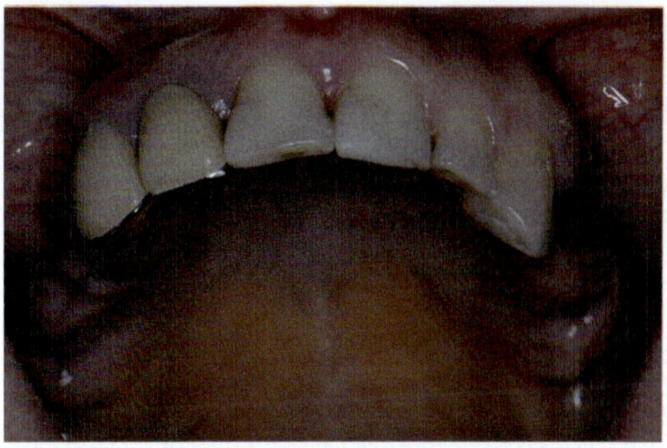

Fig. 16.35 Occlusal view of the entire maxillary alveolar ridge

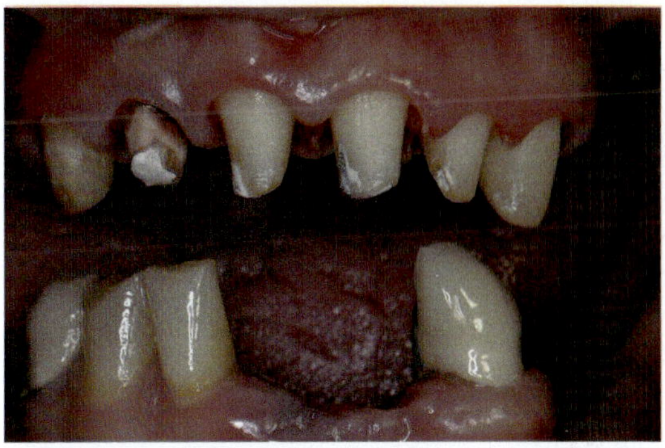

Fig. 16.36 Six or less remaining anterior teeth should be prepared to form one rigid abutment

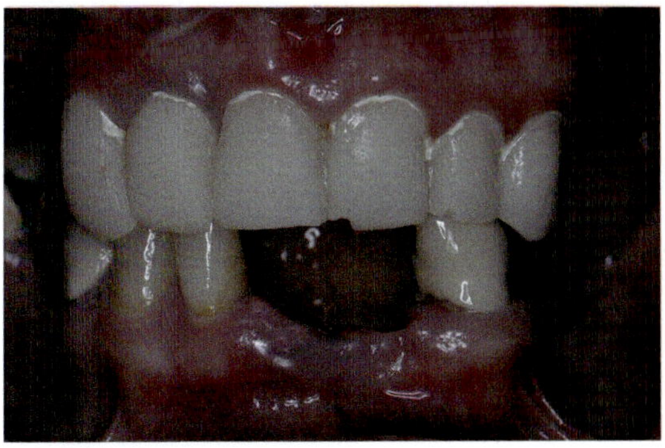

Fig. 16.37 Temporary crowns are made and cemented

Clinical Procedures of Extracoronal Attachments

1. Abutment teeth are prepared. It has been reported that at least two abutment teeth should be splinted (the number of the splinted

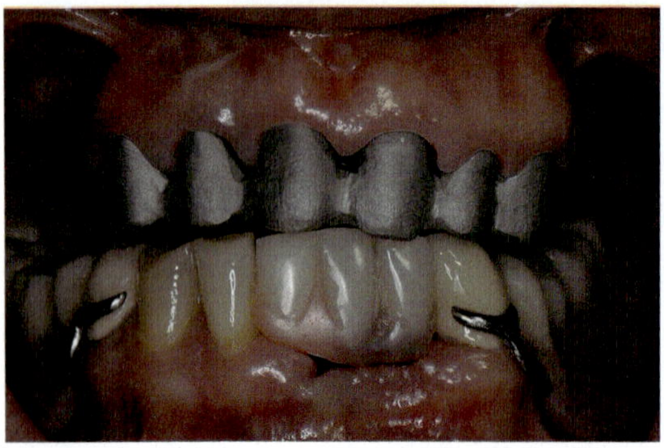

Fig. 16.38 The close-up view of extracoronal part of the metal ceramic crowns

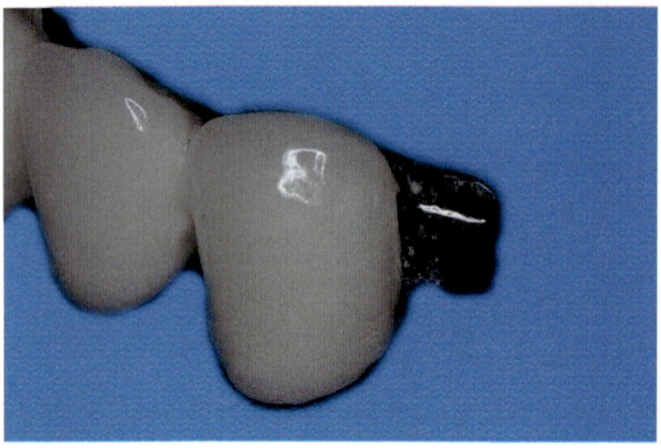

Fig. 16.39 The male part of the ASC 52

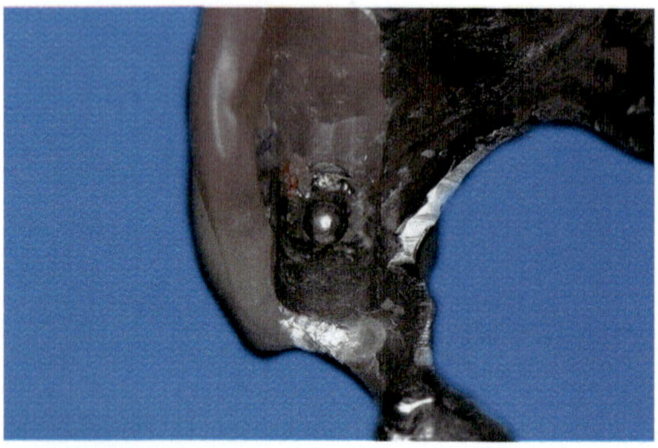

Fig. 16.40 ASC 52 is fixed to RPD with cold curing acrylic resin

teeth should be considered according to the condition and location of the teeth in the mouth, taking into account the biomechanical rules) if they will retain an attachment for an RPD. Preserving tooth structure, retention and resistance form, marginal integrity, and conservation of periodontal structures are essential for tooth preparation.

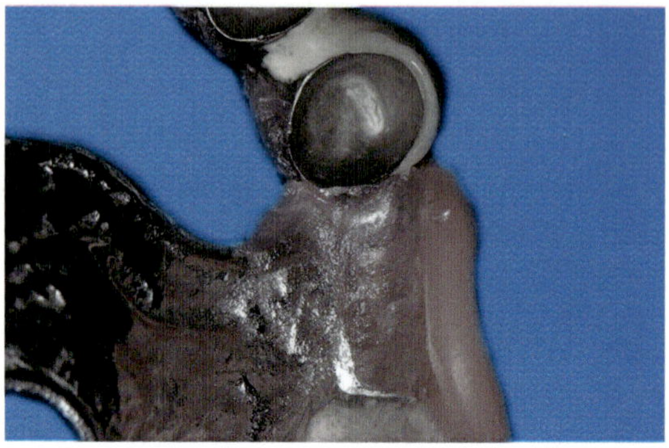

Fig. 16.41 The attachment parts are covered with cotton pellets or petroleum jelly in order to avoid cement escape between the attachments and the soft tissues

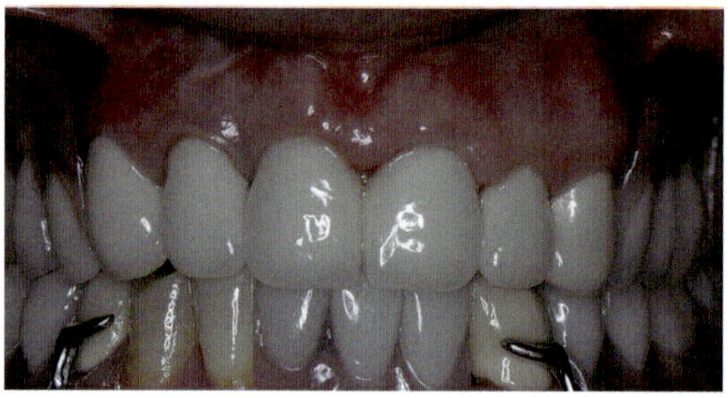

Fig. 16.42 The view of maximum intercuspidation of the RPD

2. Impressions are made with appropriate elastomeric impression material and sent to the laboratory to fabricate cast frameworks. Provisional crowns are prepared and cemented until the next appointment.
3. Try-in of the metal framework of the crowns is performed with marginal integrity; passivity, occlusion, and substructure design are inspected. The distance between the gingival tissues and the bottom part of the extracoronal attachments should be inspected. Attachments should touch the gingival tissues slightly and should not apply pressure, and there should not be a big gap in between in order not to cause subsequent gingival hyperplasia. Bite registration and centric relation position are established by using wax or an elastomeric registration material. Color, hue, and shade selection is completed, and the metal frame-

works are sent to the laboratory to apply veneering materials.

4. An aesthetic try-in of the veneering materials is performed. During the try-in, the size and tightness of proximal contacts, marginal integrity, and occlusion are checked and verified. An impression is made using a reversible hydrocolloid or a polyether impression material with the crowns in place for the RPD framework. The impression is poured with dental stone, but the intaglio surfaces of the crowns are poured using auto-polymerizing acrylic resin (pattern resin) using retentive dies to provide extra resistance while milling the crowns for refining shoulders acting as occlusal rests.
5. RPD framework is cast and attached to the crowns and tried in the mouth. After the harmony of a major connector with the soft tissues is evaluated, occlusal vertical dimension and centric relation position are determined, and the framework is sent to the laboratory for artificial tooth setup.
6. Aesthetic try-in is performed considering the occlusal contacts, centric relation, and occlusal vertical dimension.
7. Glazed crowns and finished RPDs are attached together and applied to the mouth. Any misfit of the crowns or the RPDs is inspected. Except for the intaglio surface of the crowns, petroleum jelly is applied to every other part of the crown-RPD assembly in order to avoid cement escape between the attachments and the soft tissues. If the crowns are not cemented with adhesive cement, the excess visible cement is cleaned after setting and a day after appointment is given to the patient instructing not to remove the RPD. One day after, the RPD is removed and excess cement is cleaned. Occlusal contacts and RPD borders are checked using pressure-indicating paste and articulating papers with different thicknesses. RPDs are delivered to the patients after describing the insertion and removal of the prosthesis.

Stud Attachments

Stud attachments are one of the most preferred attachments in prosthodontics and are currently mostly used in implant-assisted removable prostheses. Stud attachments are usually used after root canal treatment in order to use the root for a retaining structure (Fig. 16.43). There are two types of stud attachments: radicular or intraradicular types (Fig. 16.10). The male part is soldered or cast to a root-retained cap, and the female part is embedded in the denture base for the radicular ones. The male part is embedded in the denture base, and the female part is prepared on the abutment teeth for the intraradicular ones. These attachments are either placed directly into the root or soldered/cast to a root-cap coping. The female part of the intraradicular stud attachment is placed within the root shape. Better oral hygiene and reduction of crown-root ratio are the main advantages of stud-type attachments. If the root canal is used for retention, at least 2/3 root length should be used, and the crown height should not exceed 2–3mm for the accomplishments of the ferrule. The inclination of abutment teeth will be managed by a dental technician and the production process with a dental surveyor. If there is a discrepancy of more than 15° between the trajectories of implant abutments, this type of attachment should not be chosen.

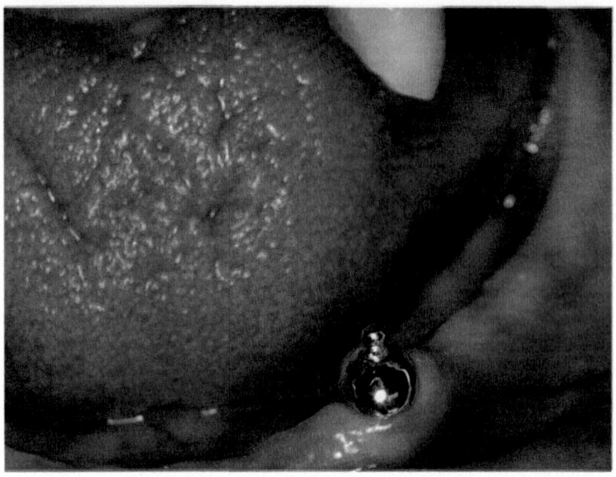

Fig. 16.43 Stud attachments are usually used after root canal treatment in order to use the root for a retaining structure

Stud attachments tolerate 5–20° of divergence from each other according to their brand. Shorter attachments have better toleration capacity. Taller attachments may need precise attention on the path of insertion. There are different types of stud attachments according to their resilience characteristics. Most of the stud attachments are class 3 hinge resilient attachments, but there are also some class 4 attachment types showing hinge and vertical resilience. Though most of the stud attachments require less space, there may be some patients who do not have sufficient space because of the eruption of teeth. Mounted diagnostic casts are very useful to determine the required space for the stud attachments, and it should be emphasized that the presence of attached gingiva around the abutment teeth provides a better prognosis. Usually, one stud attachment on each side of the dental arch will be enough, and other remaining roots may be covered with metal caps if they exist. Two adjacent roots with stud attachments will only weaken the acrylic resin of the RPD and create problems in the future.

Types of Stud Attachments

Preci-Clix

This type of attachment has a wide range of clinical indications from root-supported overdenture to extracoronal attachments. It has a 4 mm long design, which allows the female to engage all the surfaces of the ball. An audible click sound will be heard when the patient inserts the RPD in place. This attachment will tolerate 30° divergence, and females may still engage the undercut of the attachment. The system has a metal housing for the plastic clips and plastic inserts at different retention forces. There are also kits for precision and semi-precision applications. This attachment provides a class 3 hinge resilience.

Swiss Dalbo System

The Swiss Dalbo System is in use for over 40 years. The highly resistant compact shape and precious lamellar design of the female make the Dalbo System reliable and durable. The Swiss Dalbo System is easy to use and requires minimum space in the denture, and the retention force is adjusted according to patients' expectations. There is a clear nylon silicone sleeve around the female that protects the lamellae from becoming blocked by acrylic resin in the laboratory or intraoral practice. Metal lamella insert is screwed inside the housing for adjusting retention force. This attachment system tolerates 40° divergence, and the precious lamellae may be changed when needed. This attachment has a class 3 hinge resilience. Swiss Dalbo System recommends two different metal females with round and elliptic shapes. The overall height of the attachment differs from 2.9 to 3.7 mm. This attachment system also has parts for implant applications.

Gerber Unit

The Gerber Unit was originally designed by Prof. A. Gerber and is available in two sizes. The Gerber Unit is normally a rigid stud attachment with a slight vertical resilience. The system consists of five parts, and the main advantage of the Gerber Unit is the interchangeability of the parts. The interchangeability, replicability, and adjustability of the system make it reliable. On the other hand, the requirement of special accessory tools, mandrels, and the cost of the system are the main disadvantages of the Gerber Unit. The overall height of the Gerber Unit differs from 3.7 to 5.2 mm. Gerber pointed out that two attachments are sufficient to retain a denture; three or more abutments are unnecessary. A simple coping should be made for the excess roots. If two adjacent teeth are used, a resilient-type attachment should be chosen for the posterior tooth and a rigid for the anterior because of the altered displacement of the denture over the posterior teeth while chewing.

TiSi.snap

In recent years, with the developments in polymer technology, special matrix silicones have been offered in dentistry used over the stud and bar attachments as matrices.

TiSi.snap is a special form of abutment designed for silicone matrices. TiSi.snap, which has a retentive ring on a conical design, is available in high-cone (5 mm) and short-cone (3 mm) types. The high cone model provides adequate retention and stabilization for overdenture prostheses supported by two implants, while the short cone model provides adequate retention in cases where the interocclusal distance is insufficient. The plastic matrices of the locator system can be used to increase retention in patients where the retention with silicone matrices is insufficient.

In cases where the interocclusal distance is insufficient, or there is not enough space for the matrix, silicone-based soft lining materials or specially produced matrix materials can be an alternative to conventional matrices.

Matrix silicones (Retention sil.®, Bego) have three different shore hardness degrees, which results in three different retention strengths. It is recommended that the diameter of the ball attachment will be 2.5 mm or larger for stud attachments other than TiSi.snap abutments where silicone matrix will be used.

Locator

Locator is a well-known stud attachment type with its low profile and self-aligning design. Locator attachments female (matrix) part will be inserted in roots, dental implants, and milled bars and the male(patrix) part is located in the denture. This system allows 40° divergence of two abutments with extended range patrices. The most important feature of the locator attachment compared to other stud attachments is its low profile that allows easy use in cases where the interocclusal distance is insufficient. The locator system has three different retentive caps in low(blue), medium(pink), and high(clear) retention forces. Standard range male processing kit contains denture cap assembly, black processing male, block-out spacer, and three different retentive caps. The angle between locator abutments exceeds 30° extended range male processing kit should be ordered. After insertion of attachment into its place put block-out spacer onto the abutment. Put the black processing male-inserted denture cap onto the abutment. Leave enough space between the abutment-cap assembly in the dentures by grinding. Pour auto-polymerized Polymethylmethacrylate (PMMA) into the slot prepared in the denture and insert the denture into the mouth. Be sure that the denture is seated in the correct place and guide the patient to clench their denture at centric relation. After setting the PMMA, remove the denture from the mouth, remove the block-out spacer from the abutment, grind the excess PMMA and take the black processing male, and insert the retentive cap with the Locator core tool which is suitable for your patient's demands. A clinical case of implant-borne Locator is shown in the figures (Fig. 16.44, 16.45, 16.46, 16.47, 16.48, 16.49, 16.50, 16.51, and 16.52).

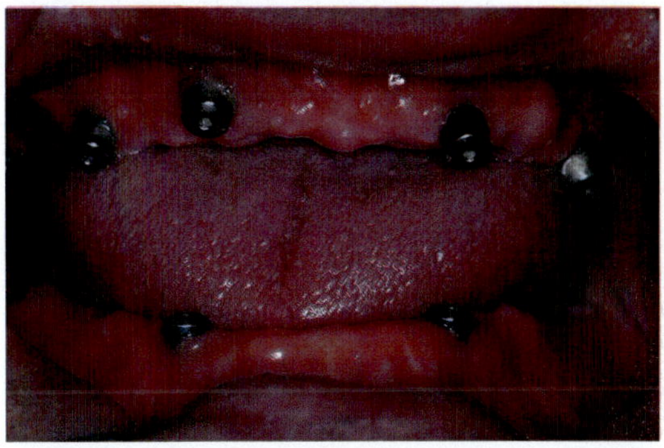

Fig. 16.44 Intraoral view of dental implants with gingiva formers

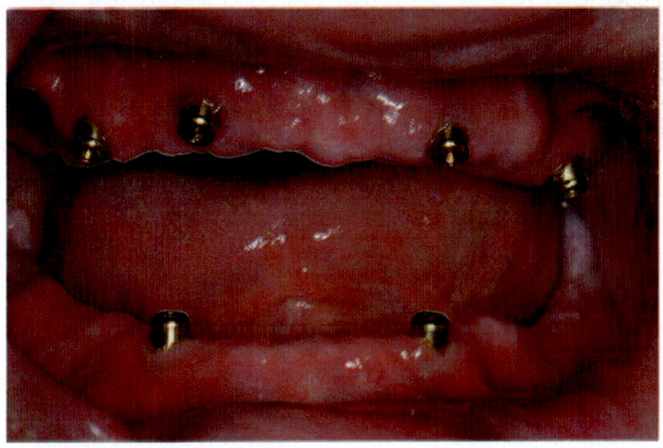

Fig. 16.45 Locator abutments are screwed and torqued in to the dental implants

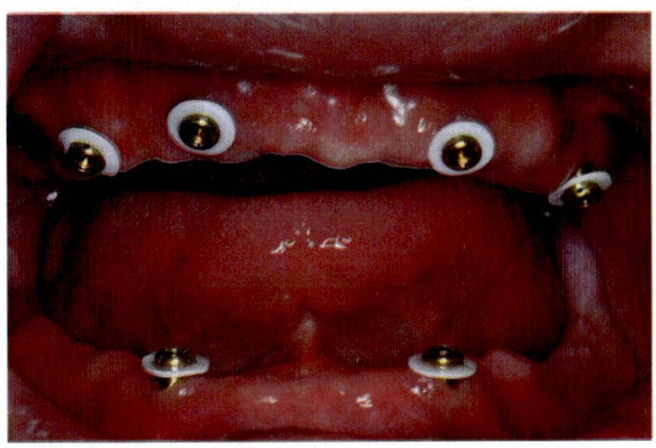

Fig. 16.46 Block-out spacers inserted

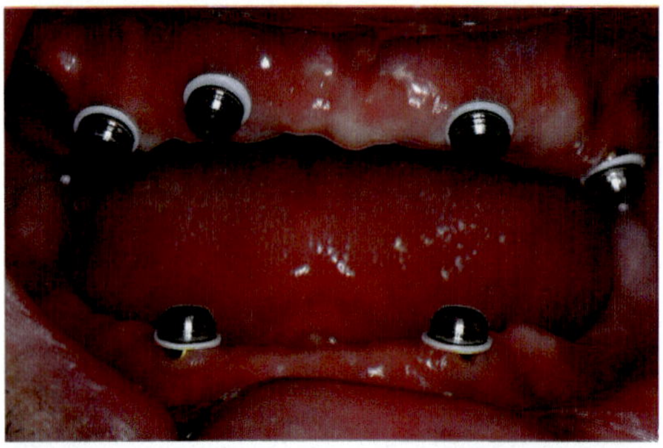

Fig. 16.47 The black processing male-inserted denture cap seated onto the abutment

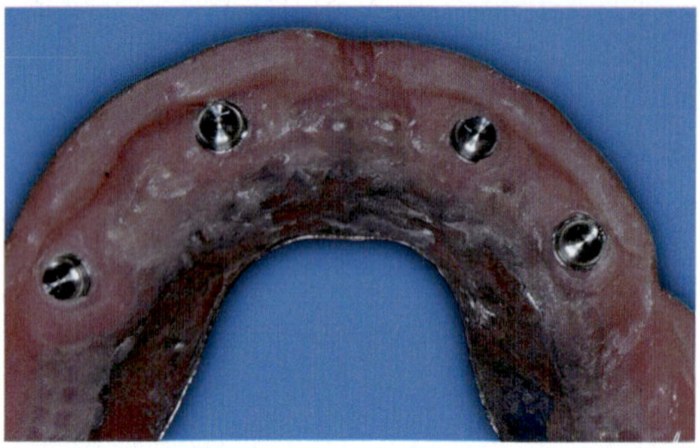

Fig. 16.48 After setting the autopolymerizing PMMA denture, black processing caps in maxillary denture are removed

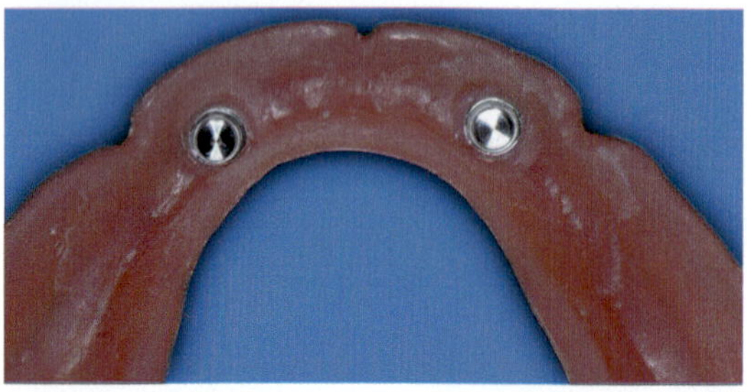

Fig. 16.49 After setting the autopolymerizing PMMA denture, black processing caps in mandibular denture are removed

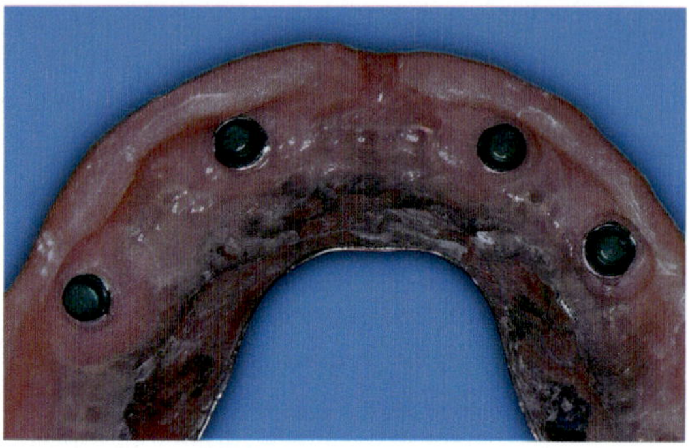

Fig. 16.50 Extended range retentive caps are inserted in maxillary denture in order to compensate the angular divergence

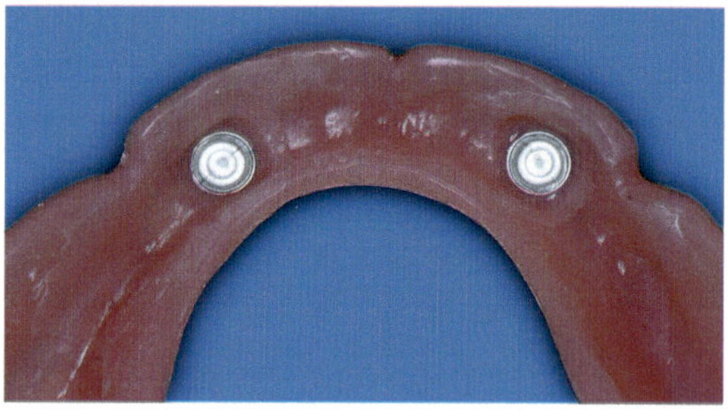

Fig. 16.51 Standard retentive caps with high retention force are chosen for mandibular denture

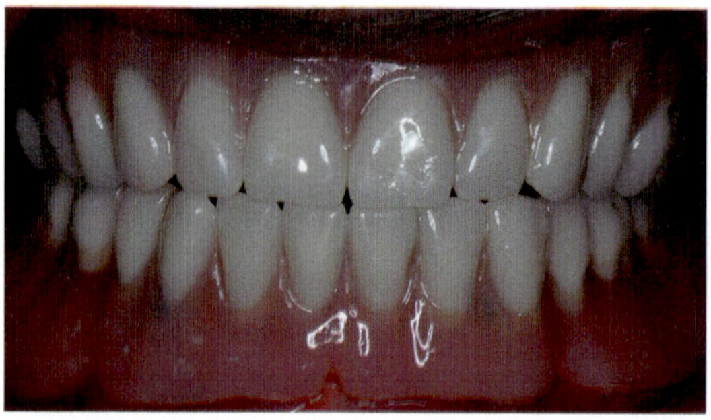

Fig. 16.52 Intercuspidation of maxillary and mandibular dentures in situ

Clinical Procedures of Stud Attachments

1. Abutment teeth are prepared. If necessary, crown height is adjusted to 2 mm, and the root canal should be enlarged up to 2/3 of the root canal length. After the light consistency elastomeric impression material is sent to the enlarged root canal using a paste carrier, a used file is inserted as a reinforcement for the root canal impression, and the final impression is made with polyvinylsiloxane or polyether impression material. The impression is poured with dental stone, and record bases with occlusal rims are prepared.
2. The occlusal vertical dimension and centric relation position are determined with the guidelines described in Chap. 13.

3. After the aesthetic try-in appointment, a silicone index is prepared to check for adequate space for the stud attachment and the matrix and to decide their position.
4. The stud attachment is fabricated with an appropriate alloy, and an individual tray is prepared.
5. The passive fit and the accuracy of the stud attachment on the abutment teeth are checked. If the stud attachment does not fit the abutment tooth passively, put some light consistency elastomeric impression over the casted post and insert with gentle pressure. The passivity is rechecked in the mouth, and a functional impression is made with the prepared individual tray by using zinc oxide eugenol or polyether impression materials with the attachments in place.
6. Another aesthetic try-in is performed with the stud attachments in place. After the occlusal vertical dimension and centric relation position are verified, the denture is processed using conventional laboratory methods.
7. The stud attachment and the denture assembly are seated on the abutment teeth to check the centric relation position and occlusal contacts before cementation. Petroleum jelly is applied to the stud attachments except for the intaglio surface of the crowns. Cementation procedures are performed afterward. If adhesive cement is not used, the denture is removed the day after (Figs. 16.53, 16.54, 16.55, and 16.56).

Bar Attachments

Bar attachments have been used for nearly 100 years in dentistry. The general advantages of the bar attachments are favorable retention, increased stability, reduced crown-root ratio, splinting of the remaining abutments, and correcting their divergence. On the other hand, vertical and sagittal space requirements show aesthetic and technical problems. Plaque accumulations, mucosal hypertrophy, the requirement of technical skills with clinical expertise, and the complexity of the relining/rebasing and repair procedures are the main disadvantages of bar attachments. Bar attachments are used to join

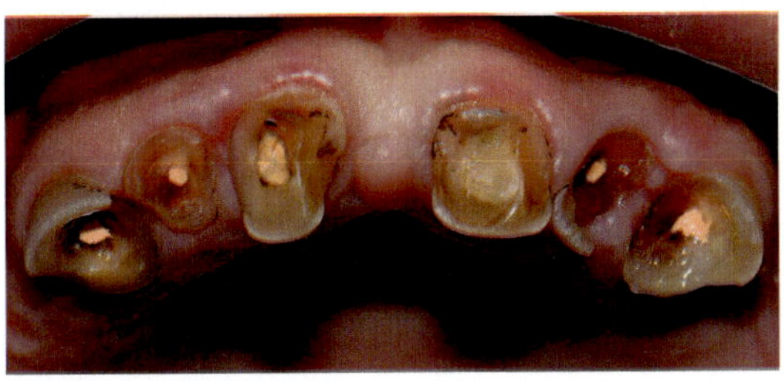

Fig. 16.53 Intraoral view of maxillary teeth showing excessive material loss

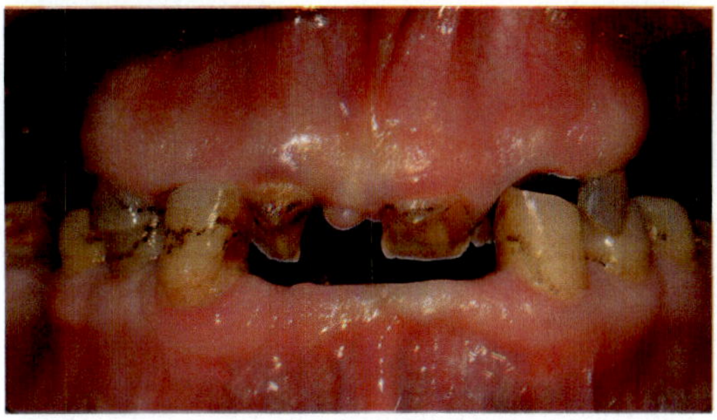

Fig. 16.54 Occlusal relation of teeth with excessive material loss

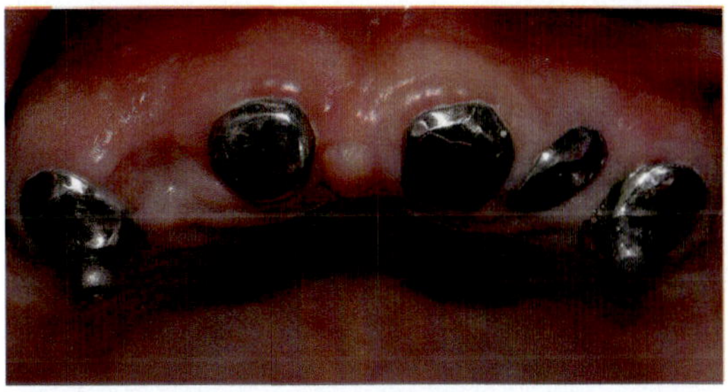

Fig. 16.55 Intraoral view of stud attachments and metal covers over the roots

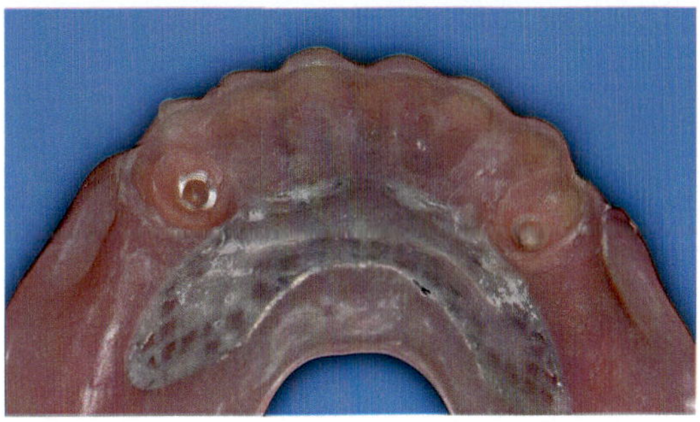

Fig. 16.56 The impression surface of the RPD after the matrices are attached

roots, teeth, crowns, and implants. Bar attachments are cast with hard precious, semiprecious, or non-precious alloys or may be prefabricated gold. Some bar types, such as Dolder bars, may be soldered to root caps or crowns. Most abutment teeth need root canal treatment, and placing dowels in the root canal can give extra retention to bar attachment. Plastic and metal clips are both available for different types of bar attachments. Nowadays special matrix silicones have been offered in dentistry used over the bar attachments as matrices (Figs. 16.57, 16.58, 16.59, and 16.60). It has been reported that matrix silicone materials increase patient satisfaction and comfort, and provide increased retention. Also, it maintains the health of peri-implant soft tissues by covering all the gaps between the bar and the denture and reduces microbial dental plaque accumulation. The use of silicone matrices over the rigid bar matrix system as a retainer provides a resilient character to the attachment system.

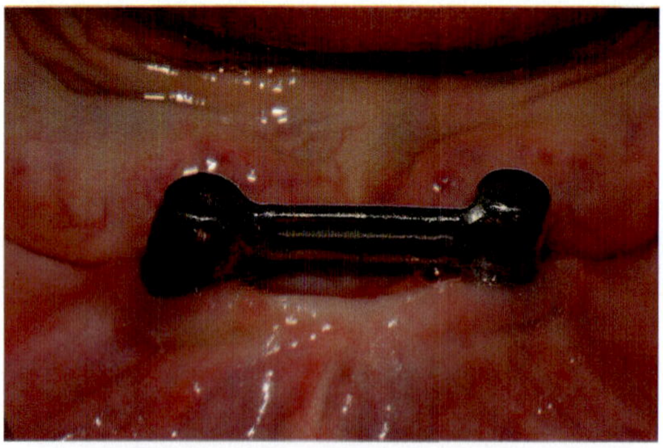

Fig. 16.57 Intra-oral view of the two implant-supported bar attachment

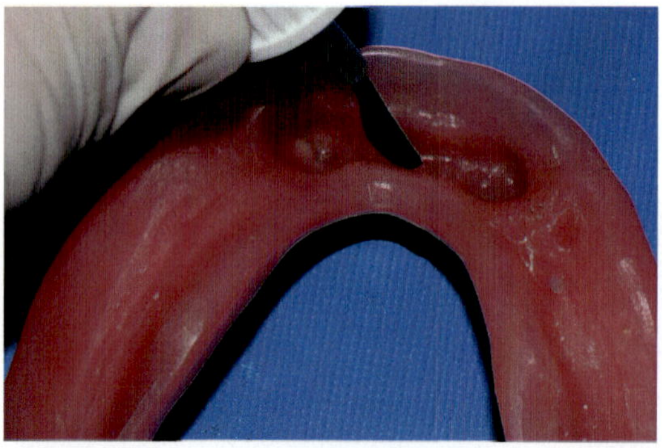

Fig. 16.58 Bonding application to the cavity prepared for retention silicones

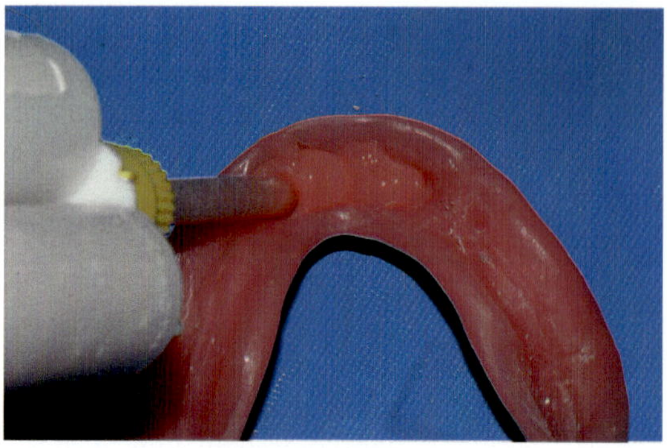

Fig. 16.59 Application of retention silicones in the cavity with auto-mix dispenser gun

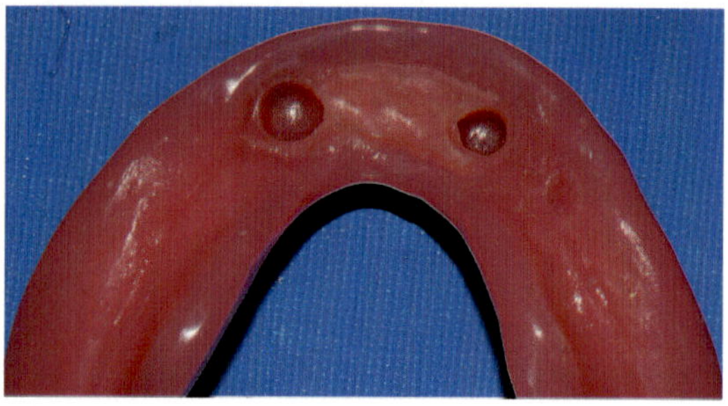

Fig. 16.60 The impression surface of overdenture after setting of the retention silicone

Bar attachments are divided into two groups: resilient bars (bar joints) and rigid bars (bar units). Resilient bars (bar joints) provide class 2 (vertical) and/or class 3 (hinge) resilience according to the number of abutment teeth used in the prosthetic restoration. Bar attachments are constructed on at least two abutments. Periodontally compromised teeth require root canal treatments and crown shortening for a better prognosis. There are different types of bar profiles such as round, pear-shaped, and parallel-sided "U" shaped.

There is also another classification of bar joints:

- Single-sleeve bar joints
- Multi-sleeve bar joints

Dolder bar is a very good example of single-sleeve bar joints. However, this type of bar joint has to be made straight which may be regarded as a disadvantage. The roots or teeth have to be in a straight line, and a bar may be located lingually to gain more space for the arrangement of the artificial teeth.

There is no need for the bar to run straight when multi-sleeve bar joints have been chosen and can follow ridge curvature. On the other hand, a bar with a big curvature may cause excessive load to abutment teeth or roots and may cause periodontal problems. When multi-sleeve bar joints are chosen, the bar must be cast with a rigid alloy.

Metal or plastic clips are available for single- or multi-sleeve applications.

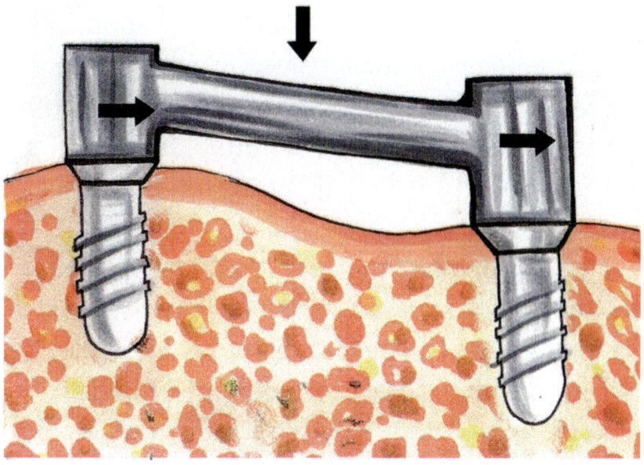

Fig. 16.61 If the levels of abutment teeth are not aligned at frontal plane, bar should be placed parallel to the hinge axis

Fundamentals of Bar Designs

As a general rule, if the levels of abutment teeth are not aligned at the frontal plane, the bar should be placed parallel to the hinge axis (Figs. 16.61 and 16.62). There should be at least a 2 mm or more gap between the bottom of the bar and the mucosa. This space allows easy cleaning of the food particles by saliva or cleaning tools. If the space is narrow, this will cause plaque and calculus accumulation, and oral hygiene management will be problematic. If the bar slightly compresses the mucosa, this will cause hyperplasia of the gum. The bar should be placed directly above the alveolar ridge. If the bar is positioned lingually, it may restrict the tongue space. If the bar is located buccally, this may disturb the lips. These scenarios complicate the fabrication of dentures. Bars should follow a straight line between the abutments. In case the curvature of the alveolar crest does not allow a straight design, the prognosis of the abutment teeth may become unclear.

If there are two abutment teeth connected with a bar attachment, the borders of the denture should be like a conventional complete denture. But in the presence of four or more abutment teeth, flanges of the denture may be shortened. If the distance between the abutment teeth is long, the resilient bar should be used. Rigid alloys should be used to construct multi-sleeve bars, which follow the curvature of the alveolar crest.

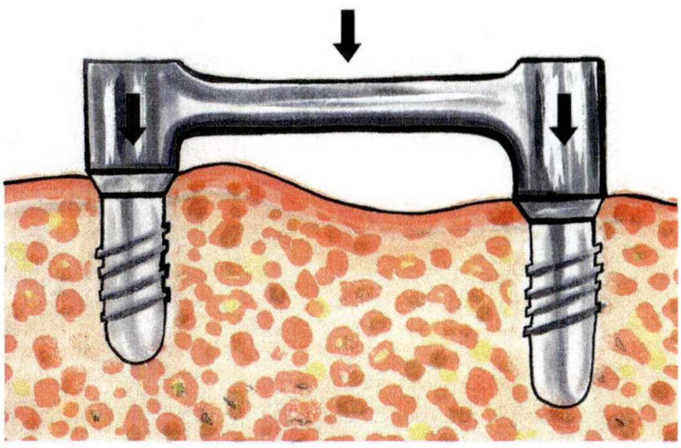

Fig. 16.62 The arrangement of the levels of the implants provides balanced load transfer

Rigid bars are also used as auxiliary components to extracoronal attachments. Two canines of a Kennedy Class I Mod 1 case is a typical example of the concept. The canines are not reduced to gingival level to serve under an overdenture; instead, they are kept as abutment teeth, restored with single crown restorations, for an RPD. A rigid bar is used to splint the two canines. The bar provides indirect retention to the RPD as the axis of rotation is moved posteriorly with the help of distal extension extracoronal attachments; however, it does not contribute to direct retention actively. This design offers a support polygon from two teeth with posteriorly extended support points. The distal extensions establish a lever arm that exerts torque forces on the splinted abutment teeth when the saddles make dislodging movements. To minimize any harmful effects, distal attachments should be chosen among resilient types. In many aspects, the advantages of this design over other alternatives, like an overdenture, are quite questionable, but occasionally, it may be preferred for selected cases.

Metal and plastic sleeves will be available, and the advantages of the metal sleeve are that it has more wear resistance, retention force can be adjustable, and total bar dimensions can be smaller; on the other hand, replacing a metal clip is more difficult and needs more chairside effort. The advantages of plastic clips are as follows: they are easy to change, clips with different retention forces are available, they need less time at the chairside but need more space, they do not allow adjustment, and they can be worn easily. Silicone matrices also have the advantage of the ease of rebasing and relining. The retention force of the silicone matrix materials is superior to metal and plastic riders. They have resilience capacity and better force distribution compared to metal or plastic riders.

Hader Bar

Helmut Hader, a master technician, developed a semi-precision attachment bar system in 1973. The Hader bar and rider system is one of the most popular bar systems due to its cost-effectiveness and simplicity. This system allows hinge movement when a single Hader bar is used with a plastic female rider and has a mechanical snap retention mechanism. The Hader bar system is a semi-precision bar system with a castable bar replica. The Hader bar is available in two sizes: standard (8 mm height) and short (4.5 mm height). The Hader bar will be shortened up to 2.5 mm. A common application is processing the Hader Metal Housings into the denture utilizing the Hader Processing Spacers and then using one of the four plastic female riders in the metal housings. The system has four different color-coded female riders with different retentive strengths: yellow standard, white decreased, red increased, and a new blue rider for worn bars. Using metal housing for female riders is highly recommended in clinical usage for easy maintenance. The Hader bar and plastic rider normally allow only rotational movement when two abutment teeth are used. The Ackerman gold and stainless steel clips with vestibular-lingual retentions and with mesial-distal retention are also available with a spacer, which will allow vertical resilience to dentures.

Dolder Bar

Dr. Eugene Dolder in Switzerland developed this bar system. The main point of the Dolder bar design is to allow a remarkable amount of both vertical and rotational movements around the long axis of the bar. The Dolder bar works best where the remaining teeth or roots are in a square arch and can be joined by a straight line. Patients with adequate inter-alveolar distance and when maximum retention is expected are the main indications. On the other hand, patients with poor oral hygiene and decreased manual dexterity are the main contraindications. The Dolder bar system is originally based on wrought wire pear-shaped precious metal bar and metal precious rider. Plastic replicas for waxing up between natural abutments and implant plastic cylinders are also available for non-precious bar systems. Dolder bars have either pear-shaped or U-shaped cross sections and are available in two sizes: standard (diameter 2.2 mm, height 3 mm) and mini (diameter 1.6 mm, height 2.3 mm). The pear shape is used for a resilient prosthesis and is called a bar joint. The U shape is for a rigid or non-resilient prosthesis and is called a bar unit. Resilient pear-shaped bars are normally ideal for tooth (implant)- and mucosa-supported dentures. The pear-shaped bar and rider will provide vertical and rotational resilience. There is a spacer between the bar and rider, which will be removed after the acrylic resin has been polymerized. The spacer will allow the denture vertical and rotational freedom over the pear-shaped bar. The retention force of the metal rider will be fully adjusted according to the patient's expectations. The Dolder bar system does not offer plastic riders.

Ackermann Bar

Dr. Ackermann's bar is similar to the Dolder bar with different cross sections and a semi-precision bar system that is cast of gold. This is also a multi-sleeve bar system, which can follow the ridge contour. Oval and round cross-sectioned bars are available with metal riders and a spacer. Round bars are the most versatile and can be set in all planes. The riders of the Ackermann bar have retention parts placed in acrylic resin that lies buccolingually. This rider requires more space so be careful when removing the rider for rebasing. When using the Ackermann bar unit, it is recommended that a 5 mm extension from the most distal root will be made for extra retention.

Clinical Procedures of Bar Attachments

1. Abutment teeth are prepared. If necessary, the crown height is adjusted to 2 mm. The final impression is made with polyvinylsiloxane or polyether impression material. The impression is poured with dental stone, and record bases with occlusal rims are prepared.
2. The occlusal vertical dimension and centric relation position are determined with the guidelines described in Chap. 13.
3. After the aesthetic try-in appointment, a silicone index is prepared to check if there is adequate space for the bar and the rider and additionally to decide their position.
4. The bar is fabricated with an appropriate alloy, and an individual tray is also prepared.
5. The passive fit and the accuracy of the bar on the abutment teeth are checked. If the bar does not fit the abutments passively, it is cut with an appropriate bur between the abutments and joined together with an autopolymerizing acrylic resin (pattern resin), and the passivity is checked again in the mouth and a new impression is made and the cut bar parts are welded in the laboratory. The cast is resent to the laboratory and veneering materials are applied to the crowns. A functional impression is made with the prepared individual tray by using zinc oxide eugenol or polyether impression materials with the bar in place.
6. Another aesthetic try-in is performed with the bar in place. After the vertical dimension of occlusion and centric relation position are verified, the RPD is processed using conventional laboratory methods.
7. The bar and the RPD assembly are seated on the abutment teeth to check the centric relation position and occlusal contacts before cementation. Petroleum jelly is applied to the bar except for the intaglio surface of the crowns and the bar seated on the RPD. Cementation procedures are performed afterward. If adhesive cement is not used, the RPD is removed the day after.

16.3 Double Crown Systems

The terminology used in the description of double crowns is unclear. In 1886, R. Walter Starr first described telescopic crowns which have proven an effective means of retaining RPDs. The similarity of double crowns to a collapsible optical telescope urged him to define the system as the "telescope system." All double crown systems are called telescopic crowns, but a telescopic crown precisely represents a double crown that achieves retention by the friction of parallel-sided surfaces (Fig. 16.63). Double crown systems transfer forces along the direction of the long axis of the abutment teeth thereby protecting them from the dislodging movements of the RPDs and providing support and guidance which is worthy for patients having neuromuscular coordination problems. Thin metal primary

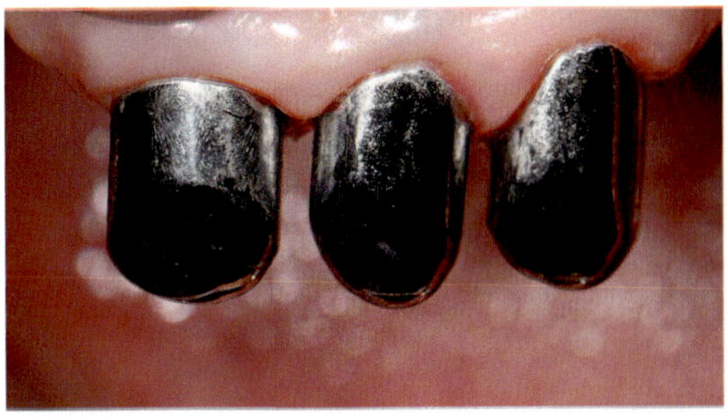

Fig. 16.63 A telescopic crown precisely represents a double crown that achieves retention by friction of parallel-sided surfaces

crowns do not intrude on the periodontal tissues, and oral hygiene is provided easily by removing the RPD. Loss of retention is one of the most common technical failures and is independent of the friction-fit concept which is used to retain the denture. A common disadvantage of all double crown systems is the need for more extensive tooth reduction to provide enough space for the primary and secondary crowns, which may cause a requirement for root canal treatment, especially in younger patients.

The properties of the alloy chosen for double crowns are very important. The elastic modulus of a Co-Cr-Mo alloy is about twice as high as the elastic modulus of a type IV alloy with a high gold content. Therefore, if a high gold content alloy is used, appropriate major and minor connectors delivering the rigidity of the RPD should be planned. Base metal alloys provide enough rigidity to fabricate a framework without major connectors. The outer crowns are able to serve as minor connectors between the bases. The fabrication of cast double crown-retained RPDs is a technique-sensitive process and requires a qualified laboratory. Today, primary crowns may also be manufactured with zirconia or laser-sintered base metals, and the secondary crowns or the retentive part may be manufactured by electroforming afterward (Figs. 16.64, 16.65, 16.66, 16.67, and 16.68). With the widespread use of developing computer-aided design and manufacturing CAD/CAM technologies in dentistry, improved ceramics and polymer-based materials

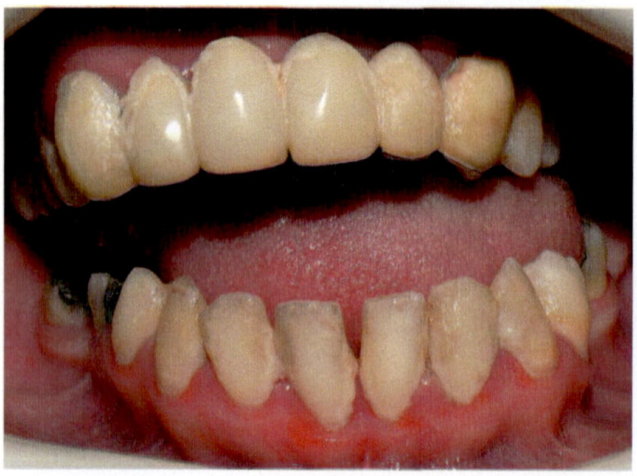

Fig. 16.64 Intraoral view of a patient with hemimandibular elongation

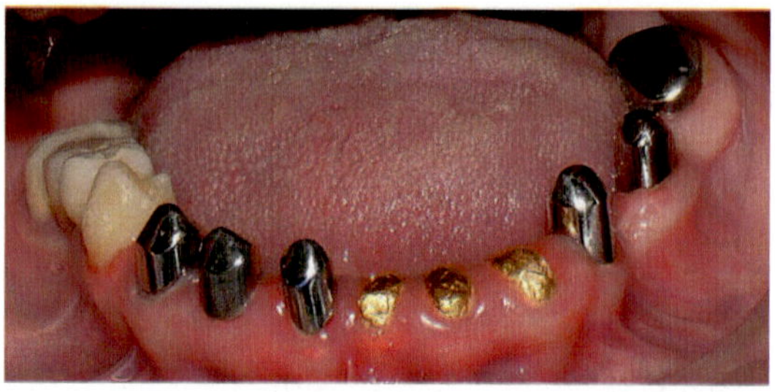

Fig. 16.65 Telescopic primary crowns are made with base metal alloy and root caps are made by using an electroforming technique

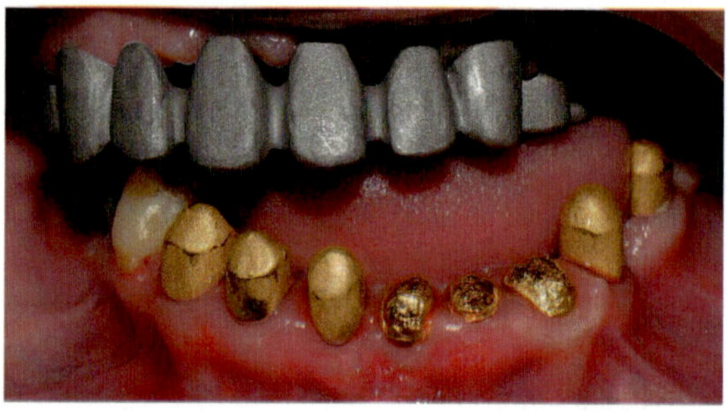

Fig. 16.66 Secondary crowns are made by using an electroforming technique

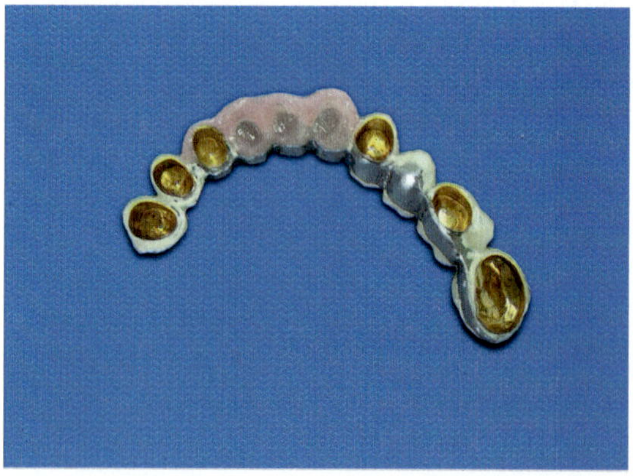

Fig. 16.67 Bridge-like framework without a major connector

(Polyetheretherketone (PEEK)and polyetherketoneketone (PEKK)) can be produced faster, and cost-effectively, eliminating conventional casting errors (see Part V). Easy establishment of higher retention forces may be regarded as the advantage of the electroformed secondary crowns, whereas high costs and requirement of extra equipment as the disadvantages compared to con-

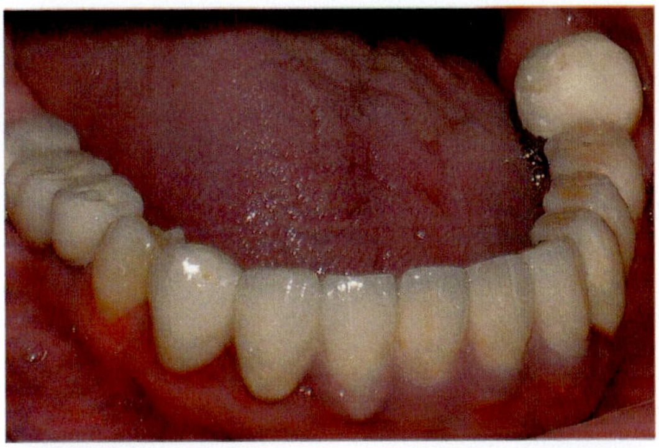

Fig. 16.68 Esthetic, functional, and hygienic RPD in situ

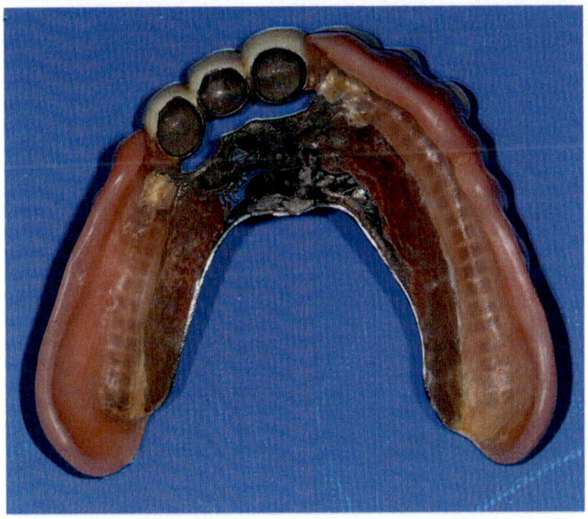

Fig. 16.69 Framework with a conventional major connector

ventional methods. The technically demanding and time-consuming manufacturing process of secondary crowns produced using electroforming leads to an expensive dental restoration and in vitro studies have shown that milled PEEK or PEKK copings can be an affordable alternative to electroplated ones. In case of loss of retention in PEEK or PEKK secondary crowns produced as CAD/CAM, it may be an advantage to continue using the same prostheses by replacing only these parts without the need to change the entire restoration. Longer-term in vivo studies are still needed to prove the clinical success of such polymer-based double crown systems.

The framework of an RPD with a double crown system can be constructed in two methods: with a conventional major connector (Fig. 16.69) and a bridge-like framework without a major connector (Fig. 16.67). If the number of abutment teeth is insufficient or the location of the remaining teeth is not suitable, and there is a significant amount of soft tissue loss, bridge-like frameworks should not be preferred.

Framework with a conventional major connector is indicated in the following situations:

- Replacement of bilateral posterior and anterior missing teeth with supporting weakened abutments
- Bilateral splinting of the posterior missing teeth supported by one telescopic crown from each side
- Absence of unilateral abutment teeth
- Several abutment teeth with unclear periodontal prognosis

Bridge-like framework without a major connector is indicated in the following situations:

- Numerous periodontally healthy abutment teeth can enable the reduction of the unnecessary bulk of the denture.
- Abutment teeth with sufficient crown heights.
- A unilateral edentulous area with natural teeth both anterior and posterior to the area.

There are three different double-crown systems for retaining RPDs:

1. Telescopic crowns having parallel milled surfaces that achieve retention by frictional forces.
2. Conical or conus crowns exhibiting friction only when completely seated using a "wedging effect."
3. The double crowns with clearance fit accomplish no friction or wedging during insertion or removal. Retention is generated by using additional attachments.

16.3.1 Telescopic Crowns

Telescopic crowns have been used for more than a 100 years in dentistry. Telescopic crowns have parallel milled surfaces which achieve retention by frictional forces. The system consists of one inner (primary) and one outer (secondary) crown. The primary crown should have at least 4 mm vertical height, and it is cemented to prepared abutment teeth, and the secondary crown is soldered to the RPD framework (Fig. 16.70). The retention force is activated when the secondary crown contacts the primary crown and continues until the RPD is inserted. Noble alloys (Fig. 16.71) are the first choice when manufacturing telescopic crowns, but nowadays due to economic reasons, base alloys (Fig. 16.72) are also used. Abutment teeth may require root canal treatment in order to avoid over-contoured restorations. Cross-arch stabilization, improved oral hygiene, less wear compared to other attachments, reasonable retention force, and aesthetic appearance are the main advantages of the telescopic crowns (Fig. 16.73a–c). Cross-arch stabilization of periodontally involved teeth can alter the prognosis of abutment teeth. If an abutment tooth is lost, secondary crowns are converted to pontics by filling the hollow with acrylic resin. The retention force decreases but remains acceptable as the abutment teeth are lost until one tooth is left. Abutment teeth, which are not used for retention purposes, are also used for stabilization and support. Telescopic crown-retained RPDs

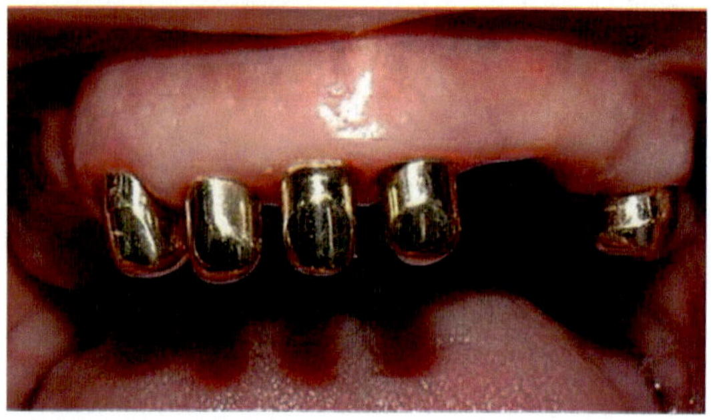

Fig. 16.71 Noble alloys are the first choice when manufacturing telescopic crowns

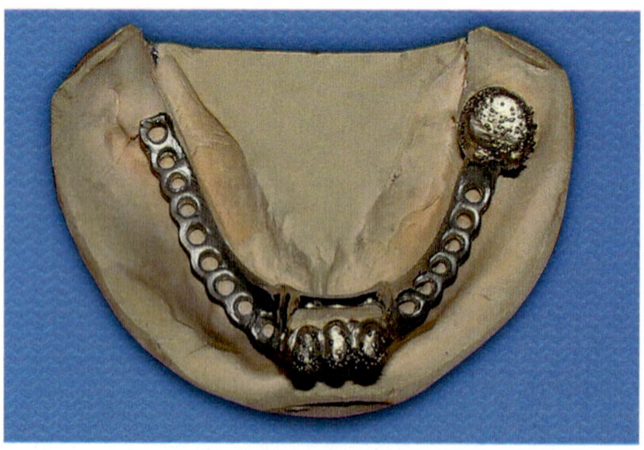

Fig. 16.70 Secondary crown is soldered to the RPD framework

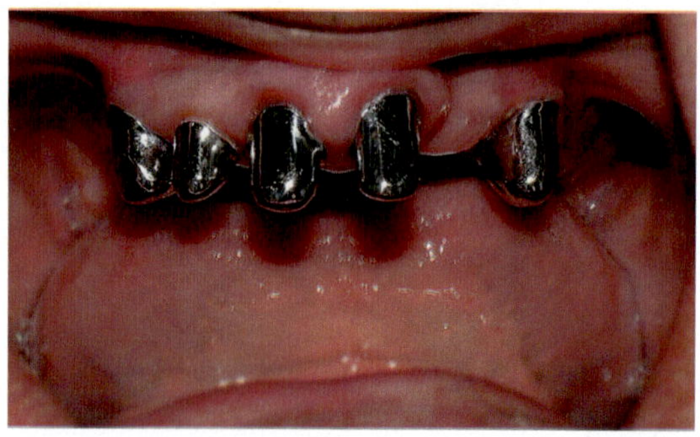

Fig. 16.72 Base alloys can be used due to economic reasons

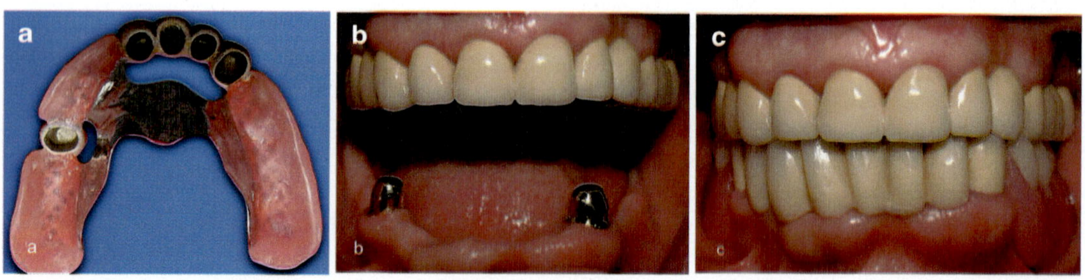

Fig. 16.73 The main advantages of telescopic crowns are (**a**) the cross-arch stabilization of the abutment teeth, (**b**) improved oral hygiene, (**c**) esthetic appearance

Table 16.1 Advantages and disadvantages of telescopic crown-retained RPDs when compared to conventional RPDs

Advantages	Disadvantages
Adjustable retention force	Double crowns sometimes generate over-contoured teeth
Long-term retention force stability	Metal may be exposed in cervical region
Splinting effect of abutment teeth	Requirement of root canal treatments when necessary
Good periodontal health	Requirement of increased vertical and buccolingual space
Good aesthetic results	Wear easily
Retention of the RPD is acceptable until one abutment tooth remains	High frictional forces acting on abutment teeth while removing the RPD

Table 16.2 Advantages and disadvantages of conus crown-retained RPDs when compared to conventional RPDs

Advantages	Disadvantages
Adjustable retention force	Double crowns sometimes generate over-contoured teeth
Long-term retention force stability	Metal may be exposed in the cervical region
Splinting effect of abutment teeth	Requirement of root canal treatments when necessary
Good periodontal health	Requirement of increased vertical and buccolingual space
Good aesthetic results	Rigid connection
	When an abutment tooth is lost, the retention of the RPD is compromised

have rigid and resilient types. The difference between the two systems is that the resilient telescopic crowns have a very small gap between the occlusal surfaces of the primary and secondary crowns, and this gap allows movements of the denture toward the oral mucosa by the functional occlusal forces to provide maximum soft tissue support. The advantages and disadvantages of telescopic crown-retained RPDs are listed in Table 16.1.

16.3.2 Conical Crowns

Conical crowns or conus crowns were first described by Körber in 1958 and exhibit friction only when the RPD is completely seated using a "wedging effect." The magnitude of the wedging effect is mainly determined by the convergence angle of the inner (primary) crown. This convergence angle can be adjusted from 4° to 8° to afford the adequate retention force to retain an RPD. When the convergence angle becomes smaller, retentive force becomes high. The taper angle of the inner (primary) crown depends on the clinical crown height and periodontal mobility.

The number and location of the abutment teeth are the other factors affecting the taper angle, and the total retention force is calculated according to this number. Conus crown-retained RPDs provide all the requirements, such as restoration of phonetic functions, arrangement of occlusal stability, preservation of the residual alveolar ridge, stabilization of the temporomandibular joint, and good aesthetics as well as continuous retention and splinting effect on abutment teeth. Conus crown-retained RPDs are rigid and provide respectable support in maintaining periodontal health. The advantages and disadvantages of conus crown-retained RPDs are listed in Table 16.2.

Abutment teeth with periodontal problems and compromised soft tissues are the contraindications of conus crown-retained RPDs because of their rigid behavior. When the retention of the RPD is lost because of the wear of conus crowns, grinding from the occlusal surfaces of primary crowns with a silicone polishing disc may increase the wedging effect and improve retention.

16.3.3 Double Crowns with Clearance Fit (Marburg Double Crown System)

Clearance fit double crown system, which is also called Marburg double crown system (MDC system), was first described by Lehmann and Gente in 1988. The double crown with clearance fit exhibits no friction or wedging during the insertion or removal of the prosthesis. Retention is achieved by using additional attachments. This system may be used to retain both tooth-supported and distal-end RPDs. The secondary crown fits onto the primary crown without any friction or wedging. This clearance fit is precise, allowing a minimal, invisible lateral movement and a smooth, effortless gliding along the axis of the path of insertion. The inner crown is fabricated with a groove for the production of resilience. A 0.3–0.5 mm tinfoil is inserted between the primary and secondary crowns before the RPD is processed. After the laboratory procedures, tinfoil is removed, and the denture base contacts the denture-bearing mucosa, while there is an additional space between the inner and outer crowns. When an occlusal load is applied, the RPD moves vertically through the mucosa, depending on the resilience of the denture-bearing mucosa, and returns to its former position after the load is removed. The MDC system provides a rigid metal framework, including the secondary crowns. Retention is achieved by using the TC-SNAP system which is an auxiliary attachment. To avoid unfavorable leverage and overloading of the periodontal tissues, the abutment teeth must be shortened until achieving a balanced crown-root ratio. This equalization of the crown-root ratio may require root canal treatment followed by post and core restorations. Using a single type of alloy for the fabrication of primary and secondary crowns, and the framework of the RPD, provides enough rigidity and decreased manufacturing cost.

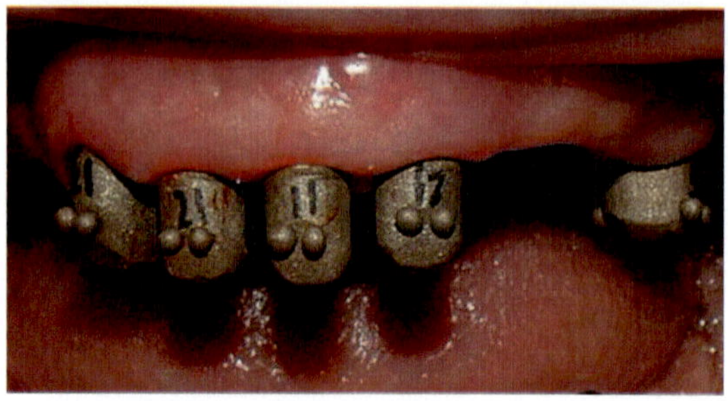

Fig. 16.74 Primary crowns with proper retentive elements for functional impression

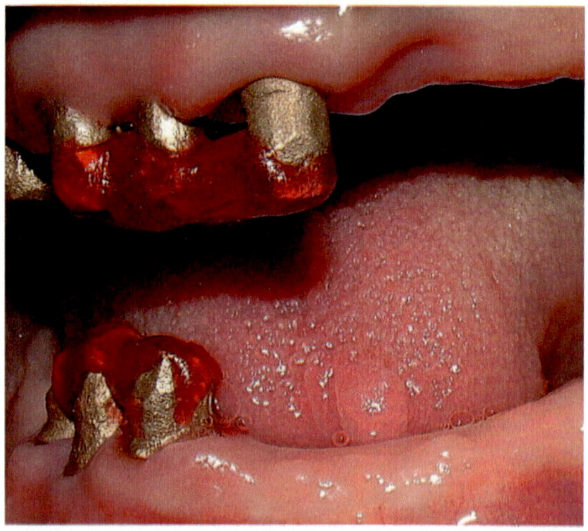

Fig. 16.75 Primary crowns without retentive elements should be attached together with autopolymerizing acrylic resin (pattern resin) before the functional impression

Clinical Procedures of Double Crown Systems

1. Abutment teeth are prepared with a chamfer margin and minimum taper angle. Reduction from the occlusal and buccal surface should be done carefully to prepare enough space for metal and aesthetic materials.
2. Impressions are made using elastomeric impression materials, and a dental stone cast with dies is fabricated.
3. Primary crowns are cast with appropriate alloy, and an individual tray is fabricated with auto-polymerizing acrylic resin over the crowns. If the interocclusal distance is insufficient, the occlusal vertical dimension should be established before the production of primary crowns, and therefore occlusal scheme of the secondary crown can be made with metal.
4. Primary crowns are tried in the mouth (Fig. 16.74). If the primary crowns are cast without retentive elements, they are attached together with auto-polymerizing acrylic resin (pattern resin) before the functional impression (Fig. 16.75).
5. The functional impression is made by polyether or polyvinylsiloxane impression materials having hydrophilic properties by using the individual tray.

6. The dies of primary crowns are poured with auto-polymerizing acrylic resin (pattern resin) using retentive pins. This procedure should be done for milling the primary crowns for the path of insertion and adjusting the retention force.
7. After milling and polishing the primary crowns, secondary crowns and major connectors are fabricated. The passive fit of the primary and secondary crown assemblies is checked in the mouth. The occlusal vertical dimension is established (Fig. 16.76).
8. Try-in of the RPD with double crowns is performed checking and ensuring accurate aesthetics and phonetics of the patient.
9. The RPD is processed, finished, and polished.
10. Petroleum jelly is applied around the primary crowns and major connectors. Primary crowns are seated into the secondary crowns on the RPD and cemented with zinc polycarboxylate or adhesive cement. During cementation, the RPD should be settled in place completely.
11. After setting the cement, excess cement is cleaned using appropriate instruments. The RPD is removed preferably the next day to avoid the risk of decementation of the primary crowns if the primary crowns are not cemented with adhesive cement (Fig. 16.77).
12. The day after, the RPD is removed and excess cement is cleaned. Occlusal contacts are arranged. Maintenance and cleaning procedures are described to patients in detail and the RPD are delivered to the patients.

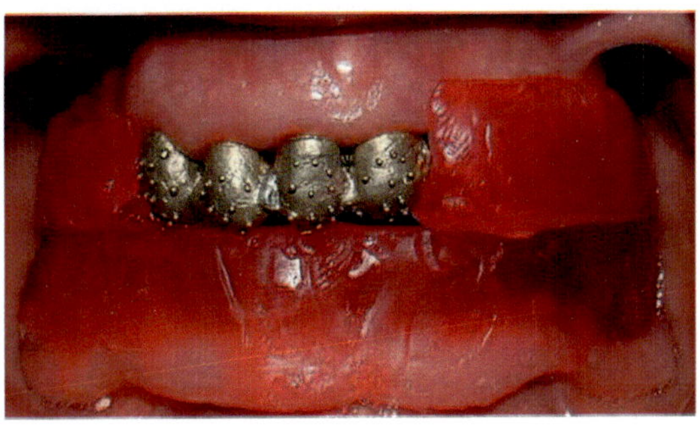

Fig. 16.76 Occlusal vertical dimension is established with primary and secondary crowns attached to framework of the RPD

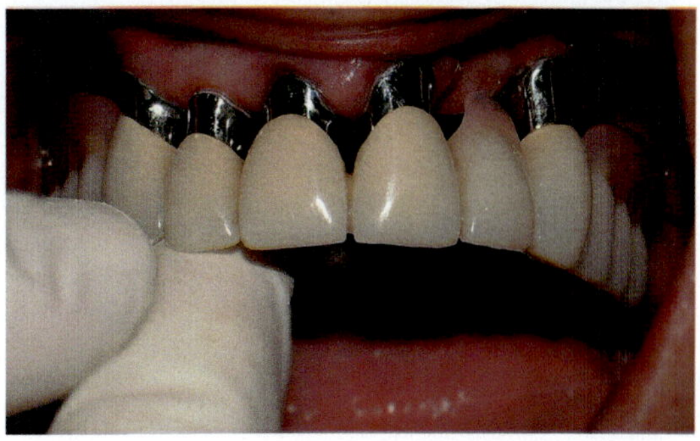

Fig. 16.77 RPD is removed preferably next day to avoid the risk of decementation

Further Reading

Behr M, Kolbeck C, Lang R, Hahnel S, Dirschl L, Handel G. Clinical performance of cements as luting agents for telescopic double crown-retained removable partial and complete overdentures. Int J Prosthodont. 2009;22:479–87.

Brudvik JS, Shor A. The milled surface as a precision attachment. Dent Clin N Am. 2004;48:685–708.

Herpel C, Springer A, Puschkin G, Zimmermann L, Stober T, Rammelsberg P, Schwindling FS. Removable partial dentures retained by hybrid CAD/CAM cobalt-chrome double crowns: 1-year results from a prospective clinical study: CAD/CAM cobalt-chrome double crowns: 1-year results. J Dent, 2021;115:103847.

Igarashi K, Katagiri H, Abou-Ayash S, Schimmel M, Afrashtehfar KI. Double-crown prosthesis retention using Polyetherketoneketone (PEKK): an in vitro study. J Prosthodont. 2023;32:154–61.

Kimura T, Yang T-C, Maeda Y. Influence of rigid Bar and nonrigid double crown attachments on maxillary implant overdentures: an in vitro study with differential bone quality. Int J Oral Maxillofac Implants. 2018;33:764–9.

Korber KH, Huber K. Retention correction of conical crowns with a preadjusted conus angle. Dent Labor (Munch). 1982;30:1027–33.

Kubo K, Koike T, Ueda T, Sakurai K. Influence of the mechanical properties of resilient denture liners on the retention of overdenture attachments. J Prosthet Dent. 2018;120:431–8.

Micovic Soldatovic D, Bitter M, Meinen J, Huth KC, Liebermann A, Stawarczyk B. Impact of material combinations and removal and insertion cycles on the retention force of telescopic systems. Clin Oral Investig. 2023;27:4007.

Owall B. Precision attachment retained removable partial dentures: 1 technical long-term study. Int J Prosthodont. 1991;4:249–57.

Owall B. Precision attachment-retained removable partial dentures: part 2. Long-term study of ball attachments. Int J Prosthodont. 1995;8:21–8.

Owall B, Jönsson L. Precision attachment-retained removable partial dentures. Part 3. General practitioner results up to 2 years. Int J Prosthodont. 1998;11:574–9.

Preiskel HW. Precision attachments in prosthodontics v. 1. The applications of intracoronal and extracoronal attachments. Batavia, IL: Quintessence; 1984. p. 318.

Preiskel HW, Harold W. Precision attachments in prosthodontics v. 2: overdentures and telescopic prostheses. Batavia, IL: Quintessence; 1984. p. 365.

Sakar O, Sanli Y, Marsan G. Prosthodontic treatment of a patient with hemimandibular elongation: a clinical report. J Prosthet Dent. 2006;96:150–3.

Seo JG, Cho JH. Clinical outcomes of rigid and non-rigid telescopic double-crown-retained removable dental prostheses: an analytical review. J Adv Prosthodont. 2020;12:38–48.

Shafie HR. Clinical and laboratory manual of implant overdentures. Copenhagen: Blackwell Munksgaard; 2007. p. 247.

Sherring-Lucas M, Martin P. Attachments for prosthetic dentistry: introduction and application. Quintessence. 1994;4:84.

Shiba A. The conical double-crown telescopic removable periodontic prosthesis. St Louis, MO: Ishiyaku Euro America; 1993. p. 56.

Stober T, Bermejo JL, Beck-Mussoter J, Seche AC, Lehmann F, Koob J, Rammelsberg P. Clinical performance of conical and electroplated telescopic double crown-retained partial dentures: a randomized clinical study. Int J Prosthodont. 2012;25:209–16.

The glossary of prosthodontic terms: ninth edition. J Prosthet Dent. 2017;117(5S):e1–105.

Turp I, Bozdağ E, Sünbüloğlu E, Kahruman C, Yusufoğlu İ, Bayraktar G. Retention and surface changes of zirconia primary crowns with secondary crowns of different materials. Clin Oral Investig. 2014;18:2023–35.

Uludağ B. Hassas Tutucular İmplant Vakalarında Sorunlar ve Çözümler. Ada Ofset. 2012:264.

Wenz HJ, Hertrampf K, Lehmann KM. Clinical longevity of removable partial dentures retained by telescopic crowns: outcome of the double crown with clearance fit. Int J Prosthodont. 2001;14:207–13.

Wenz HJ, Lehmann KM. A telescopic crown concept for the restoration of the partially edentulous arch: the Marburg double crown system. Int J Prosthodont. 1998;11:541–50.

Wöstmann B, Balkenhol M, Weber A, Ferger P, Rehmann P. Long-term analysis of telescopic crown retained removable partial dentures: survival and need for maintenance. J Dent. 2007;35:939–45.

Yalisove IL, Dietz JB. Telescopic prosthetic therapy: periodontal prosthesis, fixed and removable. Philadelphia: University of Pennsylvania. School of Dental Medicine; 1977. p. 352.

Yılmaz E, Gencel B, Geckili O, Sakar O. Comparison of the retention of conventional and polyvinyl siloxane matrix materials with different Patrices for implant-retained overdentures: an in vitro study. Int J Prosthodont. 2022;35:311–8.

17 The Role of the Dental Implant in Removable Partial Dentures

Hakan Bilhan

Abstract

Dental implants, as a helpful adjunct of prosthodontics, may have a key role in retention as well as stability and support of partial dentures, too. Not only being a step back solution after loss of several implants, having been placed for a fixed solution, but also as a less invasive method providing a very comfortable remedy, especially for patients with impaired systemic condition hindering greater surgical interventions. A variety of different attachments or abutments can be used ranging from single standing to splinted or resilient to rigid. Position of the implant to be placed depends on the relevant indication. The main aim is to reduce the length of the edentulous space, move the fulcrum to more distally, and if possible, eliminate a clasp via a suitably positioned dental implant. Implants may additionally offer the advantage of not requiring the use of teeth as prosthetic abutments, thus play a protective role on the remaining natural dentition. It may also be speculated that strategically situated implants may help preserving the residual bone especially around the implants. The indications/contraindications, advantages/disadvantages, and clinical approach related to implant-assisted removable partial dentures is presented in this chapter.

17.1 Dental Implants and Removable Partial Dentures

Several factors associated with removable prostheses, such as impaired function and uncomfortable use force the majority of patients to prefer fixed prosthetic solutions. Most of the time, undeservedly, factors such as esthetics, higher risk of periodontal disease, alveolar crest resorption, and development of decays on abutment teeth are asserted as an excuse to quit wearing removable dentures. On the other hand, loss of teeth especially in the posterior, has to be somehow compensated by a prosthetic restoration, since symptoms such as reduced masticatory efficiency, loss of vertical dimension of occlusion, and attrition of anterior teeth may accompany partial edentulism. Clinical studies have shown that partially edentulous patients complained mostly about dissatisfaction, discomfort, occlusal instability, chewing difficulty, and temporomandibular joint (TMJ) disorders. Nevertheless, it is clear that dentures with less mobility will give a better comfort feeling and thus be better accepted.

The implant-assisted removable partial denture (IARPD) represents a cost-effective prosthetic solution for patients with partial edentulism not being immediate candidates for extensive,

H. Bilhan (✉)
Department of Periodontology, Faculty of Dentistry, University of Witten/Herdecke, Witten, Germany
e-mail: hakan.bilhan@uni-wh.de;
http://www.ruhrweiss.de

O. Şakar (ed.), *Removable Partial Dentures*, https://doi.org/10.1007/978-3-031-47083-7_17

fixed implant-supported restorations. Including dental implants for improvement of removable partial denture (RPD) support and retention as well as to enhance patient satisfaction should be considered when planning the treatment with RPDs. Large long-term benefits may be expected using a few implants for the support of partial dentures. Even a few implants have been reported to enhance the retention of the denture, thus being very precious from the patients' point of view. In a very recent meta-analysis, it was concluded that IARPDs significantly improved quality of life and patient satisfaction. The main reason for this improvement seems to be the increased occlusal force and masticatory efficiency in comparison to those with conventional removable dentures.

Although not a routine treatment modality, a few strategically placed dental implants combined with the remaining dentition can help to achieve a more favorable RPD design. In cases where fixed rehabilitation is not possible, a few dental implants placed in strategically important positions could help preventing the movement around a fulcrum axis and bring biomechanic advantages by providing vertical support, as well. Rotation around the fulcrum axis created between the abutment teeth closest to the edentulous area, namely the distal abutments, against tissues as well as away from tissues may be prevented by a proper positioned implant.

In some patients the mandibular bilateral distal-extension RPD situations opposing a maxillary complete denture, resorption of the anterior part of the maxilla causing a flabby ridge may appear from time to time. Although the relation between the above-mentioned symptoms and distal-extension RPD is still controversial, it may be suggested that the proper placement of one or more implants in combination with the RPD may overcome some of the possible problems. A destabilization of the occlusion, however, following the resorption of the residual ridge below distal extension saddles and not only wear of the denture should be expected. The placement of an implant beneath a distal extension denture base could be a way to slow down the bone resorption and maintain ridge height. By the elimination of clasps the esthetic expectations of patients can be satisfied, while reduced displacement of the dentures have ended up in better tissue tolerability and options for RPD use have increased.

As in individual teeth, being evaluated for best use in RPD design to control prosthesis movement, use of an implant should be directed in a similar manner toward the most beneficial movement control. Implant use subsumes all three desired principles demonstrated by prostheses, namely support, stability, and retention. The major functional demand on RPDs is chewing, thus the greatest benefit of implant use could be considered as the improved support and stability of the prosthesis. Additionally, the use of implants as a rest, taking advantage of the vertical stiffness characteristic they possess, will mostly eliminate compression of supporting soft tissues, control vertical movement of the denture base, and alter fulcrum lines (Figs. 17.1, 17.2a, b, and 17.3). Implants may be considered useful for retentive needs as well and as mentioned above, implants can effectively alter rotation around a fulcrum line, eliminating it if applied to the most distal end of a denture base. In a more mesial position it is to be expected to reduce the effects by decreasing the effective lever arm. A recent numerical study showed that when compared with complete dental arch restoration, RPDs supported by a single implant unit demonstrated decreased stress values and mucosa displacements under vertical and oblique loading conditions. The first report about an implant in combination with a conventional removable partial denture (CRPD) is from 1974, where the authors treated a bilateral distal extension situation with an endosseous blade implant, while the

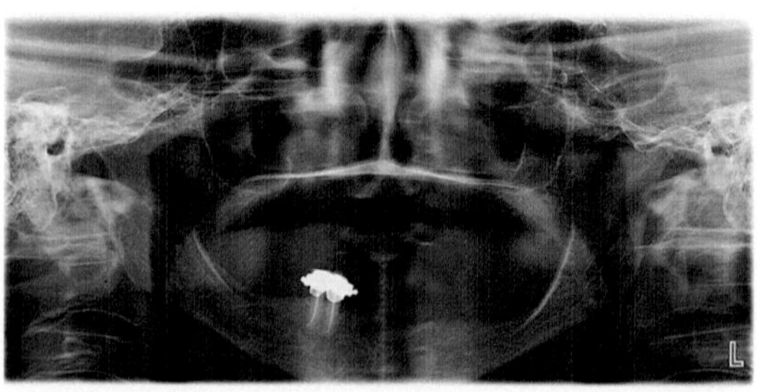

Fig. 17.1 Kennedy Class I situation with a very unfavorable fulcrum

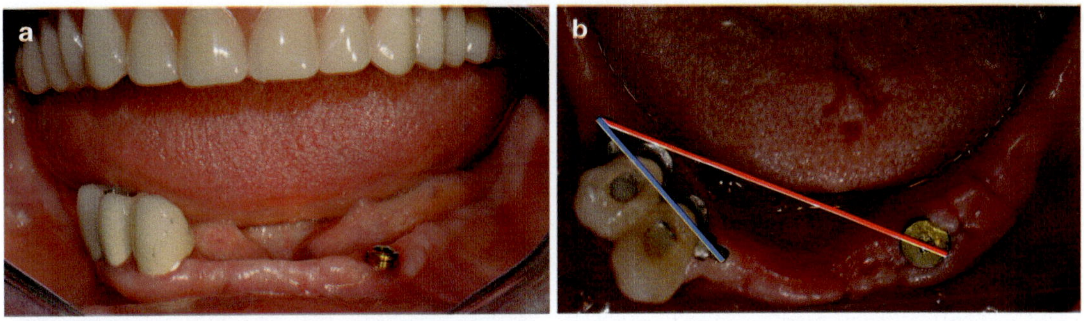

Fig. 17.2 (**a**) A strategically positioned implant for the improvement of the fulcrum position. (**b**) Occlusal view of the altered fulcrum line

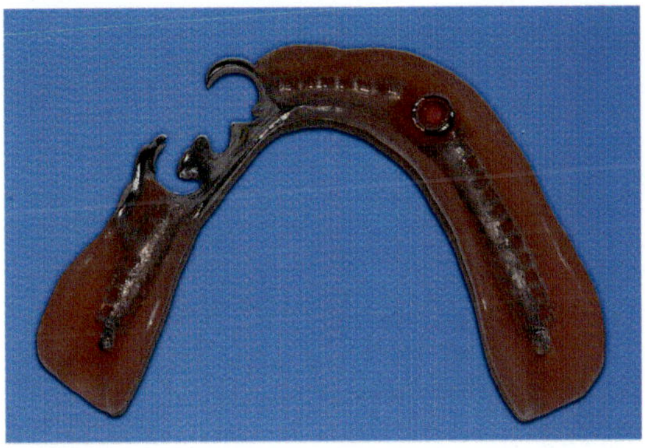

Fig. 17.3 The strategic implant attachment in the denture

other side of the partially edentulous mandible was used as a control. The follow-up was only seven months, but improved patient satisfaction had been presented.

One of the greatest advantages of implant use in conjunction with RPDs is that their position can be determined by the clinician in order to find the best suitable location for an abutment. While decision-making for the strategic implant position, anatomic characteristics of bone availability should be considered, too, since it would not be a great advantage to a patient if extensive augmentation procedures were required to allow implant placement in conjunction with an RPD. If anatomic needs are met, placement of an implant within the edentulous gap requires consideration of most mesial, mid, or most distal placement.

In distal extension spaces, where no support of teeth at each end can be expected, only two options may be considered primarily: the CRPD or the fixed/removable implant-supported prosthesis.

Solutions such as the cantilevered bridge or the shortened dental arch (SDA) can be regarded, in case of patient medical factors, concerns for the risk of surgical morbidity, increased time required for treatment, and costs, hindering the selection of implant therapy, as a compromise.

Today the SDA concept is widely accepted and practiced by prosthodontists and needs to be considered in the treatment planning of partially edentulous patients as an option (see Chap. 5). This approach provides an affordable treatment method that may provide an acceptable result, improving both oral hygiene and patient satisfaction. On the other hand, there are a minimum number of teeth needed to satisfy patients' functional demands and achieve SDA. When compared with CRPDs, the SDA showed a long-term comfort and oral function. Nevertheless, it should be pointed out that long-term randomized controlled studies are needed to compare IARPDs with the SDA situation.

The cantilevered solution is without a doubt an option giving a patient a comfortable solution in the beginning. In a case where molars are missing, the clinician can provide a fixed prosthetic alternative with a chewing surface reaching the molar area, without an implant. Here again the principle of prevention must be respected. The cantilevered option using the teeth neighboring to the edentulous area is a risky alternative and not preferred by the author of this chapter. Damage varying from secondary caries to overloading can lead to loss of the related teeth. A recent evidence-based review article evaluating the long-term success of cantilever cases reported that estimated survival and success rates of cantilever fixed partial dentures (FPDs) were lower than previously reported rates for typical end-abutment supported FPDs.

There are several classification systems of partially edentulous situations having been proposed and still in use as mentioned in Chap. 3. It has been estimated that there are over 65,000 possible combinations of teeth and edentulous gaps in opposing arches. The most familiar classification originally proposed by Kennedy is probably the most widely accepted system for categorizing of partially edentulous arches today.

The most commonly encountered patient complaints related to RPDs especially in Kennedy Class I (bilateral free end) and II (unilateral free end) cases are missing stability, minimal retention, discomfort upon loading, and esthetic problems caused by clasps and reciprocal arms. Obviously, the Kennedy Class IV in extremely long anterior edentulous spans creates a challenge for the prosthodontist, too. A limited number of implants can help preventing visible retentive elements.

The choice of IARPD treatment is often a useful escape from multiple surgeries or extensive and complicated surgical procedures such as sinus lifting. The demand for prosthodontic treatment is influenced more by esthetic expectations in most industrialized countries. In this manner, a very helpful treatment alternative is the placement of a few interforaminal implants (Fig. 17.4) supporting an anterior fixed bridge with extra coronal precision attachments (Fig. 17.5) and an RPD, thus reducing implant costs as well as the need for extensive surgery. This treatment modality brings the advantage that an edentulous patient feels confident even when the removable denture is taken off, since the anterior part is fixed and the edentulism is less visible. There are studies showing a not different force distribution in comparison to the single or splinted implant attachment solutions and concluding that patients may benefit of the fixed anterior part.

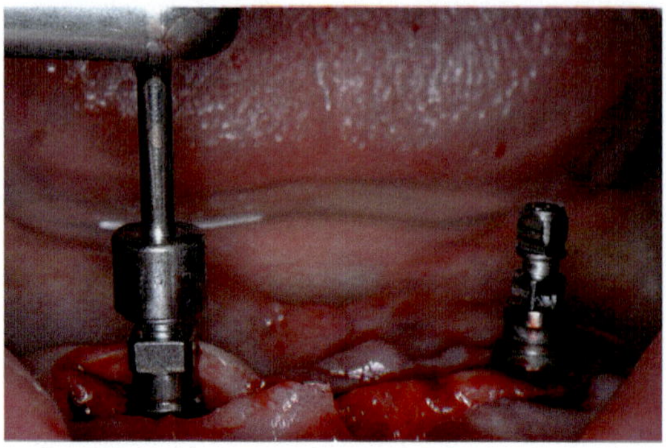

Fig. 17.4 Two interforaminal implants (mandible)

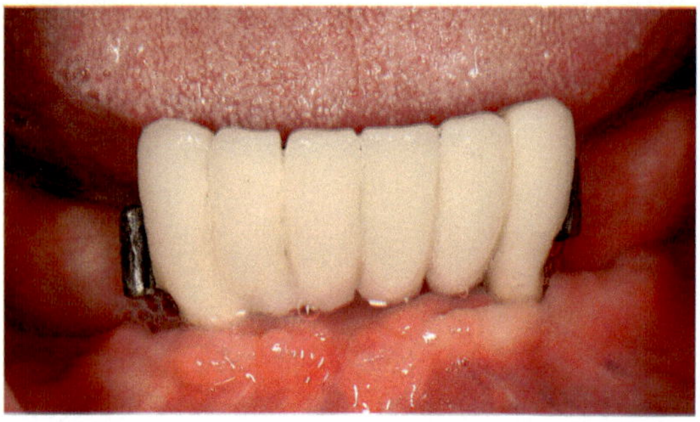

Fig. 17.5 An implant-supported anterior fixed bridge with extra coronal precision attachments

Dental implants can play a major role in terms of biomechanical support. A dental implant would act as a terminal abutment in a Kennedy Class III situation. As pointed out earlier, one of the most challenging situations is the Kennedy Class II when there are abutments on only one side of the arch and the long lever arm to the unilateral edentulous side causes insufficient stability, an implant placed strategically convenient would improve the fulcrum line position.

Before making the decision the oral condition of the patient and the exigency for implant use must be thoroughly overthought and justifiable indications should be determined. As an example, in a Kennedy Class I situation, where only molars are missing, it would be an unnecessary attempt to place implants for RPD support, since the patient could receive a fixed solution with the two implants. Similarly, a short edentulous gap would be a weak indication for an implant placement. Implants offer the advantage of not requiring the use of teeth as prosthetic abutments, and thus do not increase the functional burden on the natural dentition. Implants can eliminate the necessity of involving adjacent teeth in the reconstruction, but when nonetheless the adjacent teeth are in need of restoration, a conventional prosthesis should be considered primarily, especially in short-span spaces. The costs as well as the invasiveness of the surgical intervention associated with implants must always be considered. On the other hand, for longer span modification spaces with four or more missing teeth, a greater challenge for natural tooth–supported fixed prostheses is existing. In these cases, the tooth supported fixed partial denture is not an alternative any more. The clinician will aim either a CRPD or an implant-supported solution. As mentioned in several studies, the residual ridge resorption can be greater with longer spans, which will increase the need for augmentation procedures if implants are intended. Besides the additional costs with implants, the increased morbidity associated with augmentation procedures can also limit universal application. Only for this reason an implant manufacturer has developed an implant material with a much higher strength, namely a titanium-zirconium alloy, allowing the use of narrow diameter implants in the posterior. Although not an evidence-based fact yet, short implants are much more often successfully used compared to a decade ago, in cases with insufficient bone volume, thus avoiding the necessity of invasive augmentation procedures. Looking at this issue from another point of view, it must be pointed to the information that implants in large edentulous spans may promote bone preservation owing to peri-implant remodeling stimulus; thus it could be discussed that implants do not only bring additional costs and morbidity, but also long-term benefit. A troublous feature of IARPDs is the need for an osseointegration period, thus the need to fabricate an interim prosthesis. The provisional brings additional costs and a relatively uncomfortable time interval for the patient. It is important to design the provisional, even in a Kennedy Class III situation without a modification, cross-arch stabilized. The tiny design in comparison (Fig. 17.6) might appear more comfortable due to smaller volume, but during use, it will be difficult to keep stable. In the planning of an interim removable partial denture the author of this chapter prefers the Adams or ball clasps, since it guarantees a certain support, because there are no occlusal rests keeping the denture from tissueward movement. The alternative would be immediate loading of the implants in order to avoid an additional denture for provisionalization of the partial edentulism situation. Immediate loading in the edentulous mandible has been well documented. Although the maxilla is still showing a question mark, there are good data showing that immediate loading of the edentulous maxilla may also be feasible if bone quality is suitable. There are a lot of techniques described in literature offering possibilities to achieve good stability even in cancellous bone. In spite of these facts, the immediate loading is not a routine clinical application and should be considered with caution.

It should be kept in mind that the use of implants as a valuable help for RPDs does not allow to leave main principles of design such as the necessity of seats or rigid rests and major connectors.

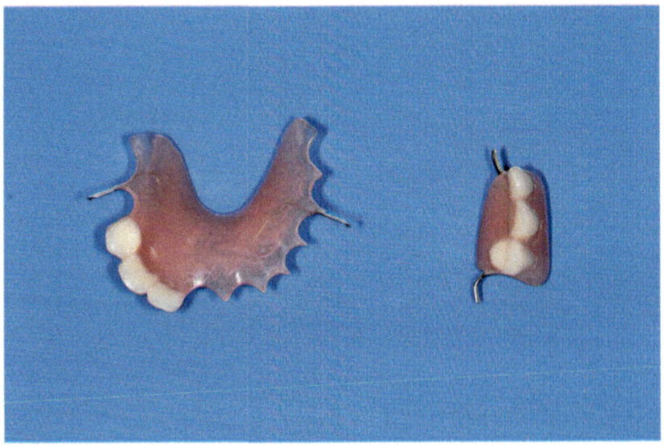

Fig. 17.6 It is important to design the provisional, even in a Kennedy Class III situation without a modification, cross-arch stabilized. The tiny design in comparison might appear more comfortable due to smaller volume, but during use it will be difficult to keep stable

17.2 Important Hints for Clinicians

17.2.1 Main Indications for IARPDs

- In order to help out the patient after loss of several dental implants with a step back solution (from fixed to removable).
- When the remaining dentition is not suitable to be used as abutment teeth and/or patient does not wish to lose all teeth, even when these are not strategically suitable.
- In cases where implants are placed gradually in a certain time period and there is a time interval where a transitional RPD is needed.
- Advanced ridge resorption in edentulous areas, making additional stability and retention measures necessary.
- In cases where surgical augmentation procedures for placement of all needed implants are contraindicated.
- In cases where the clasps should not be visible and the denture base is desired to be smaller.
- In cases where the jaw relation is inconvenient and the placement of the artificial teeth in intercuspal position (e.g. too far buccally) threatens the denture stability.
- In a few cases where extremely angulated implants cannot be treated by conventional methods.
- Patient desires.

17.2.2 Contraindications for IARPDs

- Cases where no surgery may be performed.
- Patients not able to use any removable denture.
- Situations where interocclusal or interarch distance does not allow the placement of an implant attachment.

17.2.3 Advantages of IARPDs

- Enhanced esthetics by elimination of clasps and compensation for loss of supporting tissues (assuring better lip support).
- Change of the fulcrum axis position possible.
- The forces on remaining teeth may be reduced.
- In free-end partially edentulous arch situations vertical support may be increased.
- Improved retention and stability.
- The arrangement of the insertion path is less problematic with implant abutments.
- Depending on attachment type, the maintenance may be easier.
- Reduced pressure or trauma on supporting tissues.
- Preservation of the bone around implants through delayed alveolar atrophy in edentulous areas.
- Compared to complete edentulism the remaining teeth help preserving the proprioception.
- It may reduce the need for indirect retention.

17.2.4 Disadvantages

- Increased cost.
- Additional surgical interventions.
- Increased treatment time.
- Multidisciplinary approach necessary.
- The treatment is more technique sensitive.
- Depending on attachment type, the maintenance may be more difficult.
- In some instances the denture production stages may be more complicated.
- Osseointegration period.

17.3 Main Alternatives and Different Treatment Modalities with Dental Implant Use as RPD Support

17.3.1 Edentulism

Two or three implants placed in the mandibular interforaminal region for a canine-to-canine bridge (Fig. 17.4) and support of a posterior RPD. This solution can be a valuable remedy in case of loss of one or more implants in a fixed planning. In a conservative approach the remaining implants can be used for a step back solution and for support of an RPD. The advantage of this modality is the transformation of the edentulous situation to a more favorable Kennedy Class I. The permanent presence of a fixed anterior bridge (Fig. 17.5) even after removal of the removable denture can give an esthetical confidence feeling and may be preferred by a not-to-be underestimated number of patients.

In partial edentulism, is a well-known fact that the remaining teeth, especially directly neighboring the edentulous area, may be periodontally compromised and threatened by overloading. Exactly at this point, dental implants can be a valuable aid in distributing the forces and relieving the rest dentition.

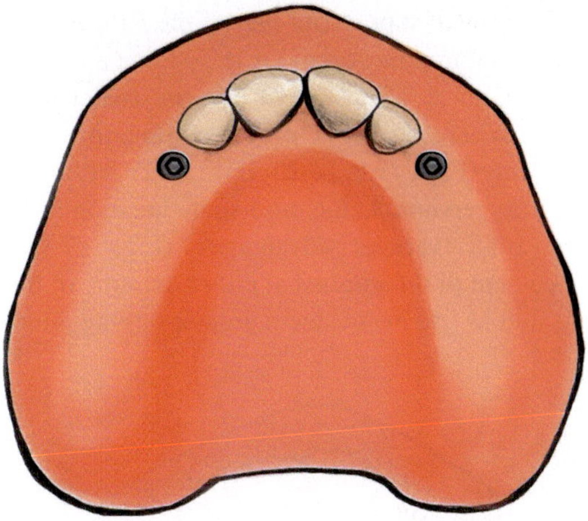

Fig. 17.7 In case of a Kennedy Class I situation, where canines are missing and only the central and lateral incisors are present, implants in the canine positions can have several important roles: support, retention without visible elements, and protection of the remaining teeth

17.3.2 Kennedy Class I and/or II Situation

There is no consensus on the position of the implants to be placed in order to achieve stability and retention in free-ending situations such as the Kennedy I and Kennedy II classifications. A popular location for the placement is in the posterior end, around the second molar area. On the other hand, there are clinicians who prefer the location next to the tooth neighboring to the free end as the most suitable position.

The distal extension mandibular RPD comprises some difficulties in use, partly due to the varying resilience characteristics of abutment teeth and mucosa, thus transfer of occlusal load. These difficulties can decrease patient satisfaction and even cause patients to quit the use of removable dentures. In case of a Kennedy class I situation, where canines are missing and only the central and lateral incisors are present, implants in the canine positions can have several important roles: support, retention without visible elements, and protection of the remaining teeth (Fig. 17.7). The placement of implants adjacent to distal abutment teeth, in general (Fig. 17.8) is additionally useful if a future fixed restoration is intended. This solution allows delivery of a provisional or permanent RPD without clasp showing and later changing to a fixed bridge after adding the necessary implants in the posterior. The Kennedy Class II partially edentulous situation is characterized by a unilateral extension. Clinicians should be aware that frequently RPDs prescribed especially for patients with a Kennedy Class II situation are not being used. It is well known that the Kennedy II cases represent a difficult group from planning as well as use point of view. One of the reasons is the insufficient indirect retention causing the

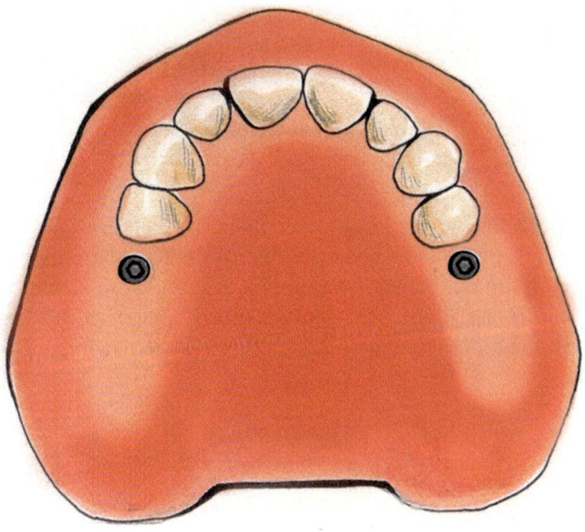

Fig. 17.8 This solution allows delivery of a provisional or permanent RPD without clasp showing and later changing to a fixed bridge after adding the necessary implants further posteriorly

shift of the most posterior part of the RPD resulting in food trapping or giving the patient a feeling of discomfort. The use of one or two dental implants here may be helpful in eliminating these problems (Figs. 17.9, 17.10, and 17.11). Although not very common, the mid-span location may also offer various advantages (Fig. 17.12). Placement of the implant at either extreme of the edentulous gap may cause a greater tipping effect and should be taken into consideration. However, it may be discussed that the ideal indirect retention effect could fail and the implant attachment will be subject to larger torsion movement, eventually causing more frequent complications. This alternative with the interim positioned implant would be probably valuable as a step back solution after loss of several implants, having been placed for a fixed solution. All discussed considerations apply to both situations, Kennedy Class

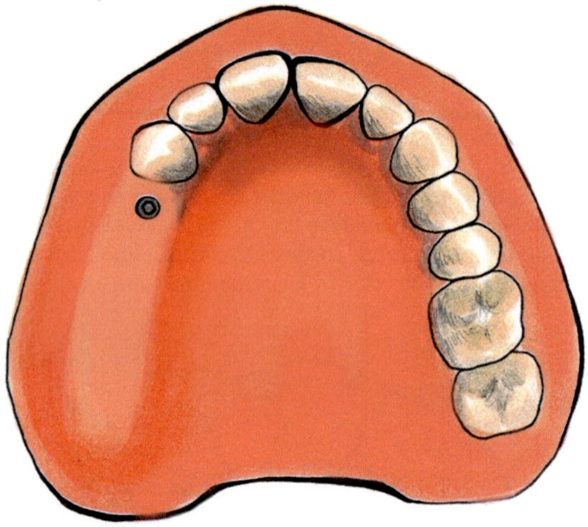

Fig. 17.9 Due to insufficient indirect retention causing the shift of the most posterior part of the RPD resulting in food trapping, patients may feel a discomfort in Kennedy Class II situations. An implant placed distal to the last abutment tooth may help preventing this inconvenience

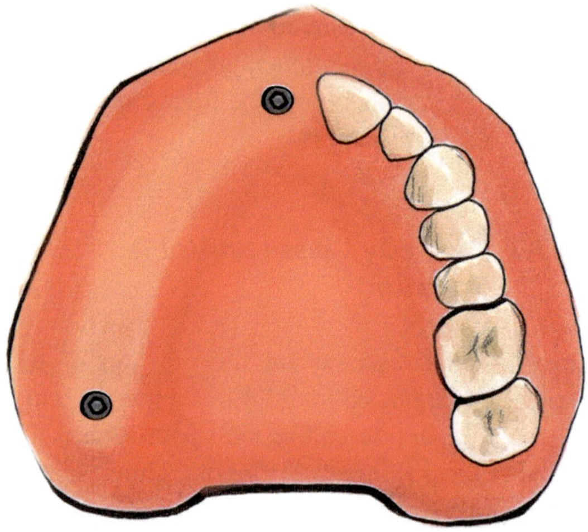

Fig. 17.11 In cases where the edentulous span is wide and covers unilaterally a whole quadrant, two implants should be taken into account

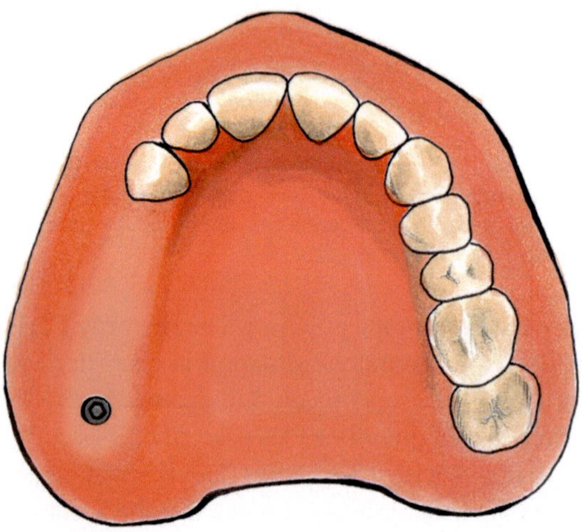

Fig. 17.10 If the visible clasp is not an issue and the distal abutment is a dependable tooth such as the canine, the implant can also be placed in the second molar position

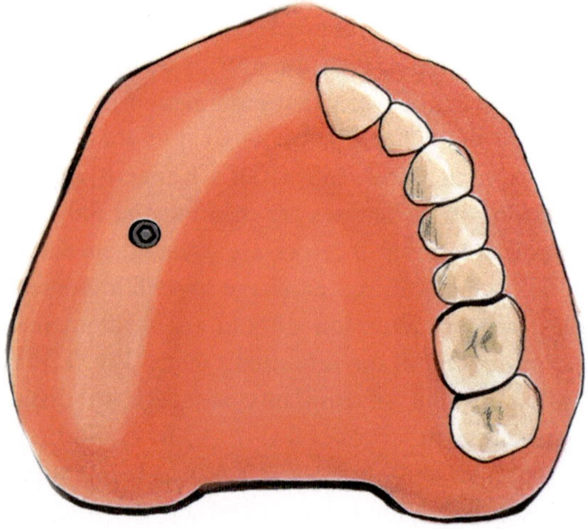

Fig. 17.12 The mid-span location is not common, but it may also be considered

I as well as Kennedy Class II. Placing four implants (Fig. 17.13) may be considered a bit too luxurious in a Kennedy Class I situation and can be criticized, but delineates a very good transitional situation for a later fixed solution. In case of Kennedy I and II situations, the fulcrum axis can be moved to distal by implants placed in the molar region, and additional support and retention may be obtained in order to increase patient comfort. Implants placed in the area of the second molars would change the Kennedy Class I situation to a more favorable Kennedy Class III (Fig. 17.14a, b). The results of a finite element analysis study, however, showed a tendency to more displacement of the denture, when implants were placed in a second molar position. Accordingly, a more central position in the arch, such as the first molar region was suggested. In another study, where a bi-dimensional finite element method had been used, it was found that approximating the implant to the abutment tooth caused the best distribution of stresses on the analyzed structures. On the other hand, a more central position, e.g. the first molar position, had decreased the dislodging of the denture, compared to the further distal or most mesial positions. In case of inadequate posterior alveolar ridge, the placement adjacent to the distal abutment tooth, at the most mesial location is recommended. As above mentioned this position can also be advantageous for possible future use in fixed implant-supported prosthesis or in order to improve aesthetics by avoiding the use of a retentive clasp.

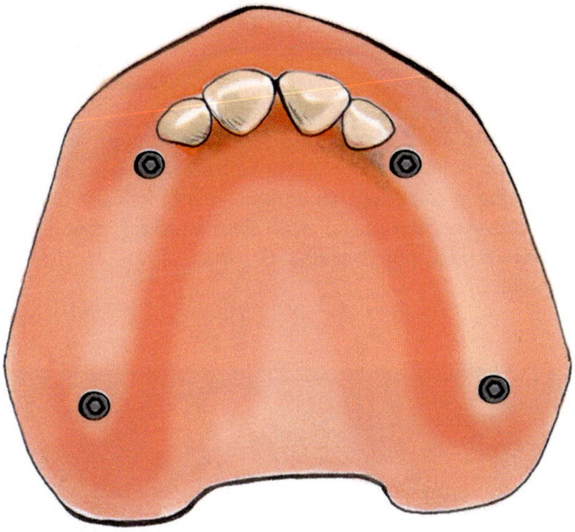

Fig. 17.13 Placing four implants may be considered a bit too luxurious in a Kennedy Class I situation and can be criticized, but delineates a very good transitional situation for a later fixed solution

Although the optimal length and diameter of the implants associated with RPD have not been determined yet, a probable disadvantage could be that short implants must be used in case of lack of sufficient bone height, when located as distally as

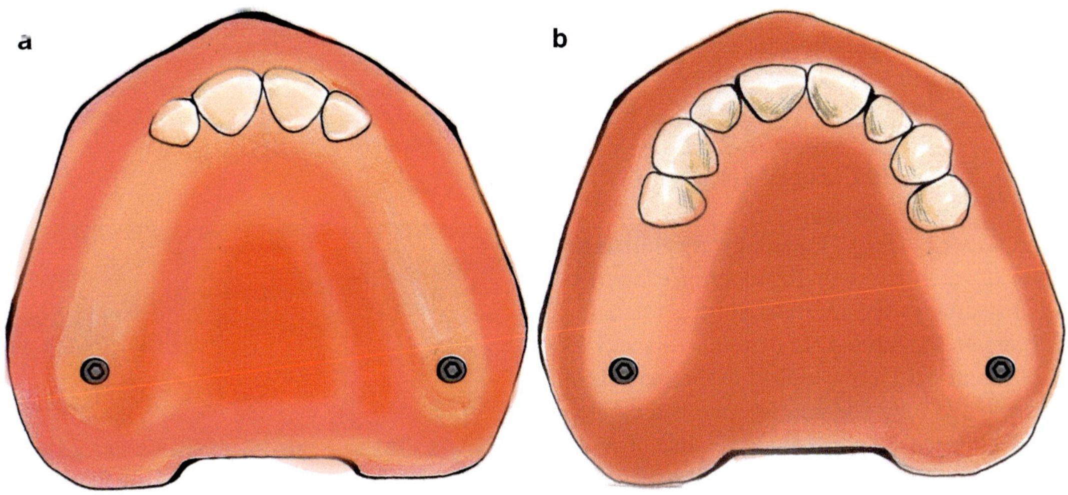

Fig. 17.14 (**a**, **b**) Implants placed in the area of the second molars would change the Kennedy Class I situation to a more favorable Kennedy Class III

possible to provide maximal support and stability, in Kennedy I or Kennedy II cases, due to local anatomy. In many Kennedy Class I or II cases, the remaining alveolar bone height above the mandibular canal is insufficient for implant placement of conventionally accepted length. The frequency of the use of short implants is growing and today implants of even 4 mm length are available on the market. However, the long-term success will have to be shown in clinical studies in the coming years. This treatment modality would be even more suitable for cases with existing canines, where clasps can be placed more securely because of better support from their stronger roots. Otherwise, e.g. when canines are missing and lateral incisors or weakened premolars are aimed, avoiding direct retainers applying unfavorable lateral displacing forces, especially in endodontically treated abutments, would be specifically beneficial.

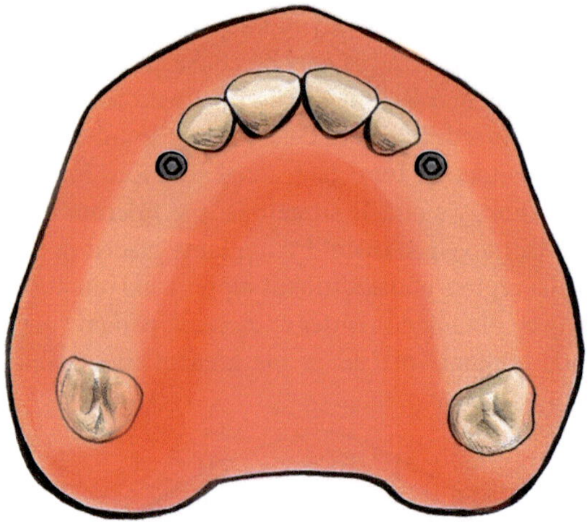

Fig. 17.15 If a Kennedy Class III situation already exists, implants can be used for several purposes, such as shortening a too long edentulous space, in case of not dependable compromised weak abutments (e.g. root canal treated or post-cored teeth) or when clasps are to be eliminated

17.3.3 Kennedy Class III Situation

If a Kennedy Class III situation already exists, implants can be used for several purposes, such as shortening a too long edentulous space, in case of not dependable compromised weak abutments (e.g. root canal treated or post-cored teeth) or when clasps are to be eliminated (Fig. 17.15). The best position for the implants in these cases is adjacent to the abutment teeth. However, it should be known that implants are only used seldom in Kennedy III cases.

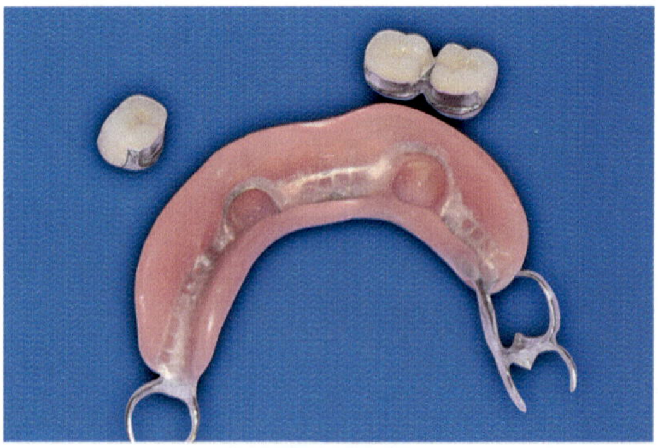

Fig. 17.16 In extreme Kennedy IV cases where only a few molars in the most distal exist and the long edentulous span can create a challenging fettle complicating the use of a partial denture

17.3.4 Kennedy Class IV Situation

In the Kennedy Class IV partially edentulous situation the arch has a single, anterior edentulous gap that crosses the midline and the remaining teeth create the butting. In extreme Kennedy IV cases where only a few molars in the most distal exist and the long edentulous span can create a challenging fettle complicating the use of a partial denture (Fig. 17.16). In such cases a few dental implants, e.g. two implants in the canine positions (Figs. 17.17 and 17.18) could give the

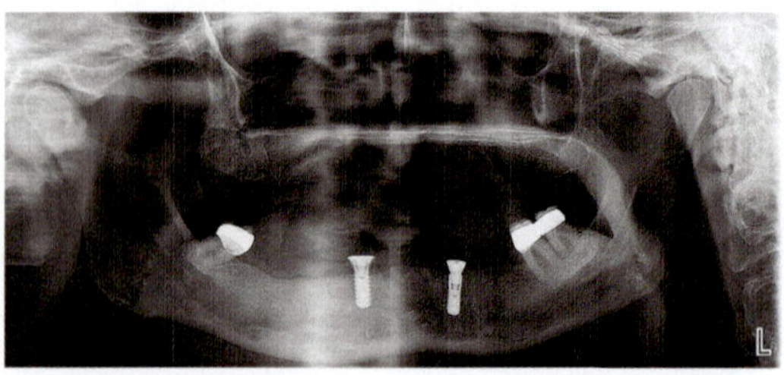

Fig. 17.17 A panoramic radiography showing two interforaminal implants in an extreme Kennedy Class IV situation

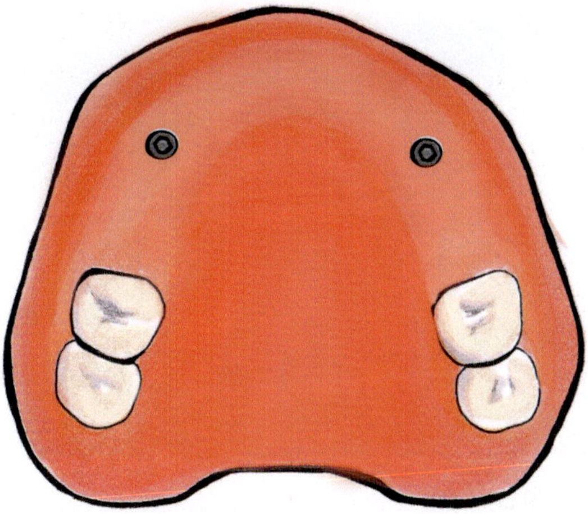

Fig. 17.18 In extreme Kennedy Class IV cases a few dental implants could give the dentures a very reliable stability as well as retention

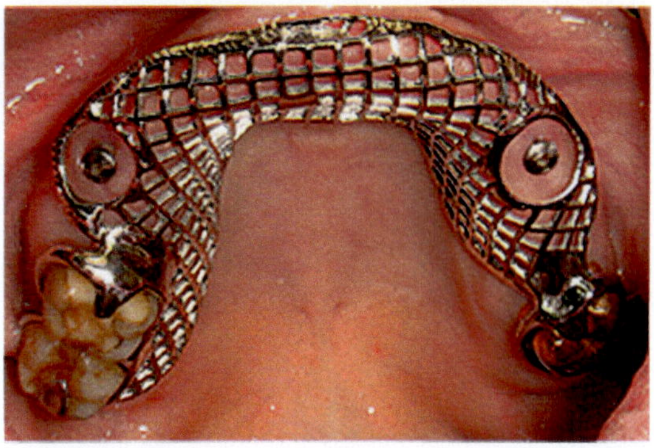

Fig. 17.19 Two anterior implants giving anterior support and retention in a maxillary Kennedy IV situation

dentures a very reliable stability as well as retention. The position of the two implants to be placed is a subject of discussion. In general clinicians use preferably symmetrically the canine positions for the two interforaminal implants, perhaps still as the result of experience with overdentures (OVDs) supported by natural teeth, since the mandibular canines frequently are the last natural teeth remaining due to better intrabony support and are suitable as OVD abutments. However, other arguments should be kept in mind, too. Moving the implants slightly anterior, to the lateral incisor position, could create several advantages in certain situations. When using a bar connecting the two implants in a situation with a tapering arch form, the canine positioned implants could cause cantilevering to the anterior to avoid encroaching on the tongue space and floor of the mouth, which may increase the risk of screw loosening or fracture due to bending moments involved with cantilever loading. In this manner, the implant placement slightly more to the anterior will definitely reduce the potential need for off-center bar placement. It is enunciated that another advantage of a more anterior placement of the two implant OVD abutments is that this placement reduces the tendency for the mandibular denture to rotate around the fulcrum created between the two implant abutments. It is claimed that if the implants are placed in the canine position, there may be a tendency for the distal denture bases to lift when the patient incises with the anterior teeth. This could be particularly problematic when the retentive components of the OVD attachment system are designed to permit rotational freedom of movement around the implant fulcrum. Implant placement in the lateral incisor position could reduce the anteroposterior distance from the incisal edges to the rotational axis between the implants, which would be a factor inhibiting the tendency for the denture to lift to the posterior and thereby increasing its stability. In the author's opinion, if single attachments are planned to be used, this argument is not eligible any more. On the contrary, there are clinical studies showing the trend for better patient satisfaction scores the more distal the two implants are placed. Independent from the position the anterior support and retention via implants should not be neglected as a viable option in mandibular as well as maxillary Kennedy IV situations (Figs. 17.19 and 17.20a, b). As very well known, an important factor in the decision-making of attachments is the space needed for the retentive components. If there is insufficient interarch (interocclusal) space, a locator is a better choice compared to a bar-and-clip type of attachment. A controversial issue worth to study further as a treatment modality would be the use of a single mandibular midline implant as an OVD abutment to increase mandibular denture retention and stability, especially inhibiting the tendency for the posterior extensions of the OVD to lift during incising. A single

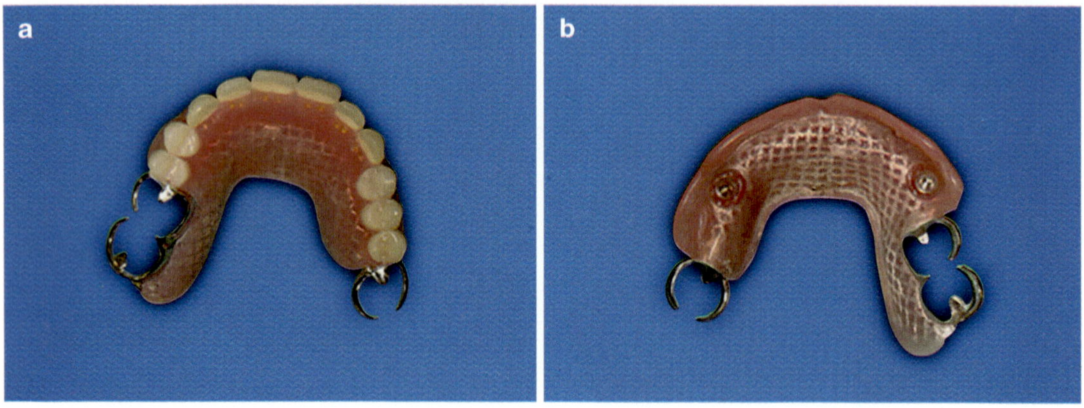

Fig. 17.20 (**a**) Implant-supported anterior retention elements embedded in a removable partial denture. (**b**) Occlusal view of the maxillary Kennedy IV removable partial denture

implant may be nearly as effective as two anterior implants in this regard and could reduce treatment costs considerably.

Another argument is that if later a fixed solution in the form of interforaminal five implants supporting a detachable denture is aimed or should the patient desire additional implant therapy in future in a severely resorbed mandible, the placement of two implants in the lateral incisor positions allows for future placement of implants in midline and as far distally as the mental foramina allow bilaterally. It is often stated that placement of three additional implants is feasible when the original two implants are placed in the lateral incisor positions. This, of course, does not comply in a mandibular edentulism case, where there is sufficient bone volume for implant placement in the posterior. Here the ideal implant positions (if six implants are planned) would be bilaterally the canines, first premolars, and first molars and the canine position would be very convenient.

In cases of severe alveolar atrophy hindering even the placement of two interforaminal implants, a single symphiseal implant was pointed out in a study, to play a pivotal role to improve the integrity of the principle abutments and alveolar bone support in long span Kennedy Class IV cases. The symphiseal region is generally known to have the greatest available bone height, thick dense cortical plates, and dense trabecular bone making it an ideal location for an implant treatment.

Different than the other Kennedy classifications, in a Kennedy IV situation, an RPD has superiority vs. fixed solutions; especially in cases with severely resorbed alveolar ridges, the buccal flanges of the dentures are capable to give better lip support and assure a better esthetic result. If the retention and stability in these critical cases can be improved by dental implants, it is to be expected that patients often prefer the removable alternative.

Long-term studies evaluating the success of dental implants used for RPD support, revealed very high survival rates, minor prosthetic complications, and superior patient satisfaction. On the other hand, there are generally only poorly reported clinical studies in the literature and quantitative systematic reviews or meta-analyses are missing due to lack of randomized or non-randomized controlled trials. For this reason, there are no settled guidelines dictating the number and location of RPD-supporting dental implants yet and the clinicians have to act obeying their sense of clinic and own experience. As an example, there is no consensus on the most favorable implant position in a Kennedy Class I or II situation. While some authors recommend the second molar position (most distally possible position) to transform the situation to a much more comfortable Kennedy Class III case, others suggest a more central position such as the first molar position against a tendency to displacement. The author of this chapter advises to choose the implant position, taking cognizance of the available bone volume for optimal implant size. In a distally placed implant situation a clasp has to be used at the most distal abutment tooth. If the most distal abutment tooth is an incisor, the strategy of transforming to a Kennedy Class III situation has to be given up and the implant position chosen at the most mesial part of the edentulous span. This brings an esthetic advantage and protects the generally weaker roots of incisors from lateral overload. The use of an implant to support a distal extension removable partial dental prosthesis is potentially effective in preserving the remaining teeth, soft tissues, and alveolar ridges by reducing excessive stress in patients with mandibular free-end partial edentulism. As shown in case reports, distal implants with retention elements provide additional support and retention and stability to a distal extension RPD. Favorable outcome of such scenarios is shown in very recent systematic reviews of the literature. IARPDs to convert a Kennedy class I to class III denture may be beneficial for the patient's enhanced comfort and function. In this manner, the problem of intrusive movements of the free-end part of the RPD may be resolved. In a recent study where the implants had been virtually placed in three different positions (most distal, central, and most mesial), it was shown that the load on the abutment tooth was greatest with the distally placed implant, followed by the central and mesial. On the other hand, the load on the residual ridge was lowest with the distally placed implant, followed by the mesially and centrally placed implant.

17.4 Useful Facts Concerning Implant-Assisted Removable Partial Dentures

Evidence from long-term clinical follow-up is needed, but it can be speculated that the frequency of complications and maintenance requirements of IARPDs are to be expected similar in number as in CRPDs. Mainly the most often encountered complications are related to the retention mechanism. Generally, there is an agreement about no observable effect of the attachment design on the incidence of maintenance requirements. Other maintenance requirements would be periodic adjustment of occlusal contacts, changing of artificial teeth, and elimination of possible sore spots. Additionally, in implant-assisted prostheses peri-implant complications such as peri-implantitis may occur from time to time. Although there is a very high success rate, it would be advisable to inform patients thoroughly from the beginning about probable complications as well as expected maintenance requirements and the costs to avoid unpleasant confrontations. Possibilities and recommendations related to attachment selection as well as probable complications and maintenance requirements will be reviewed and explained in the coming paragraphs.

17.4.1 Attachments and Different Strategies

The details of the precision attachments are described in Chap. 16. Attachments may be classified in very different ways. A popular one is dividing them in two groups as "single" and "splinted." Currently there is no scientific evidence showing the need for splinting. However, it would rather be advisable to splint the implants in situations of insufficient bone quality and quantity, especially when narrow implants had been placed. As stated in a paper, attachment selection should be directed by the available interarch distance and rather be evaluated at the diagnostic phase. Suitable attachments/abutments for implant retention of RPDs are:

- Bar attachments
- Ball attachments (retentive anchors)
- Locator (Zest Anchor)
- Locator abutments may be recommended because of their availability in different heights in addition to their resiliency and retention. Locator abutment can also be easily repaired and replaced which enhance their durability. For the solution of the wear problem of the abutment parts (patrices) several

manufacturers have developed meanwhile products such as the Novaloc® System, where the surface hardness is sufficient to resist early retention loss due to wear.

- Telescopic attachments (Figs. 17.21 and 17.22)
- Magnets
- Crown and bridge abutments
- These are used in combination with precision attachments fabricated for use with tooth crowns. To avoid often decementation, abutments with occlusal screw retention system may be preferred. An implant-supported crown is also reported as an alternative to be used unilaterally to replace a primary abutment tooth. The crown may also be used without a precision attachment, serving solely as an abutment tooth, having the suitable retention area for a clasp.
- Innovative solutions
- Titanium shock absorber from Bonecare Dynamics NV (Belgium) suggests a slightly improved load-damping feature on the implants for highly resilient mucosa supported by the edentulous alveolar crest. This feature may be of special value in cases where short or narrow implants have been used, to protect from biomechanical overloading.

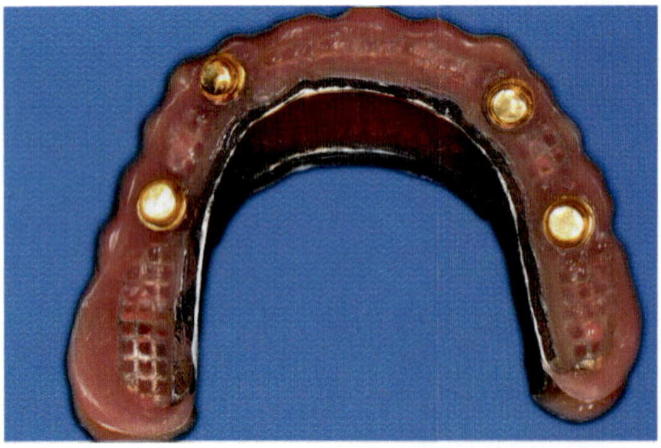

Fig. 17.21 Telescopic gold attachments in the denture

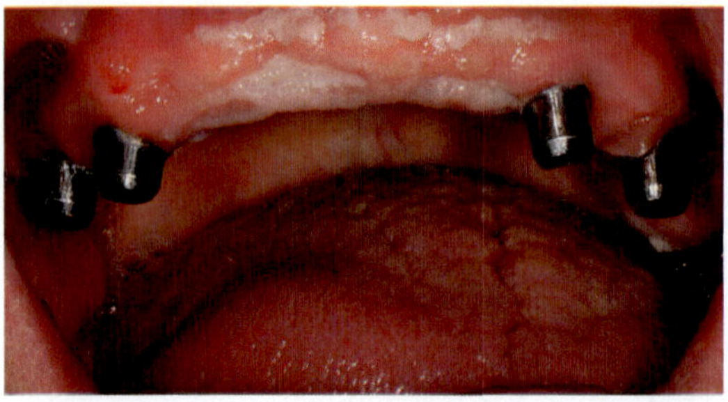

Fig. 17.22 Telescopic abutments intraorally

As several other issues are related with IARPDs, such as the ideal implant location and size of the implant, the choice of the most suitable attachment system remains mainly dependent on the clinicians' preferences and needs more evidence from research to build up a guideline. A very recent systematic review has reported overall that different attachment systems did not influence the implant survival rate and patient satisfaction.

In addition to several above-mentioned classification methods of partially edentulous arches, a classification system depending on the Applegate-Kennedy system was described by Misch & Judy, with emphasis on the available bone in the edentulous area for implant placement. This proposed classification had involved four divisions. Divisions A and B were indicating that bone is available for implant placement, while division C was pointing that there is not sufficient bone for implant placement, and finally division D, where only basal bone is available due to severe atrophy of the edentulous area. A more recent article was suggesting a new classification method with the name "Implant-Corrected Kennedy (ICK) Classification System." The authors used the Applegate-Kennedy system for the explanation of the partial edentulism situation and added the location of the placed or planned implant(s) using the American Dental Association (ADA)'s numbering between parentheses (Fig. 17.23). In this book the FDI (Federation Dentaire Internationale) system was preferred for numbering the dentition (see Chap. 3).

17.4.2 Complications and Maintenance Requirements

Long-term studies having evaluated the success of dental implants being used for RPD support

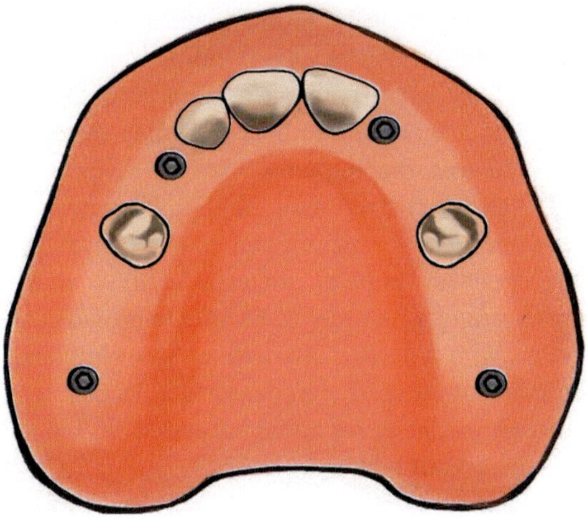

Fig. 17.23 ICK I mod 2 (# 2, 6, 10, 15); if modified to FDI dental numbering system it would correspond to: ICK I mod 2 (# 17, 13, 22, 27)

revealed very high survival rates, minor prosthetic complications, and superior patient satisfaction. On the other hand, it should be pointed out that there are generally only poorly reported clinical studies in the literature and quantitative systematic reviews, or meta-analyses are missing due to lack of randomized or non-randomized controlled trials in these cases.

The forces at the pivot points such as the abutments are at maximum level, being even higher with increased occlusal force and base length. In this manner, distal extension RPDs may show a risk of failures more frequently in the supporting elements of denture or abutments. Shear forces lead to a bending moment as a function of distance, thus leading to instability of distal extension RPDs. Although it was reported that implants might tolerate higher forces than abutment teeth, complications will inevitably occur in time.

Additional to general partial denture complications, the IARPD complications or maintenance needs tend to concentrate more in the retention mechanism. Similarly, the most frequent complications related to implant OVDs that have been reported in the literature are loss of retention or damage to the retention mechanism, fractures of the restorative material and need of rebasing or relining.

There is an ongoing debate about the influence of attachment type on later technical complications in implant OVDs, although only a few studies have compared treatment outcomes with different attachment systems of OVDs. It is well recognized that attachments of OVDs on implants lose retention after some time. Fatigue and wear of the material could be another factor causing complications with retention loss. While food chewing, forces from three directions appear and may cause rotation or rocking, thus clinically leading to plastic deformation of the matrices, resulting in a reduction of retention or dislodgement of the clip. Most frequently the wear happens in the female part of the retention mechanism; however it is not rare that the male part is subject to detrition.

Although there is no unanimous opinion, generally, there is an agreement about no observable effect of the attachment design on the incidence of maintenance requirements. On the other hand, several authors have reported that prosthodontic maintenance requirements with ball attachments were higher, particularly during the first year. In a review it was pointed out that a dislodged, worn, or loose matrix or its respective housing was more common after the first year with ball retainers and the most common repair was retentive component replacement. The results of another study focusing mainly on the comparison of the retention mechanism complications showed that with resilient attachments, the frequency of broken, loose, or lost bar clips and female retainers of ball anchors had been significantly higher. The rigid bar, on the other hand, had required significantly more retightening of the female part during the first five years. Another maintenance requirement is the need of relining of the denture base of the RPD. It is speculated by several authors that OVDs with rigid attachments show less need to be relined. In the same way, it could be speculated that the implant could help preserving the surrounding alveolar bone and reducing the need for relining. In the author's view, the choice of attachment system should be left to the predilection of the clinician, if the path of denture insertion is parallel to the implant axis. Otherwise, a system such as the telescopic attachment, being able to compensate the angle differences, is to be recommended, in order to avoid early wear of the retentive parts. If there are several implants, bar attachments may help to compensate for severely malpositioned implants, too. Although the manufacturer and some authors praise the locator abutment and attachment system for allowing compensation of up to 40°, our clinical experience shows else. In case of angular deviation from the path of insertion, the matrice as well as the patrice can undergo severe wear and lose retentive properties in a very short time. Too often maintenance requirements of a prosthesis can damage the confidence of the patient and may lead to giving up its use.

Other maintenance requirements would be periodic adjustment of occlusal contacts, changing of artificial teeth, and elimination of possible sore spots. A high incidence of periodontal disease and tooth decay has been reported in CRPD wearers, attributed mainly to a lack of motivation and compliance with adequate oral hygiene. Patients should be advised of their role in the maintenance of the IARPD, and a definite follow-up protocol is mandatory to obtain satisfactory long-term results. It must be discussed what influence the missing proprioception in IARPD patients may provoke. The missing feedback may cause the patients to bite or chew stronger, whereas this overload could have a more detrimental effect on these cases since implants will inhibit the resilience and forces will concentrate at certain sites. Weak parts of the IARPD such as the acrylic junction with the attachment matrice then are more prone to fracture. Long-term clinical follow-up studies will give valuable data concerning the difference between IARPD and CRPD complications.

It could be expected from learned clinical notion that the placement of short and/or narrow implants may create a biomechanical handicap, but long-term clinical follow-up studies are necessary to be able to draw reliable conclusions. The width of the implant could be a decisive factor, too. It is known that manufacturers do not recommend the use of implants with diameters less than 3.5 mm in the posterior region or as single standing attachment support because of the danger of fracture. In this manner, the author exhorts the use of stronger implants having a width of at least 4.0 mm for this purpose. On the other hand, there are authors affirming that it is expected that the implants used to support an RPD can be shorter with smaller diameter. As mentioned above, an implant manufacturer has developed an implant material with a much higher strength, in order to be able to provide clinicians with a narrow alternative. Short implants are more often used, compared to a decade ago, although evidence for equal success as in longer implants is still lacking.

In some scientific research articles resilient attachments in combination with IARPDs have been recommended. A low-profile attachment may be preferred to decrease the off-load forces to the implants. At the most distal of the denture flange where the base thickness is limited, a high abutment could cause a bulge.

The technical complexity of an IARPD may increase the probability of technical complications and some costs. On the other hand, the provided stability and different retention mechanism is capable to reduce the often-mentioned high incidence of periodontal disease and dental caries, extending the survival period of the remaining dentition. Additional research and long-term clinical follow-up studies will be able to give valuable data concerning the influence of dental implants on the prognosis of the abutment teeth, supporting soft tissue and alveolar bone, due to decreased loading.

Although no scientific data is available yet, there are still a huge group of scientists and clinicians believing that the biomechanical behavior of teeth and implants under functional loading is similar. However, the majority of in vitro, in vivo, and clinical follow-up studies indicate that the reaction of implants to load is different than traditionally taught in textbooks. Issues such as the influence of crown-implant ratio, cantilevers, and lateral forces are to be debated from a different point of view in implant dentistry. The efficacy of stress-breaking on tooth-implant supported prosthesis was evaluated in a numerical simulation study and it was reported that the stress-breaker keyway device function becomes obvious only when occlusal forces act on the natural tooth. In the opinion of the author of this chapter, the supporting implants do not need to be protected from functional loading forces with special measures. The implants seem to tolerate a great amount of load unless they are underdimensioned in size or having been placed in inadequate bone. The prejudices from the 1980s concerning implant length have been revolutionized by clinical experience and scientific, evidence-based data and today implants of down to 6 or even 4 mm length are being used instead of 16–17 mm earlier. Literature clearly defines that functional loading forces do not have a detrimental effect on osseointegration process, and it was shown that in single implants off-axial loads do not lead to marginal bone loss. The knowledge regarding the response of the peri-implant bone when the dental implant is excessively loaded is limited and the level of evidence is poor. With animal experimental studies showing conflicting results, it is unclear whether occlusal overload might cause marginal bone loss or total loss of osseointegration to already osseointegrated dental implants when the applied load exceeds the biologically acceptable limit. This biological limit is also unknown. Furthermore, higher remodeling activity of the peri-implant bone is found around implants subjected to high loading forces. In this manner, we do not necessarily need to recommend a resilience mechanism to protect the RPD-supporting implants from overloading during denture function.

Although there is a very high success rate, it would be advisable to inform patients thoroughly from the beginning about probable complications as well as expected maintenance requirements and the costs to avoid unpleasant confrontations.

Further Reading

Abou-Ayash S, Rudaz AC, Janner S, Kraus D, Schimmel M, Enkling N. Converting bilateral free-end removable partial dentures to implant-assisted removable partial dentures using 6 mm short implants: patient-reported outcomes of a prospective clinical study. Int J Environ Res Public Health. 2022;19:8998.

Al-Johany SS, Andres C. ICK classification system for partially edentulous arches. J Prosthodont. 2008;17:502–7.

Allen PF, McMillan AS, Smith DG. Complications and maintenance requirements of implant-supported prostheses provided in a UK dental hospital. Br Dent J. 1997;182:298–302.

Arat Bilhan S, Geckili O, Cilingir A, Bozdag E, Bilhan H. Evaluation of two interforaminal implants and implant-assisted removable dentures on stress distribution: an in vitro study. J Korean Assoc Oral Maxillofac Surg. 2019;45:199–206.

Arita S, Gonda T, Togawa H, Maeda Y, Ikebe K. Influence of mandibular distal extension implant-supported removable partial dentures on the force exerted on maxillary anterior teeth. J Prosthodont Res. 2021;65:541–5.

Bandiaky ON, Lokossou DL, Soueidan A, Le Bars P, Gueye M, Mbodj EB, Le Guéhennec L. Implant-supported removable partial dentures compared to conventional dentures: a systematic review and meta-analysis of quality of life, patient satisfaction, and biomechanical complications. Clin Exp Dent Res. 2022;8:294–312.

Bilhan H, Geckili O, Mumcu E, Bilmenoglu C. Maintenance requirements associated with mandibular implant overdentures: clinical results after first year of service. J Oral Implantol. 2011;37:697–704.

Bilhan H, Geçkili O, Mumcu E, Bozdag E, Sünbüloğlu E, Kutay O. Influence of surgical technique, implant shape and diameter on the primary stability in cancellous bone. J Oral Rehabil. 2010;37:900–7.

Budtz-Jørgensen E, Bochet G, Grundman M, Borgis S. Aesthetic considerations for the treatment of partially edentulous patients with removable dentures. Pract Periodontics Aesthet Dent. 2000;12:765–74.

Budtz-Jörgensen E. Restoration of the partially edentulous mouth—a comparison of overdentures, removable partial dentures, fixed partial dentures and implant treatment. J Dent. 1996;24:237–44.

Carr A, Brown D. Mc Cracken's removable partial prosthodontics. 12th ed. Elsevier Mosby; 2010.

Cehreli MC, Karasoy D, Kokat AM, Akca K, Eckert SE. Systematic review of prosthetic maintenance requirements for implant-supported overdentures. Int J Oral Maxillofac Implants. 2010;25:163–80.

Chang M, Chronopoulos V, Mattheos N. Impact of excessive occlusal load on successfully-osseointegrated dental implants: a literature review. J Investig Clin Dent. 2013;4:142–50.

Chee WW. Treatment planning: implant-supported partial overdentures. J Calif Dent Assoc. 2005;33:313–6.

Chikunov I, Doan P, Vahidi F. Implant-retained partial overdenture with resilient attachments. J Prosthodont. 2008;17:141–8.

Chronopoulos V, Sarafianou A, Kourtis S. The use of dental implants in combination with removable partial dentures: a case report. J Esthet Restor Dent. 2008;20:355–65.

Cunha LD, Pellizzer EP, Verri FR, Falcón-Antenucci RM, Goiato MC. Influence of ridge inclination and implant localization on the association of mandibular Kennedy class I removable partial denture. J Craniofac Surg. 2011;22:871–5.

Cunha LD, Pellizzer EP, Verri FR, Pereira JA. Evaluation of the influence of location of osseointegrated implants associated with mandibular removable partial dentures. Implant Dent. 2008;17:278–87.

de Carvalho WR, Barboza EP, Caúla AL. Implant-retained removable prosthesis with ball attachments in partially edentulous maxilla. Implant Dent. 2001;10:280–4.

de Freitas RF, de Carvalho Dias K, da Fonte Porto Carreiro A, Barbosa GA, Ferreira MA. Mandibular implant-supported removable partial denture with distal extension: a systematic review. J Oral Rehabil. 2012;39:791–8.

Dudic A, Mericske-Stern R. Retention mechanisms and prosthetic complications of implant-supported mandibular overdentures: long-term results. Clin Implant Dent Relat Res. 2002;4:212–9.

Enkling N, Nauli J, Kraus D, Wittneben JG, Schimmel M, Abou-Ayash S. Short strategic implants for mandibular removable partial dentures: one-year results from a pilot randomized crossover abutment type study. Clin Oral Implants Res. 2021;32:1176–89.

Fields H Jr, Campfield RW Jr. Removable partial prosthesis partially supported by an endosseous blade implant. J Prosthet Dent. 1974;31:273–8.

Geckili O, Cilingir A, Erdogan O, Kesoglu AC, Bilmenoglu C, Ozdiler A, Bilhan H. The influence of interimplant distance in mandibular overdentures supported by two implants on patient satisfaction and quality of life. Int J Prosthodont. 2015;28:19–21.

Gharehchahi J, Asadzadeh N, Mirmortazavi A, Shakeri MT. Maximum dislodging forces of mandibular implant-assisted removable partial dentures: in vitro assessment. J Prosthodont. 2013;22:543–9.

Gonçalves TM, Campos CH, Garcia RC. Implant retention and support for distal extension partial removable dental prostheses: satisfaction outcomes. J Prosthet Dent. 2014;112:334–9.

Grossmann Y, Nissan J, Levin L. Clinical effectiveness of implant-supported removable partial dentures—a review of the literature and retrospective case evaluation. J Oral Maxillofac Surg. 2009;67:1941–6.

Jensen C, Raghoebar GM, Kerdijk W, Meijer HJA, Cune MS. Implant-supported mandibular removable partial dentures; patient-based outcome measures in relation to implant position. J Dent. 2016;55:92–8.

Jensen C, Ross J, Feenstra TL, Raghoebar GM, Speksnijder C, Meijer HJA, Cune MS. Cost-effectiveness of implant-supported mandibular removable partial dentures. Clin Oral Implants Res. 2017;28: 594–601.

Jones JD, Garcia LT. Dental implants in RPDs. In: Removable partial dentures—a clinician's guide. Singapore: Wiley-Blackwell; 2009. p. 156–61.

Kang SH, Kim SK, Heo SJ, Koak JY. Survival rate and clinical evaluation of the implants in implant assisted removable partial dentures: surveyed crown and overdenture. J Adv Prosthodont. 2020;12:239–49.

Keltjens HM, Kayser AF, Hertel R, Battistuzzi PG. Distal extension removable partial dentures supported by implants and residual teeth: considerations and case reports. Int J Oral Maxillofac Implants. 1993;8:208–13.

Klein MO, Schiegnitz E, Al-Nawas B. Systematic review on success of narrow-diameter dental implants. Int J Oral Maxillofac Implants. 2014;29:43–54.

Kobayashi E, Matsumoto S, Doi H, Yoneyama T, Hamanaka H. Mechanical properties of the binary titanium-zirconium alloys and their potential for biomedical materials. J Biomed Mater Res. 1995;29:943–50.

Kono K, Kurihara D, Suzuki Y, Ohkubo C. Pressure distribution of implant-supported removable partial dentures with stress-breaking attachments. J Prosthodont Res. 2014;58:115–20.

Kuzmanovic DV, Payne AG, Purton DG. Distal implants to modify the Kennedy classification of a removable partial denture: a clinical report. J Prosthet Dent. 2004;92:8–11.

Lee DW, Lee DW, Park KH, Moon IS. The effects of off-axial loading on periimplant marginal bone loss in a single implant. J Prosthet Dent. 2014;112:501–7.

Lin CL, Wang JC, Kuo YC. Numerical simulation on the biomechanical interactions of tooth/implant-supported system under various occlusal forces with rigid/non-rigid connections. J Biomech. 2006;39:453–63.

Ma M, Qi M, Zhang D, Liu H. The clinical performance of narrow diameter implants versus regular diameter implants: a metaanalysis. J Oral Implantol. 2019;45:503–8.

Matsudate Y, Yoda N, Nanba M, Ogawa T, Sasaki K. Load distribution on abutment tooth, implant and residual ridge with distal-extension implant-supported removable partial denture. J Prosthodont Res. 2016;60:282–8.

McAndrew R. Prosthodontic rehabilitation with a swing-lock removable partial denture and a single osseointegrated implant: a clinical report. J Prosthet Dent. 2002;88:128–31.

Mijiritsky E, Karas S. Removable partial denture design involving teeth and implants as an alternative to unsuccessful fixed implant therapy: a case report. Implant Dent. 2004;13:218–22.

Mijiritsky E, Ormianer Z, Klinger A, Mardinger O. Use of dental implants to improve unfavorable removable partial denture design. Compend Contin Educ Dent. 2005;26:744–50.

Mijiritsky E. Implants in conjunction with removable partial dentures: a literature review. Implant Dent. 2007;16:146–54.

Minoretti R, Triaca A, Saulacic N. The use of extraoral implants for distal-extension removable dentures: a clinical evaluation up to 8 years. Int J Oral Maxillofac Implants. 2009;24:1129–37.

Misch CE, Judy KW. Classification of partially edentulous arches for implant dentistry. Int J Oral Implantol. 1987;4:7–13.

Mitrani R, Brudvik JS, Phillips KM. Posterior implants for distal extension removable prostheses: a retrospective study. Int J Periodontics Restorative Dent. 2003;23:353–9.

Mohamed GF, El Sawy AA. The role of single immediate loading implant in long class IV Kennedy mandibular partial denture. Clin Implant Dent Relat Res. 2012;14:708–15.

Murakami K, Ayukawa Y, Ogino Y, Nakagawa A, Horikawa T, Yamaguchi E, Takaki K, Koyano K. Clinical effectiveness of implant support for distal extension removable partial dentures: functional evaluation using occlusal force measurement and masticatory efficiency. Int J Implant Dent. 2021;7:101.

Naert I, Alsaadi G, van Steenberghe D, Quirynen M. A 10-year randomized clinical trial on the influence of splinted and unsplinted oral implants retaining mandibular overdentures: peri-implant outcome. Int J Oral Maxillofac Implants. 2004;19:695–702.

Nickenig HJ, Spiekermann H, Wichmann M, Andreas SK, Eitner S. Survival and complication rates of combined tooth-implant-supported fixed and removable partial dentures. Int J Prosthodont. 2008;21:131–7.

Oh WS, Oh TJ, Park JM. Impact of implant support on mandibular free-end base removable partial denture: theoretical study. Clin Oral Implants Res. 2016;27:e87–90.

Oh YK, Bae EB, Huh JB. Retrospective clinical evaluation of implant-assisted removable partial dentures combined with implant surveyed prostheses. J Prosthet Dent. 2021;126:76–82.

Owall B, Bieniek KW, Spiekermann H. Removable partial denture production in western Germany. Quintessence Int. 1995;26:621–7.

Putra Wigianto AY, Goto T, Iwawaki Y, Ishida Y, Watanabe M, Ichikawa T. Treatment outcomes of implant-assisted removable partial denture with distal extension based on the Kennedy classification and attachment type: a systematic review. Int J Implant Dent. 2021;7:111.

Rodrigues RC, Faria AC, Macedo AP, de Mattos Mda G, Ribeiro RF. Retention and stress distribution in distal extension removable partial dentures with and without implant association. J Prosthodont Res. 2013;57:24–9.

Saito M, Miura Y, Notani K, Kawasaki T. Stress distribution of abutments and base displacement with precision attachment- and telescopic crown-retained removable partial dentures. J Oral Rehabil. 2003;30:482–7.

Sato M, Suzuki Y, Kurihara D, Shimpo H, Ohkubo C. Effect of implant support on mandibular distal extension removable partial dentures: relationship between denture supporting area and stress distribution. J Prosthodont Res. 2013;57:109–12.

Shahmiri RA, Atieh MA. Mandibular Kennedy class I implant-tooth-borne removable partial denture: a systematic review. J Oral Rehabil. 2010;37:225–34.

Taylor TD. Indications and treatment planning for mandibular implant overdentures. In: Feine JS, Carlsson GE, editors. Implant overdentures: the standard of care for edentulous patients. Chicago, IL: Quintessence; 2003. p. 71–81.

Telles LH, Portella FF, Rivaldo EG. Longevity and marginal bone loss of narrow-diameter implants supporting single crowns: a systematic review. PLoS One. 2019;14:e0225046.

Turkyilmaz I. Use of distal implants to support and increase retention of a removable partial denture: a case report. J Can Dent Assoc. 2009;75:655–8.

Vahidi F, Pinto-Sinai G. Complications associated with implant-retained removable prostheses. Dent Clin North Am. 2015;59:215–26.

van Kampen F, Cune M, van der Bilt A, Bosman F. Retention and postinsertion maintenance of bar-clip, ball and magnet attachments in mandibular implant overdenture treatment: an in vivo comparison after 3 months of function. Clin Oral Implants Res. 2003;14:720–6.

Verri FR, Pellizzer EP, Rocha EP, Pereira JA. Influence of length and diameter of implants associated with distal extension removable partial dentures. Implant Dent. 2007;16:270–80.

Walls AW. Cantilever FPDs have lower success rates than end abutted FPDs after 10-years of follow-up. J Evid Based Dent Pract. 2010;10:41–3.

Walton JN. A randomized clinical trial comparing two mandibular implant overdenture designs: 3- year prosthetic outcomes using a six-field protocol. Int J Prosthodont. 2003;16:255–60.

Wismeijer D, Tawse-Smith A, Payne AG. Multicentre prospective evaluation of implant-assisted mandibular bilateral distal extension removable partial dentures: patient satisfaction. Clin Oral Implants Res. 2013;24:20–7.

Witter DJ, van Elteren P, Käyser AF, van Rossum MJ. The effect of removable partial dentures on the oral function in shortened dental arches. J Oral Rehabil. 1989;16:27–33.

Xiao W, Li Z, Shen S, Chen S, Wang Y, Wang J. Theoretical role of adjunctive implant positional support in stress distribution of distal-extension mandibular removable partial dentures. Int J Prosthodont. 2014;27:579–81.

Zancopé K, Abrão GM, Karam FK, Neves FD. Placement of a distal implant to convert a mandibular removable Kennedy class I to an implant-supported partial removable class III dental prosthesis: a systematic review. J Prosthet Dent. 2015;113:528–33.e3.

Zhang H, Ramos V Jr, Bratos M, Liu PP, He W. Effect of the attachments on clinical outcomes of mandibular distal extension implant-supported removable partial dentures: a systematic review. J Prosthet Dent. 2022;128:1211–20.

Part V

Digital Workflow of Removable Partial Dentures

Data Acquisition and Designing 18

Süleyman Çağatay Dayan, Sina Saygılı, and Gökçen Ateş

Abstract

Digital technology, as well as the rapid development of computer-aided manufacturing methods and novel materials, has given rise to alternatives to traditional methods of casting removable partial denture (RPD) frameworks. New technologies are being evolved to address the shortcomings and errors of casting. The further advantages of incorporating digital technologies into the fabrication of the RPD framework are the automated decision of a preferred placement path, the quick elimination of undesired undercuts, and the equally rapid recognition of favorable undercuts. In addition, intraoral scanners (IOSs) can minimize patient discomfort associated with conventional impression making, allergies to impression materials, and inaccuracies associated with impression distortion. Digital technologies not only save time, but they also let you make as many trials or combinations of designs as you want without harming the cast or fabricating the final product. By implementing this method, the potential for human error can be reduced and quality control can be improved within the dental laboratory. This chapter describes the data acquisition and design of digital RPDs.

Supplementary Information The online version contains supplementary material available at https://doi.org/10.1007/978-3-031-47083-7_18.

S. Ç. Dayan (✉)
Dental Laboratory Technology Program, İstanbul University-Cerrahpaşa, İstanbul, Türkiye
e-mail: suleyman.dayan@iuc.edu.tr

S. Saygılı · G. Ateş
Faculty of Dentistry, Department of Prosthodontics, İstanbul University, İstanbul, Türkiye
e-mail: sinasaygili@istanbul.edu.tr; gokcenates@istanbul.edu.tr

18.1 Definitions

CAD-CAM: acronym for Computer-aided design-computer-aided manufacturing (or Computer-Asisted Machining): the Computer Numerical Control (CNC) subtractive fabrication of a 3D object; in dentistry, it is a CAD-CAM technology used to produce different types of prostheses, including crowns, veneers, inlays, onlays, fixed dental prostheses, removable dental prostheses, dental implant prostheses, and orthodontic and other devices.

Digital scan: (1) Capturing the computer numerical format of raster images (bitmap) of a geometric object that can be viewed on a monitor screen (two-dimensional [2D]) or hologram (3D). (2) In dentistry, capturing the optical image directly of the patient's anatomy or indirectly of a definitive cast of the anatomy.

O. Şakar (ed.), *Removable Partial Dentures*, https://doi.org/10.1007/978-3-031-47083-7_18

Digitally fabricated denture: A removable complete or partial denture created with automation by using CAD-CAM technology.

Digital light processing: It is another type of stereolithography (SLA). The major difference of digital light processing (DLP) from laser-based SLA is that DLP uses a projection of ultraviolet (UV) light (or visible light) from a digital projector to flash a single image of the layer across the entire resin at once.

Direct metal laser sintering: acronym is DMLS; an additive CAM technique which uses a sintering of metal alloy powder to develop 3D objects.

Fused deposition modeling: acronym is FDM; a computer-aided manufacturing (CAM) by additive modeling using a layering of a thermoplastic material.

Rapid prototyping: A general term used for several additive layer manufacturing techniques.

Selective laser melting: acronym is SLM; an additive CAM continuous layering buildup process in which elemental metal or alloy powder deposition is closely followed by laser melting to create a finished shape under computer control.

Selective laser sintering: acronym is SLS; an additive CAM technique by sintering plastics, glass, or ceramics into 3D structures.

Standard tessellation language (STL): a digital file used in stereolithographic display and printing; the 3D image surface is interpreted by a series of triangles.

Stereolithography: acronym is SLA; a computer numerical control (CNC) additive fabrication of an object; in dentistry, it relates to the laser initiation of light-reactive resin layering to make replicas of casts and devices; alternative to processes of casting, injection molding and vacuum thermoforming; orig, the photo sculpturing principle is credited to Francois Willeme, 1860; the term and manufacturing process is credited to Charles Hull, 1986.

Three-dimensional (3D) printing: It is used as a synonym for rapid prototyping, selective laser scanning, and stereolithography.

18.2 Background

The traditional RPD framework manufacturing method is complicated, time-consuming, expensive, and prone to mistakes. In recent years, CAD-CAM-based digital dentistry has gained prominence, and the workflow for RPD manufacturing has altered dramatically. While the Glossary of Prosthodontic Terms, ninth edition, limits CAD-CAM terminology to subtractive fabrication, this book uses it more broadly as an umbrella term for "digital fabrication," which encompasses both subtractive and additive methods for creating a 3D object. There are two types of digital manufacturing technologies: subtractive manufacturing (milling) and additive manufacturing, such as selective laser sintering (SLS), direct metal laser sintering (DMLS), fused deposition modeling (FDM), selective laser melting (SLM), and stereolithography (SLA).

The digital technology has several benefits, including accurate planning of the framework's components, a reduction in manufacturing time, enhanced functional and esthetic outcomes, and an improvement in the fit quality of RPD frameworks. Furthermore, unlike traditional methods, a virtual master cast and final design can be archived for later use in a digital library, making planning much more efficient. Its inherent reproducibility helps the dental prosthetic laboratory maintain high quality standards and avoid the inconsistencies that can arise between different operators. Even though digital technology is used to make frameworks, it is important to remember that technicians are still needed for many steps, such as running software, removing support structures, and polishing frameworks. As a result, even using digital technologies, it is not feasible to completely automate the process of manufacturing the RPD framework.

Clinicians have three options for collecting data for RPDs: conventional functional impressions, laboratory scanning of the master cast, or intraoral digital scanning. After data collection, clinicians can choose between the indirect technique, which involves traditional lost-wax casting or manufacturing castable resin or wax patterns by subtractive milling or additive techniques and then casting them, or they can fabricate a metal framework directly using subtractive milling or additive techniques. RPD frameworks' intricate design, including clasps, connentors, and rests, makes subtractive milling manufacture difficult, and it has been shown to be costly and time-consuming because of the durability of RPD alloys, which causes the milling burs to wear rapidly. Furthermore, although commercially available milling wax or resin patterns exist, they have not gained widespread acceptance. Recently, SLA has been employed to produce castable resin or wax patterns for RPD frameworks. This approach produces accurately fitting frameworks and reduces the relatively high price and potential errors associated with dental technicians manual waxing.

Research into the feasibility of producing RPD frameworks using the aforementioned methods began in the early 2000s. Bibb et al. manufactured frameworks using the indirect SLA technique with sacrificial patterns and traditional casting, and claimed that the RPD framework required adjustments due to lengthy and difficult production times. Almost simultaneously, Williams et al. employed SLM for the production of RPD frameworks; however, they reported that the frameworks necessitated adjustments and highlighted the associated increment in production cost. Both studies utilized the same software for planning RPD frameworks. However, a limitation of this software was its reliance on physical sculptors to construct the framework virtually. A physical sculptor refers to a haptic device that enables individuals to interact with objects in a 3D virtual space through touch. This constraint has been noted in the literature and may hinder the accessibility and ease of use of the software. Although the use of physical sculptors in the software enabled technicians to mimic the hand movements used in traditional framework wax-up, it also resulted in increased time, expense, and complexity of the operations. Consequently, several software alternatives were explored to allow for the virtual planning of RPDs without the need for a sculptor. Subsequently, Han et al. introduced specialized RPD framework design software in 2010, which addressed these limitations. The automated calculation of insertion and removal pathways, as well as the practical identification and management of undercuts, are some of the advantages of contemporary software. Today's CAD software utilized in the dental laboratory or clinic has a library of RPD components, and an RPD could well be intuitively designed utilizing a haptic input device. The tactile feeling of an object's 3D location in virtual space was thus enabled.

Modern software solutions can automatically eliminate undesired undercuts and choose suitable components from a pre-existing library, thereby reducing working time and removing operator variability through digital planning. As a result, master cast block-out can be accomplished by pressing a single button, and the block-out region can be viewed from all sides simultaneously. Moreover, the need for refractory cast has been eliminated as the framework can be fabricated without the need for a manual wax-up process. Both the researchers and clinicians have shown a greater interest in digital RPDs as a result of breakthroughs with new generations of intraoral scanners as well as enhancements made to design software.

18.3 Data Acquisition

18.3.1 Digital Scan

Both IOS and laboratory digital scanners can be used to collect digital data for master cast of the partially edentulous arch and remaining teeth in order to design RPDs (Table 18.1). If a laboratory scanner is used, impressions can be made conventionally, scanned directly using the laboratory scanner, or poured into master casts before being scanned. These methods are collectively known as the hybrid technique. According to previous studies, IOS may be less reliable than dental laboratory scanners when scanning a larger region, and inaccuracies apparently rise when scanning more than half of the dental arch. Furthermore, in partially edentulous cases, the accuracy of IOS seems to be related to the width and length of the

Table 18.1 Digital workflow of removable partial dentures

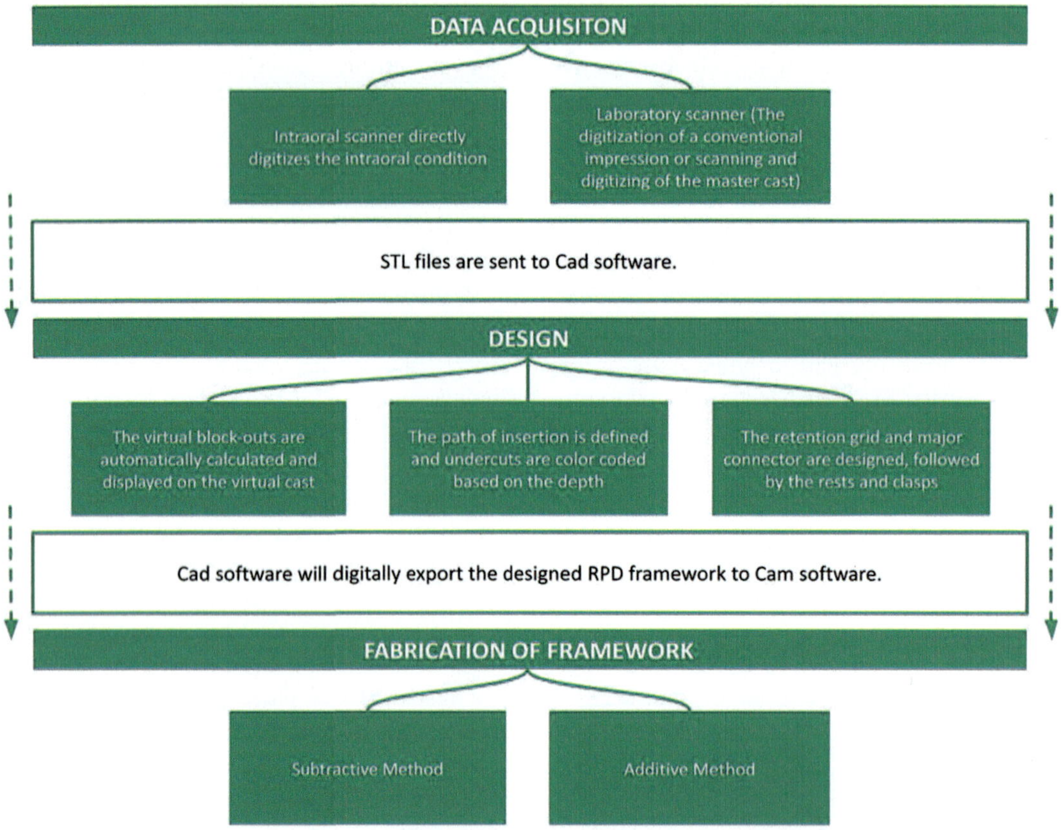

edentulous region, with more mistakes being made when scanning larger edentulous regions. On the other hand, Tregerman et al. compared conventional, hybrid (conventional-digital), and entirely digital approaches for the fabrication of RPD frameworks and concluded that the sole IOS-based method demonstrated a significantly better RPD framework fit than the conventional and hybrid workflows, irrespective of Kennedy's classification. Moreover, surprisingly, the conventional method of framework manufacturing was superior to the hybrid method. The authors linked this result to making an analogue impression, pouring it into the stone, and then scanning that to make a digital cast, all of which contribute to an increase in inaccuracies.

There has been an inconclusive debate about whether a full digital workflow is a suitable option for RPD fabrication. Literature on full digital processes for fabricating RPDs is overflowing, and it shows that IOS-based digital scans give enough information. It should be remembered that both hard and soft tissues must be recorded for an RPD to provide the most accurate impression possible. Capturing a functional impression of non-attached mucosa during intraoral scanning in edentulous areas is a significant challenge. The functional depth and width of the edentulous region, the shape of the remaining tooth, and the arch should also be recorded. Despite the fact that IOS save time, require less materials, simplify clinical procedures for clinicians, make the impression procedure more patient-friendly, eliminate stone casts, and improve communication with the dental laboratory, they are not appropriate for every partial edentulous case. The primary reason behind this is that it is practically impossible to make a functional impression with an IOS. Due to the fact that IOS devices are image-based, the digital

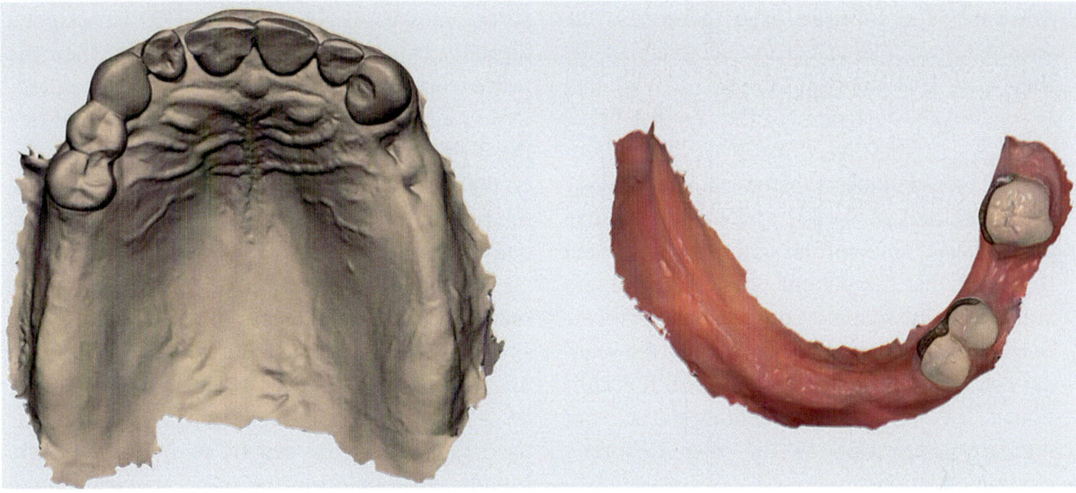

Fig. 18.1 Colored and colorless intraoral scan images for partially edentulous patients

scans are performed in passive mucostatic circumstances (Fig. 18.1).

There is overwhelming evidence for the notion that, unlike the teeth, which have a complex geometric shape, the residual ridge of edentulous jaws is flat, and its digital 3D data is readily affected and apparently displays poor precision and trueness. It is possible to stitch together, with less potential for error, the scan obtained from the teeth. However, because the process of stitching is more difficult with longer edentulous regions that have smoother surfaces, it is harder to collect reliable scans from such areas because of the lack of clear anatomical landmarks and poorly differentiated structures. A previous study by Shimizu et al. suggested that the accuracy of making an impression of the residual ridge using an IOS might be enhanced by employing a novel scanning technique that employs markers that can be positioned in the oral cavity. They showed that the placement of markers on the residual ridge for clinical usage seems to improve intraoral scanning precision. It is challenging to place markers in the edentulous region, which is the major drawback of this recommended strategy. To overcome this, the authors attempted to secure the marker with denture adhesive. The clinical practicability and application of this technique are encouraging for the future of the digital scan of the long edentulous regions, notwithstanding the need for more in vivo studies (Fig. 18.2).

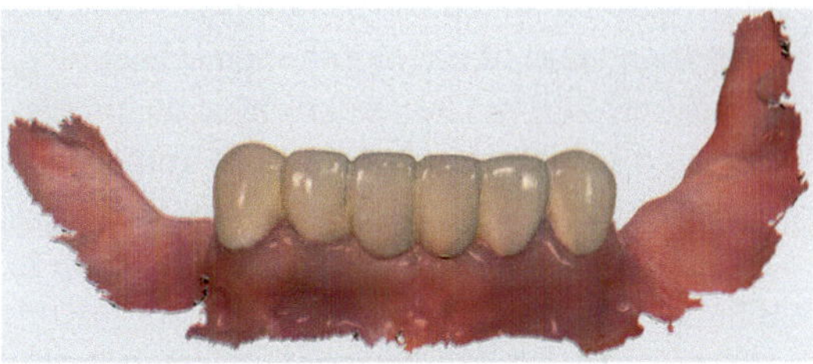

Fig. 18.2 Intraoral scan of long edentulous regions

There was no comprehensive long-term clinical study that evaluated RPDs fabricated based on IOS data. Even so, many clinical reports have shown that the results of using IOS to manufacture RPDs are clinically acceptable. Even though most of the clinical reports that use IOS to manufacture RPDs are for patients in Kennedy Classes III and IV with partial edentulism, reports of cases in Kennedy Classes I and II with partial edentulism have started to be published using the newly developed, next-generation IOS.

Finally, several issues should be taken into consideration when using IOS. Numerous factors may affect the accuracy of digital scans made using an intraoral scanner.

- Technique: The accuracy of the scan is highly dependent on the operator's method. Proper technique, such as maintaining proper angulation and positioning of the scanner, can help ensure accurate results.

- Software: The software used to process the scan data can also affect the accuracy of the final scan. It is important to use software that is specifically designed for the scanner being used.
- Patient factors: Patient factors such as salivary flow, intraoral moisture, and movement can affect the accuracy of the scan. It is important to ensure that the patient is comfortable and still during the scanning process.
- Scanner calibration: The accuracy of the scanner can also be affected by how well it is calibrated. It is important to calibrate the scanner regularly according to the manufacturer's recommendations.
- Scanner design: The design of the scanner can also play a role in its accuracy. Some scanners may be better suited for certain types of scans or certain areas of the mouth than others.
- Image resolution: The resolution of the images captured by the scanner can also impact the accuracy of the scan. Higher resolution images generally provide more detail and can result in a more accurate scan.
- Operator experience: The experience and skill level of the operator can also play a role in the accuracy of the scan. Proper training and experience can help ensure that the scanner is used correctly and that accurate results are obtained.

There seems to be a compelling reason to argue that the intention of collecting data by IOS and then digitally fabricating a framework was more beneficial than utilizing a traditional framework manufactured by casting from a framework wax pattern onto a refractory cast. On the basis of the evidence currently available, it seems fair to suggest that the digital scan method can be effective in Kennedy Class III cases when there is enough tooth support. However, the data appears to suggest that, in the situation of distal extension in a Kennedy class I or II, conventional impressions may provide better results than direct digital scans. Therefore, an altered cast technique might be applied using a digitally manufactured framework for such situations. A digital master model is produced after intraoral scanning of the patient's hard and soft tissues using an IOS. An RPD is designed digitally by a dedicated program, and then the framework is manufactured by either subtractive or additive manufacturing processes. When the RPD fabrication process is complete, the components should be clinically tested to ensure retention and fitting accuracy. Then, as with the conventional method, acrylic saddles are placed on the retentive gridwork of the framework to make an impression of the free-end edentulous space(s) (see Chap. 8). At this point, the 3D-printed master cast, which is fabricated by SLA through initial digital scan STL data, is used to connect the acrylic to the framework. Finally, as detailed in the previous chapter, the functional impression is made and the definitive master cast is updated in the laboratory (Fig. 18.3).

Wu et al. suggest using altered casting techniques in the digital workflow in a different way. After getting a digital scan, instead of manufacturing a digital framework right away, they use SLA to make a custom tray with record rims and a window, which is different from the previous method. The remaining natural teeth are uncovered, and occlusal rests are constructed for the window. Consequently, the clinician can obtain an altered cast impression and maxillomandibular relationship record at the same visit. After making the impression, the dental stone is poured. A laboratory scanner or IOS is used to scan the altered cast. The right software is used to carefully match the original cast image with the new one with the best fit alignment, using data from the remaining teeth as common points of refer-

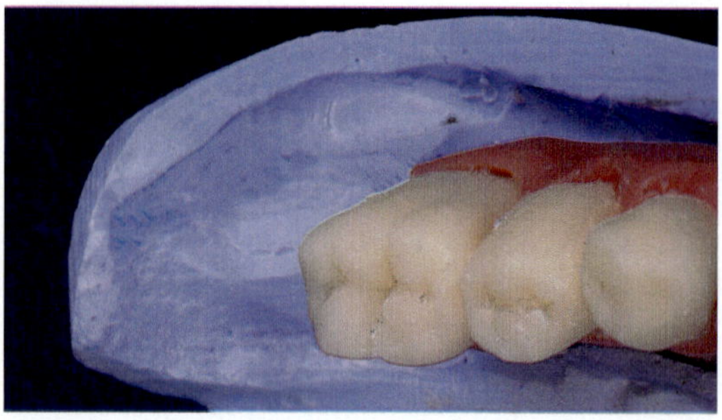

Fig. 18.3 Functional impression is made after digitally fabricated RPD framework. The definitive master cast is updated in the laboratory for further steps

ence. The data for the distal extension is taken off of the master cast and replaced with data images from the revised cast. Even though the data for the natural teeth on the secondary cast was incomplete, it was similar enough to the data for the primary cast that the two virtual casts could be superimposed. The data is recreated as an altered digital STL file. At the end of all these processes, the master model is obtained for both framework fabrication and finishing procedures.

18.3.2 The Advantages of Digital Scan in Removable Partial Denture Manufacturing

Moving from the current conventional/analog impression method to a digital scan may be a challenge, so it is important to know the benefits of this change and how it differs from the old method. Technology makes our lives simpler, better, and more efficient in every way. Dental workflows benefit from digital scans in the same way. During the data collecting phase, digital scanners accurately and precisely detect surface points and determine surface topography. While IOS has been mentioned in some studies as being used in the fabrication step of RPDs, there are far fewer reports for RPDs than for fixed prostheses and complete dentures because of the huge variety in missing tooth patterns and the intricacy of denture components.

The adoption of a digital process in removable partial denture (RPD) manufacturing offers numerous essential and potentially substantial advantages. With the use of a scanner, the risk of defective impressions, which might occur with a conventional approach, is eliminated as the scanner can add scans as required. The scanner stitches pictures together in real time, enabling the clinicians to detect and rectify any ambiguous regions with more scanning instantly. Digital scanning may record tissues in a passive condition, resulting in a mucostatic impression that may be advantageous in some circumstances. Screenshots may make it easier for the dental lab and clinic to communicate with each other, and designs can be approved and changed before the framework is fabricated.

The advantages of digital data collection over conventional methods:

- Prevents distortion from occurring during impression removal from the oral cavity.
- Allows scan results to be easily corrected and repeated.
- Improves visualization since the size of the picture on the computer screen is far greater than what can be viewed intraorally, even with loupes.
- Prevents the formation of air bubbles during the plaster injection.
- Establishes objective and simple communication between patients and the dental laboratory.
- Maintains strong data storage reliability and repeatability.
- Avoids damage to the plaster model.
- Reduces model transportation costs and time.
- Improves patients' comfort, vomiting reflex, and breathing at the time of impression.
- Ensures safety from the standpoint of infection control.
- Avoids the risk of data loss associated with conventional impression-digital design-manufacture or other combined workflows.

18.3.3 The Disadvantages of Digital Scan in Removable Partial Denture Manufacturing

While there are various benefits to adopting digital scans for RPD impressions, there are some drawbacks. The main disadvantage of a digital scan is that it cannot capture the soft tissue condition and border molding during functional movements for RPD fabrication. Unfortunately, making functional impressions with IOS is currently impossible. The classification of Kennedy and the number and length of modification spaces have an influence on the accuracy and precision of the collected data. In addition, it is tough to get clear scans of the hamular notches and the retromolar pad. Under such circumstances, after a framework is fabricated digitally, conventional functional impression making may be necessary. This means more chair time, laboratory procedures, and prolonged manufacturing time.

Kennedy Class III/IV partly edentulous arches represent the majority of cases having full digital RPD fabrication. In order for digital RPDs to become more widely used, several challenges need to be addressed. These include developing an algorithm that accounts for pressure displacement of the mucosa in denture-bearing areas, improving impression techniques along the border of the denture base, and creating methods for recording maxillo-mandibular relationships in cases without occlusal support.

Also, to acquire a stable focus, it is sometimes required to apply certain coatings to the teeth and to place the camera wand on a tooth. Furthermore, the 3D virtual model is often rebuilt by post-processing individual photos; as a result, the reconstruction is not completed in real time with continuous data acquisition. Additionally, data on the accuracy of the available equipment are often lacking. Another problem is that the functionality of an IOS is not sufficient in distally extended and large edentulous areas.

Furthermore, the learning curve for digital scanning technology can be steep, which can cause delays in the production process. Additionally, the accuracy of digital scans can be affected by factors such as moisture and the presence of reflective surfaces, which can result in inaccuracies in the final RPD design. Another potential issue with digital scanning is the need for regular software updates and maintenance to ensure optimal performance, which can also add to the cost of using this technology. Finally, some dental professionals may be resistant to using digital scanning technology due to their preference for traditional impressions and the associated workflow.

18.3.4 Scanning Strategy

Scan pathways or strategies may be described as the precise motions of IOS throughout the scanning phase that improve the precision and trueness of digital scan. Previous studies have shown that the scanning approach influences the accuracy of digital scan. Each manufacturer offers a different scanning technique that may be used to capture a whole dental arch. Still, during a complete-arch scan, manufacturers have not supplied any recommendations for which quadrant to start with. There is no consensus in the literature on whether digital scans are affected by which quadrant the scan begins in. Hayama et al. stated that deviations were smaller in the quadrant where scanning started for the mandibular Kennedy Class I and III models, whereas Diker and Tak demonstrated that deviations were present in both the maxillary Kennedy Class I and Kennedy Class IV models regardless of where scanning started for the specific IOS type. This variation may be a result of the various lengths of edentulous areas employed in the study models. Furthermore, since these studies were conducted in vitro, intra-oral variables such as saliva, patient movement, differing reflecting qualities of the teeth and gingiva, and soft tissue movement were not taken into account. In practical practice, however, it may be advantageous to consider the scanning sequence while scanning the whole arch with IOS since the accuracy varies depending on the scanning order.

The quality of the digital image depends on how close the IOS's scanning tip is to the surface being scanned. The distance between the patients and the head of the IOS should be kept as close as possible during IOS management. Rotar et al. findings lend support to the claim that the best results are achieved when the scanning tip is kept at a distance of 10.0 mm from the recording region. However, their study was an in vitro study that only analyzed the "scanning distance factor" of the prepared molar teeth. The study did not evaluate the effect of other possible clinical parameters such as the presence of edentulous areas, humidity, or ambient lighting conditions. Due to the fact that edentulous regions are normally uniform and devoid of characteristics, and also because saliva is commonly present, this distance may alter. It should be guaranteed with future studies.

Manufacturers of IOS devices usually suggest a pattern of scanning for the best performance with their devices. Scanning may start in the left anterior quadrant, progress to the distal region, and then return to the right anterior quadrant by scanning the right dental arch. Scanning may be conducted in a zig-zag pattern in the sequence of the occlusal surface, buccal surface, and lingual surface for remaining teeth. In addition, the edentulous ridge mucosa can be scanned in a zig-zag pattern without losing the continuity of the image. Alternatively, the scanning route may be constructed to capture data for the remaining teeth first, followed by the remaining ridge. Missing areas must be rescanned after final evaluation. In practically every scanning technique, the highest deviation occurs on the buccal side of the most distal tooth, which is the initial turning point of the scanning sequence. Clinicians must exercise caution at this stage since the buccal side of the most distal tooth is often designed as a clasp to facilitate retention in distal extension RPDs.

Of course, the scanning method may alter according to the partial edentulism scenario. For example, in a mandibular Kennedy Class I partially edentulous arch with only molars and second premolars missing, before moving on to the lingual side of the front teeth or the labial side of the front teeth, the remaining teeth are first scanned from the point of the right first premolar to the tip of the left first premolar via the incisors' edge. The residual ridge is first scanned from the right side, then from the left. The retromolar pad, the buccal portion of the residual ridge, the lingual section of the first premolar, and then the buccal part of the residual ridge are all scanned.

In another case, consider a patient with a Kennedy Class IV partially edentulous maxillary arch, with anterior teeth and first premolars missing on both sides. The scan can start on the occlusal side of the right molars and move to the occlusal side of the left molars through the entire arch, then continue on the buccal side in the opposite direction, then move to the palatal side, and end with a zigzag path through the soft tissues. It can also start on the left side and move in the opposite direction.

18.3.5 Maxillomandibular Relationship Record

To establish clinically effective restorations with the proper occlusal morphology and minimize the need for chairside occlusal adjustment, it is essential to precisely transfer the maxillomandibular relationships (MMRs) into the digital software, exactly as it is in the traditional technique. Digital MMR record consists of one or more 3D images that depict the relationship between the jaws in the maximal intercuspal position or centric relation. With digital MMRs, virtual maxillary and mandibular casts acquired from IOS can be repositioned in CAD software using a best-alignment technique that aligns several 3D files by matching related data. The majority of IOSs require bilateral digital MMRs to determine the relative location of the maxillary and mandibular virtual casts, and each digital MMR consists of opposing maxillary and mandibular teeth. However, the technique of occlusal alignment for digital casts becomes challenging when teeth are missing. Ren et al. conducted an in vitro study to investigate if the accuracy of digital MMRs varies with the size of simulated edentulous regions or the position of missing teeth. It has been demonstrated that the trueness and precision of digital MMRs were influenced by the size and location of edentulous regions. The trueness and precision of digital MMRs were also influenced by the presence of unilateral or bilateral long edentulous spans, the absence of three or more posterior teeth, and the presence of an extended edentulous span in the anterior area. According to their findings, a fully digital process may not be a reliable method in clinical circumstances including extensive edentulous space.

In the workflow of digitally fabricated dentures, digital MMR records were obtained in two ways: with or without using record bases and occlusion rims. While digital scans for MMR can be accomplished without the use of record bases with occlusion rims in patients with molar occlusal supports and a limited number of missing teeth, record bases with occlusion rims are necessary for digital MMR recording in situations of distal extended RPDs for the replacement of many teeth. On the other hand, clinicians generally choose to proceed without a physical model for reducing the number of clinical appointments. In this respect, clinicians can either use a 3D printer to fabricate a record base from digital scans made with an IOS and record the MMR using the IOS, or they can use bite registration silicone and record the MMR using the IOS if they prefer to proceed with a model-free approach (Fig. 18.4).

Another method begins with a silicone impression of the patient using a prefabricated tray. Then, the impression is removed from the tray, and the silicone impression's anterior section is cut off so it can be used as a basis and scanned with the teeth. A minimally mobile construction is created because thick silicone, which was only trimmed anteriorly, fits well on the lingual surfaces. The silicones are combined after the bite registration silicone has been applied to the impression and the bite registration has been completed at the centric relation position. After that, the lower teeth are scanned while the silicone impression is in the mouth, and the upper teeth have been scanned. After that, the bite registration is completed. Returning to the lower jaw impression in the software, areas where the silicone has been erased can be seen. Scanning is restarted from this area, and edentulous areas of the lower jaw are scanned, referencing only the anterior teeth of the lower jaw. However, the clinical acceptability of MMR accuracy recorded without the support of a record base remains uncertain, owing to the limited number of studies conducted in this particular context (Figs. 18.5, 18.6, 18.7, 18.8 and 18.9).

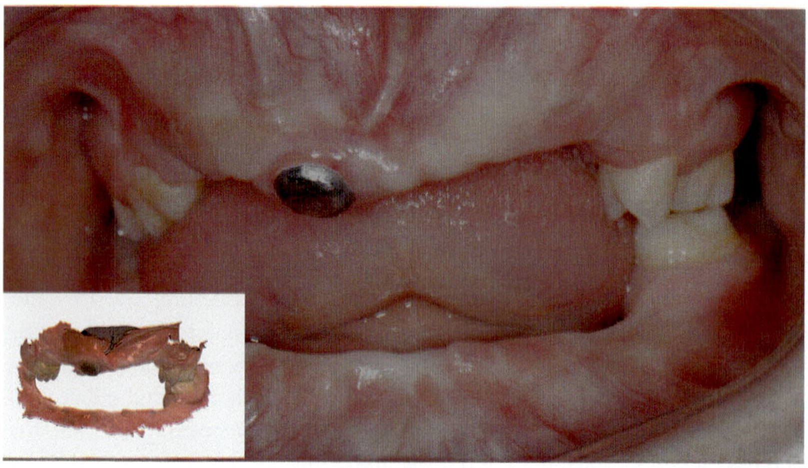

Fig. 18.4 Intraoral scanning and recording of the MMR using the IOS. It is possible to proceed with a model-free approach in such cases where dentist can capture MMR with reference on existing tooth

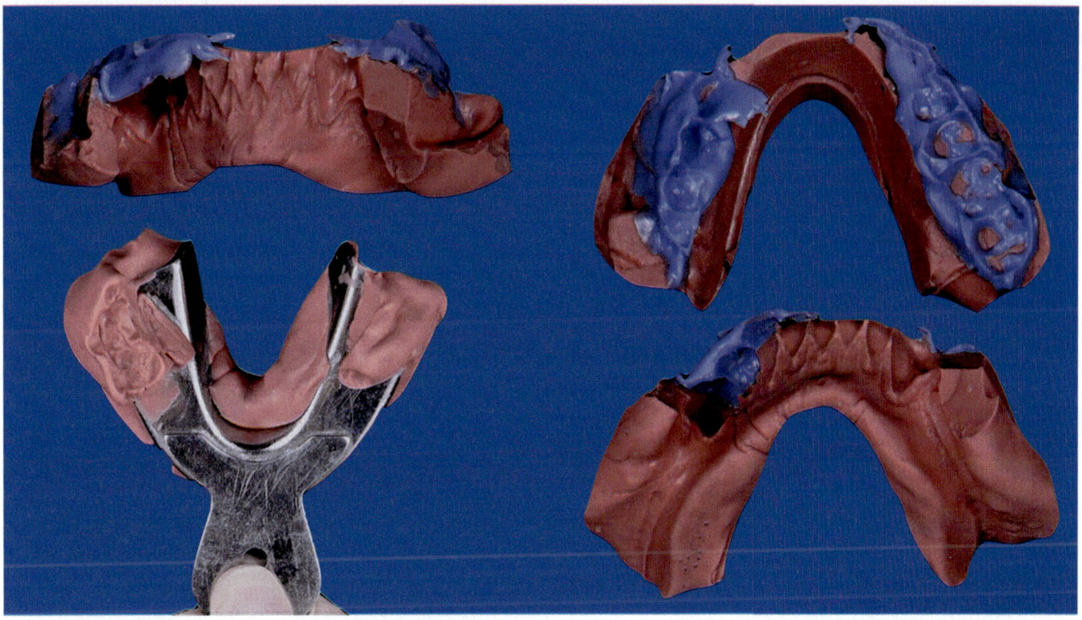

Fig. 18.5 Creating silicone index for MMR record

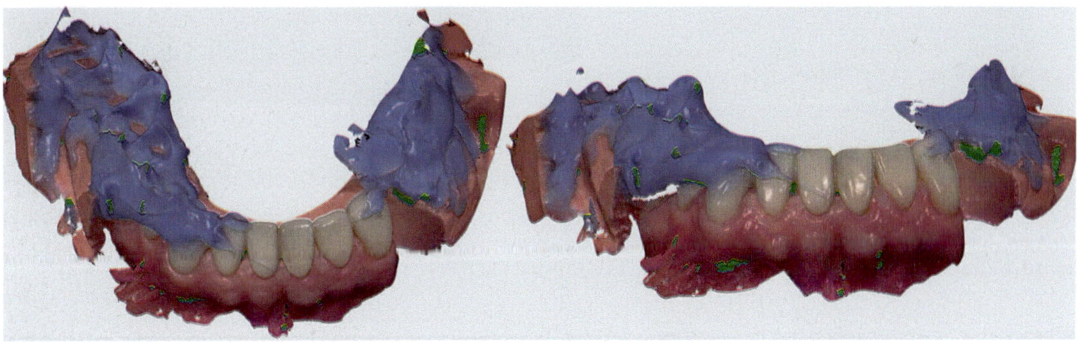

Fig. 18.6 Lower jaw scan with bite record and silicone index

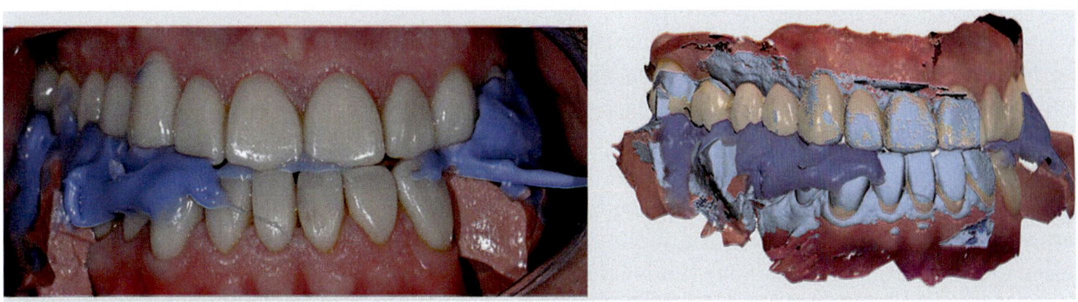

Fig. 18.7 Intraoral scanning and recording of the MMR using the IOS

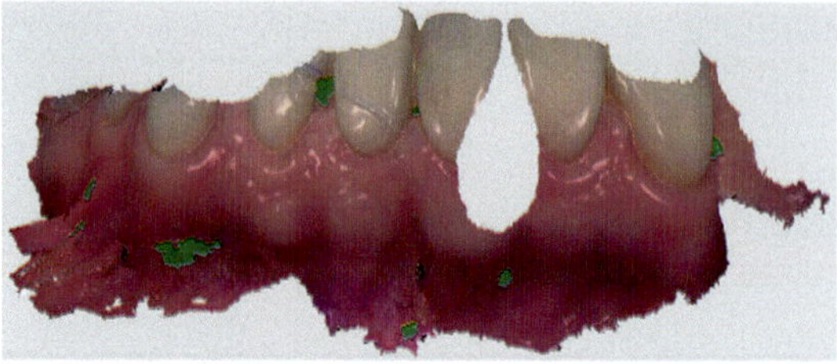

Fig. 18.8 Deleting silicone index area and leaving anterior teeth as reference to complete the scan for rest of the arch

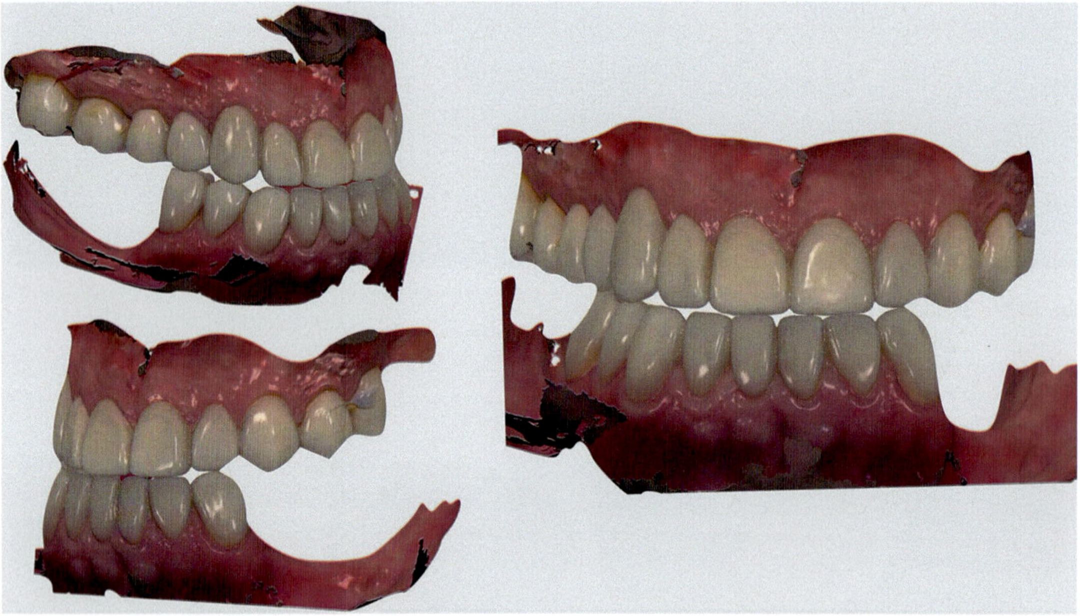

Fig. 18.9 Intraoral scanning and recording of the MMR using the IOS

18.4 Design of Digital Removable Partial Dentures

Digital workflow requires the digitalization of the real world into a virtual world. Initial acquisition can be performed either conventionally or digitally; however, in a digital environment, designs must be generated in software, which can be free 3D software or software designed specifically for dentistry. Recorded and digitalized diagnostic cast of high quality are essential for a successful design and production process. This is crucial for the mesh structure and design of the final product. Both traditional impressions with lab scanners and digital impressions can be utilized by dental practitioners, as described above.

CAD softwares are very common in daily life. Photoshop and Word, for example, operate on the X and Y axes and can only edit files in two dimensions. The third dimension is mandatory to rotate, scale, manipulate, and edit in all three dimensions. Architecture, aerospace, cartography, engineering, automobile, etc. benefit from 3D software. Dental products have also been manufactured using 3D software for decades. Nowadays, virtually every human-made item is initially conceived in some sort of CAD software. To design 3D objects in dentistry, open softwares such as Meshmixer and Freeform can be used; however, companies, like any other industry, invest in coding special tailored software to ease the design process and create a smoother CAD-

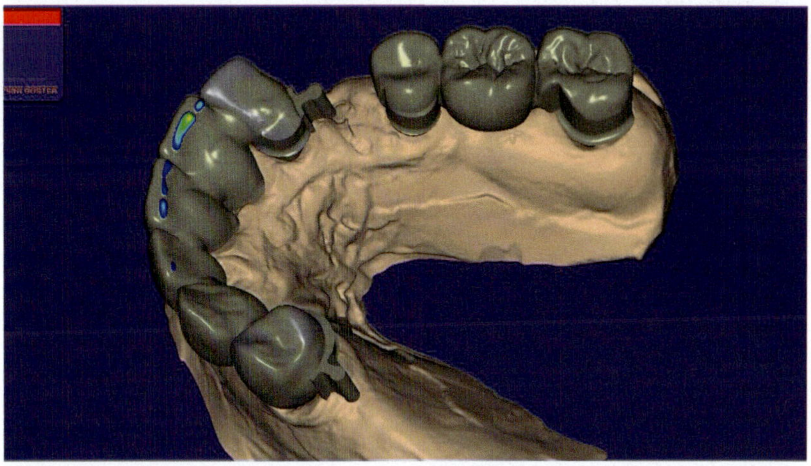

Fig. 18.10 Precision attachments and many removable partial denture parts are possible to place in virtual model on dental design softwares

CAM dental world. Dedicated dental software has the major advantage that most of the steps are done automatically, simplifying complex algorithms. Terms and geometries for the dental world, for example, attachments, virtual articulators, clasps, major connectors, etc., are coded and ready for use in dental 3D software (Fig. 18.10). However, for complex and intricate designs for special applications, a professional software program is a considerable option.

Not only the framework but also the teeth and bases of the RPD can be designed in dental 3D software. According to biomechanical principles and indications, the user can modify any component of the RPD. Design requires selecting and deciding on major and minor connectors, rests, clasps, and other components, which can be placed and modified on a virtual model. Clinicians require a diagnostic model to examine the guiding planes, the preparation of the abutment teeth for the rest seats, the formation of the retentive area, and the crowning of the abutment tooth or teeth before starting an RPD (see Chap. 5). Thus, clinicians can consider making any necessary modifications before finalizing the design. The advantages and disadvantages of designing RPD digitally are summarized in Table 18.2.

Digital workflows can be used not only for RPD design but also for rest seat preparations and guiding plane preparations for RPDs. The technique is efficient, requires no additional laboratory steps, and provides an objective display of preparation parameters. When compared to a freehand procedure, CAD-CAM-assisted procedures can improve plane preparation. CoCr alloy guides (metal templates) can assist in preparing accurate guiding planes for RPDs without the need for direct vision. Resin guides are also possible to use for complex guiding structures, but they may lead to more imprecise guiding plane preparation than those with single-plane guiding structures. A previous study that compared the trueness of CAD-CAM-assisted and freehand

Table 18.2 Advantages and disadvantages of digital design

Advantages	Disadvantages
Increase in interdisciplinary communication Detects path of placement is easily determined by automatic undercut detection Identifies retentive areas rapidly Saves time and reduces preparation time for removable prosthesis Demonstrate pre-production design to the clinician in 3D, errors may be avoided Works with large scales Enables endless trial possibilities Detects problems that may arise in production before manufacturing Eliminates handmade failures Assists with artificial intelligence Creates back up files, if needed, for reproduction without any impression or redesign of the case	Loses perception of reality Requires advanced equipment, Needs improved computer skills Demands different software knowledge

procedures for making guiding planes for RPDs found that the CAD-CAM template-assisted procedure can significantly improve tooth preparation of the guiding planes compared to freehand preparation. The CAD-CAM template could help clinicians prepare parallel guiding planes in a predictable manner (Figs. 18.11, 18.12 and 18.13).

RPD requires intense care in the design step. Recent advancements in denture materials, both teeth and bases, have resulted in a shift in RPD philosophy (see Chap. 19). Tracing the lateral crest profile (see Chap. 14) can be performed using virtual articulators, and the tooth alignment and suprastructure of the denture design can be completed in time for production. Various workflows are presented. Framework and suprastructure production and application for RPD have been presented many times. Patients with microstomia are treated with both conventional

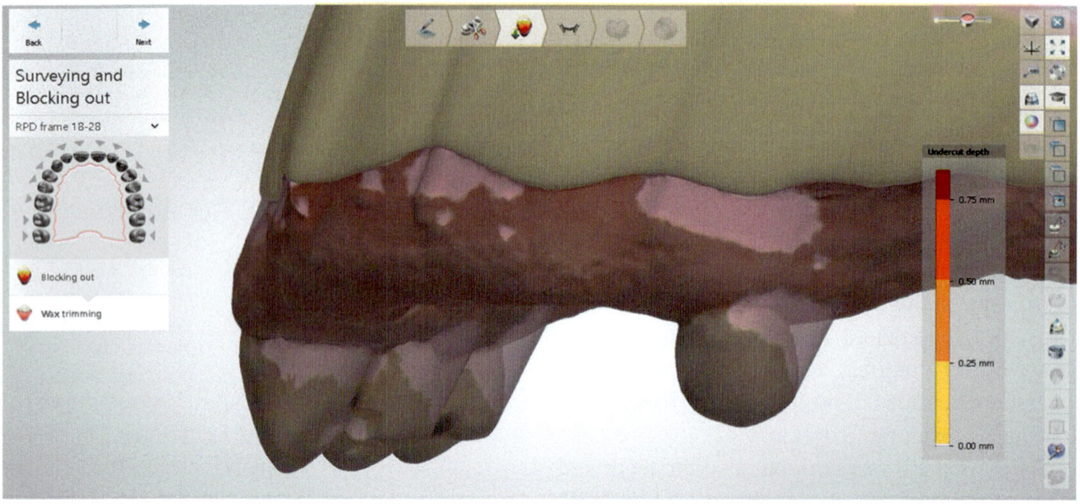

Fig. 18.11 Virtual surveying can show the undercut areas, where block out is needed. Before changing the insertion axis of RPD

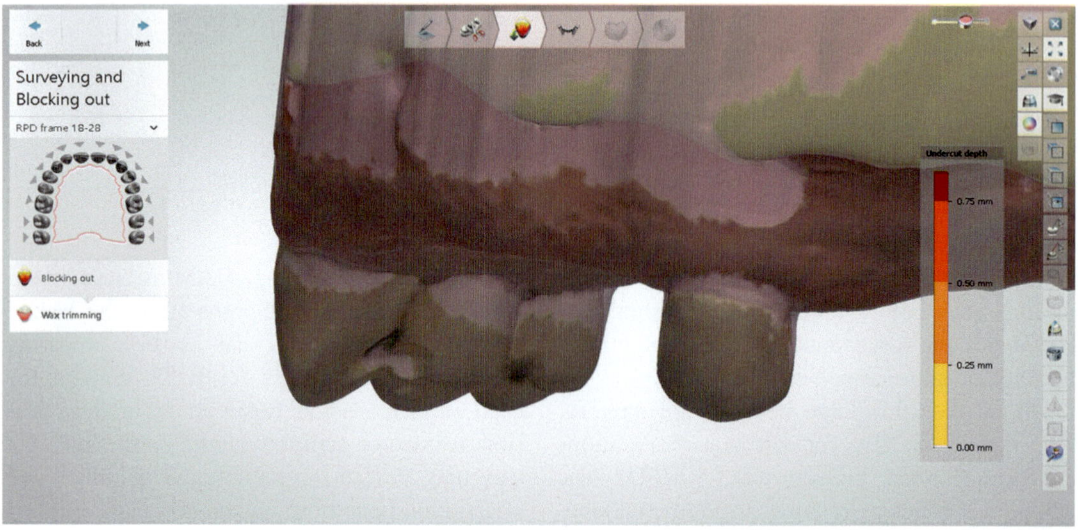

Fig. 18.12 Virtual surveying can show the undercut areas, where block out is needed. After changing the insertion axis of RPD

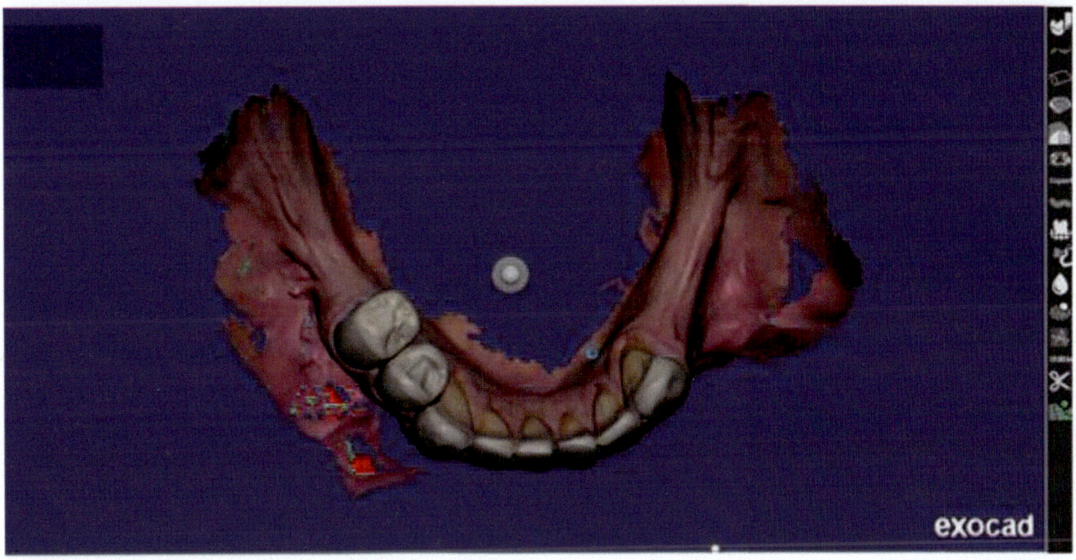

Fig. 18.13 Editing block out areas (Video 18.1)

and digital workflows for designing special trays. One of the challenges is producing an abutment tooth crown for an existing RPD. Digital design and manufacturing with monolithic materials make this process much easier and error-free. RPDs are also used as immediate applications after tooth extractions. Virtual extractions can be performed in software, and a denture can be designed and manufactured accordingly.

Dental professionals might have some problems regarding laboratory prescriptions, which involves the designing and manufacturing of RPDs. Incomplete design decisions lead to shortcomings in final prostheses. Such errors in prescribing are very expensive in terms of patients being dissatisfied and repeating the prosthesis process once again with a precious time loss. To prevent these difficulties, the dental team should focus more on creating an accurate design and production process for RPDs. These conditions are identical for complete dentures as well. Digital design improves communication between the dentist and technician. The design process can be cooperative, either with screenshots or video chat programs. The virtual cast will not be damaged, many variations can be performed, and the best decision can be made by both professionals, which prevents deviations in designs. With digital software, dental technicians can now design all structures and send a web link to the dentist to control or ask questions before manufacturing. Dentists can control this design either on a web browser or a designated application on smart phones or tablets (Figs. 18.14 and 18.15).

Traditionally, the steps involved in the manufacture of a removable partial denture (RPD) are confined to manual design, waxing, and casting processes. Analog data acquisition is employed to produce a stone cast, which is then used to create a metal framework through conventional casting of the wax structures made by the dental technician. However, dental software has introduced various material options that allow the user to adjust settings such as casting thickness, major connector width, and others based on the material used. At this stage, a consistent design can be achieved without the potential for human error (Figs. 18.16, 18.17, 18.18, 18.19, 18.20, 18.21, 18.22, 18.23, 18.24, 18.25 and 18.26), (Video 18.3).

Development of digital design softwares created much smoother workflow over conventional prosthesis, also valid for RPDs, also might lower costs for frameworks production. However, in digital workflow devices such as milling units, laser sintering, digital design softwares and hard-

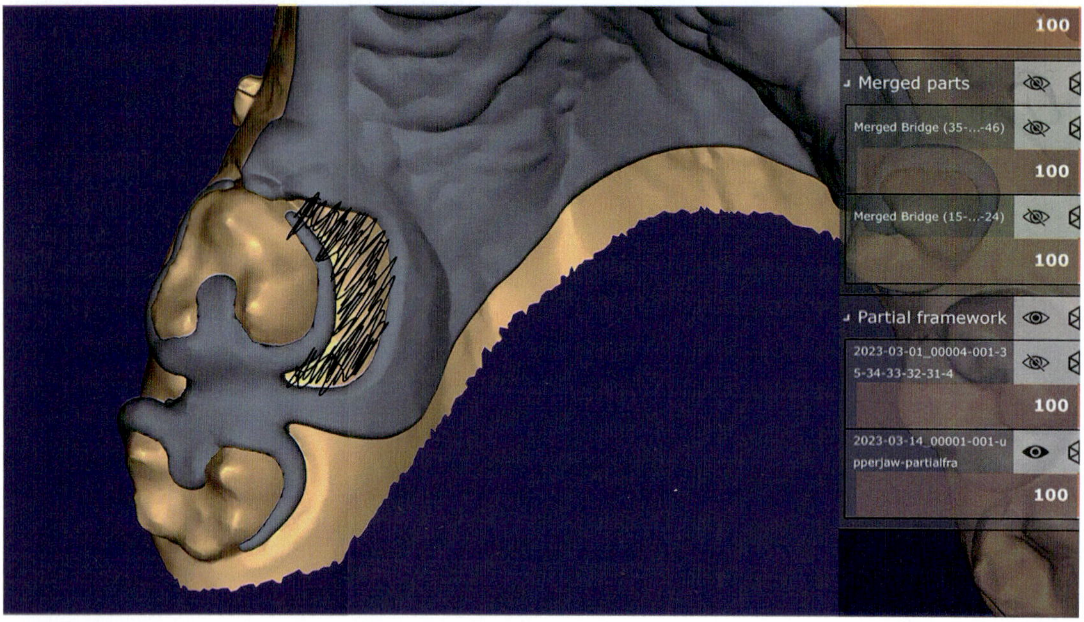

Fig. 18.14 As the same principle on paper drawing, clinicians can edit existing design on virtual file, send a picture or video to dental technician on dental software applications or web view

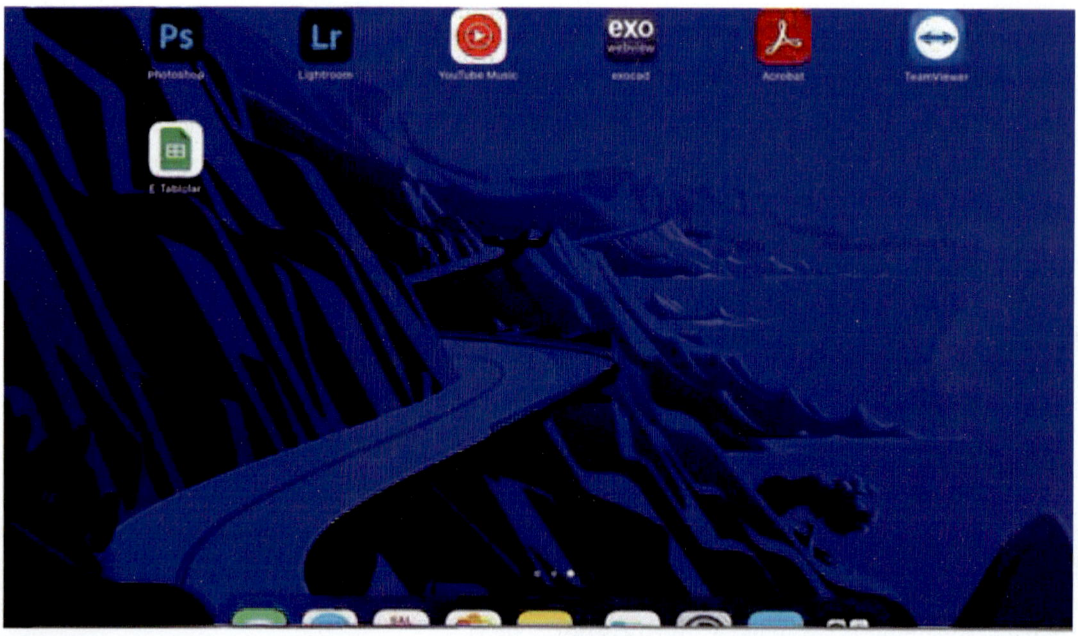

Fig. 18.15 Creating a screenshot and drawings on HTML file (Video 18.2)

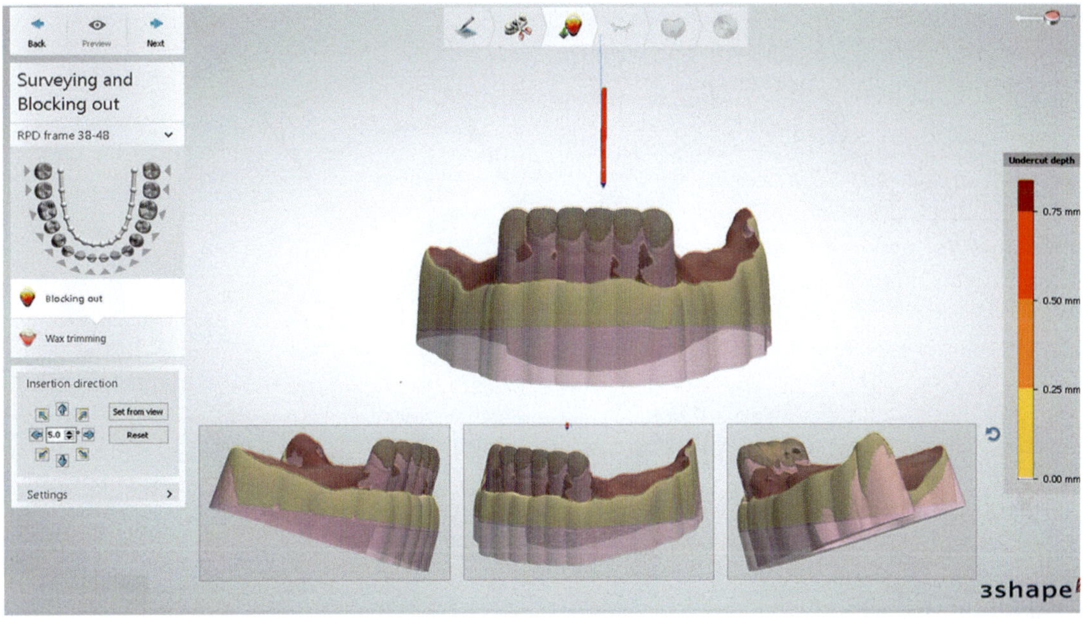

Fig. 18.16 Digital design process is an advanced option regarding the visibility against conventional workflow. Surveying and blocking out can be done in minutes and can be changed in seconds with a more efficient workflow

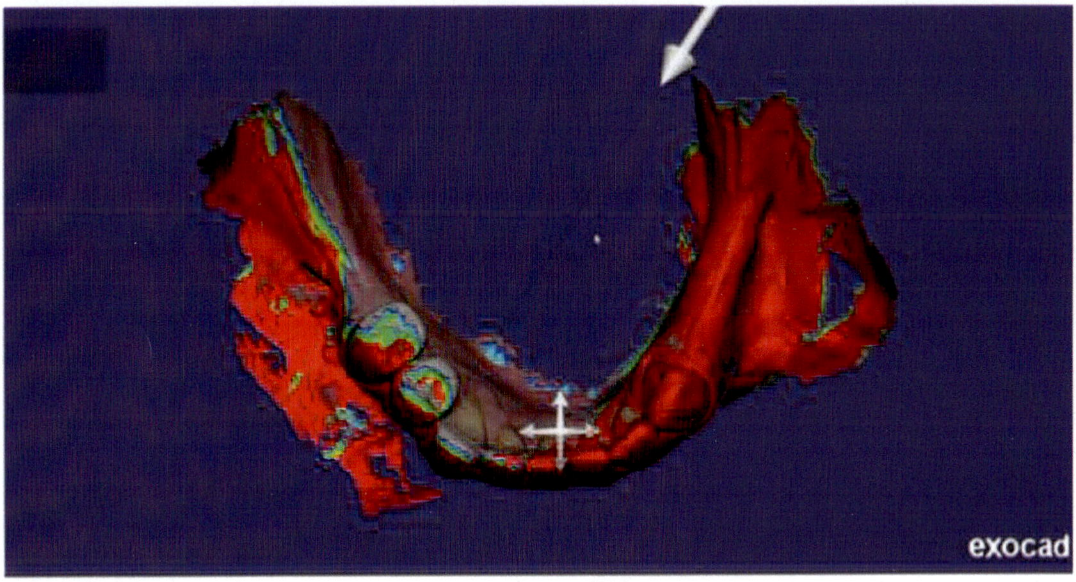

Fig. 18.17 Correction of insertion axis of RPD (Video 18.3)

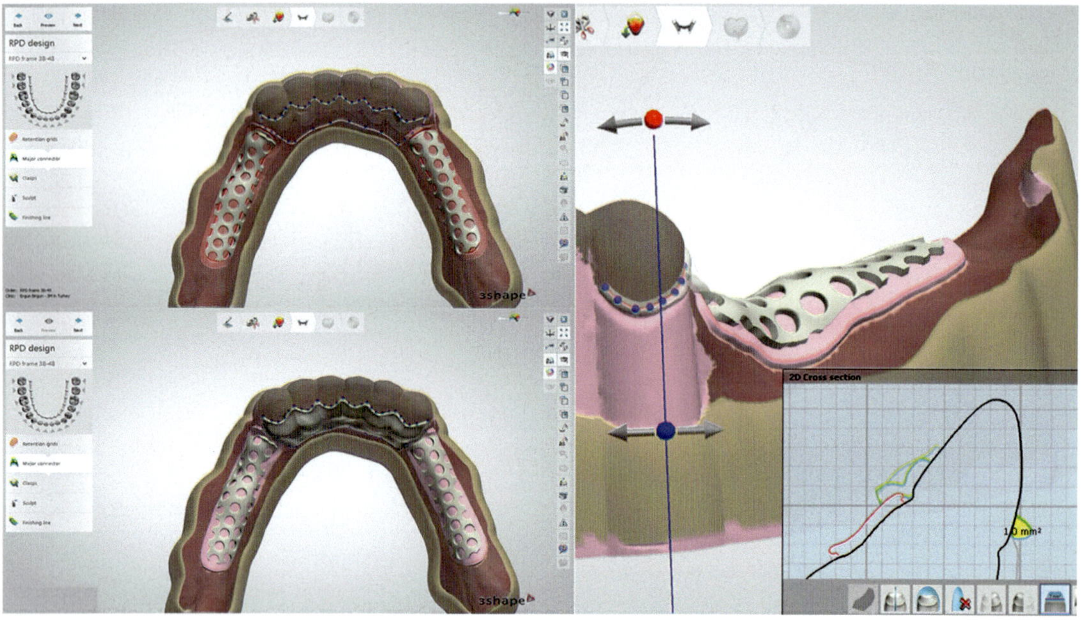

Fig. 18.18 Digital design of RPD framework

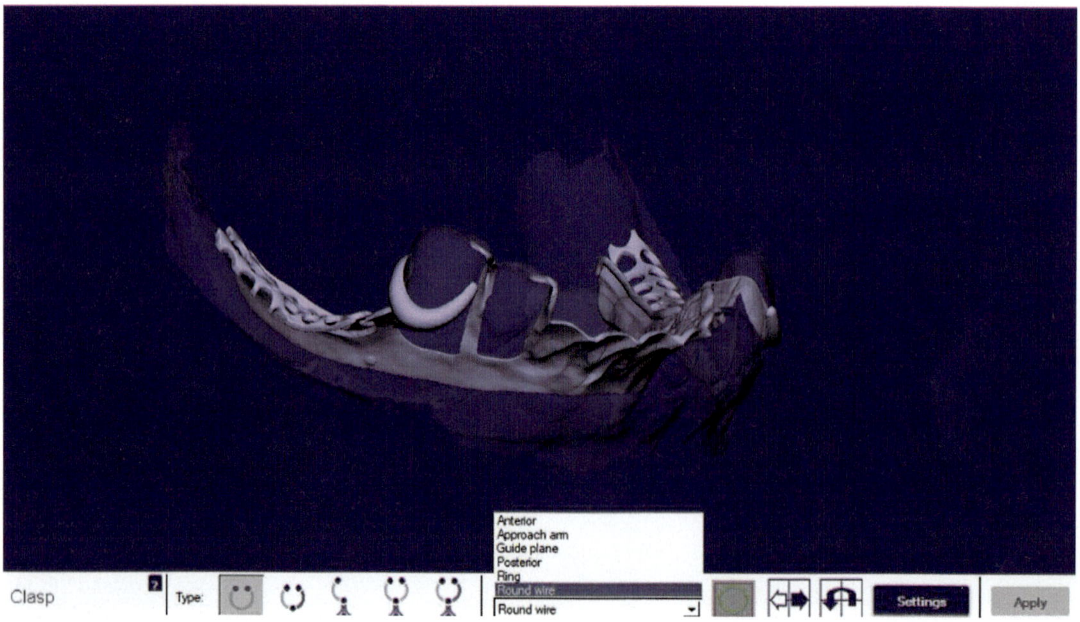

Fig. 18.19 Clasp options, design of metal framework

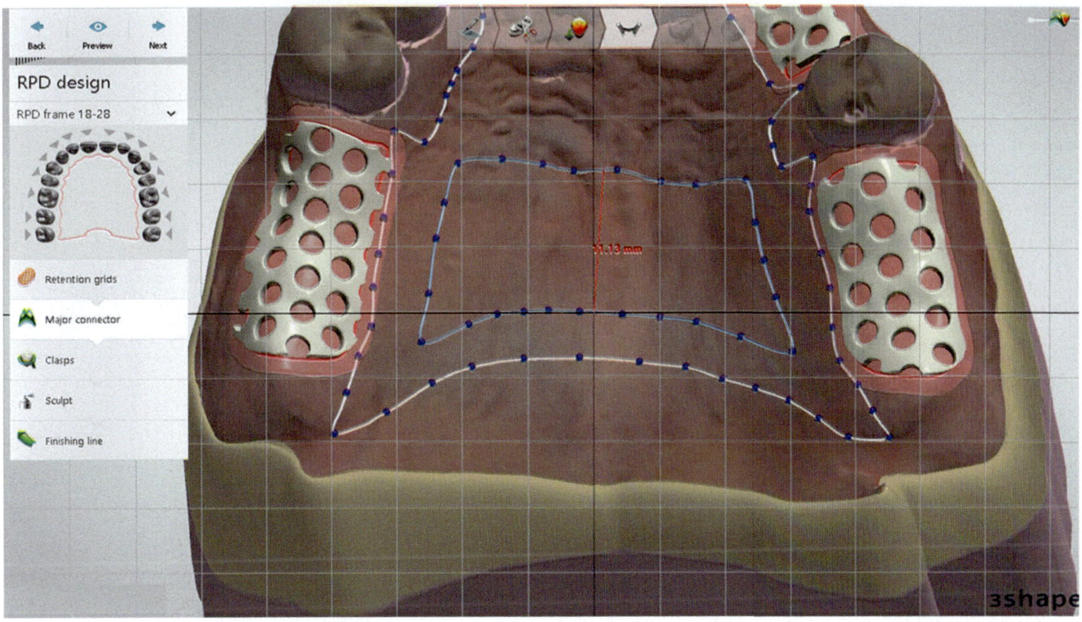

Fig. 18.20 Measurement of RPD Framework width. Incorrect design of aperture for mid part of RPD

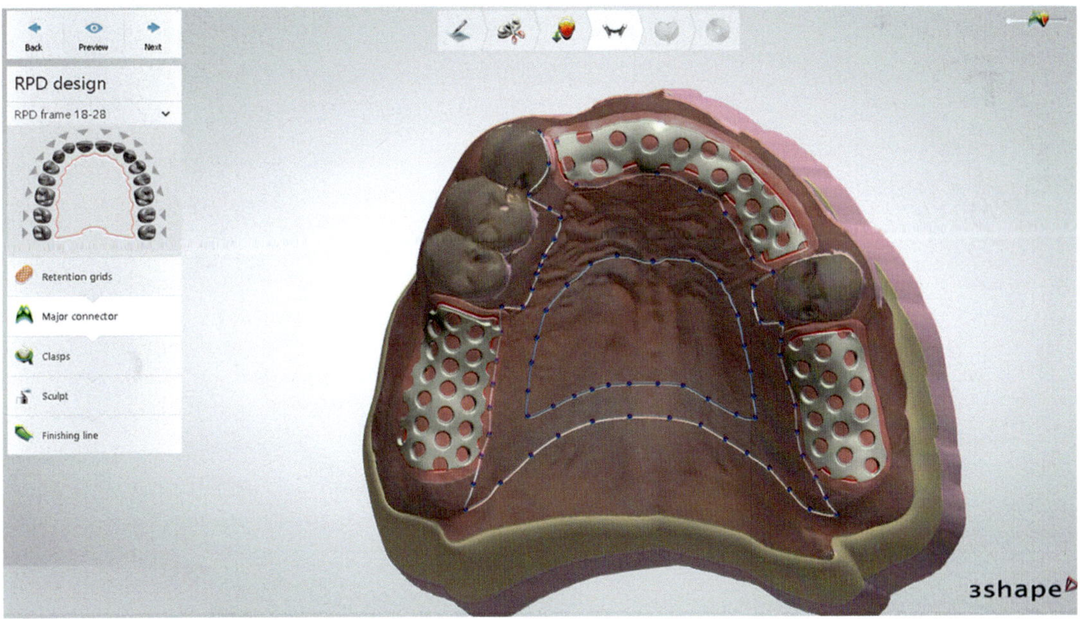

Fig. 18.21 Correction of design according to adequate width for metal framework

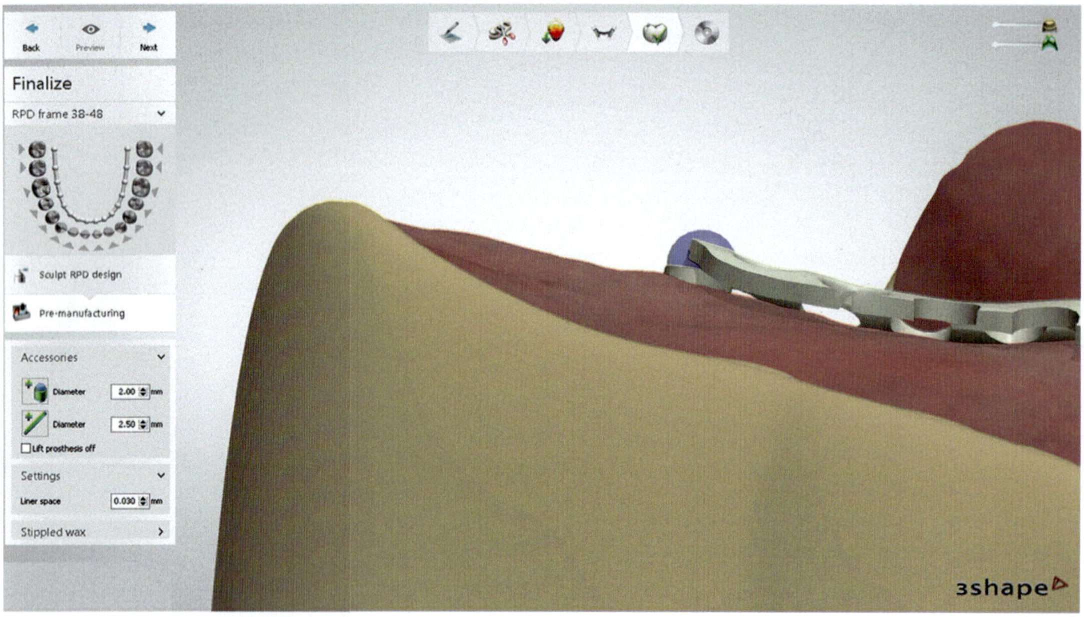

Fig. 18.22 Cast stop for free-end saddle partial denture framework

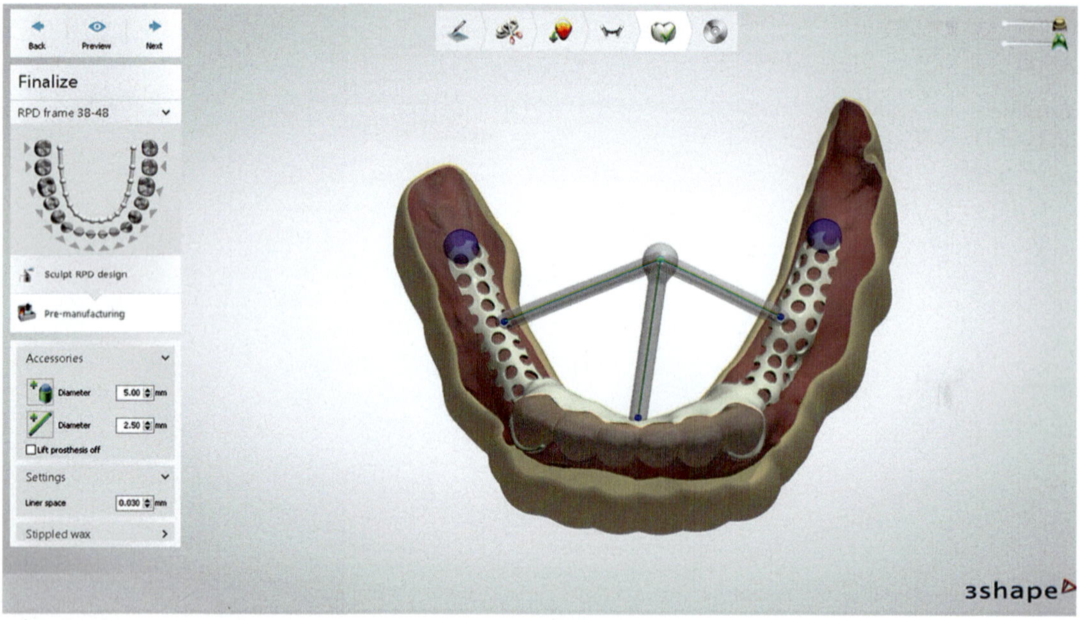

Fig. 18.23 Metal framework final design and accessories placed for wax production

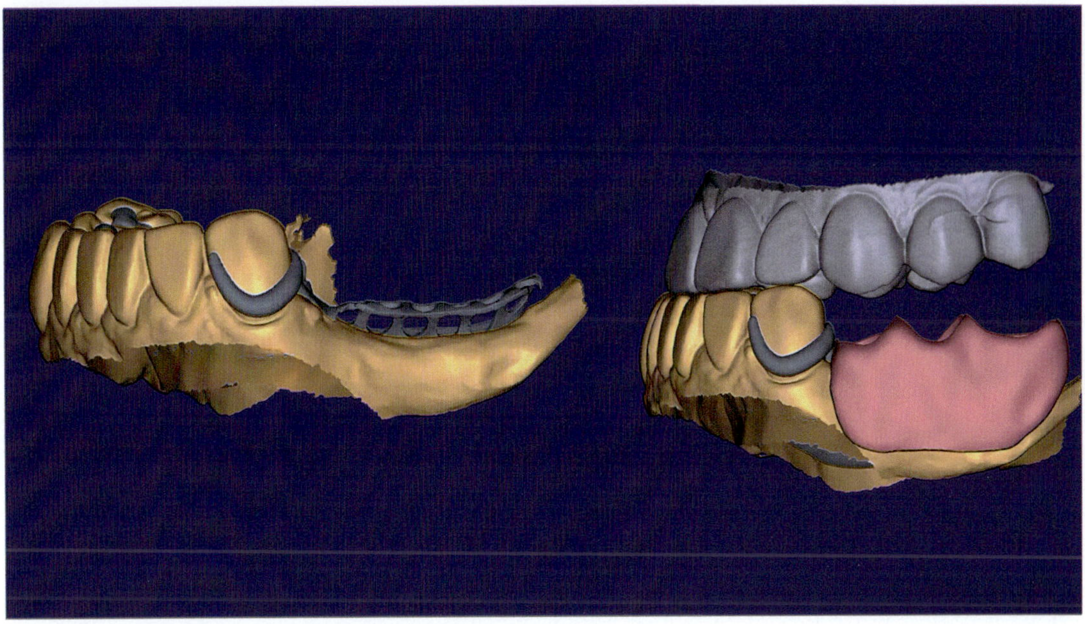

Fig. 18.24 Final design of a metal framework and denture base

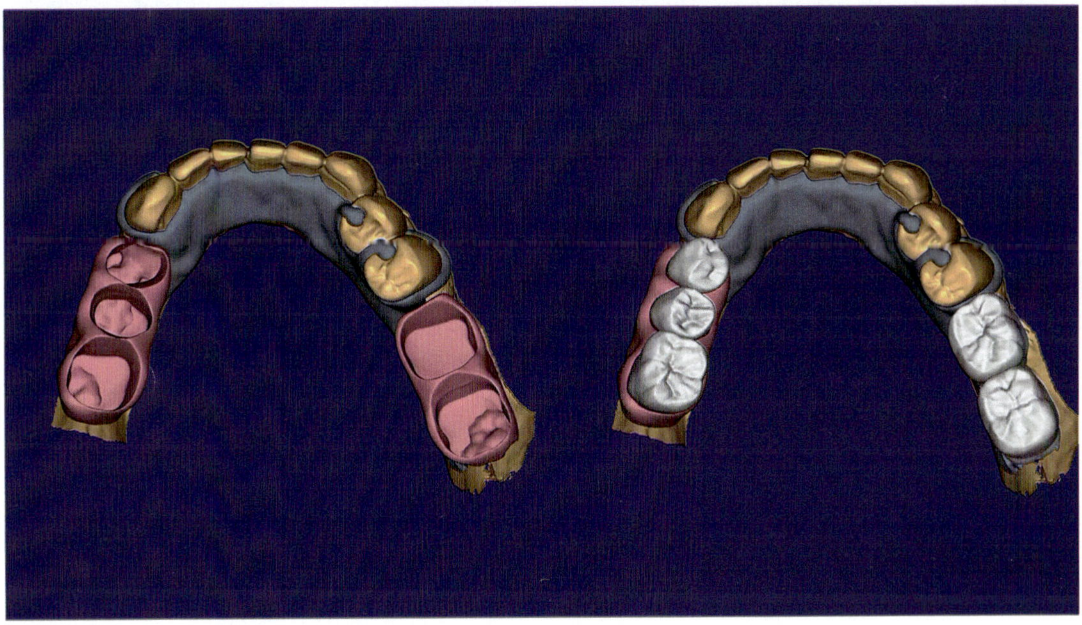

Fig. 18.25 Final design of denture base and teeth setup. Missing intraoral scan on retromolar area will be completed with functional impression or intraoral relining

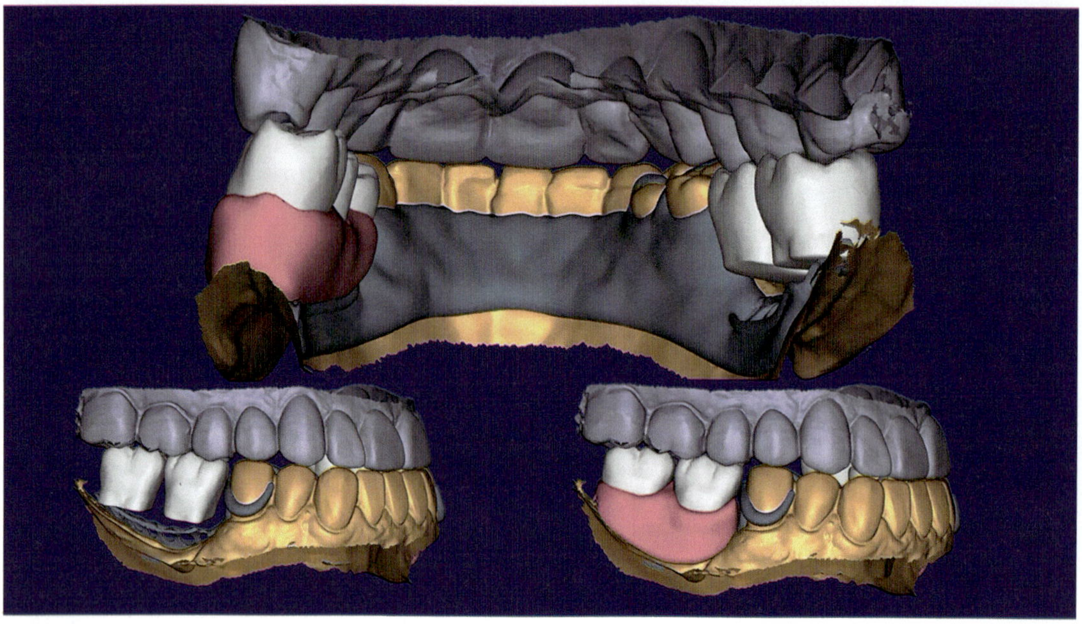

Fig. 18.26 Final design of all RPD components

wares are quite expensive. Conventional techniques will still be in action in developing economies and in transition countries, where hand work is cheaper. Beside this aspect, digital workflows are already accepted and valid option for designing and production for RPDs. In addition, a variety of novel polymer materials that may be utilized to create digitally designed RPDs have just introduced on the market and have been demonstrated to be more accurate than traditional RPDs.

Simplest way for prescribing a RPD design is to draw on a paper or stone cast, which has to be followed by dental technician during wax application before casting of framework. Less experienced operators, especially students face difficulties cause of visualization on hand, there is a possibility for conflicts between them and dental technicians in design process. Digital design possibilities allow students or less experienced operators to understand different design options, expand their knowledge and perspective about framework design. This workflow should also be available and implemented as a teaching module in dental faculties. From a clinical perspective, digital workflow improves fit for prosthesis adjustments and more efficient correction. Automated workflows create standardized quality for lowering laboratory costs, time spend, inaccuracies for design and most importantly need for clinical skills and experience for treating each specific patient. Effective and predictable workflow is much more needed now and in the future from the point of aging population, increase for treatment numbers, reducing necessary steps, which are minimum of four or five visits, post insertion controls, as well high laboratory expenses and time spend during all treatment process.

Presently, common dental design softwares impose framework shapes. On the other hand, the final design of RPD must examine case specific, oral habits and esthetic requirements, not only the abutment teeth and the edentulous ridges. The virtual system explained above integrated criteria into artificial intelligence (AI) and object to create automatically RPD design; however, a gigantic amount of clinical data was needed, and it is hard to bring this workflow in daily use. Chen et al. tried a simplified workflow for a better prediction workflow; as mentioned, AI-supported digital design requires enormous data. In order to manipulate AI machine learning, researchers created 112 different case scenarios. Software successfully automates the design of RPD diagrams for both upper and lower arch cases. As demonstrated, the Kennedy classification had no effect on the success rate of the result; however, for upper denture designs, the shape of the major connectors or boundaries varies because there are many design options available and AI requires more raw data to estimate the ultimate design. This study is for a 2D design workflow; in the future, however, clinical trial results stored on a personal computer will be able to be fully integrated with the RPD design by being linked to the software.

Artificial intelligence applications growing each day. Soon biomechanical principles and case scenarios will be in database of softwares and AI will give design automatically. One study develops a software which detect a fine fully automatical perception for the RPD design. Software can formulate required design by dentist in a basic scheme and transfer this file to laboratory. Next step would be implementing this feature in dental softwares to design dentures full automatically.

Further Reading

Abduo J, Elseyoufi M. Accuracy of intraoral scanners: a systematic review of influencing factors. Eur J Prosthodont Restor Dent. 2018;26:101–21.

Al-Haj Husain N, Özcan M, Schimmel M, Abou-Ayash S. A digital cast-free clinical workflow for oral rehabilitation with removable partial dentures: a dental technique. J Prosthet Dent. 2020;123:680–5.

AlRumaih HS. Clinical applications of intraoral scanning in removable prosthodontics: a literature review. J Prosthodont. 2021;30:747–62.

Asaka A, Uekubo Y, Mitsui T, et al. Applying intraoral scanner to residual ridge in edentulous regions: in vitro evaluation ofinter-operator validity to confirm trueness. BMC Oral Health. 2019;19:264.

Bibb RJ, Eggbeer D, Williams R, Woodward A. Trial fitting of a removable partial denture framework made using computer-aided design and rapid prototyping techniques. Proc Inst Mech Eng H J Eng Med. 2006;220:793–7.

Cameron AB, Evans JL, Robb ND. A technical and clinical digital approach to the altered cast technique with an intraoral scanner and polyvinyl siloxane impression material. J Prosthet Dent. 2022;S0022-3913:00357-2.

Campbell SD, Cooper L, Craddock H, Hyde TP, Nattress B, Pavitt SH, Seymour DW. Removable partial dentures: the clinical need for innovation. J Prosthet Dent. 2017;118:273–80.

Chang I-C, Hung C-C, Du J-K, Liu T-C, Lai P-L, Lan T-H. Accuracy of intraoral scanning methods for maxillary Kennedy class I arch. J Dent Sci. 2023;18:747–53.

Chen Q, Lin S, Wu J, Lyu P, Zhou Y. Automatic drawing of customized removable partial denture diagrams based on textual design for the clinical decision support system. J Oral Sci. 2020;28:236–8.

Diker B, Tak Ö. Accuracy of digital impressions obtained using six intraoral scanners in partially edentulous dentitions and the effect of scanning sequence. Int J Prosthodont. 2021;34:101–8.

Eggbeer D, Bibb R, Williams R. The computer-aided design and rapid prototyping. Eng Med. 2005;219:195–2.

Fueki K, Inamochi Y, Wada J, Arai Y, Takaichi A, Murakami N, Ueno T, Wakabayashi N. A systematic review of digital removable partial dentures. Part I: clinical evidence, digital impression, and maxillomandibular relationship record. J Prosthodont Res. 2022;66:40–52.

Gan N, Ruan Y, Sun J, Xiong Y, Jiao T. Comparison of adaptation between the major connectors fabricated from intraoral digital impressions and extraoral digital impressions. Sci Rep. 2018;11:529.

Han J, Wang Y, Lü P. A preliminary report of designing removable partial denture frameworks using a specifically developed software package. Int J Prosthodont. 2010;23:370–5.

Hayama H, Fueki K, Wadachi J, Wakabayashi N. Trueness and precision of digital impressions obtained using an intraoral scanner with different head size in the partially edentulous mandible. J Prosthodont Res. 2018;62:347–52.

Hu F, Pei Z, Wen Y. Using intraoral scanning technology for three-dimensional printing of Kennedy class I removable partial denture metal framework: a clinical report. J Prosthodont. 2019;28:473–6.

Kattadiyil MT, Mursic Z, AlRumaih H, Goodacre CJ. Intraoral scanning of hard and soft tissues for partial removable dental prosthesis fabrication. J Prosthet Dent. 2014;112:444–8.

Kihara H, Hatakeyama W, Komine F, Takafuji K, Takahashi T, Yokota J, Oriso K, Kondo H. Accuracy and practicality of intraoral scanner in dentistry: a literature review. J Prosthodont Res. 2020;64:109–13.

Kim EY, Wada J, Sakamoto K, Ishioka Y, Arai Y, Murakami N, Yamazaki T, Hayama H, Utsumi M, Inukai S, Wakabayashi N. Effect of scanning origin location on data accuracy of abutment teeth region in digital impression acquired using intraoral scanner for removable partial denture: a preliminary in vitro study. J Clin Med. 2022;11:7392.

Kontis P, Güth JF, Keul C. Accuracy of full-arch digitalization for partially edentulous jaws—a laboratory study on basis of coordinate-based data analysis. Clin Oral Investig. 2022;26:3651–62.

Lee JH, Yun JH, Han JS, Yeo IL, Yoon HI. Repeatability of intraoral scanners for complete arch scan of partially edentulous dentitions: an in vitro study. J Clin Med. 2019;8:1187.

Majeed-Saidan A, Dutra V, Levon JA, Chu TG, Morton D, Alfaraj A, Lin WS. The trueness of scans using one intraoral scanner in different partially edentulous conditions. J Prosthodont. 2022;32:588.

Nishiyama H, Taniguchi A, Tanaka S, Baba K. Novel fully digital workflow for removable partial denture fabrication. J Prosthodont Res. 2020;64:98–103.

Rasaie V, Abduo J, Hashemi S. Accuracy of intraoral scanners for recording the denture bearing areas: a systematic review. J Prosthodont. 2021;30:520–39.

Ren S, Morton D, Lin WS. Accuracy of virtual interocclusal records for partially edentulous patients. J Prosthet Dent. 2020;123:860.

Rotar RN, Faur AB, Pop D, Jivanescu A. Scanning distance influence on the intraoral scanning accuracy-an in vitro study. Materials. 2022;15:3061.

Schimmel M, Akino N, Srinivasan M, Wittneben JG, Yilmaz B, Abou-Ayash S. Accuracy of intraoral scanning in completely and partially edentulous maxillary and mandibular jaws: an in vitro analysis. Clin Oral Investig. 2021;25:1839–47.

Shimizu T, Tasaka A, Wadachi J, Yamashita S. A new proposal for improving the accuracy of intraoral scanning for partially edentulous residual ridge. J Prosthodont Res. 2023;67:246–54.

Suzuki Y, Harada N, Watanabe KI, Maruo R, Shimpo H, Ohkubo C. Clinical application of an intraoral scanner and CAD/CAM system for a Kennedy class I partially edentulous patient. J Oral Sci. 2022;19:109–11.

Takaichi A, Fueki K, Murakami N, Ueno T, Inamochi Y, Wada J, Arai Y, Wakabayashi N. A systematic review of digital removable partial dentures. Part II: CAD/CAM framework, artificial teeth, and denture base. J Prosthodont Res. 2022;66:53–67.

Tamanaka I, Isshi K, Takahashi Y. Fabrication of a nonmetal clasp denture supported by an intraoral scanner and CAD-CAM. J Prosthet Dent. 2018;120:9–12.

Tasaka A, Uekubo Y, Mitsui T, Kasahara T, Takanashi T, Homma S, Matsunaga S, Abe S, Yoshinari M, Yajima Y, Sakurai K, Yamashita S. Applying intraoral scanner to residual ridge in edentulous regions: in vitro evaluation of inter-operator validity to confirm trueness. BMC Oral Health. 2019;19:264.

The glossary of prosthodontic terms: ninth edition. J Prosthet Dent. 2017;117(5S):e1–e105. https://doi.org/10.1016/j.prosdent.2016.12.001. PMID: 28418832.

Tregerman I, Renne W, Kelly A, Wilson D. Evaluation of removable partial denture frameworks fabricated using 3 different techniques. J Prosthet Dent. 2019;122:390–5.

Williams RJ, Bibb R, Rafik T. A technique for fabricating patterns for removable partial denture frameworks using digitized casts and electronic surveying. J Prosthet Dent. 2004;91:85–8.

Williams RJ, Bibb R, Eggbeer D, Collis J. Use of CAD/CAM technology to fabricate a removable partial denture framework. J Prosthet Dent. 2006;96:96–9.

Wu J, Cheng Y, Gao B, Yu H. A novel digital altered cast impression technique for fabricating a removable partial denture with a distal extension. J Am Dent Assoc. 2020;151:297–302.

Manufacturing and Materials

19

Süleyman Çağatay Dayan, Gökçen Ateş, and Sina Saygılı

Abstract

Recent years have seen a meteoric rise in the widespread use of digital technologies in dental practice. It is now possible to use a greater variety of materials and techniques in the fabrication of removable partial denture (RPD) framework, denture bases, and artificial teeth because of advancements in CAD-CAM technologies. When compared to frameworks fabricated using conventional casting processes, those produced using CAD-CAM and rapid prototyping exhibit greater improvements in the mechanical strength of the metal framework. Lab work, time, and materials required to fabricate the denture's base and framework might be reduced as a result of these innovation. Studies have demonstrated that RPDs may be produced with clinically acceptable precision and accuracy using digital technology. Furthermore, in vivo studies revealed that these cutting-edge technologies are positive in terms of patient satisfaction and suitable biomechanical performance. There are several machines available for both subtractive and additive manufacturing processes. Each technique differs in its method and materials employed, as well as its benefits, limitations, and applications. In the first chapter of this part, it is described that the data acquisition and design of a digital RPD. The second chapter draws attention to the fabrication process and materials of the digital RPD.

S. Ç. Dayan (✉)
Dental Laboratory Technology Program, İstanbul University-Cerrahpaşa, İstanbul, Türkiye
e-mail: suleyman.dayan@iuc.edu.tr

G. Ateş · S. Saygılı
Faculty of Dentistry, Department of Prosthodontics, İstanbul University, İstanbul, Türkiye
e-mail: gokcenates@istanbul.edu.tr; sinasaygili@istanbul.edu.tr

19.1 Definitions

Binder jetting: An additive manufacturing process in which a liquid bonding agent is selectively deposited to join powder materials. In metal binder jetting (MBJ) the metal powder is bound using a polymer binding agent.

CAD-CAM: acronym for Computer-aided design-computer-aided manufacturing (or Computer-Asisted Machining): the Computer Numerical Control (CNC) subtractive fabrication of a 3D object; in dentistry, it is a CAD-CAM technology used to produce different types of prostheses, including crowns, veneers, inlays, onlays, fixed dental prostheses, removable dental prostheses, dental implant prostheses, and orthodontic and other devices.

Digital light processing: It is another type of stereolithography (SLA). The major difference of digital light processing (DLP) from laser-based SLA is that DLP uses a projection of ultraviolet

O. Şakar (ed.), *Removable Partial Dentures*, https://doi.org/10.1007/978-3-031-47083-7_19

(UV) light (or visible light) from a digital projector to flash a single image of the layer across the entire resin at once.

Direct metal laser sintering: acronym is DMLS; an additive CAM technique which uses a sintering of metal alloy powder to develop 3D objects.

Fracture toughness: Describes resistance of brittle materials to the propagation of flaws under an applied stress, and it assumes that the longer the flaw, the lower is the stress needed to cause fracture.

Fused deposition modeling: acronym is FDM; a computer-aided manufacturing (CAM) by additive modeling using a layering of a thermoplastic material.

Rapid prototyping: A general term used for several additive layer manufacturing techniques.

Selective laser melting acronym is SLM; an additive CAM continuous layering buildup process in which elemental metal or alloy powder deposition is closely followed by laser melting to create a finished shape under computer control.

Selective laser sintering: acronym is SLS; an additive CAM technique by sintering plastics, glass, or ceramics into 3D structures.

Standard tessellation language (STL): A digital file used in stereolithographic display and printing; the 3D image surface is interpreted by a series of triangles.

Stereolithography: acronym is SLA; a computer numerical control (CNC) additive fabrication of an object; in dentistry, it relates to the laser initiation of light-reactive resin layering to make replicas of casts and devices; alternative to processes of casting, injection molding and vacuum thermoforming; orig, the photo sculpturing principle is credited to Francois Willeme, 1860; the term and manufacturing process is credited to Charles Hull, 1986.

Tensile strength: The maximum stress that a material can bear before breaking when it is allowed to be stretched or pulled.

Three-dimensional (3D) printing: It is used as a synonym for rapid prototyping, selective laser scanning, and stereolithography.

Yield strength: Refers to an indication of maximum stress that can be developed in a material without causing plastic deformation.

19.2 Manufacturing Techniques

Digital dentistry consists of three systems: data acquisition, data processing, and data manufacturing. Subtractive manufacturing (SM) and additive manufacturing (AM) are the two main types of data manufacturing technology. SM relies on computer numerical control (CNC) and milling equipment, whereas AM builds layers upon layers. AM is a more contemporary technique than SM and is often known as "rapid prototyping." These technologies allow for simpler and more predictable fabrication of RPDs by reducing the likelihood of faults occurring during traditional steps such as waxing, casting, and investment. There are several machines available for both SM and AM processes. Each technique differs in its method and materials employed, as well as its benefits, limitations, and applications.

19.2.1 Subtractive Manufacturing

SM is a method for producing three-dimensional objects by meticulously removing layers of the appropriate material from a block of the desired composition. The manufacturing process begins after the final design phase has been completed using proper CAD software and the CAD model is created. After completing the task, the dedicated software will simulate the milling unit's performance to verify its ability to process the designated RPD components effectively. Following software verification of the planned RPD component's viability, the CNC machine may be started. Milling machines have multiaxis units with either 3, 4, or 5 axes. In clinic practice, the number of axes does not affect the quality of the restoration. Rather, it depends on how effectively the demand is matched with the appropriate production technique and material. Complicated 3D structures, such as denture bases and RPD frameworks, need five-axis milling machines.

Milling can be used in two ways: direct production and indirect production. Direct production allows for metal or non-metal RPD frameworks to be fabricated from a block of the specified composition. For indirect production, a castable pattern manufactured from resin or wax must be milled, and then it is ready to be cast. When compared to direct production, the results of hybrid procedures, which is also called "indirect production," are much less accurate. So far, this approach has failed to acquire popularity in the field of dentistry. In fact, there have been effective studies conducted on this subject. Arnold et al. demonstrated in an in vitro study that milled castable wax patterns had a similar or better retentive clasp fit accuracy than those fabricated using standard wax-up and lost wax techniques. Under a microscope, however, samples from the milled castable wax pattern groups showed flaws like rough surfaces, minor discontinuities, pores, and holes that should be taken into account. In another study, RPD frameworks were first milled and printed (using DLP, which will be explained in paragraphs below) into a castable pattern before being casted. The results demonstrated a significant difference in accuracy between the two manufacturing techniques, with SM producing more precise RPDs than AM.

By manufacturing the framework from a solid block of the same material, milling reduces the likelihood of defects such as porosities and inhomogeneous consistencies. In addition to the advantages already mentioned, milling allows for the use of non-metallic materials in the framework's manufacturing, including polyetheretherketone, aryl ketone polymers, acetyl copolymers, and polyethylene terephthalate. However, at the moment, subtractive milling has a few limitations that must be taken into account when fabricating RPD frameworks:

- requiring considerable time to process the framework,
- cutting complicated shapes and/or undercut areas is difficult,
- deformation or breaking might happen in thin or narrow regions,
- significant amounts of milling chips are not recycled,
- due to the difficulty in locating an appropriate connecting point for the milling machine, components may be distorted,
- milling accuracy suffers after cutting tools become worn out.

Manufacturers produce Cobalt Chromium (CoCr) prefabricated blocks, which enable soft metal milling with manufacturing processes comparable to presintered zirconia, to eliminate the possible issues associated with hard metal milling. Desktop milling machines may be used to process CoCr soft metal milling alloys, making them a cost-effective choice. Soft CoCr blank fabricated by dry-milled and metal powder is combined with a binder. The ensuing procedure for sintering in the furnace, which varies among manufacturers and usually entails temperatures ranging from 1200 to 1350°C, eliminates the binder and triggers the sintering of metal particles. This process causes a reduction in volume of approximately 10% until the material reaches full density. The microstructure and mechanical characteristics of the CoCr alloy after sintering are equivalent to those of CoCr alloys prepared using other procedures. Hong et al. showed encouraging results with soft milling and subsequently sintering milled CoCr alloy frameworks, but no clinical studies have been conducted to determine if it is appropriate for RPD framework. It is well known that milling frameworks for RPDs from metal blocks is technically complex and costly, especially when working with base metals. Noble metal alloys are not utilized since they are expensive. Due to the emergence of resin-based polymers as a replacement for CoCr in RPD frameworks, the milling technique has gained widespread acceptance. Most contemporary polymers are produced as discs that are milled to form the ultimate denture frameworks. Following the milling process, these frameworks generally necessitate minor adjustments, finishing touches, and polishing.

19.2.2 Additive Manufacturing

The aforementioned challenges can be overcome with the use of AM technology. It is more suited for manufacturing metal RPD framework since it can generate huge objects with surface imperfections including undercuts, voids, and hollow morphologies. Rapid prototyping is another name for AM technology, which is a technique for rapidly fabricating scale replicas of physical components or assemblies using CAD data. Rapid prototyping allows for the production of delicate and thin structures since no force is applied and no machine vibration occurs during production. This process wastes fewer raw materials than subtractive. The manufacturers assert that AM-produced CoCr alloys exhibit elevated yield strength and tensile strength in comparison to traditional cast alloys, in addition to increased density and hardness. However, when fabricating RPD frameworks, metals produced with the AM method have a rougher surface than those made with the subtractive or conventional lost-wax methods. Many different AM techniques and procedures are now employed for the fabrication of frameworks, either in part or in whole. Surface roughness is affected not just by the specific AM processing technology utilized, but also by the parameters chosen for the build.

There are various types of 3D printing technologies that include Binder Jetting, Directed Energy Deposition, Material Extrusion, Material Jetting, Powder Bed Fusion, Sheet Lamination, and Vat Photopolymerization. In addition, these AM techniques, like the SM technique, may be divided into two sub-categories for RPD framework fabrication: direct and indirect methods. Direct AM does not necessitate castable pattern resin because it allows for the direct manufacturing of metal frameworks using a novel machine, in contrast to the so-called "indirect" AM method, which creates a castable pattern resin and continuously casts the metal framework using the conventional method.

No matter how many or how complex the dimensions of an object are, AM technology makes it possible to produce anything. AM has various benefits over milling for RPD frameworks, including the following:

1. no milling chips are generated;
2. free-form curves, undercuts, and hollow structures may be constructed;
3. blunt milling tools have no effect on precision;
4. several frameworks can be prepared at once;
5. the price is kept to a minimum.

Although the advantages of utilizing AM technology in clinical settings are alluring, it is essential to contemplate specific factors to guarantee successful implementation. These factors include the tolerance of the AM machine, which depends on its x-y resolution and stacking pitch, as well as the z-axis. Additionally, the material and powder particle size, amount of warping and shrinkage, supporting structures used, and the geometrical orientation of the manufacturing process can all affect the accuracy of AM frameworks.

19.2.2.1 Indirect Additive Manufacturing Techniques

"Vat-polymerization" techniques, namely Stereolithography (SLA) and digital light processing (DLP), are popular methods for producing castable pattern resin using additive manufacturing (Fig. 19.1). In these approaches, printers leverage coordinates from a digital file to guide the projection of light through a clear resin tank. The castable pattern resin is constructed in stages as curing continues. SLA printers use an ultraviolet laser beam to cure the photopolymers, while DLP printers cure the resin layers with precisely directed short-wavelength light through a digital micromirror device or liquid crystal screen. Dental casts, interim restorations, resin RPD frameworks, removable denture-base materials, denture teeth, and surgical guides are a few instances of products that can be produced using the SLA method. Compared to SLA printers, DLP printers are faster, make less waste, and cost less to run. To ensure maximum polymerization and biocompatibility, both DLP and SLA require postprint polymerization using a UV light-emitting diode. Material jetting technology is

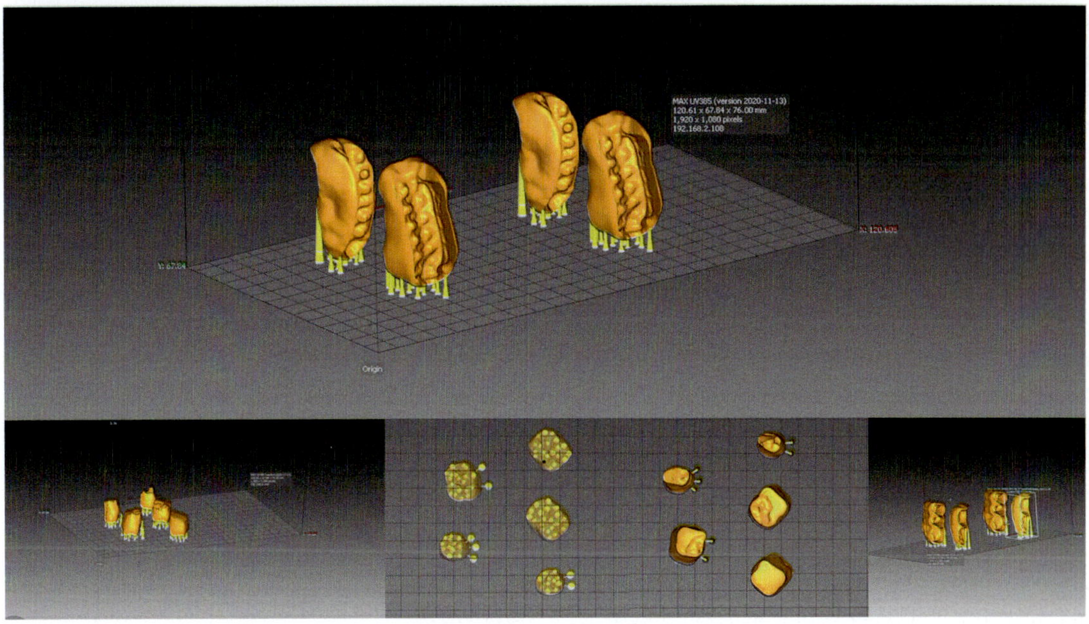

Fig. 19.1 Placing the denture base and teeth setup on designated printer bed in 3D printer software

another type of photopolymerization process that could be used to manufacture resin or wax RPD frameworks for investment casting. This method enables users to achieve a precision of 29–32 μm when printing on a smooth surface. Jet printing involves the utilization of multiple resin-jet print heads that dispense tiny streams of resin material onto the build platform for each layer of construction. A UV light source is subsequently used to polymerize each jetted layer. Due to the material's curing process using UV radiation, deterioration from direct sunlight may create deformation. This effect may be avoided by immediately investing the casting pattern once it has been printed.

The "staircase" surface texture effect that often results from SLA fabrication of framework designs may have a negative impact on the framework's overall fit and feel. Using SLA, the operator may define or adjust the layer thickness, which has major effects on the accuracy, build time, adaptability, and surface roughness of the framework of the RPDs. As of right now, the SLA method typically uses a layer thickness setting between 15 and 150 mm. The layer thickness setting may be reduced to achieve the clinical demand for greater trueness and precision. The layer thickness setting, on the other hand, may be raised to reduce manufacturing time. Because of this, when using SLA to make an RPD framework, the layer thickness of the castable resin pattern must be set correctly. You et al. tested varied layer thicknesses of 16, 50, and 100 μm in the fabrication of SLA framework patterns to evaluate this impact and advised a 50 μm layer thickness for effective RPD framework fit.

Although indirect manufacturing methods can produce frameworks with acceptable fit, it is important to note that errors may occur during casting. Therefore, careful consideration should be given before selecting this approach. In the context of RPD metal frameworks, SLS fabrication is noted to provide superior precision in comparison to the SLA-cast technique. In an in vitro study, SLA-printed pattern casting and SLS were used to compare the accuracy of CoCr frameworks in a Kennedy class II mod. 1 maxillary reference model with deep and medium palate vault depths. These findings align with an analysis by Tasaka et al., which found that clasps and rests made using SLS technology exhibited reduced total discrepancies in comparison to those generated by Material Jetting-printed pattern casting.

While the aforementioned research using technical comparisons suggest that direct manufacturing is superior, other investigations have shown that indirect approaches are not without benefits. The Kennedy Class III Mod I maxillary reference model was utilized by Rokhshad et al. to evaluate the accuracy of DLP-cast frameworks vs. those manufactured using traditional methods. The findings suggest that the fit of frameworks manufactured using DLP-printed patterns was not significantly different from that of frameworks manufactured using the traditional method. Lee et al. presented data from a clinical study in which patients with SLA-cast RPDs were monitored for up to 2 years and 8 months and no occurrences of denture failure were discovered. According to their findings, the internal discrepancy acquired from the major connector was much higher than those obtained from the rest, the clasp, and the minor connector. Similarly, the edentulous region reported a higher discrepancy than the rest and the minor connector. Additionally, they observed that the precision of the periphery surpassed that of the central portion when examining discrepancies beneath the cingulum rest.

Polymerization shrinkage might occur during the indirect AM process because the castable patterns are not entirely polymerized. Thus, it is crucial to follow the post-processing techniques that the manufacturer recommends. Polymerizing for 30 min after soaking in 95% ethanol for 10 min and then drying at room temperature is often sufficient for post-processing processes. It is also possible for the distortion to occur during the procedure of removing the partly polymerized design from the building platform. Finally, some parameters that might influence the accuracy of 3D printed objects should be known and understood by clinicians and lab technicians. These variables are categorized as follows:

- 3D printer technology: The type of 3D printer and its printing technology can influence the accuracy of the printed framework. Different Technologies have different resolution capabilities and accuracy.
- Printing parameters: Printing parameters such as layer thickness, exposure time, and curing settings can all affect the accuracy of the printed framework.
- Material shrinkage: Resin materials used for printing can undergo shrinkage during the curing process, which can affect the accuracy of the printed framework.
- Scanning technology: The quality of the digital scan used to design the framework can also affect its accuracy.
- Design software: The software used to create the framework can have an impact on the end product's accuracy. The precision of the software and the accuracy of the CAD file can influence the accuracy of the printed framework.
- Post-processing: Post-processing procedures such as sandblasting, polishing, and finishing can all impact the accuracy of the final product.

19.2.2.2 Direct Additive Manufacturing Techniques

Powder bed fusion (PBF) technologies are commonly used for 3D metal printing as they enable direct additive manufacturing. Among PBF technologies, three types have been introduced, namely SLS, selective laser melting (SLM), and electron beam melting (EBM). While EBM uses an electron beam as an energy source, SLS and SLM technologies use a laser beam to achieve sintering and melting. Both SLM and EBM have shown promise in studies comparing their use in the fabrication of titanium-based alloy prostheses. When compared to SLM frameworks, however, the surfaces that EBM generates are rougher, weaker, and less well fitted. It is probable that this is due to the fact that EBM employs a hot powder bed and, as a result, does not create a fine microstructure as SLM does, which works in an inert environment with a cold powder bed.

The most used AM method for fabricating RPD frameworks is SLM, which allows for layer-by-layer construction of the object. Process optimization uses support structures, which are typical in metal melting designs. These components enable a solid foundation and aid in heat transfer during melting. The SLM method allows for the production of complex objects made from a variety of materials, each with their own unique resistance and refined features. The melting parameters, which are determined at the beginning of the SLM, require careful attention. This is because the mistaken process parameters can cause micropores, which can lead to cracks when mechanical stress is applied. SLM-manufactured materials have residual stress that causes them to distort. During SLM, large residual stresses build up between layers, which cause the product to change shape. The final fused top layer shrinks to a degree that depends on the material below it. Heat processing has been utilized to minimize deformation and distortion to the greatest extent possible, along with the use of support structures to limit distortion. In addition, metals' crystal flaws may be eliminated with heat treatment, allowing for a more stable microstructure and less residual stress. Therefore, the framework has to be annealed at 800–1100°C for 30–60 min, as recommended, and then chilled in an argon environment before the support structure is removed. Yan et al. evaluated the mechanical characteristics of SLM CoCr metal-ceramic alloys designed for the manufacture of thin RPDs to the impacts of two heat treatments. Despite the fact that the 0.2% yield strength of the two heat treatment groups exceeded 500 MPa and elongation exceeded 2%, satisfying the minimum ISO requirements, they reported that the heating process at 1100°C is more appropriate for manufacturing RPDs due to the improved fracture toughness compared to that at 880°C. In addition to post-processing heat treatment, the scanning paths for laser melting, the flow of inert gas in the chamber, the design of the support (whether it is independent or dependent), and the build orientation of the part (whether it is in transverse or horizontal directions) all affect the physical and mechanical properties of AM-made RPD frameworks.

There is enough data in the literature to use SLM-manufactured frameworks safely in clinical applications. In their study, Zhou et al. compared the microstructures and mechanical characteristics of SLM CoCr dental alloys to those generated by milled and cast methods. They reached the conclusion that the SLM method provided superior microstructures and mechanical qualities. Tasaka et al. carried out a study in which they examined the fitting accuracy of two digitally designed and manufactured RPD frameworks. In one study group, they used traditional lost-wax casting of a printed resin design, whereas the other utilized RPD frameworks manufactured by SLM. Fit differences were reduced in SLM-fabricated frameworks, indicating that this fabrication approach is preferable. Chen et al. studied different types of maxillary frameworks fabricated by SLM and observed internal gaps ranging from 150 to 330 μm (an internal discrepancy in the range of 69–426.3 μm has been shown to be clinically acceptable in previous studies), concluding that the adaptation of SLM-manufactured frameworks is equivalent to that of cast frameworks, with the exception of complicated designs. An in-vitro study comparing the trueness of powdered CoCr or titanium-6 aluminum-4 vanadium (Ti-6Al-4V) alloy frameworks for RPDs manufactured by SLM indicated that the RPD frameworks generated by SLM had the greatest trueness when compared to the traditional cast method. Furthermore, the authors proved that there was no statistical difference between the CoCr and Ti-6Al-4V groups in the SLM-fabricated groups.

The process for SLS is the same as the process for SLM. The procedure is referred to as direct metal laser sintering (DMLS) rather than SLS when the material being printed is metal. Since the highest temperature reached during DMLS is much below the melting point, powder materials are not completely melted or sintered. Sintering is advantageous over the traditional casting method because it reduces thermal distortion and increases yield and accuracy. Heat treatments for postprocessing should be performed according to the manufacturer's recommendations, often at 450°C for 45 min and 750°C for 60 min, and then cooled. A randomized, controlled clinical trial with a within-subjects design was conducted to find out how satisfied patients were with SLS-fabricated RPDs. The participants were much more satisfied with SLS RPDs than with traditional cast RPDs in terms of overall satisfaction, the ability to clean and speak, comfort, chewing ability, chewing efficiency, and oral condition. However, the follow-up period was just 4 weeks; this should be kept in mind when evaluating the findings. In their study, Alageel et al. evaluated the precision error, biocompatibility, and physical and mechanical behaviors of RPD CoCr alloys produced by DMLS systems and compared them to those made by the traditional casting method. They found that, because of their higher homogeneity and fine grain size, CoCr alloys used to produce DMLS are more accurate and have better fatigue resistance and mechanical qualities for RPDs than cast alloys. Furthermore, the biocompatibility of DMLS and cast CoCr alloys is comparable. As a result, DMLS RPDs may provide clinical advantages over cast ones in terms of mechanical stability. In another study, Oh et al. compared the accuracy of CoCr 3D-printed frameworks by DMLS for RPDs by digital superimposition in a partially edentulous maxillary Kennedy Class II, modification I master cast to that of frameworks manufactured by traditional and 3D printing with DLP and then casting workflows.

The metal powder's particle size that is used in the SLM and DMLS processes can affect the final product's surface quality or the precision of the product's fit. While working with AM methods, it is essential to take into account the layer thickness as well as the laser scan speed and the building orientation. Even if there is a lack of information on these parameters, it would appear that a layer thickness of 30 mm, a scan speed of 5–7 m/s, and a construction direction of 45 or 90° are all feasible alternatives based on the current scientific knowledge.

Metal binder jetting (MBJ) is another direct AM technique that might theoretically manufacture metal frameworks, although very limited research on MBJ as a kind of direct AM to produce RPD metal frameworks could be identified. As no particles are melted during the MBJ process, its underlying operating principle is fundamentally different from that of the powder bed fusion techniques. MBJ enables the creation of complete polymer composite and metal powder products. In this process, heat treatment, or sintering, is required as a subsequent process if the printed material is metal. From a technical point of view, the MBJ manufacturing method is more efficient and quicker than the SLM procedure. Unfortunately, the MBJ method has gotten less attention in dentistry and the scientific community than powder bed fusion-based AM techniques, so the literature is scarce.

19.3 The Advantage of Digitally Fabricated Removable Partial Denture Frameworks

- The electronic sharing of digital framework designs may ease communication between the dentist and laboratory technician.
- Unlike traditional methods, the digital casting and design of a component can be kept in a digital library for later use.
- Industrial processing of stock materials, rather than laboratory preparation of castable materials, may result in more consistent material qualities.
- Enables the dental prosthesis laboratory to keep quality control consistent across operators.
- Enables the use of a variety of materials, including polymer-based materials, to overcome the limits of metal PRDPs.
- The elimination of lost wax casting and refractory cast pattern waxing has reduced manufacturing times.
- It is friendly for the environment because there is less waste of wax, alloy, and investment ingredients. The uncured metal powder that remains after laser sintering may be recycled and reused.

19.4 The Disadvantage of Digitally Fabricated Removable Partial Denture Frameworks

- Since RPD consist of a denture base and a framework, a fully digital process is often not possible.
- Possible factors affecting RPD structure quality include the type of software used and the practitioner's degree of expertise.

- There may be a scarcity of experienced digitally ready labs.
- Special supports are necessary to retain the framework throughout the 3D-printing process, which necessitates extra procedures for designing these supports and removing them after manufacturing.
- Both the dentist and the laboratory technician encounter a considerable and ultimately significant learning curve.
- The staircase effect that comes from the layered structure of 3D printing is greatly reduced when the layers are made thinner. Yet, reducing layer thickness may cause a rise in manufacturing time.
- The clinical efficacy of digitally manufactured RPDs has not been studied over the long term.

19.5 Denture Base and Denture Teeth

At the present, it seems challenging to manufacture RPDs using a model-free digital method. Given its limitations, the authors of this book consider that the traditional approach is still preferable to the digital one when it involves fabricating the denture base and artificial teeth. Recent studies mentioned a framework, a denture base, and teeth that were bonded together with an adhesive product. Nevertheless, more time is required for more technical effort and skill growth in order to use this approach. When the framework has been manufactured digitally, a printed master model for the arrangement of artificial teeth and the design of denture bases may be produced. In this way, clinicians and lab professionals may benefit from using both digital and analog techniques.

All denture components may be developed using intraoral scans and digitally manufactured, then constructed without the use of physical casts in appropriate circumstances. In this way, clinicians are significantly accelerating the laboratory workflow. After framework design completed, the teeth setup and denture base designed over the framework. All designed STL files exported from software.

If the technician and clinician are sure that the design is appropriate and that validation is not required, the prosthesis can be manufactured immediately. It would be reasonable to prioritize evaluating this design if there are doubts regarding the framework design and MMR records. Similar to the conventional treatment workflow, by verifying the final situation with the patient, dentists can prevent mistakes in the treatment workflow.

The final version of the design can be produced from biocompatible temporary restoration resins in order to evaluate esthetic, functional, and phonetic parameters. The prototype obtained from the framework design can be controlled alone, just like the fit of a conventional framework. However, it should be noted that the flexibility of these resins is higher than that of the materials used as the main connector. In terms of accuracy, the flexibility features of these resins might occasionally be deceiving. A misfit framework might appear to be an appropriate fit. If the try-in of the resin framework is successful, the version of the tooth setup produced can also be adhered to this framework with a flowable composite and controlled in together intraorally. Corrections to be made can be applied to the teeth together with leveling or composite resins, and changes in parameters such as tooth dimensions and the occlusal plane can be transferred to the laboratory. Taking pictures before and after alterations will help to improve communication. These provisional resins can also be used to evaluate the occlusion and maxillomandibular relation record before to fabrication.

Two methods are commonly used for fabricating RPDs. The first method involves creating the artificial teeth and denture base as a single structure, while the second method involves producing them independently. The choice of fabrication method is influenced by various factors, such as the visibility of the gingiva and the amount of soft tissue loss. When the teeth and denture base are fabricated separately, they must be bonded together in the laboratory. The compatibility of the RPD framework and dental files produced from design files can be assessed and resolved using different methods after alignment. After designing the RPD components, the STL files are transmitted to the desired device for production. The denture base and artificial teeth files are 3D printed, while the framework is created using rapid prototyping with CoCr. In the first step of combining the denture base and teeth, hard reline material is used, which is a commonly used method in the literature. Alternatively, autopolymerizing or heat polymerized acrylic resin can also be used during 3D printing to achieve this combination. However, using intraoral reline material can offer an advantage since it can close the space under the retention mesh, thereby increasing success due to the same chemical structure of the resin that binds different materials together. 3D printer resin is primarily utilized in situations where the retention mesh of RPD is created without holes or when the resin will remain between two materials, such as in complete denture fabrication. To achieve better adhesion of both materials, a bonding agent can be applied per the manufacturer's instructions before combining them, and a metal primer can be applied to the metal framework. Again, the same reline material is applied on the metal and denture base to combine all pieces of the RPD (Figs. 19.2, 19.3, and 19.4).

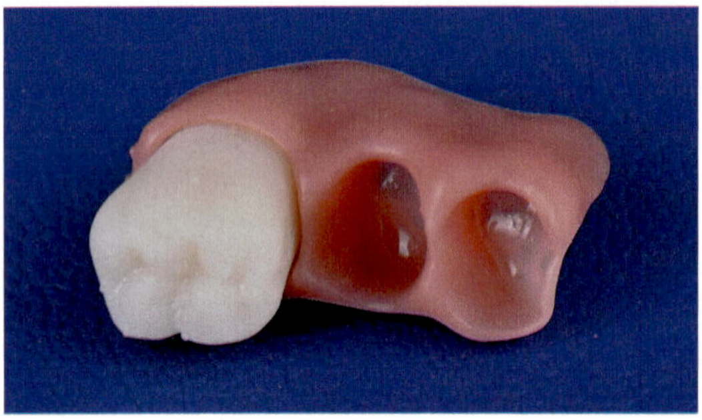

Fig. 19.2 3D printed denture base and permanent resin restoration material

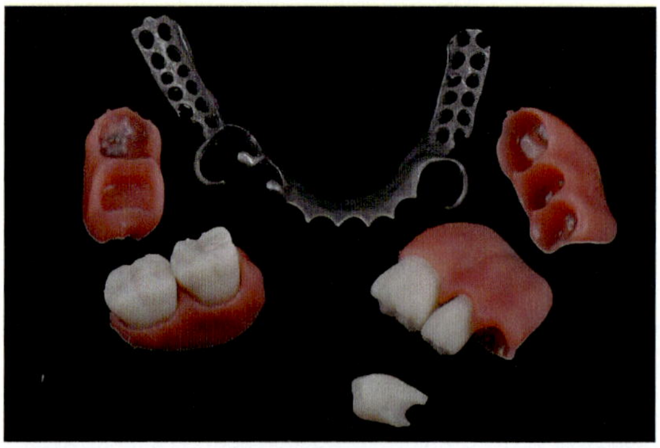

Fig. 19.3 Fabricated parts of RPD, model free workflow

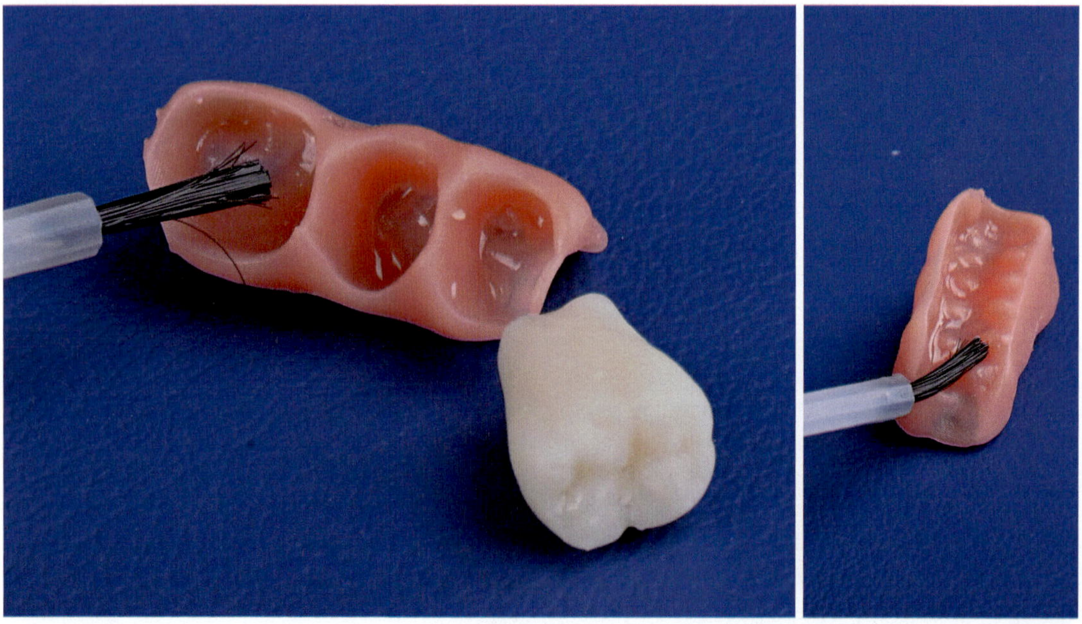

Fig. 19.4 Cementation of RPD parts

19.6 Materials for Digital Removable Partial Dentures Framework

The choice of framework material is essential for RPDs. Frameworks are the structures that support the artificial teeth and anchor the RPD to the remaining natural teeth or implants. Two main categories of framework materials are used in digital RPDs: metal-based and metal free-based.

19.6.1 Metal-Based Frameworks

Metal-based frameworks are made of alloys that are known for their strength, durability, and biocompatibility. Two of the most commonly used metal alloys in RPDs are CoCr and Titanium.

19.6.1.1 Cobalt Chromium

CoCr alloys are often utilized for the framework of RPDs, due to their safety and strength. The emergence of digital technology has revolutionized the fabrication of CoCr frameworks for RPDs, making it possible to employ milling, additive, and hybrid methods. Digital technology offers significant advantages in the fabrication of CoCr frameworks for RPDs, such as increased efficiency, reduced laboratory procedures, and enhanced accessibility for a larger patient population (Figs. 19.5 and 19.6).

The conventional method of manufacturing CoCr frameworks for RPDs is still widely used, but milling and printing techniques are now considered clinically acceptable alternatives. Each method has its unique advantages and challenges, which may affect the fit and clinical performance of the final RPDs. Milling is a subtractive manufacturing technique that uses CAD-CAM technology to produce CoCr frameworks from a solid block of alloy. This method offers high precision and excellent fit, which can lead to improved clinical outcomes. However, the milling process can be time-consuming and may generate waste material. AM techniques, such as SLS and SLM, utilize 3D printing technology to build CoCr frameworks layer by layer. AM methods offer the ability to create complex geometries and reduce material waste. However, Snosi et al. reported that subtractive manufacturing resulted in a better framework fit and more accurate RPDs than AM. Moreover, the effect of AM methods on biocompatibility, as well as the physical and mechanical characteristics of CoCr alloys, raises questions that could potentially impact the clinical performance of RPDs. The fabrication process of CoCr alloys can be significantly affected by various factors, including metal powder size, laser beam power, scanning speed, layer thickness, and molding angle. These aspects are crucial in assessing the quality, durability, and clinical efficacy of RPD frameworks created through additive manufacturing approaches like SLM. Kobayashi et al. carried out a research project to examine the influence of the molding angle on RPD frameworks produced through the SLM process. The results demonstrated that the SLM molding angle influences the trueness, or the accuracy of the RPD framework in replicating the desired design, as well as the presence of defects. These defects may include internal

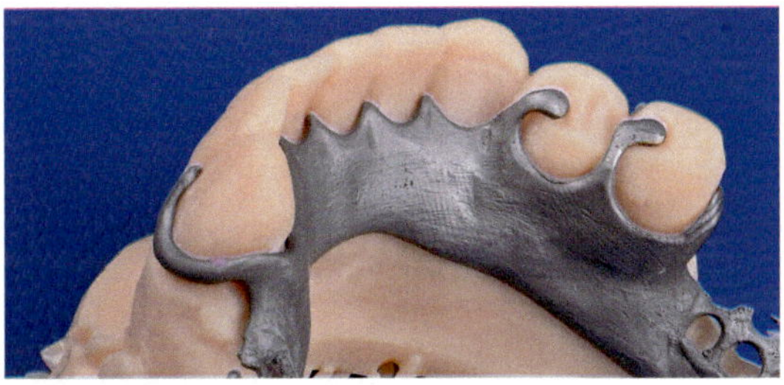

Fig. 19.5 Production of metal framework via laser melting according to digital design

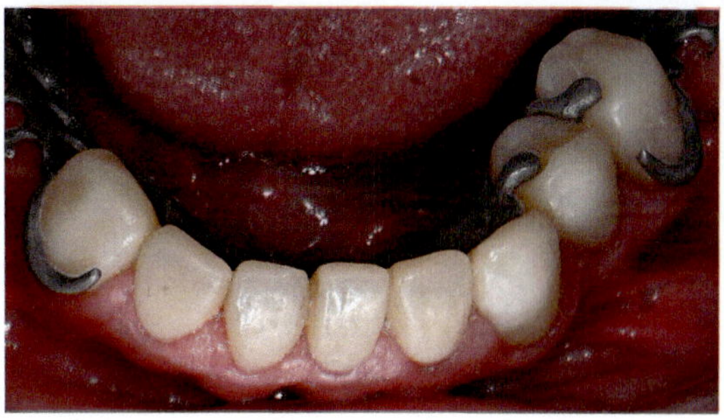

Fig. 19.6 Metal framework intraoral situation

imperfections and surface roughness, which can affect the overall fit, longevity, and clinical performance of the RPD. In another study, Alageel et al. compared the properties of RPD CoCr alloys produced by two different laser-sintering systems with those made using the traditional casting method. The researchers found that laser-sintering techniques resulted in RPDs with greater strength and improved properties compared to conventionally cast RPDs. This improvement can be attributed to the precision and uniformity of laser-sintering methods, which produce a smaller grain size and more consistent microstructure in the CoCr alloy. These studies highlight the importance of carefully controlling the manufacturing process of CoCr alloys for RPD frameworks, particularly when using AM like SLM. The molding angle, among other factors, can significantly impact the trueness and presence of defects in the final product. These findings suggest that the fit of SLM-produced RPD frameworks compared to conventionally prepared ones is not consistently better or worse and may be influenced by various aspects related to the design and components of the RPD. Dental professionals should weigh these factors when choosing the fabrication method for RPD frameworks, keeping in mind the unique requirements and features of each patient's case.

Retentive clasps in RPDs are essential components that secure the prosthesis to the remaining teeth. These clasps are subject to flexure stress, which can lead to deformation and fatigue failure, affecting the overall performance and longevity of the RPD. SLS CoCr frameworks have been introduced to improve clasp performance in RPD manufacturing. However, research indicates that the fit and accuracy of connectors, such as clasps, can be affected by the manufacturing technique. It is recommended to build the clasps with their longitudinal axes parallel to the build platform to achieve optimal fatigue resistance. Additionally, incorporating support structures intentionally can enhance the clasp's fatigue strength, although removing these structures may require extra effort. However, when creating components at this specific angle, it is important to note that the manufacturing capacity may be limited. This limitation arises because the framework occupies a larger area than when it is manufactured at a tilted angle relative to the platform. Consequently, fewer frameworks can be produced simultaneously, potentially affecting production efficiency. In summary, while AM can produce unique microstructures and textures in metallic components, it is crucial to carefully consider the manufacturing process's orientation and support structures to optimize the mechanical properties of elements like clasps in RPDs. Although this approach may limit production capacity, it ensures the best possible performance and fatigue resistance for the final product.

While there is no consistent evidence to suggest that frameworks designed and manufactured digitally are superior. RPD frameworks produced using CAD-CAM technology exhibit greater mechanical strength compared to those made with conventional casting methods. However, it is noted that the fitting accuracy of CAD-CAM frameworks might not always surpass that of conventionally produced RPDs. This is because human, technical factors can still have an impact on the quality of the framework. For instance, errors in the initial scanning process, inaccuracies in the design, or imperfections introduced during the finishing and polishing stages can affect the overall fit of the framework. Ensuring that all stages of the CAD-CAM process are performed with care and precision can help mitigate these potential issues and optimize the final product's fit and quality. Future research should focus on both CAM technology and CAD software to enhance the design and manufacturing of RPD frameworks.

19.6.1.2 Titanium

Titanium has gained prominence in dentistry thanks to its numerous beneficial properties, a significant portion of which bear a resemblance to the attributes of cobalt chromium. As a biocompatible, corrosion-resistant, ductile, and lightweight metal, titanium offers excellent mechanical strength while maintaining a lower density than other metals. Grade IV titanium, in particular, is the recommended choice for fabricating RPD frameworks. Despite initial challenges in casting titanium, recent advancements in material science and technology have enabled the fabrication of RPD frameworks using commercially pure titanium. Research indicates that cast CoCr and cast titanium frameworks perform similarly in terms of porosity, surface roughness and clinical fit. With the advent of CAM, SLS/SLM and milling methods have been employed to produce titanium frameworks. Nonetheless, titanium's low machinability compared to other dental alloys requires extended milling durations, leading to considerable wear and tear on the cutting instruments. This wear leads to decreased milling accuracy and increased material waste, making the process highly inefficient. Regarding additively manufactured titanium RPD frameworks, there is a limited body of research available. Studies that have investigated laser-sintered titanium clasps have reported varying results, potentially due to differences in handling and polishing protocols. A particular research study observed that clasps produced using SLM displayed greater initial retentive forces; however, retention notably decreased after laboratory cycling. The researchers determined that laser sintering of titanium needs additional refinement before it can be employed in clinical environments. On the other hand, another study found that retention of laser sintered titanium clasps was comparable to that of cast titanium clasps, with the latter experiencing a more significant decline in retentive capacity after multiple insertions and removals.

In clinical practice, additive manufacturing (AM) can sometimes result in rough surfaces due to larger particle sizes (greater than 50 μm). Şahin et al. investigated the impact of different manufacturing techniques on the corrosion resistance, surface hardness and ion release of Ti-6Al-4V and CoCr alloys produced through SLS and CAD-CAM milling. They discovered that the Ti-6Al-4V alloy exhibited the highest corrosion density. These findings have implications for clinical practice. As different manufacturing techniques can influence the metal ion release, surface hardness, and electrochemical corrosion of dental prosthetics, it is essential for dental professionals to be aware of the potential consequences when choosing a fabrication method. The presence of rough surfaces or increased corrosion can lead to increased plaque accumulation, reduced biocompatibility, and possible allergenic reactions. To address these concerns, clinicians may need to implement additional steps in the fabrication process, such as polishing and finishing, to achieve a smoother surface and minimize the risk of complications. Furthermore, the selection of the appropriate manufacturing technique should be carefully considered to ensure the optimal balance between the desired mechanical properties and biocompatibility of the dental prosthetic. By understanding the influence of manufacturing techniques on the properties of dental alloys, dental professionals can make informed decisions on the most suitable fabrication method for their patients' needs, ultimately improving the quality and longevity of dental prosthetics.

Despite the promising nature of titanium as a dental material, additional research and development are necessary to optimize its use in RPD frameworks, especially when employing additive manufacturing techniques. As it stands, clinical practitioners must weigh the benefits and drawbacks of using titanium for RPD frameworks, considering factors such as cost, efficiency, and the current state of the technology. While titanium has the potential to revolutionize dental prosthetic fabrication, ongoing studies, and technological advancements are essential to fully realize its capabilities in clinical practice.

19.6.2 Metal Free-Based Frameworks

Digital RPDs have gained popularity in recent years due to their superior accuracy, efficiency, and aesthetics compared to traditional RPDs. One of the significant developments in digital RPDs is the use of metal-free frameworks, which can be fabricated using various methods. Regardless of the method used, metal-free frameworks offer several advantages over traditional metal frameworks, such as improved aesthetics, biocompatibility, and reduced weight. However, some limitations are also to consider, such as reduced strength and durability compared to metal frameworks. You can see more detailed information on traditional methods of metal free-based frameworks in RPDs (see Chap. 12). Overall, developing metal-free frameworks in digital RPDs represents an exciting advancement in dental technology that offers several benefits for patients and practitioners alike. Several materials can be used as a base framework for digital metal-free removable partial dentures (RPDs). Some common options:

1. **Polyaryletherketone polymers (PAEK)**
    - **1.1. Polyetheretherketone (PEEK)**
    - **1.2. Polyetherketoneketone (PEKK)**
2. **Polyamide (Nylon)**
3. **Polyoxymethylene (Acetal resin)**
4. **Aryl ketone polymer (AKP)**
5. **Graphene-based polymers (GBP)**
6. **Zirconia**

19.6.2.1 Polyaryletherketone Polymers (PAEK)

Polyaryletherketones (PAEK) are a group of high-performance, semi-crystalline thermoplastics. Different members of this family have varying ether and keto groups. The more keto groups they have, the more rigid the glass and polymer chain, and the higher the melting temperature. In modern dentistry, two polymers from the PAEK family are widely used: polyetheretherketone (PEEK) and polyetherketoneketone (PEKK). These materials are highly biocompatible, corrosion-resistant, durable, and characterized by low shrinkage, making them ideal for use in the construction of removable and fixed prosthetic frameworks, as well as dental implant applications. Additionally, they can be processed using extrusion, milling, compression-molding, injection-molding methods due to their versatility.

Polyetheretherketone (PEEK)

New materials have been developed due to advances in technology. PEEK belongs to the PAEK family of high-performance thermoplastic polymers. PEEK is an alternative to metal for dental procedures, including implants, abutments, and prosthetic frameworks (Fig. 19.7). PEEK has superior physical and mechanical properties, is resistant to high temperatures, is biocompatible, lightweight, and chemically stable. This makes it less stressful for teeth and abutments and less likely to accumulate plaque compared to metals and other resins.

The manufacturing methods of PEEK frameworks for RPDs generally involve either milling or pressing. Milling involves machining the PEEK material with a CAD-CAM system, while pressing involves the application of heat and pressure to form the material into the desired shape. In comparison to the other fabrication methods, such as the lost wax technique or selective laser melting (SLM), milling offers greater accuracy, while pressing provides improved adaptation. Milling PEEK frameworks involves a CAD program and a CAM system. The CAD program first creates a 3D model of the framework and then the CAM system uses a mechanized tool (often a milling machine) to cut the material into the desired shape. This technique allows for high accuracy in detail, flexibility in design, and most importantly, reduced distortion in the framework compared to other methods. In vitro study evaluating producing method PEEK frameworks concluded that the milling technique is more accurate than the pressing technique, and the pressing technique has better adaptation than milling.

PEEK frameworks have a natural appearance, making them an ideal material for RPD frame-

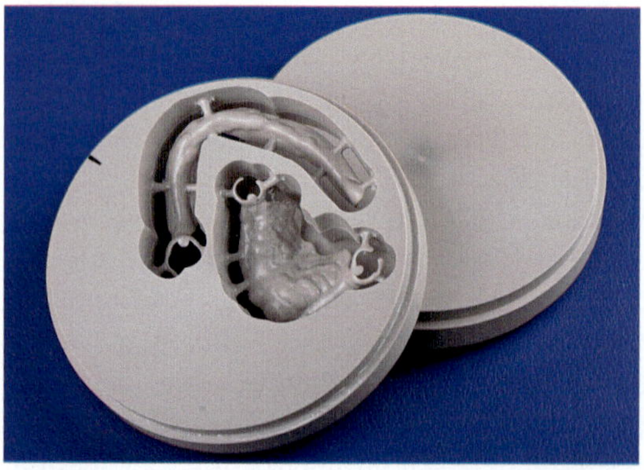

Fig. 19.7 Alternative materials for RPD frameworks

works. PEEK's translucency allows it to blend in seamlessly with the surrounding teeth and tissues, providing a natural and aesthetic appearance. This feature is particularly important for patients who are concerned about the appearance of their dental prosthesis, as it ensures that the prosthesis is discreet and virtually invisible Studies have found that PEEK frameworks fabricated with CAD-CAM systems provide improved aesthetics and require fewer adjustments. However, a randomized controlled experimental crossover study conducted by Ali et al. on 26 patients evaluated the performance of PEEK and CoCr frameworks for RPDs in terms of oral health-related quality of life, patient preference, periodontal indices, and denture satisfaction. The study results were comparable for both materials, indicating no significant preference for either, or improvement in denture satisfaction. There are several factors that may explain why the PEEK framework did not demonstrate superiority over the metal framework in RPDs. The study included a relatively small sample size of 26 patients, which may limit the generalizability of the findings to a larger population. Additionally, the study only evaluated the performance of the two materials in the short term, and it is possible that longer-term studies may yield different results. Such studies will help to ensure that the use of PEEK frameworks in RPDs is safe, effective, and produces favorable patient outcomes.

Another advantage of PEEK frameworks is their biocompatibility. PEEK is an inert material, which means it does not react with the surrounding tissues, reducing the risk of adverse reactions or inflammation. This feature makes PEEK an ideal material for patients with allergies or sensitivities to metals commonly used in dental prostheses. Furthermore, PEEK's biocompatibility and lack of toxicity make it a suitable material for use in contact with oral mucosa, making it an excellent choice for RPD frameworks. Patients have reported higher levels of satisfaction with PEEK clasps compared to metal, and fewer complications such as gingival irritation. Moreover, PEEK clasps show resistance to plaque buildup, making them easier to maintain. However, to date, there is no established standard for the design of PEEK frameworks with regard to factors such as the choice of clasps, depth of support, thickness, or biomechanics. Additional clinical research is required to obtain a more comprehensive understanding of the most effective planning and restoration approaches when utilizing PEEK frameworks in RPDs. Additionally, PEEK clasps distribute the patient's chewing forces more evenly, thus reducing the amount of stress placed on the periodontal ligaments. Furthermore, PEEK clasps are found to help prevent the overloading of the teeth that may be caused by other materials. Finally, studies suggest that the height and shape of the gums remain unchanged by PEEK-based RPDs over a short period of 1 year. In comparison to other materials, PEEK clasps offer a number of advantages for fabricating RPD frameworks. A different research investigation aimed to assess the bonding between the clasp surface and connectors fabricated from PEEK, as well as the connection with the resin base. The study found that pre-treatment of the PEEK surface with airborne-particle abrasion using 50-mm Al203 particles improved the union with the resin base. The study also reported no clinical complications related to the resin part after a 2-year follow-up. These findings indicate that the use of PEEK in combination with resin may be a viable alternative to traditional metal and resin frameworks. Additional studies are necessary to validate these results and to refine the design and manufacturing processes of PEEK frameworks intended for utilization in RPDs.

3D printing has emerged as a viable option for the fabrication of customized PEEK frameworks for RPDs. The most commonly used additive manufacturing methods for producing PEEK frameworks in RPDs include fused deposition modeling (FDM) or fused filament fabrication (FFF) and selective laser sintering (SLS). Utilizing a nozzle that heats and melts PEEK filament, FDM constructs the desired object by depositing material in layer by layer. Conversely, SLS relies on a laser that selectively melts and binds PEEK powder particles to fabricate the intended framework. These approaches both deliver high accuracy and precision while enabling the creation of elaborate structures and personalized designs. Another advantage of 3D printing PEEK RPD frameworks is the ability to customize the prosthesis to the patient's specific needs and preferences. Considerations encompass aspects like the framework's dimensions and form, the positioning of clasps and retentive components, as well as the prosthesis's hue and surface. 3D printing PEEK RPD frameworks, by enabling the creation of highly precise and customized prostheses, 3D printing technology can significantly improve patient outcomes and quality of life.

In terms of relining methods, heat-processed acrylic resin denture bases are typically used for cobalt chromium RPDs as these materials offer excellent bond strength and longevity. For PEEK frameworks, however, there are fewer relining options available due to the difficulty of bonding with acrylics or composites. Studies have shown that preparing the polymer material by sandblasting and priming before bonding with denture acrylic can result in significantly increased shear bond strength. This technique involves sandblasting the PEEK material with either alumina or aluminum oxide particles, followed by a priming procedure with a special adhesive. However, there is not yet a standard clinical guideline or suggestion for relining PEEK frameworks as this is an evolving technology. In addition, self-curing acrylics may also be used for relining PEEK frameworks, although the bond strength may be relatively weaker than that of heat-processed acrylics. Despite its numerous advantages, using PEEK in RPDs also presents some challenges. One of the main challenges is the difficulty of polishing of PEEK frameworks. PEEK is a highly crystalline material, which makes it challenging to achieve a smooth surface finish using traditional polishing techniques. To overcome these challenges, clinicians may need to use specialized polishing tools and techniques, as well as innovative approaches to adjusting the fit of the prosthesis. In addition, ongoing research is required in order to identify new ways to improve the surface finish of PEEK frameworks to optimize patient outcomes.

Based on the literature, PEEK appears to be a promising material for use in removable dental prostheses, with several studies reporting satisfactory clinical outcomes. Although studies have shown promising results regarding the use of PEEK in dental prosthetics, it is important to note that many of these studies have been relatively small in scale and short in duration. Large-scale, controlled studies with more extended follow-up periods will be necessary to fully assess the clinical benefits and limitations of PEEK as a framework material for removable dental prostheses. Such studies can help to establish best practices for PEEK use in RPDs and provide clinicians with more confidence in the material's long-term clinical performance (Figs. 19.8 and 19.9).

Polyetherketoneketone (PEKK)

PEKK is a type of material used in dentistry. It comes in two forms: crystalline and amorphous. Crystalline PEKK is strong and resistant to chemicals, used for bridges and crowns. Amorphous PEKK is more flexible and easier to work with, so it is often used for removable pros-

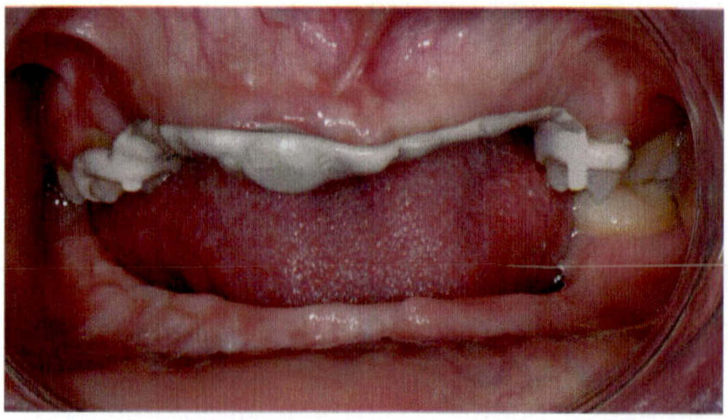

Fig. 19.8 Alternative materials for RPD frameworks. Intraoral situation

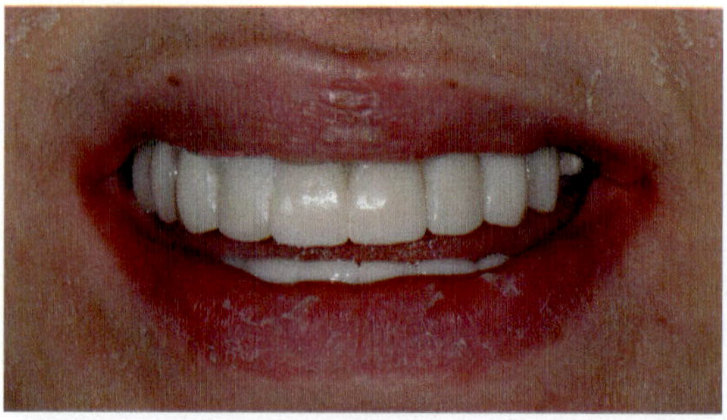

Fig. 19.9 Model-free workflow with PEEK framework and permanent restorative resins. Final result

theses. Overall, PEKK is a better material than other PAEK materials because it has superior physical and chemical properties. As per the manufacturer's claims, PEKK exhibits superior long-term fatigue and up to 80% greater compressive strength properties in comparison to unreinforced PEEK. PEKK has a similar modulus of elasticity to bone and dentine, facilitating stress distribution, shock absorption, and stress reduction at the terminal abutment in dental prosthetics, ultimately enhancing their performance and longevity.

The advantages of using PEKK frameworks in RPDs include superior mechanical strength and fatigue resistance, excellent dimensional accuracy, good corrosion and chemical resistance, and biocompatibility. However, there are a few disadvantages to using PEKK. It is a relatively expensive material and the fabrication process is relatively complex, which may increase the overall cost. Additionally, PEKK is a thermoplastic material, which makes it difficult to polish and requires special processes.

PEKK frameworks are manufactured using CAD-CAM methods. The production time for PEKK frameworks is significantly reduced compared to traditional casting methods, and the cost of production is relatively low, making it an attractive option for both dentists and patients These methods allow PEKK frameworks to be precisely fabricated in complex geometrical shapes with high dimensional accuracy and repeatability. 3D printing is also being used as an additive manufacturing process for PEKK frameworks in RPDs. The primary difference between digital manufacturing PEKK frameworks and digital manufacturing PEEK frameworks in RPDs is the material used. Whereas PEEK frameworks are typically made from a combination of polymers and ceramics, PEKK frameworks are milled from a single block of PEKK (a high-strength polymer). This offers higher accuracy and strength to the framework, as well as greater durability in the mouth. Additionally, PEKK frameworks can be designed with more precision and tailored to fit a patient's exact dentition, unlike PEEK frameworks which cannot. Despite the differences between PEEK and PEKK, both materials have shown promising results in short-term studies for use in RPD frameworks. The choice between PEEK and PEKK depends on each patient's specific requirements and the dental practitioner's preferences. Factors such as occlusal force, flexibility, biocompatibility, and aesthetic appeal should be considered when choosing between PEEK and PEKK frameworks. Further research and development in this field are likely to increase the use of both materials in dentistry.

19.6.2.2 Polyamide (Nylon)

Polyamide belongs to the nylon family and is a popular choice for replacing acrylic resins. It has been used in the dental market since the 1950s. Polyamides are heat-resistant and less soluble in solvents due to their crystalline structure. The success of these prostheses is largely attributed to their high flexibility, low elastic modulus, and fracture resistance, in addition to a substantial resistance to acid and alkalis. These unique characteristics allow for reliable denture retention due to their ability to extend into undercuts of abutment teeth. However, they require a specific design and greater undercut, and are flexible, which makes them comfortable especially for older patients.

Polyamides can be produced using CAD-CAM, especially for RPDs without clasps, in a completely digital process. Polyamides based RPDs are manufactured through a combination of subtractive and additive techniques. Subtractive manufacturing involves removal of material from a single block of plastic to create the base of the denture, while additive manufacturing utilizes 3D printing and laser sintering to form the denture layer-by-layer. Each process has its own advantages and disadvantages, depending on the individual needs of the patient and the dentist. For RPDs, subtractive manufacturing offers the benefit of simplifying the manufacturing process and reducing the amount of manual labor needed to achieve accurate shapes.

Additive manufacturing provides the benefit of creating highly precise and anatomically-accurate components. The two most common additive manufacturing processes used for polyamides in RPDs are SLS and FFF. FFF is a rapid process which involves melting and extruding plastic filaments onto each layer of an object, creating intricate designs and geometries. SLS utilizes a laser to sinter powder materials, fusing them together to produce an object. These processes are ideal for producing high precision and complex structures, such as small medical devices and large aerospace components. FDM is another type of AM process used for producing polyamides in RPDs. This process is similar to FFF and utilizes the same nozzle-based method, but uses a continuous filament of plastic material instead of plastic filaments. FDM is ideal for creating large projects with high-density filament, making it a great choice for creating RPDs.

Recent studies have explored the use of FDM printing method and polyamide material for creating temporary solutions for small gaps, particularly for non-metal clasp RPD fabrication. The effectiveness of intraoral scanning and FDM printing of a gingiva-colored polyamide non-metal clasp RPD was evaluated in a clinical study, with promising results as a temporary solution until the patient underwent implant placement.

Polyamide material has gained attention recently as a suitable material for clasps in RPDs due to its excellent mechanical properties and biocompatibility. Polyamide clasps have several benefits over traditional metal clasps. They are lightweight, flexible, and more natural, making them more aesthetically pleasing. Polyamide clasps also provide a more comfortable fit for patients as they distribute forces more evenly and are less prone to irritating soft tissues. While polyamide clasps offer many benefits, they do have some limitations. The material may be inclined to wear and discoloration over time, and the clasp may need to be stronger than traditional metal clasps. However, these limitations can be addressed through the addition of reinforcing fibers or other additives.

19.6.2.3 Polyoxymethylene (Acetal Resin)

Polyoxymethylene (POM), also known as acetal resin, is created by polymerizing formaldehyde. It has become a popular material in the automotive industry due to its high crystallinity, which results in stiffness, fatigue resistance, and good appearance. Compared to Polymethylmethacrylate (PMMA), POM has higher wear resistance, fracture toughness, and microhardness. It is also chemically and thermally stable, making it a good choice for medical implants. This material has since gained traction in the field of dentistry, gaining popularity for its numerous benefits. Since the 1980s, POM has been used by dentists as an alternative to metal for constructing denture bases and clasps, due to its desirable esthetic qualities and increased strength.

The production of RPDs, based on POM, can be achieved through both subtractive and additive fabrication methods. Digital production methods such as CAD-CAM technology can also be utilized to produce POM-based RPDs, offering high-accuracy digital imaging and fabrication that results in more lightweight and aesthetically pleasing designs compared to conventional production methods. A clinical case report by Teeranuwat et al. described a partially edentulous patient who sought a lightweight and aesthetically pleasing denture. The report evaluated the success of the patient's denture, which was produced using CAD-CAM technology with POM blocks. The report concluded that the denture provided a secure and comfortable fit, with no considerable deterioration after 1 year. The patient expressed satisfaction with the denture's appearance and weight. The use of CAD-CAM technology in producing POM-based RPDs has several advantages. Digital imaging and fabrication provide high accuracy and precision, resulting in a more comfortable and secure fit for the patient.

POM clasps are an alternative to metal clasps in RPDs. One of the benefits of POM clasps is that they do not suffer from deformation, unlike metal clasps, which may experience a loss of retention due to their malleability. Previous studies have suggested that POM clasps have lower retention properties when compared to metal clasps. However, the addition of increased thickness and an undercut of the POM clasp can render it capable of providing sufficient retention in clinical applications. The use of POM clasps in

RPDs has several advantages. They are biocompatible and have a low friction coefficient, which reduces wear and tear on the abutment teeth. POM clasps are also aesthetically pleasing and can be matched to the color of the teeth and gingiva, which is important for patients' confidence and self-esteem. One limitation of POM clasps is that they may not be suitable for patients with allergies to plastic materials. Additionally, POM clasps may require more frequent adjustments due to their lower rigidity compared to metal clasps.

Water and color staining are undesirable qualities that can affect the aesthetics of a restoration. When a POM material is exposed to water, it can absorb and trap moisture, leading to damage to the restoration due to corrosion or discoloration. Additionally, color staining occurs when certain colors are absorbed by the POM, resulting in an alteration in its appearance. This can lead to a diminished esthetic effect of the restoration. Both water and color staining can reduce the longevity of the restoration, which is why it is important to choose a POM material that is highly resistant to these effects. CAD CAM technology has allowed for the creation of high-quality parts made from POM materials that are highly resistant to water and color staining. This is due to the precision and accuracy of the digital manufacturing process, which enables the parts to be made to tighter tolerances and finer structural features. This results in a POM with reduced porosity, creating a more impervious surface that is less susceptible to water and color staining. As such, digital manufacturing can offer POM parts that are extremely resistant to such effects, offering improvements in the longevity and aesthetic of the restoration. A laboratory study by Kamal compared the staining susceptibility of three CAD-CAM milled denture base materials (Polyoxymethylene (POM), Polyetheretherketone (PEEK) and Polymethylmethacrylate (PMMA), when exposed to various storage media. The results showed that the POM denture base material had the lowest color changes, followed by the PEEK denture base material. The acrylic resin denture base material had the most notable differences in color.

To ensure their long-term success and patient satisfaction, denture base materials must possess superior physical and mechanical properties that enable them to function effectively in the unique environment of the oral cavity. These properties include durability, strength, and biocompatibility, among others, which are crucial for ensuring the stability and performance of dental prosthetics. Cracking or fracturing of the denture base is a common issue in dental practice, often arising from heavy biting forces or accidental impact, which can cause significant discomfort to the patient and require costly repairs or replacements. Additionally, incorrect denture design or improper fabrication methods can also contribute to denture fracture. Kamal also conducted a study evaluating the fracture toughness and surface micro-hardness of PMMA and POM denture base materials constructed using either the heat polymerized conventional method (lost wax method) or the CAD-CAM milling method. The results of the study indicate that denture base materials constructed using the CAD-CAM method possess superior mechanical properties compared to those constructed using conventional methods.

19.6.2.4 Aryl Ketone Polymer (AKP)

Aryl Ketone Polymer (AKP) is a recently developed high-performance material. Ultaire AKP was created to address a gap in the market by offering dentures. AKP does not contain monomer or nickel, which makes it fully biocompatible and suitable for patients with nickel sensitivity. In vitro tests have also shown that AKP supports less biofilm growth of C. albicans and cariogenic Streptococci than CoCr, making it more hygienic. Clinical trials have also demonstrated that AKP RPDs are preferred to CoCr RPDs, with improved oral health-related quality of life recorded for 78.9% of patients. They can also be autoclave-disinfected because they are heat-resistant. AKP is a polymer that has been found to have improved cleaner-induced surface roughness compared to other polymers.

AKP is milled on five-axis milling machines, presenting superior mechanical and retention qualities compared to other materials, as well as greater aesthetics and comfort. The digital production process allows for greater precision and accuracy in the fabrication of RPD frameworks. The use of five-axis milling machines enables precise milling of AKP blocks according to the digital design, resulting in a customized framework that fits the patient's dental arches and remaining teeth accurately. Furthermore, superior fatigue properties enable the RPD to withstand non-ideal removal conditions without deformation.

19.6.2.5 Graphene-Based Polymers (GBP)

Graphene is a new material made through nanotechnology that is used to develop other materials. Graphene-based polymer composites are used in many dental applications, such as orthodontics, restorative dentistry, prosthodontics, and implant dentistry, where they can enhance the mechanical properties and antimicrobial characteristics of PMMA. The material is composed of two components: graphene oxide (GO) and its reduced form (GOr), which are milled and processed using CAD-CAM to produce discs for use in milled parts that have previously been 3D-designed.

Digital manufacturing of GBP frameworks for RPDs offer several potential benefits over traditional fabrication methods. GBP frameworks represent a combination of graphite particles and polymer resins, typically employed to produce a denture base with greater strength and flexibility. The exact composition of these materials can be adapted to a patient's specific needs to ensure the production of a device with the necessary mechanical properties. When used in RPDs, these materials can significantly reduce the thickness of the framework and help to create an aesthetically pleasing prosthesis. Another advantage of GBP frameworks is their accuracy. When digitally designed and milled, the frameworks can be accurately fitted to a patient's oral cavity for improved adaptation. This increased accuracy also leads to improved fit and easier insertion of the prosthesis. The material is also biocompatible and exhibits good wear characteristics. The primary disadvantage of GBP frameworks is their cost. Also, due to the material's relatively low mechanical properties, according to an in vitro study conducted by Hussein et al., GBP frameworks may not be suitable for all RPD applications. In the study, PEEK and GBP materials were tested for insertion and removal, as well as resistance to temperature changes. The researchers produced all the clasps with CAD-CAM and compared the performance of the two materials. They concluded that PEEK was a better option for esthetic clasps due to its superior properties.

Graphite-based polymers have lower strength and rigidity than other materials, which makes them more suitable for lightweight structures and applications. On the other hand, digital PEEK frameworks are better suited for structural applications that require high strength, rigidity, and durability. The complex synthesis of PEEK provides superior performance in high-stress environments. It is important to note that while GBP frameworks may not be suitable for all RPD applications, they still have their own advantages and can be used in certain situations.

19.6.2.6 Zirconia

Zirconia is a material made of zirconium dioxide that has properties similar to metal and teeth. Zirconia is also known as "ceramic steel" and is strong, stable, and chemically resistant. The material exhibits mechanical characteristics similar to stainless steel, with a Young's modulus resembling CoCr alloys. However, zirconia may be more likely to break under tension because of natural imperfections in the material.

Zirconia frameworks are used in RPDs. Zirconia can be used to create rests, major connectors, minor connectors, and artificial teeth. The manufacturing process traditionally includes milling a pre-sintered material, sintering the milled material in a furnace, and polishing the final product. The zirconia framework provides numerous advantages, such as being highly biocompatible. Unlike metal-based RPDs, zirconia-based RPDs do not contain nickel or other metals that can cause allergic reactions. This makes them a safer and more comfortable option for patients with metal allergies or sensitivities, including other advantages of having excellent mechanical properties, and being resistant to staining and wear. Zirconia is a highly durable material that can withstand repeated chewing forces and is highly resistant to wear and corrosion. This makes it an ideal material for use in RPDs, which must withstand daily use over an extended period of time. It also has a wide range of strength and can tolerate extreme temperatures. Despite these advantages, zirconia frameworks also have disadvantages, such as a potential for delamination and breakage, inconsistent glaze during sintering, and bland aesthetics.

Zirconia and PEEK both can be used as occlusal rests in RPD. Lyu et al. analyzed the performance of PEEK versus zirconia occlusal rests in RPDs, employing FEA for comparison. The study found that PEEK occlusal rests with a thickness of 1.5 mm and a width of 3.0 mm were the strongest, while a zirconia rest with a width of 2 mm and thickness of 1 mm was sufficiently strong based on stress analysis. Although zirconia is capable of withstanding repeated chewing for long-term use, it may not be as safe as traditional metals in a clinical setting. This is because zirconia restorations have been associated with the potential risk of fracture, particularly when used in thin sections or in areas of high stress. On the other hand, PEEK has been shown to be a safer and more biocompatible material, making it a suitable alternative to zirconia for occlusal rests in RPDs. However, PEEK rests also have disadvantages, such as having a high sensitivity to temperature, being prone to fracturing, and being sensitive to staining. Nevertheless, there is no consensus agreed-upon design for PEEK and zirconia occlusal rests.

Further Reading

Aarts JM, Choi JJE, Metcalfe S, Bennani V. Influence of build angulation on the mechanical properties of a direct-metal laser-sintered cobalt-chromium used for removable partial denture frameworks. J Prosthet Dent. 2021;126:224–30.

Agarwalla SV, Malhotra R, Rosa V. Translucency, hardness and strength parameters of PMMA resin containing graphene-like material for CAD/CAM restorations. J Mech Behav Biomed Mater. 2019;100:103388.

Ahmed N, Abbasi MS, Haider S, Ahmed N, Habib SR, Altamash S, Zafar MS, Alam MK. Fit accuracy of removable partial denture frameworks fabricated with CAD/CAM, rapid prototyping, and conventional techniques: a systematic review. Biomed Res Int. 2021;6:3194433.

Alabdullah SA, Hannam AG, Wyatt CC, McCullagh APG, Aleksejuniene J, Mostafa NZ. Comparison of digital and conventional methods of fit evaluation of partial removable dental prosthesis frameworks fabricated by selective laser melting. J Prosthet Dent. 2022;127:478.e1–478.e10.

Alageel O, Abdallah MN, Alsheghri A, Song J, Caron E, Tamimi F. Removable partial denture alloys processed by laser-sintering technique. J Biomed Mater Res B Appl Biomater. 2018;106:1174–85.

Ali Z, Baker S, Sereno N, Martin N. A pilot randomized controlled crossover trial comparing early OHRQoL outcomes of cobalt-chromium versus PEEK removable partial denture frameworks. Int J Prosthodont. 2020;33:386–92.

Almufleh B, Emami E, Alageel O, de Melo F, Seng F, Caron E, et al. Patient satisfaction with laser-sintered removable partial dentures: a crossover pilot clinical trial. J Prosthet Dent. 2018;119:560–7.e1.

Alsheghri AA, Alageel O, Caron E, et al. An analytical model to design circumferential clasps for laser-sintered removable partial dentures. Dent Mater. 2018;34:1474–82.

Arnold C, Hey J, Schweyen R, Setz JM. Accuracy of CAD-CAM-fabricated removable partial dentures. J Prosthet Dent. 2018;119:586–92.

Bajunaid S, Altwaim B, Alhassan M, Alammari R. The fit accuracy of removable partial denture metal frameworks using conventional and 3D printed techniques: an in vitro study. J Contemp Dent Pract. 2019;20:476–81.

Barraclough O, Gray D, Ali Z, Nattress B. Modern partial dentures—part 1: novel manufacturing techniques. Br Dent J. 2021;230:651–7.

Bibb RJ, Eggbeer D, Williams RJ, Woodward A. Trial fitting of a removable partial denture framework made using computer-aided design and rapid prototyping techniques. Proc Inst Mech Eng H. 2006;220:793–7.

Carneiro Pereira AL, Bezerra de Medeiros AK, de Sousa Santos K, Oliveira de Almeida É, Seabra Barbosa GA, da Fonte Porto Carreiro A. Accuracy of CAD-CAM systems for removable partial denture framework fabrication: a systematic review. J Prosthet Dent. 2021;125:241–8.

Chen H, Ma K, Zhou Y, Wang Y, Sun Y. Effects of selective laser melting process parameters on the accuracy of the intaglio surface of maxillary removable partial denture frameworks. Rapid Prototyp J. 2022;28:1625–35.

Chen X, Mao B, Zhu Z, Yu J, Lu Y, Zhang Q, Yue L, Yu H. A three-dimensional finite element analysis of mechanical function for 4 removable partial denture designs with 3 framework materials: CoCr, Ti-6Al-4V alloy and PEEK. Sci Rep. 2019;9:13975.

Chen H, Li H, Zhao Y, Zhang X, Wang Y, Lyu P. Adaptation of removable partial denture frameworks fabricated by selective laser melting. J Prosthet Dent. 2019;122:316–24.

Chia VAP, See Toh YL, Quek HC, Pokharkar Y, Yap AU, Yu N. Comparative clinical evaluation of removable partial denture frameworks fabricated traditionally or with selective laser melting: a randomized controlled trial. J Prosthet Dent. 2022;5:S0022-3913(22)00011-7.

Dawson JH, Hyde B, Hurst M, Harris BT, Lin WS. Polyetherketoneketone (PEKK), a framework material for complete fixed and removable dental prostheses: a clinical report. J Prosthet Dent. 2018;119:867–72.

Di Carlo S, De Angelis F, Brauner E, Pranno N, Tassi G, Senatore M, Bossù M. Flexural strength and elastic modulus evaluation of structures made by conventional PMMA and PMMA reinforced with graphene. Eur Rev Med Pharmacol Sci. 2020;24:5201–8.

Eggbeer D, Bibb R, Williams R. The computer-aided design and rapid prototyping fabrication of removable partial denture frameworks. Proc Inst Mech Eng H. 2005;219:195–202.

Forrester K, Sheridan R, Phoenix RD. Assessing the accuracy of casting and additive manufacturing techniques for fabrication of a complete palatal coverage metal framework. J Prosthodont. 2019;28:811–7.

Gentz FI, Brooks DI, Liacouras PC, Petrich A, Hamlin CM, Ellert DO, Ye L. Retentive forces of removable partial denture clasp assemblies made from polyaryletherketone and cobalt-chromium: a comparative study. J Prosthodont. 2022;31:299–304.

Gray D, Barraclough O, Ali Z, Nattress B. Modern partial dentures—part 2: a review of novel metal-free materials and innovations in polymers. Br Dent J. 2021;230:813–8.

Grech J, Antunes E. Zirconia in dental prosthetics: a literature review. J Mater Res Technol. 2019;1:4956–64.

Guo F, Huang S, Liu N, Hu M, Shi C, Li D, Liu C. Evaluation of the mechanical properties and fit of 3D-printed polyetheretherketone removable partial dentures. Dent Mater J. 2022;30:816–23.

Hagiwara Y, Nakajima K. Use of ceria-stabilized zirconia/alumina nanocomposite for fabricating the frameworks of removable dental prostheses: a clinical report. J Prosthet Dent. 2016;116:166–71.

Hamanaka I, Isshi K, Takahashi Y. Fabrication of a nonmetal clasp denture supported by an intraoral scanner and CAD-CAM. J Prosthet Dent. 2018;120:9–12.

Hamed HAE, Hebeshi AM, Husseiny E. Effect of palatal vault depth on the trueness of metal laser-sintered and cast cobaltchromium removable partial denture frameworks. J Prosthodont. 2023;32:353–60.

Harb IE, Abdel-Khalek EA, Hegazy SA. CAD/CAM constructed Poly(etheretherketone) (PEEK) framework of Kennedy class I removable partial denture: a clinical report. J Prosthodont. 2019;28:595–8.

Hong MH, Lee DH, Hanawa T, Kwon TY. Comparison of microstructures and mechanical properties of 3 cobalt-chromium alloys fabricated with soft metal milling technology. J Prosthet Dent. 2022;127:489–96.

Hussein MO, Hussein LA. Optimization of digital light processing three-dimensional printing of the removable partial denture frameworks; the role of build angle and support structure diameter. Materials (Basel). 2022a;21:2316.

Hussein MO, Hussein LA. Trueness of 3D printed partial denture frameworks: build orientations and support structure density parameters. J Adv Prosthodont. 2022b;14:150–61.

Hussein MO. Performance of graphene-based and polyether-ether-ketone polymers as removable partial denture esthetic clasp materials after cyclic fatigue. Polymers (Basel). 2022;23:2987.

Hwang S, An S, Robles U, Rumpf RC. Process parameter optimization for removable partial denture frameworks manufactured by selective laser melting. J Prosthet Dent. 2023;129:191–8.

Kamal M. Evaluation of surface micro-hardness and fracture toughness of conventionally constructed versus CAD/CAM constructed denture base materials-an invitro study. Egypt Dent J. 2021;1:757–65.

Kamal MN. Comparative evaluation of color stability between three different CAD/CAM milled denture base materials: an In vitro study. J Int Dent Med Res. 2020;1:854–60.

Kobayashi H, Tasaka A, Higuchi S, Yamashita S. Influence of molding angle on the trueness and defects of removable partial denture frameworks fabricated by selective laser melting. J Prosthodont Res. 2022;7:589–99.

Koike M, Greer P, Owen K, Lilly G, Murr LE, Gaytan SM, Martinez E, Okabe T. Evaluation of titanium alloys fabricated using rapid prototyping technologies-electron beam melting and laser beam melting. Materials (Basel). 2011;10:1776–92.

Koutsoukis T, Zinelis S, Eliades G, Al-Wazzan K, Rifaiy MA, Al Jabbari YS. Selective laser melting technique of Co-Cr dental alloys: a review of structure and properties and comparative analysis with other available techniques. J Prosthodont. 2015;24:303–12.

Lee JW, Park JM, Park EJ, Heo SJ, Koak JY, Kim SK. Accuracy of a digital removable partial denture fabricated by casting a rapid prototyped pattern: a clinical study. J Prosthet Dent. 2017;118:468–74.

Lee JY, An J, Chua CK. Fundamentals and applications of 3D printing for novel materials. Appl Mater Today. 2017;7:120–33.

Lee WF, Wang JC, Hsu CY, Peng PW. Microstructure, mechanical properties, and retentive forces of cobalt-chromium removable partial denture frameworks fabricated by selective laser melting followed by heat treatment. J Prosthet Dent. 2022;127:115–21.

Lee WT, Chen YC. Digitally fabricated dentures for full mouth rehabilitation with zirconia, polyetheretherketone and selective laser melted Ti-6Al-4V material. Int J Environ Res Public Health. 2022;4:3021.

Li R, Malik D, Sadid-Zadeh R. Effect of adding a hard-reline material on the flexural strength of conven-

tional, 3D-printed, and milled denture base materials. J Prosthet Dent. 2023;129:796.
Lima JM, Anami LC, Araujo RM, Pavanelli CA. Removable partial dentures: use of rapid prototyping. J Prosthodont. 2014;23:588–91.
Lin L, Fang Y, Liao Y, Chen G, Gao C, Zhu P. 3D printing and digital processing techniques in dentistry: a review of literature. Adv Eng Mater. 2019;21:1801013.
Liu Y, Fang M, Zhao R, Liu H, Li K, Tian M, Niu L, Xie R, Bai S. Clinical applications of polyetheretherketone in removable dental prostheses: accuracy, characteristics, and performance. Polymers (Basel). 2022;31:4615.
Lo Russo L, Chochlidakis K, Caradonna G, Molinelli F, Guida L, Ercoli C. Removable partial dentures with polyetheretherketone framework: the influence on residual ridge stability. J Prosthodont. 2022;31:333–40.
Lo Russo L, Lo Muzio E, Troiano G, Guida L. Cast-free fabrication of a digital removable partial denture with a polyetheretherketone framework. J Prosthet Dent. 2023;129:262–6.
Lyu H, Murakami N, Yamazaki T, Wada J, Utsumi M, Wakabayashi N. Evaluation of PEEK and zirconia occlusal rest designs for removable partial dentures based on finite element analysis. J Prosthodont Res. 2023;12:196–205.
Marie A, Keeling A, Hyde TP, Nattress BR, Pavitt S, Murphy RJ, Shary TJ, Dillon S, Osnes C, Wood DJ. Deformation and retentive force following in vitro cyclic fatigue of cobalt-chrome and aryl ketone polymer (AKP) clasps. Dent Mater. 2019;1:113–21.
Martin C, Purevdorj-Gage L, Li W, Shary TJ, Yang B, Murphy RJ, Wu CD. In vitro biofilm formation on aryl ketone polymer (AKP), a new denture material, compared with that on three traditional dental denture materials. Int J Dent. 2021;2021:4713510
Maryod WH, Taha ER. Retention of removable partial denture fabricated by digital designing and 3D printing technology—a cross over study. Adv Dent Oral Health. 2019;10:101–6.
Mayinger F, Micovic D, Schleich A, Roos M, Eichberger M, Stawarczyk B. Retention force of polyetheretherketone and cobalt-chrome-molybdenum removable dental prosthesis clasps after artificial aging. Clin Oral Investig. 2021;25:3141–9.
Methani MM, Cesar PF, de Paula Miranda RB, et al. Additive manufacturing in dentistry: current technologies, clinical applications, and limitations. Curr Oral Health Rep. 2020;7:27–334.
Mostafaei A, Rodriguez De Vecchis P, Buckenmeyer MJ, Wasule SR, Brown BN, Chmielus M. Microstructural evolution and resulting properties of differently sintered and heat-treated binder-jet 3D-printed Stellite 6. Mater Sci Eng C Mater Biol Appl. 2019;102:276–88.
Muehlemann E, Özcan M. Accuracy of removable partial denture frameworks fabricated using conventional and digital technologies. Eur J Prosthodont Restor Dent. 2022;29:76–86.
Nakata T, Shimpo H, Ohkubo C. Clasp fabrication using one-process molding by repeated laser sintering and high-speed milling. J Prosthodont Res. 2017;61:276–82.
Negm EE, Aboutaleb FA, Alam-Eldein AM. Virtual evaluation of the accuracy of fit and trueness in maxillary poly(etheretherketone) removable partial denture frameworks fabricated by direct and indirect CAD/CAM techniques. J Prosthodont. 2019;28:804–10.
Nishiyama H, Taniguchi A, Tanaka S, Baba K. Novel fully digital workflow for removable partial denture fabrication. J Prosthodont Res. 2020;64:98–103.
Oh KC, Yun BS, Kim JH. Accuracy of metal 3D printed frameworks for removable partial dentures evaluated by digital superimposition. Dent Mater J. 2022;38:309–17.
Ohkubo C, Sato Y, Nishiyama Y, Suzuki Y. Titanium removable denture based on a one-metal rehabilitation concept. Dent Mater J. 2017;36:517–23.
Peng PW, Hsu CY, Huang HY, Chao JC, Lee WF. Trueness of removable partial denture frameworks additively manufactured with selective laser melting. J Prosthet Dent. 2022;127:122–7.
Peng TY, Ogawa Y, Akebono H, Iwaguro S, Sugeta A, Shimoe S. Finite-element analysis and optimization of the mechanical properties of polyetheretherketone (PEEK) clasps for removable partial dentures. J Prosthodont Res. 2020;64:250–6.
Peng TY, Shimoe S, Fuh LJ, Lin CK, Lin DJ, Kaku M. Bonding and thermal cycling performances of two (poly)aryl-ether-ketone (PAEKs) materials to an acrylic denture base resin. Polymers (Basel). 2021;12:543.
Pordeus MD, Santiago Junior JF, Venante HS, Bringel da Costa RM, Chappuis Chocano AP, Porto VC. Computer-aided technology for fabricating removable partial denture frameworks: a systematic review and meta-analysis. J Prosthet Dent. 2022;128:331–40.
Rokhshad R, Tehrani AM, Nahidi R, Zarbakhsh A. Fit of removable partial denture frameworks fabricated from 3D-printed patterns versus the conventional method: an in vitro comparison. J Prosthet Dent. 2022;18:S0022-3913(22)00210–4.
Rudd RW, Bange AA, Rudd KD, Montalvo R. Preparing teeth to receive a removable partial denture. J Prosthet Dent. 1999;82:536–49.
Scarano A, Orsini T, Di Carlo F, Valbonetti L, Lorusso F. graphene-doped poly (methyl-methacrylate) (Pmma) implants: a micro-CT and histomorphometrical study in rabbits. Int J Mol Sci. 2021;22:1441.
Schweiger J, Güth JF, Erdelt KJ, Edelhoff D, Schubert O. Internal porosities, retentive force, and survival of cobalt-chromium alloy clasps fabricated by selective laser-sintering. J Prosthodont Res. 2020;64:210–6.
Snosi AM, Lotfy SM, Thabet YG, Sabet ME, Rizk FN. Subtractive versus additive indirect manufactur-

ing techniques of digitally designed partial dentures. J Adv Prosthodont. 2021;13:327–32.

Soltanzadeh P, Suprono MS, Kattadiyil MT, Goodacre C, Gregorius W. An in vitro investigation of accuracy and fit of conventional and CAD/CAM removable partial denture frameworks. J Prosthodont. 2019;28:547–55.

Suzuki Y, Shimizu S, Waki T, Shimpo H, Ohkubo C. Laboratory efficiency of additive manufacturing for removable denture frameworks: a literature-based review. Dent Mater J. 2021;31:265–71.

Şahin M, Ünalan F, Mutlu İ. Corrosion, ion release, and surface hardness of Ti-6Al-4V and cobalt-chromium alloys produced by CAD-CAM milling and laser sintering. J Prosthet Dent. 2022;128:529.

Takahashi K, Torii M, Nakata T, Kawamura N, Shimpo H, Ohkubo C. Fitness accuracy and retentive forces of additive manufactured titanium clasp. J Prosthodont Res. 2020;64:468–77.

Takaichi A, Fueki K, Murakami N, Ueno T, Inamochi Y, Wada J, Arai Y, Wakabayashi N. A systematic review of digital removable partial dentures. Part II: CAD/CAM framework, artificial teeth, and denture base. J Prosthodont Res. 2022;11:53–67.

Tan FB, Song JL, Wang C, Fan Y-B, Dai H-W. Titanium clasp fabricated by selective laser melting, CNC milling, and conventional casting: a comparative in vitro study. J Prosthodont Res. 2019;63:58–65.

Tannous F, Steiner M, Shahin R, Kern M. Retentive forces and fatigue resistance of thermoplastic resin clasps. Dent Mater. 2012;28:273–8.

Tasaka A, Shimizu T, Kato Y, Okano H, Ida Y, Higuchi S, Yamashita S. Accuracy of removable partial denture framework fabricated by casting with a 3D printed pattern and selective laser sintering. J Prosthodont Res. 2020;64:224–30.

Teeranuwat P, Jindachua C, Rungsiyakull P, Chaijareenont P. Computer-aided design and computer-aided manufacturing fabricated polyoxymethylene used for maxillary removable partial denture framework. J Int Dent Med Res. 2022;15:306–11.

The glossary of prosthodontic terms: ninth edition. J Prosthet Dent. 2017;117(5S):e1–e105.

Torii M, Nakata T, Takahashi K, Kawamura N, Shimpo H, Ohkubo C. Fitness and retentive force of cobalt-chromium alloy clasps fabricated with repeated laser sintering and milling. J Prosthodont Res. 2018;62:342–6.

Tregerman I, Renne W, Kelly A, Wilson D. Evaluation of removable partial denture frameworks fabricated using 3 different techniques. J Prosthet Dent. 2019;122:390–5.

Tribst JPM, Dal Piva AMO, Borges ALS, Araújo RM, da Silva JMF, Bottino MA, Kleverlaan CJ, de Jager N. Effect of different materials and undercut on the removal force and stress distribution in circumferential clasps during direct retainer action in removable partial dentures. Dent Mater J. 2020;36:179–86.

Wu Q, Zhang N, Dong B, Sun M, Yang X, Yu H. Esthetic rehabilitation for a Kennedy Class IV patient using detachable 3D printing diagnostic denture and removable partial denture with polyetheretherketone framework. Heliyon. 2022;8:e10834.

Yan X, Lin H, Wu Y, Bai W. Effect of two heat treatments on mechanical properties of selective-laser-melted Co-Cr metal-ceramic alloys for application in thin removable partial dentures. J Prosthet Dent. 2018;119:1028.e1–6.

Ye H, Ning J, Li M, Niu L, Yang J, Sun Y, Zhou Y. Preliminary clinical application of removable partial denture frameworks fabricated using computer-aided design and rapid prototyping techniques. Int J Prosthodont. 2017;30:348–53.

You SG, You SM, Lee BI, Kim DY, Kim JH. Effect of layer thickness setting on the adaptation of stereolithography apparatus-fabricated metal frameworks for removable partial dentures: an in vitro study. J Prosthet Dent. 2022;127:276–81.

Zheng J, Aarts JM, Ma S, Waddell JN, Choi JJE. Different undercut depths influence on fatigue behavior and retentive force of removable partial denture clasp materials: a systematic review. J Prosthodont. 2023;32:108–15.

Zheng J, Aarts JM, Ma S, Waddell JN, Choi JJE. Fatigue behavior of removable partial denture cast and laser-sintered cobalt-chromium (CoCr) and polyetheretherketone (PEEK) clasp materials. Clin Exp Dent Res. 2022;8:1496–504.

Zoidis P, Papathanasiou I, Polyzois G. The use of a modified poly-ether-ether-ketone (PEEK) as an alternative framework material for removable dental prostheses. A clinical report. J Prosthodont. 2016;25:580–4.

Part VI

Reestablishing Normal Stomatognathic Function in Partially Edentulous Patients

Management of Temporomandibular Disorders in Partially Edentulous Patients

20

Tonguç Sülün

Abstract

Temporomandibular disorders (TMD) are a common condition that affects the temporomandibular joint (TMJ) and surrounding structures, causing pain and dysfunction. The management of TMD in these patients requires a thorough evaluation of the occlusion, TMJ, and associated musculature. Treatment options may include occlusal splints, physical therapy, medication and occlusal adjustments if needed. The success of TMD management in partially edentulous patients relies on close collaboration between the dentist, physical therapist, and other healthcare professionals. A comprehensive approach that addresses both the underlying causes of TMD and the patient's functional and esthetic needs can lead to improved quality of life and long-term success of the dental restorations.

20.1 Definitions

Centric relation: A maxillomandibular relationship, independent of tooth contact, in which the condyles articulate in the anterior-superior position against the posterior slopes of the articular eminences; in this position, the mandible is restricted to a purely rotary movement; from this unstrained, physiologic, maxillomandibular relationship, the patient can make vertical, lateral or protrusive movements; it is a clinically useful, repeatable reference position.

Grinding-in: A term used to denote the act of correcting occlusal disharmonies by grinding the natural or artificial teeth.

Maximal intercuspal position: The complete intercuspation of the opposing teeth independent of condylar position, sometimes referred to as the best fit of the teeth regardless of the condylar position.

Splint: 1: A rigid or flexible device that maintains in position a displaced or movable part; also used to keep in place and protect an injured part 2: a rigid or flexible material used to protect, immobilize, or restrict motion in a part. (synonym, **occlusal splint**)

Temporomandibular disorders: 1: Conditions producing abnormal, incomplete, or impaired function of the temporomandibular joint(s) and/or the muscles of mastication; 2: (obs) a collection of symptoms frequently observed in various combinations first described by Costen, which he claimed to be reflexes because of irritation of the auriculotemporal and/or chorda tympanic nerves as they emerged from the tympanic plate caused by altered anatomic relations and derangements of the temporoman-

T. Sülün (✉)
Faculty of Dentistry, Department of Prosthodontics, İstanbul University, İstanbul, Türkiye
e-mail: tsulun@istanbul.edu.tr

O. Şakar (ed.), *Removable Partial Dentures*, https://doi.org/10.1007/978-3-031-47083-7_20

dibular joint associated with loss of oclusal vertical dimension, loss of posterior tooth support, and/or other malocclusions; the symptoms can include headache about the vertex and occiput, tinnitus, pain about the ear, impaired hearing, and pain about the tongue.

20.2 Relationship Between Partial Edentulism and Temporomandibular Disorders

There is no universal accepted etiological factor of temporomandibular disorders (TMD) according to the recent literature. Some studies suggested that partial edentulism has only a minor role in the etiology of TMD. Although some cadaver studies are able to show the relationship between posterior tooth loss and arthritic changes in temporomandibular joint (TMJ), there is a consensus in the literature that the causal relationship between occlusion and TMD does not appear. Tooth loss and osteoarthritis (OA) is a natural progression of aging. Thus, the weak correlation between OA and tooth loss has to be reconsidered according to this fact. The historical studies especially from 70s speculated a close relationship of above-mentioned topic using mostly the biomechanical theory. Later studies however confuted this theory. The clinical signs and symptoms of TMD are not always correlated with the anatomical changes in TMJ. Therefore, the results of the clinical researches are more important compared to the cadaver and radiological studies. These studies are also not able to evaluate muscle symptoms of the patients. Consequently, recent clinical studies show weak or no correlation between TMD symptoms and lack of molar support. Additionally, the studies analyzing "shortened dental arch theory" are in consensus that the lack of molar support is not a risk for the development of TMD. This topic was explained in Chap. 5 in details.

However some studies have shown that the loss of a specific tooth may be associated with the development of TMD. One of them have shown that loss of maxillary first premolar tooth has an association with TMD. In another study it was shown that the loss of first molar tooth is related with TMD signs and symptoms. In a clinical study with better statistical analyses, the authors were able to show that not only the number of missing posterior teeth but the number of dental quadrants with missing posterior teeth has an effect on the development of TMD. These studies based their results on the premature contacts and loss of the biomechanical balance as a result of drifting and tipping of the remaining teeth.

Scientists doing research on TMD with more advanced techniques are trying to strengthen the diagnosis by jaw motion trackings, recordings of occlusal contacts, and EMG, radiological techniques. Although it may seem cool to have this information in the patient file, its benefits in clinical practice and treatments are controversial. Advanced technical diagnostic methods may also be unnecessary, especially in partially edentulous patients, due to both age and the inability to transfer this information to treatment. Treatments should be based on eliminating the symptoms caused by TMJ disorders and rehabilitating edentulousness. In cases where there is no response in standard protocol treatments or other diseases are suspected, it will be appropriate to benefit from further examinations.

In patients with partial edentulism, tooth alignment is generally far from ideal. Anterior and lateral tooth guidances have disappeared, or *as a result of early contacts, transition from centric relation to maximal intercuspal position may occur*. Adaptation of patients is a highly possible to these changes. Although it was thought in the early 1970s that patients were trying to achieve occlusal stability and create biomechanical balance by grinding these contacts, there is still no evidence of this today. Premature contacts or interferences would not lead to extraordinary muscle activity in our knowledge with current literature. Since this concept is not accepted nowadays, dentist should examine the physiological and psychological muscle activities of the patients with the multidisciplinary examination of the patients.

Although occlusion does not have a major role in the etiology of TMD, its effect cannot be ignored. This dilemma is still not resolved, experts working on this issue are divided into two as perspective. Occlusion should be evaluated on a case-by-case basis, and its involvement in treatment should be carefully examined. Selective grinding or prosthetic treatments applied to change the occlusion or to complete the missing tooth alignment can make a positive contribution to the treatment, especially in combination with the combination of treatments such as occlusal splint and physical therapy. However, there is no indication to make protective occlusal changes to eliminate TMD symptoms or to eliminate the possibility of disease in future, or to perform prosthetic treatments for same purposes. Protective occlusal changes can only prevent the development of TMD symptoms in children or adolescents for future.

In the light of all this information, the following rules should be taken into account before a prosthetic treatment.

1. If there is a natural occlusion, adaptation is valid in the physiological state and there is a patient without symptoms, no intervention should be made on the occlusion.
2. If natural occlusion is present but problematic, the patient should be followed for a long time after an occlusal splint or similar treatment as phase 1 therapy.
3. If there is an artificial (restorative) occlusion and it is non-problematic, the patient should be observed for a long time.
4. If there is an artificial (restorative) occlusion but it is problematic, the restorations must be renewed according to the ideal occlusion rules.
5. There is only one rule that applies to all situations. A simulation of the planned treatment with temporary restorations should be applied to the patient at a certain time and the patient's adaptation and the condition of the symptoms causing the complaints progress should be tested.

As a conclusion, recent literature does not support a sound relationship between partial edentulism and TMD. However, there are some good researches to point out that tooth loss and occlusal discrepancies may have an impact on the development of the functional disorder of the stomatognathic system. In future the scientists have to focus more on longitudinal studies to show the long-term effect of occlusal changes and the lack of biomechanical stability on the masticatory system disorders.

Now the question is: Should we focus on the replacement of missing posterior teeth to treat the patients with TMD, even though there is no evidence to show such a relation? First of all, we have to discuss the effect of occlusal therapy in the treatment of TMD. Longitudinal studies are not enough to demonstrate a distinction of irreversible occlusal corrections (occlusal grinding or restoration) to more conservative and simple treatment modalities like occlusal splints or physical therapies. There are however a lot of studies that support the success of occlusal splint therapy in rehabilitation of the patients with TMD. Other studies are also not able to show a positive effect of placing fixed or removable prosthesis in the treatment of TMDs, especially if the patient has lost only his/her molar teeth. Thus, there is no need to choose a sophisticated prosthodontic treatment modality for the rehabilitation of the signs and symptoms of TMD. However, in some cases with partial edentulism, there is a need of replacement of missing teeth to make a stabilization appliance. The aim of this chapter is to make clear how to construct an occlusal appliance in various partial edentulism situations.

20.3 Occlusal Splints

The occlusal splint therapy is based on changing the occlusal relations. However, that does not mean that the occlusal relations have to be restored or be adjusted in similar ways. In many cases there is no need for a definite occlusal rehabilitation after the occlusal splint therapy. The occlusal splint therapy is finished after the symptoms of the patient diminish. The treatment should be restarted when the symptoms are returned after the end of the splint therapy. If a definitive therapy with occlusal splint is not possible an irreversible occlusal rehabilitation should be evaluated. Yet, it should be kept in mind that there is no scientific evidence in dental literature that irreversible changes in dental occlusion help to reduce the symptoms of TMD.

20.3.1 How Do Occlusal Splints Rehabilitate Temporomandibular Disorders

1. **The increase of the occlusal vertical dimension**

   The occlusal splints are interocclusal devices which increase the occlusal vertical dimension of the patient for a temporary period. This is a very important characteristic of the occlusal splints. This increase elongates the masseter, temporal, and medial pterygoid muscles, which reduce the isometric contractions. It is well-known that the isometric contractions of the muscles can expose myogenic pain. In contracted muscles the blood circulation is blocked. That means the muscle cannot be nourished and purged. And the pain revealing particles collect in the muscle and expose pain. The physical therapy modalities generally function with this mechanism. The muscle is heated using infrared, laser, massage etc. and the blood circulation is regenerated. Therefore, occlusal splints achieve this goal without using any physical therapy if the patient has bruxism.
2. **The change of the condyle position**

   Placing an occlusal splint in to the mouth of the patient creates a new position of the condyles in the glenoid fossa which is more anterior and caudal to the centric position. Thus, the overload in the articular soft tissues is reduced.
3. **New occlusal relations**

   An occlusal splint should have a flat occlusal surface which eliminates the occlusal interferences and build point contacts with each antagonist teeth. These kind of splints create a harmonic slide between maximal intercuspal position (MIP) and centric relation. Additionally, a stabilization splint should have a canine guided eccentric occlusal balance. Especially the occlusal point contacts are perceived from the proprioceptif receptors in periodontium and this information is sent as an impulse to the Central Pattern Generator in brain. Thus, a decrease of muscle contraction is achieved.

Also, the cognitive awareness of the patient and the placebo effect of the occlusal devices are also important factors for the relief of the sign and symptoms of TMD.

20.3.2 Occlusal Splint Design in Partial Edentulism

First, the clinician should decide which jaw is appropriate for fabricating an occlusal splint. Therefore, the position, number, and size of the edentulous places should be analyzed. Following rules are helpful for a clinician to make the decision:

1. In cases with single (maxillary or mandibular) long, free-ending edentulous arches (unilateral or bilateral), the antagonist jaw (full dentate or with a dentition which is explained in item 3) is ideal to place an occlusal splint and the edentulous jaw should be rehabilitated using a removable partial denture (RPD) (Fig. 20.1a–c). It is not suitable to make a stabilization splint over an RPD and it is also not correct to place a splint to a dental arch with a long free-ending edentulism. It may produce a tilting force on the anterior teeth because of the resilience of the mucosa (Fig. 20.2a, b). An alternative is to make a special designed occlusal splint for only night time use (Fig. 20.3a–f).
2. In cases with both maxillary and mandibular long free-ending edentulous crest (unilateral or bilateral). The patient should be rehabilitated first with RPDs. Afterward, a special designed maxillary occlusal splint should be prepared for the nighttime use.
3. In cases with edentulous gaps or short free-ending situations (e.g., absence of second molar tooth unilateral or bilateral) the

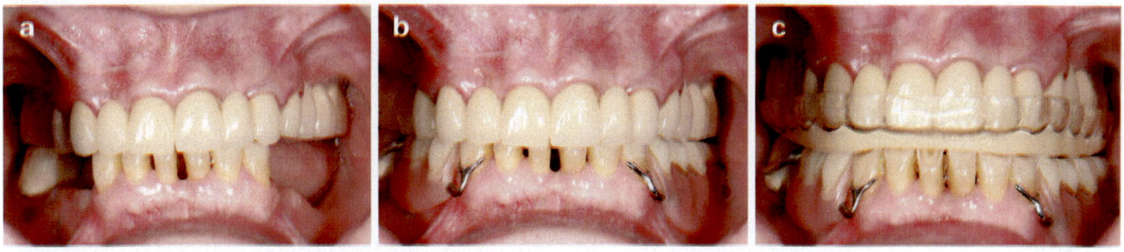

Fig. 20.1 (**a**) A TMD patient with mandibular partial edentulism. Intraoral view in occlusion. (**b**) An RPD is fabricated for the patient first. (**c**) Then a maxillary occlusal splint is fabricated

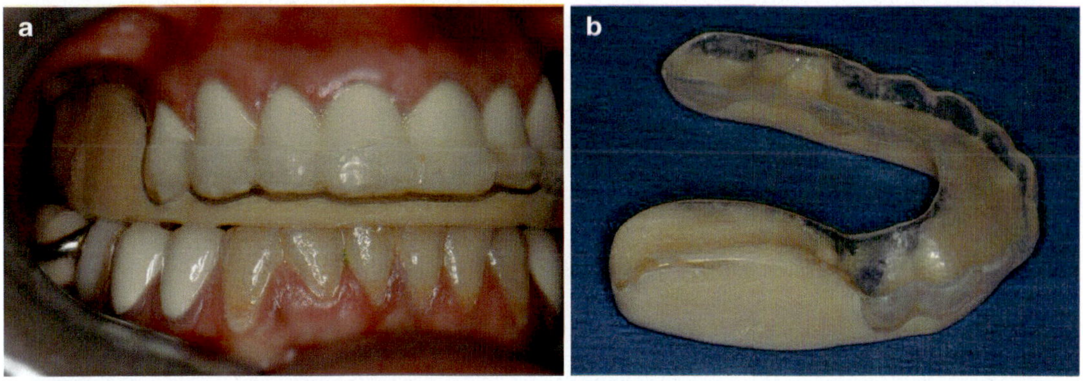

Fig. 20.2 (**a**) An occlusal splint is fabricated to a patient with a long free ending partial edentulism. (**b**) Notice the distal part of the occlusal splint

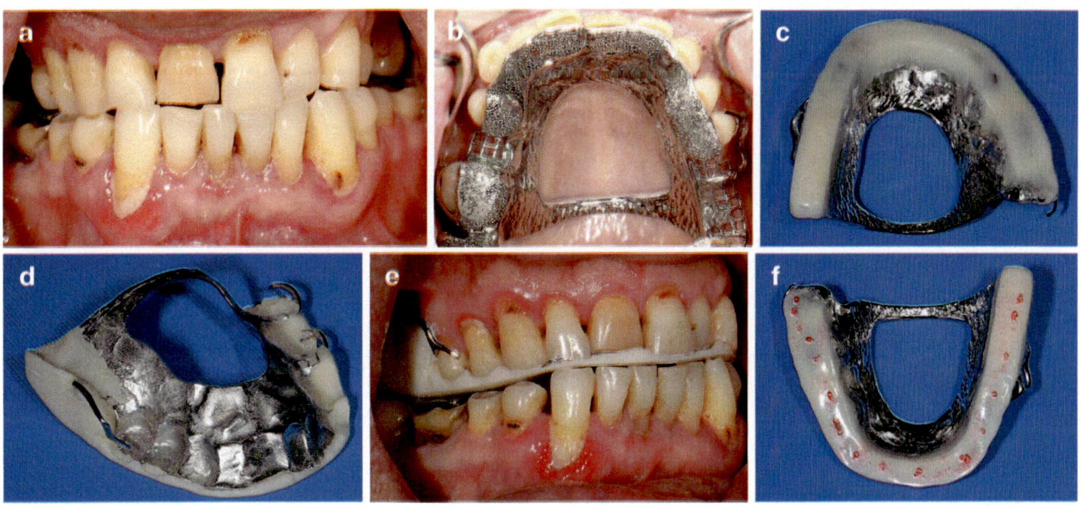

Fig. 20.3 (**a**) A TMD patient with maxillary partial edentulism. Intraoral view in occlusion. (**b**) The metal framework of the special designed occlusal splint. Occlusal view. (**c**) Occlusal splint after positioning using cold curing resin. Occlusal view. (**d**) Occlusal splint after positioning using cold curing resin. Inner view. (**e**) Special designed occlusal splint in the mouth of the patient in occlusion. (**f**) The occlusal point contacts for each antagonist teeth

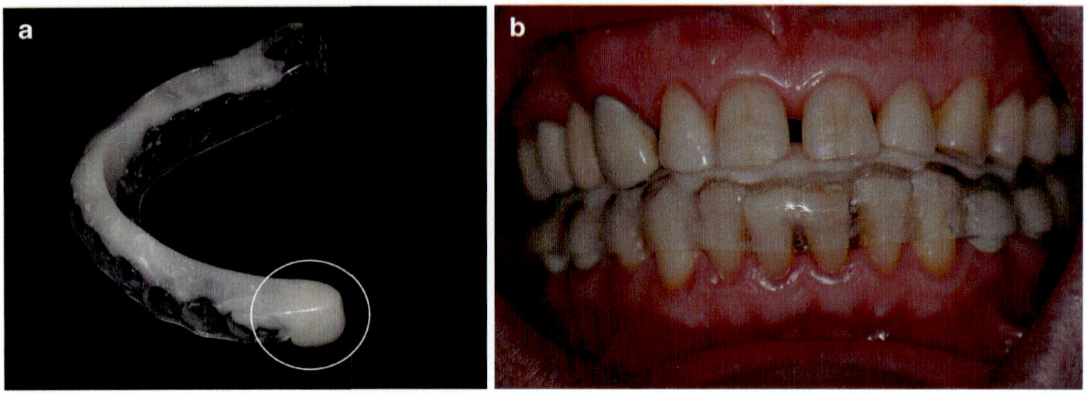

Fig. 20.4 (**a**) A mandibular occlusal splint that also replace the second molar tooth. (**b**) The occlusal splint in the mouth of the patient

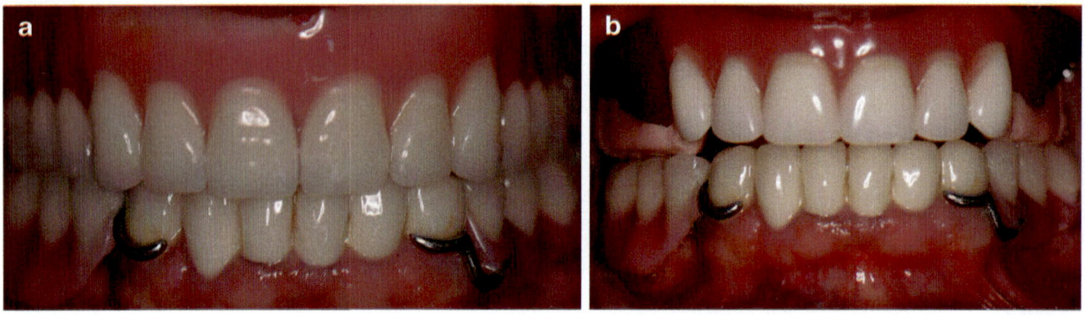

Fig. 20.5 A case with maxillary complete and mandibular partial edentulism who needs TMD management. (**a**) A maxillary complete and mandibular removable partial denture is fabricated. (**b**) A maxillary Shore prosthesis is fabricated for night time use as an occlusal splint

replacement of tooth loss can be done by using the occlusal splint. In such cases the splint should be placed to the jaw with more tooth loss (Fig. 20.4a, b).

4. In cases with mandibular partial and maxillary complete edentulism a mandibular RPD and maxillary complete denture should be prepared if the patient has no prosthesis at all. For night-time use an additionally upper denture (so-called "Shore denture") should be placed to function as an occlusal splint (Fig. 20.5a, b).
5. In cases with mandibular full edentulous arch and maxillary partial edentulism, occlusal splint therapy is contraindicated because of the poor support of mandibular alveolar crest. If the mandibular denture is supported with implants Shore prosthesis could be constructed for the lower jaw.

Further Reading

Al-Jabrah O, Al-Shumailan YR. Prevalence of temporomandibular disorder signs in patients with complete versus partial dentures. Clin Oral Investig. 2006;10:167–73.

Amorim VC, Laganá DC, de Paula Eduardo JV, Zanetti AL. Analysis of the condyle/fossa relationship before and after prosthetic rehabilitation with maxillary com-

plete denture and mandibular removable partial denture. J Prosthet Dent. 2003;89:508–14.
Aras K, Hasanreisoğlu U, Shinogaya T. Masticatory performance, maximum occlusal force, and occlusal contact area in patients with bilaterally missing molars and distal extension removable partial dentures. Int J Prosthodont. 2009;22:204–9.
Bessadet M, Nicolas E, Sochat M, Hennequin M, Veyrune JL. Impact of removable partial denture prosthesis on chewing efficiency. J Appl Oral Sci. 2013;21:392–6.
Carlsson GE. Some dogmas related to prosthodontics, temporomandibular disorders and occlusion. Acta Odontol Scand. 2010;68:313–22.
Clark GT, Tsukiyama Y, Baba K, Simmons M. The validity and utility of disease detection methods and of occlusal therapy for temporomandibular disorders. Oral Surg Oral Med Oral Pathol Oral Radiol Endod. 1997;83:101–6.
Costen JB. A syndrome of ear and sinus symptoms dependent upon disturbed function of the temporomandibular joint. 1934. Ann Otol Rhinol Laryngol. 1997;106:805–19.
Creugers NH, Witter DJ, Van 't Spijker A, Gerritsen AE, Kreulen CM. Occlusion and temporomandibular function among subjects with mandibular distal extension removable partial dentures. Int J Dent. 2010;2010:807850.
Davies SJ, Gray RM, McCord JF. Good occlusal practice in removable prosthodontics. Br Dent J. 2001;191:491–502.
De Boever JA, Carlsson GE, Klineberg IJ. Need for occlusal therapy and prosthodontic treatment in the management of temporomandibular disorders. Part I. Occlusal interferences and occlusal adjustment. J Oral Rehabil. 2000;27:367–79.
De Boever JA, Carlsson GE, Klineberg IJ. Need for occlusal therapy and prosthodontic treatment in the management of temporomandibular disorders. Part II. J Oral Rehabil. 2000;27:647–59.
Farias-Neto A, Martins AP, Sánchez-Ayala A, Rabie AB, Novaes PD, Rizzatti-Barbosa CM. The effect of posterior tooth loss on the expression of type II collagen, IL-1β and VEGF in the condylar cartilage of growing rats. Arch Oral Biol. 2012;57:1551–7.
Forssell H, Kalso E. Application of principles of evidence-based medicine to occlusal treatment for temporomandibular disorders: are there lessons to be learned? J Orofac Pain. 2004;18:9–22; discussion 23–32.
İspirgil E, Erdoğan SB, Akın A, Şakar O. The hemodynamic effects of occlusal splint therapy on the masseter muscle of patients with myofascial pain accompanied by bruxism. Cranio. 2020;38:99–108.
Krzemień J, Baron S. Axiographic and clinical assessment of temporomandibular joint function in patients with partial edentulism. Acta Bioeng Biomech. 2013;15:19–26.
Kurt H, Erdelt KJ, Cilingir A, Mumcu E, Sülün T, Tuncer N, Gernet W, Beuer F. Two-body wear of occlusal splint materials. J Oral Rehabil. 2012;39:584–90.
List T, Axelsson S. Management of TMD: evidence from systematic reviews and meta-analyses. J Oral Rehabil. 2010;37:430–51.
Mahönen KT, Virtanen KK. Occlusion and craniomandibular function among patients treated with removable partial dentures. J Oral Rehabil. 1994;21:233–40.
Marquezan M, Figueiró C. Temporomandibular disorder treatment in a patient wearing removable prostheses: a case report. Cranio. 2017;35:122–7.
Poštić SD. Specific occlusal scheme for partially edentulous patients with TMD signs-preliminary report. J Stomatol Oral Maxillofac Surg. 2018;119:337–47.
Reissmann DR, Heydecke G, Schierz O, Marré B, Wolfart S, Strub JR, Stark H, Pospiech P, Mundt T, Hannak W, Hartmann S, Wöstmann B, Luthardt RG, Böning KW, Kern M, Walter MH. The randomized shortened dental arch study: temporomandibular disorder pain. Clin Oral Investig. 2014;18:2159–69.
Rues S, Lenz J, Türp JC, Schweizerhof K, Schindler HJ. Muscle and joint forces under variable equilibrium states of the mandible. Clin Oral Investig. 2011;15:737–47.
Shroff B. Malocclusion as a cause for temporomandibular disorders and orthodontics as a treatment. Oral Maxillofac Surg Clin North Am. 2018;30:299–302.
Sulun T, Geckili O. A simple technique for increasing the occlusal vertical dimension of removable denture wearers. J Calif Dent Assoc. 2011;39:881–3.
Tallents RH, Macher DJ, Kyrkanides S, Katzberg RW, Moss ME. Prevalence of missing posterior teeth and intraarticular temporomandibular disorders. J Prosthet Dent. 2002;87:45–50.
The glossary of prosthodontic terms: ninth edition. J Prosthet Dent. 2017;117(5S):e1–e105.
Tsukiyama Y, Baba K, Clark GT. An evidence-based assessment of occlusal adjustment as a treatment for temporomandibular disorders. J Prosthet Dent. 2001;86:57–66.
Türp JC, Schindler H. The dental occlusion as a suspected cause for TMDs: epidemiological and etiological considerations. J Oral Rehabil. 2012;39:502–12.
Uchida H, Wada J, Watanabe C, Nagayama T, Mizutani K, Mikami R, Inukai S, Wakabayashi N. Effect of night dentures on tooth mobility in denture wearers with sleep bruxism: a pilot randomized controlled trial. J Prosthodont Res. 2022;66:564–71.
Wang MQ, Xue F, He JJ, Chen JH, Chen CS, Raustia A. Missing posterior teeth and risk of temporomandibular disorders. J Dent Res. 2009;88:942–5.
Weyant RJ. Questional benefit from occlusal adjustment for TMD disorders. J Evid Based Dent Pract. 2006;6:167–8.
Zoidis P, Polyzois G. Removable dental prosthesis splint. An occlusal device for nocturnal bruxing partial denture users. J Prosthodont. 2013;22:652–6.

21 Reestablishing Occlusal Vertical Dimension and Maximal Intercuspal Position in Partially Edentulous Patients

Olcay Şakar

Abstract

Reestablishing occlusal vertical dimension (OVD) and maximal intercuspal position (MIP) may be required in partially edentulous patients with decreased OVD. Also, it may be sometimes necessary to increase the OVD to gain sufficient space for a prosthetic restoration in patients without loss of OVD. Studies have shown that reestablishing the OVD can be successfully performed when an appropriate diagnosis and treatment plan is accomplished. What are the main reasons for decreased OVD? Which methods can be used to reestablish OVD and MIP? How much can OVD be increased? Are there any limitations and/or contraindications? How long is the period of adaptation and which control methods are used in this period? What is the role of overlay removable partial dentures and what are the issues to be considered in the laboratory and clinical procedures during the prosthetic treatment? This chapter will clarify all the above-mentioned questions and be a guide that can be used not only in cases of partial edentulism but also in all cases requiring OVD and MIP reestablishment.

Supplementary Information The online version contains supplementary material available at https://doi.org/10.1007/978-3-031-47083-7_21.

O. Şakar (✉)
Faculty of Dentistry, Department of Prosthodontics, İstanbul University, İstanbul, Türkiye
e-mail: osakar@istanbul.edu.tr

21.1 Definitions

Centric occlusion: The occlusion of opposing teeth when the mandible is in centric relation; this may or may not coincide with the maximal intercuspal position (synonym **Centric relation occlusion**).

Centric relation: A maxillomandibular relationship, independent of tooth contact, in which the condyles articulate in the anterior-superior position against the posterior slopes of the articular eminences; in this position, the mandible is restricted to a purely rotary movement; from this unstrained, physiologic, maxillomandibular relationship, the patient can make vertical, lateral or protrusive movements; it is a clinically useful, repeatable reference position (synonym **Centric relation position**).

Closest speaking space: The space between the anterior teeth when the patient is speaking.

Decreased occlusal vertical dimension: A reduction in the distance measured between two anatomic points when the teeth are in occlusal contact.

O. Şakar (ed.), *Removable Partial Dentures*, https://doi.org/10.1007/978-3-031-47083-7_21

Diagnostic waxing: A waxing of intended restorative contours on dental casts for the purpose of evaluation and planning restorations; a wax replica of a proposed treatment plan. Synonym: **Wax-up.**

Interocclusal rest distance: The difference between the rest vertical dimension and the occlusal vertical dimension. Synonym: **Interocclusal rest space.**

Maximal intercuspal position: The complete intercuspation of the opposing teeth independent of condylar position, sometimes referred to as the best fit of the teeth regardless of the condylar position.

Overlay removable partial denture: Overlay removable partial dentures a subset of overdentures, are often referred to as a removable partial denture that has part of their components covering the occlusal surface of the abutment teeth to restore them into a functional occlusion.

Occlusal vertical dimension: The distance between two selected anatomic or marked points (usually one on the tip of the nose and the other on the chin) when in maximal intercuspal position.

Rest vertical dimension: The postural position of the mandible when an individual is resting comfortably in an upright position and the associated muscles are in a state of minimal contractual activity. Synonym: **Physiologic rest position**, **vertical dimension at rest**.

21.2 Main Reasons for Decreased Occlusal Vertical Dimension in Dentate Individuals

Natural and artificial tooth wear, tooth loss, and migration of the teeth and/or the alveolar process may result in the loss of OVD. In addition, patients with severe dental and skeletal malocclusions and acquired and congenital anomalies may need reestablishment of OVD and MIP.

21.2.1 Tooth Wear

Attrition, erosion, and abrasion are the main reasons that the teeth become worn. In contrast to the past, dental erosion is now considered to be a major cause of tooth wear and dental wear can be seen not just in the older population but also among young people. Since tooth wear is a natural process, it generally does not need any specific treatment, especially if the patient has a proper adaptation. However, the severity of the wear according to morphological changes and the potential for progression in the context of the patient's age should be the determining factors.

In some cases tooth wear occurs, and at the same time tooth surface loss is compensated by continuous tooth eruption and alveolar bone growth. Thus, the OVD remains the same or it is still acceptable without the need to be increased (Fig. 21.1a, b). If a restoration is nec-

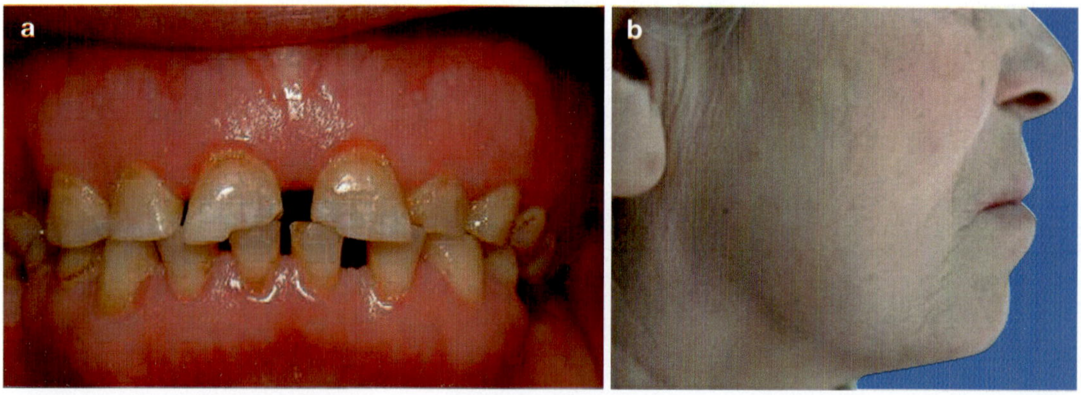

Fig. 21.1 (**a**, **b**) In some cases, tooth wear is accompanied by alveolar bone growth and continuous tooth eruption. Thus, the OVD cannot be decreased. If necessary, treatment alternatives should be applied before increasing the OVD

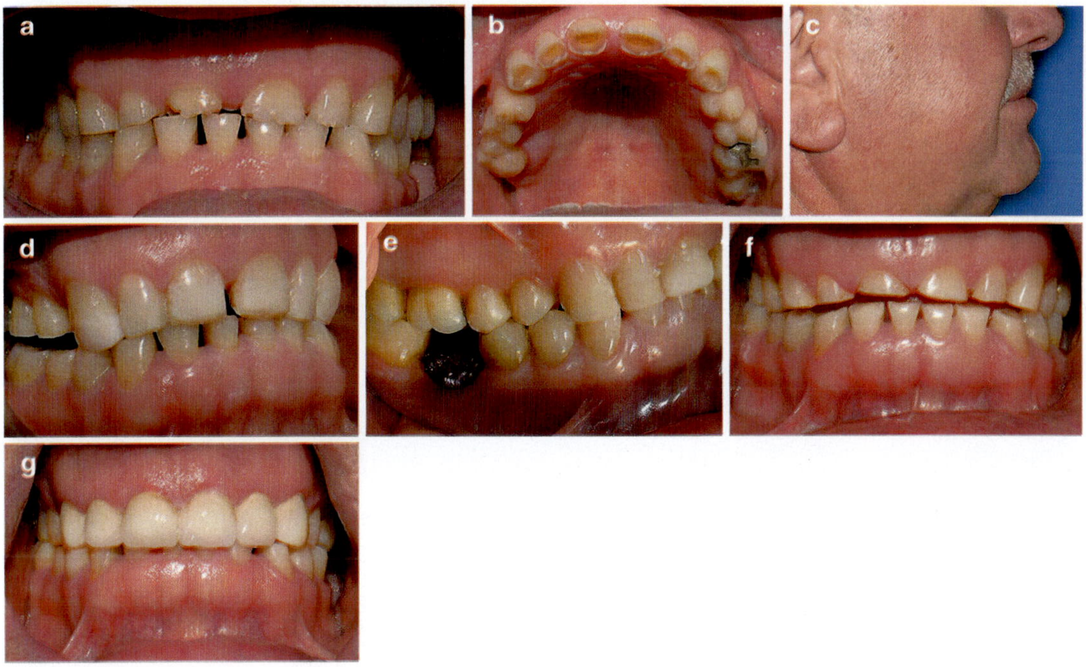

Fig. 21.2 (**a**–**g**) Intraoral examination revealed localized anterior tooth wear (**a**, **b**) and extraoral examination showed that there is no decrease in OVD (**c**). A composite Dahl restoration has been applied to gain sufficient space for prosthetic restoration and posterior disclusion was created (**d**). One year after the composite resin restorations has been applied, occlusion was reestablished (**e**). View of space gained at anterior region after the composite restorations were removed (**f**). Postoperative view with metal–ceramic restorations (**g**)

essary, the treatment options may include periodontal surgery to gain additional clinical crown length and orthodontic movement with limited intrusion. In many cases, only the anterior segments may have been worn. If there is no loss of OVD, a less radical alternative to complete restoration, the principles of combined forced intrusion of anterior teeth and supra eruption of posterior teeth, which were first described by Dahl et al. can be accomplished. An anterior cobalt-chromium removable splint, resin-bonded cast, composite restorations or temporary crowns can be used to accomplish this procedure (Fig. 21.2a–g). In addition to the "Dahl technique," space may be gained if a large horizontal discrepancy exists between centric relation position (CRP) and the MIP, but with little vertical discrepancy, occlusal adjustment of such "centric interferences" will produce a significantly more distal MIP and thereby sufficient palatal space for the full construction of anterior restorations. In cases where the natural mechanisms fail to compensate for tooth wear, the loss of OVD will occur. Consequently, the collapse of the anterior lower facial height requires an increase to restore the subjects to their original OVD. This will create the requisite interocclusal space for the restorative material. When there is general loss of vertical tooth height, careful management of the remaining tooth structure for the retention and resistance of the restoration is needed. Recommended minimal preparation height is at least 3–4 mm. If OVD is increased, it is possible to make a crown restoration with this height of clinic crown without additional treatment (such as crown-lengthening surgery).

Therapy for patients with reduced vertical tooth height includes management of gastroesophageal reflux disorder, dietary advice, fluoride application, monitoring parafunctional habits, and supporting changes in lifestyle.

After elimination of the risk factors of tooth wear, an overlay removable partial denture (ORPD) can be both an interim and permanent treatment option. It is important to be aware that erosive wear may continue under the ORPDs and the occlusal splints if the patients fail to maintain

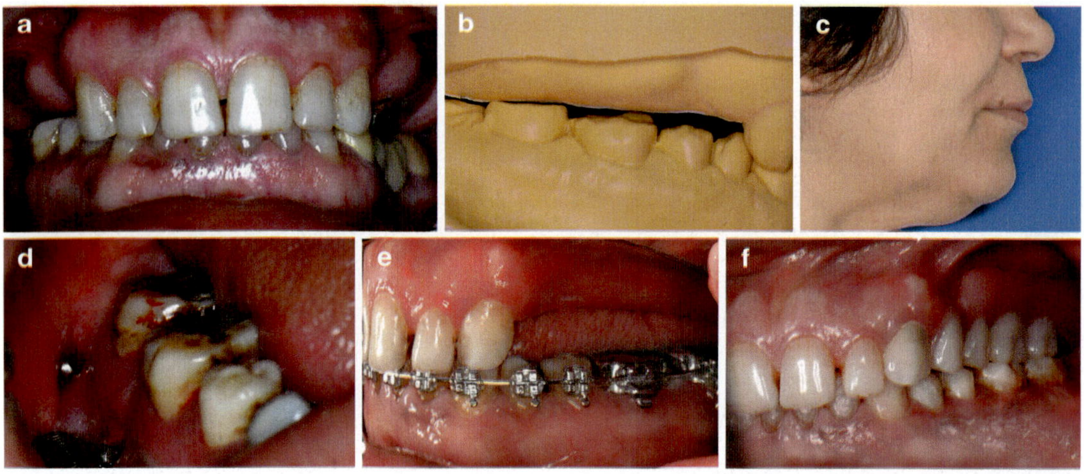

Fig. 21.3 (**a–f**) In some cases without loss of OVD, an orthodontic treatment resulting in intrusion can be an alternative to gain adequate space for prosthetic restoration

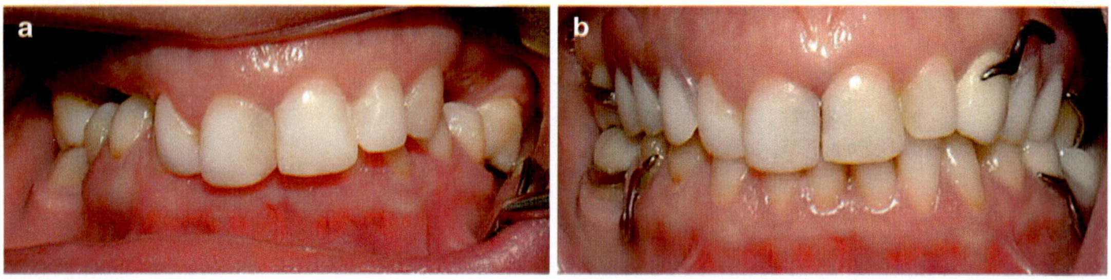

Fig. 21.4 (**a**, **b**) After 11 years of tooth loss without using any prosthetic restoration, migration of teeth accompanied by alveolar bone growth and loss of OVD were observed. ORPD was applied to reestablish OVD to provide functional and esthetic requirements

their oral hygiene. Therefore, regular observation of patients with tooth wear is necessary.

21.2.2 Tooth Loss and Migration of the Teeth and/or Alveolar Process

Occlusal interferences can be created by the overeruption caused by clinically unopposed teeth. In some patients, tooth loss may result in a decrease of the OVD. The potential restoration area may be occupied with migrated teeth and/or the alveolar process. In some cases, in spite of the presence of tooth loss and/or migrating of the teeth, decrease in OVD may not be observed. Alternative treatments such as alveoloplasty, orthodontic movement with intrusion, and crown restorations should be performed before increasing the OVD (Fig. 21.3a–f). Although it is possible to gain space for a restoration with the above-mentioned treatments, for some patients with loss of OVD, increasing the OVD enables occlusal reorganization and the establishment of an even occlusal plane (Fig. 21.4a, b). In this way, tooth or tissue structure may not need to be sacrificed.

21.2.3 Congenital and Acquired Anomalies

Congenital and acquired anomalies include amelogenesis or dentinogenesis imperfecta, cleidocranial dysostosis, and cleft palate. Patients with these congenital situations may have severely abraded or eroded dentition, stained/malformed teeth, or partial anadontia accompanied by loss of OVD. A removable partial denture (RPD) is a solution to the esthetic and functional problems faced by these patients until they reach their maximum growth. In

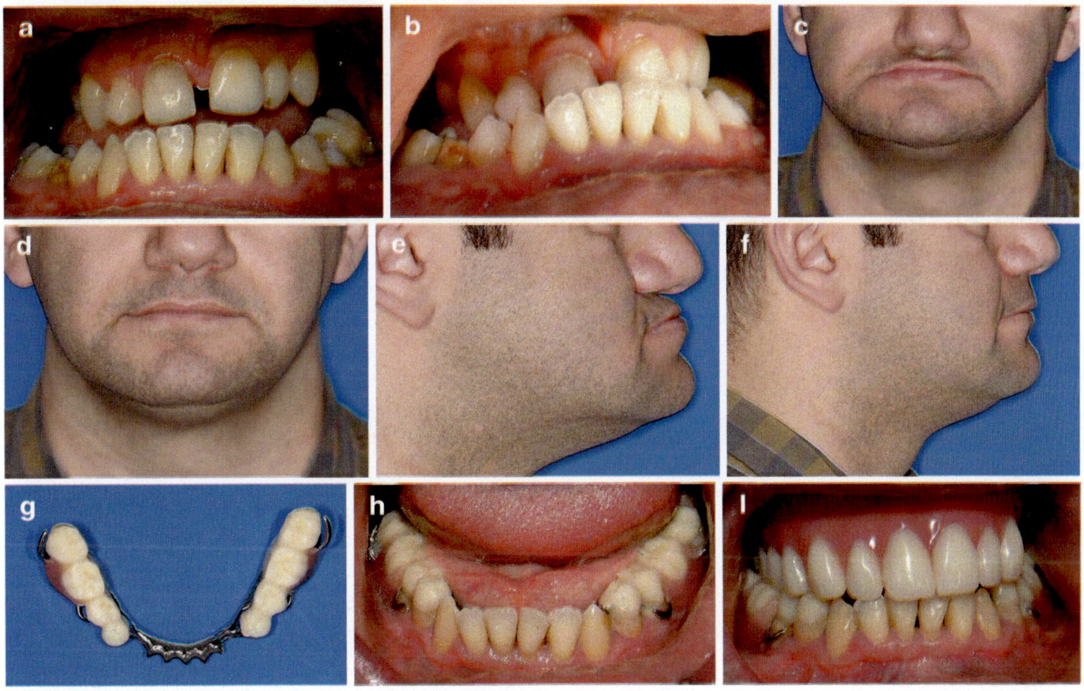

Fig. 21.5 (a–i) An ORPD and a tooth-supported maxillary complete denture have been preferred in a patient with Ehlers–Danlos syndrome, having loss of OVD with too large IORD to fabricate any other prosthetic treatment alternatives

some patients with anomalies or syndromes, an ORPD can be a final treatment if interocclusal rest distance (IORD) is too large to fabricate any other prosthetic restoration (Fig. 21.5a–i).

21.2.4 Severe Dental and Skeletal Malocclusions

A maxillary skeletal deficiency, either alone or in combination with mandibular prognathism, can be an etiological factor in Class III malocclusion development. Dentoalveolar malrelation may also result in a Class III malocclusion. Class III malocclusions are divided into two subgroups according to their characteristics: skeletal/true (deficient maxilla with a larger and prognathic mandible) and pseudo/functional Class III (deficient maxilla with a normal-sized mandible moving forward by premature contacts).

Generally, frontal and profile extraoral examinations reveal reduced vertical facial height, and intraoral examination shows the negative horizontal overlap in functional Class III patients. There is an obvious difference between MIP and CRP and the patients can rotate the mandible with help and the lower facial height can be returned to normal. In this position a bilateral posterior open occlusal relationship is observed (Fig. 21.6, Video 21.1). Prosthetic rehabilitation may be indicated to reestablish an acceptable OVD and MIP to satisfy the esthetic and functional requirements (Fig. 21.7a–f).

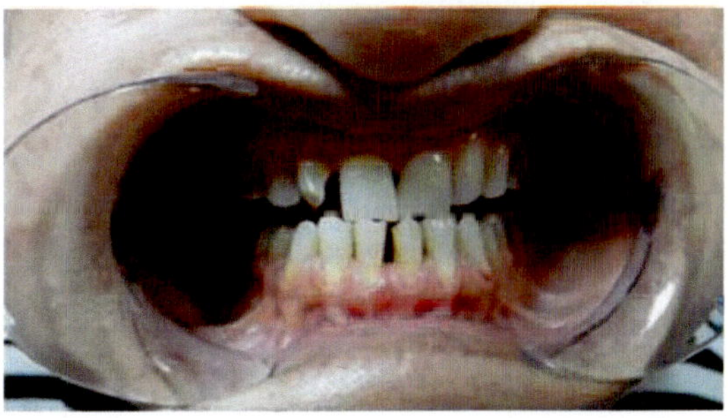

Fig. 21.6 In Angle Class III patients, generally there is a big difference between maximal intercuspal position and retruded contact position. Movie shows determining the discrepancy intraorally and extraorally. These patients are good candidates for reestablishing OVD to meet the esthetic and functional requirements. In patients not showing the discrepancy, increase in OVD should not be recommended or should be made as minimum as possible (Video 21.1)

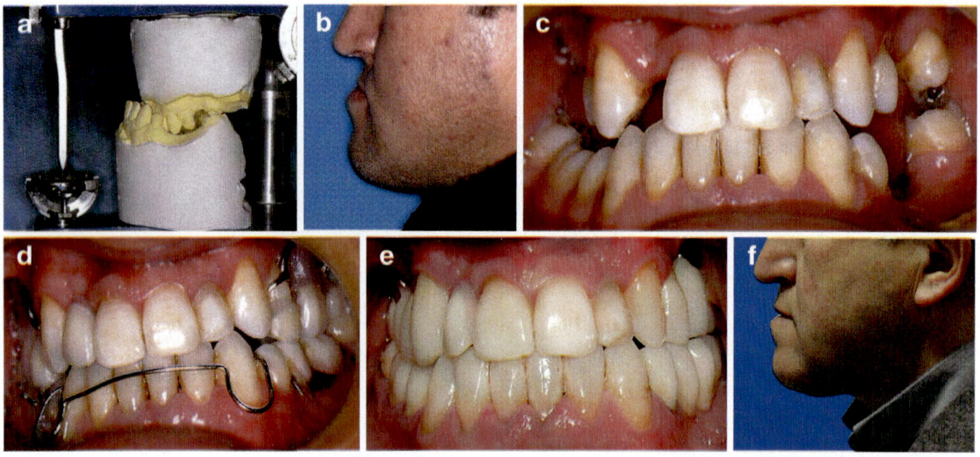

Fig. 21.7 (**a**–**f**) In Class III patient, negative horizontal overlap resulting in reduced vertical facial height (**a**, **b**). Negative horizontal overlap and reduced vertical facial height have been corrected with the aid of orthodontic treatment (**c**). An ORPD was used both in adaptation and retention period (**d**). Prosthodontic treatment was finalized with mandibular fixed and maxillary precision attachment RPD (**e**, **f**)

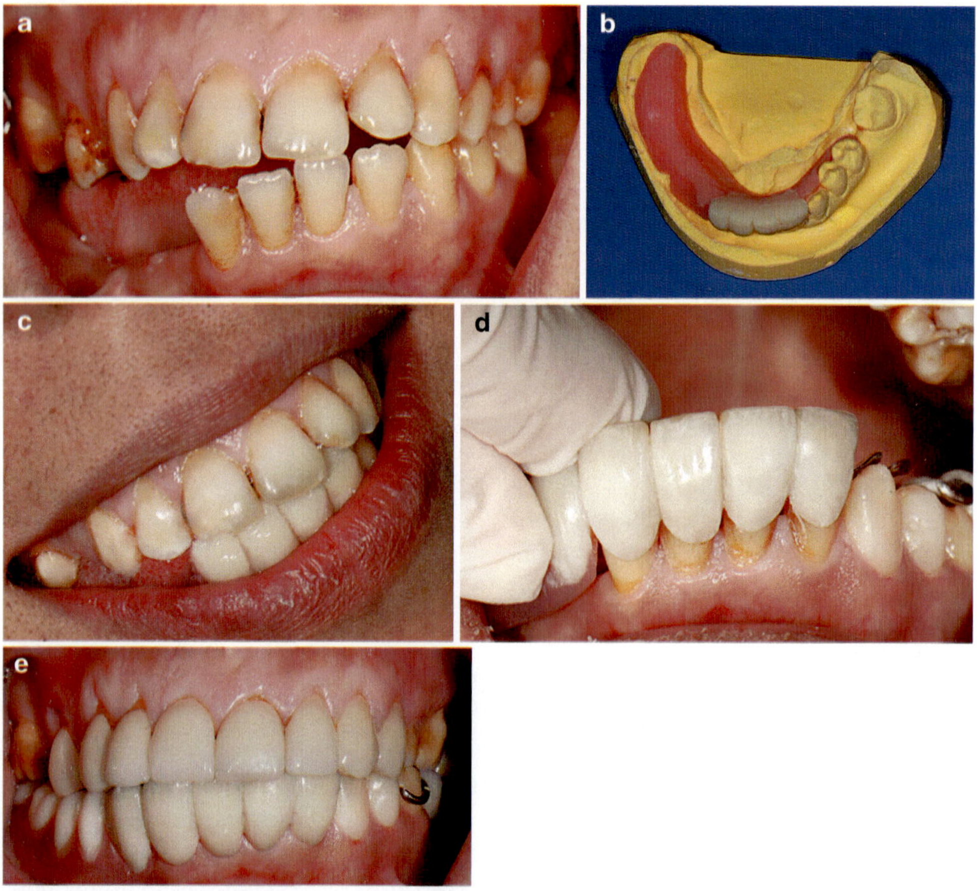

Fig. 21.8 (**a**–**e**) Maxillary laminate veneer restorations and a mandibular ORPD have been fabricated in a patient having open occlusal relationship, with the need of minimal invasive restorations because of systemic health problems. The loss of OVD is not generally observed in these cases. (**a**) Intraoral view, (**b**, **c**) base plate for esthetic verification, (**d**, **e**) final restorations

In some patients, open occlusal relationships can be observed without any discrepancy between MIP and CRP. Open occlusal relationship is defined as "the lack of tooth contact in an occluding position." It can be anterior (the lack of anterior tooth contact in any occluding position of the posterior teeth) or posterior (the lack of posterior tooth contact in any occluding position of the anterior teeth). Although the condition may occur bilaterally, unilateral situations are more frequent. The etiology is not well understood. A number of factors such as abnormal tongue function, primary failure of eruption, ankylosis of teeth, condylar trauma, or pathology have been associated with this condition. Although there is no loss of the OVD, an ORPD can be an alternative treatment option to create functional occlusion (Fig. 21.8a–e).

21.3 The Advantages and Possible Consequences of Increasing the Occlusal Vertical Dimension

In dentate individuals, the advantage of increasing the OVD is to:

1. Allow space for restorative material,
2. Improve facial appearance,
3. Rectify anterior teeth relationship,
4. Provide for reestablishment of physiologic occlusion,
5. Prevent or minimize procedures like crown-lengthening surgery and endodontic treatment, and
6. Protect tooth structure and/or to prevent sensitivity.

After increasing the OVD, some consequences may be expected such as hyperactivity of masseter muscles, elevation of bite force, bruxism, and temporomandibular disorders. However, the above consequences were not supported by evidence-based literature. It can be concluded from research findings that OVD can be increased without facing any serious complications in dentate, partially edentulous, and edentulous cases. Because of the high probability of the collapse in OVD that may have occurred in patients, such as those with pronounced antegonial notch, masseter hypertrophy, and bone exostosis in combination with an increase in alveolar bone volume, increasing OVD should be avoided.

21.4 Determination of New Occlusal Vertical Dimension and Evaluation of the Adaptation Period

Objective guidelines for the degree of increase in the OVD may not be established with any certainty. One clinical variable is the IORD. The reason for measuring the IORD is to determine how the OVD can be altered. At this point, dealing with increasing OVD in two different ways may be clinically more useful. Namely, if there is an obvious difference between OVD and rest vertical dimension (RVD) (more than 2–3 mm), OVD can be increased as much as required in order to satisfy functional and esthetic requirements. It can be termed the *reestablishment of OVD*. But if the IORD is 2–3 mm and increasing OVD is still needed to provide adequate space for the restorations, a minimal increase in OVD should be made. It can be termed the *actual increasing of OVD*. Increasing OVD should be kept to a minimum (recommended amount max: 4–5 mm inter-incisally) (Fig. 21.9a–f).

When reestablishing OVD, the method of determining the new OVD is based on complete denture fabrication procedures. Unfortunately, there is no exact means of doing this, and more than one of the following methods should be used to determine whether the OVD has been altered and the new OVD.

1. *Interocclusal rest distance*: MIP and original OVD of the existing dentition are evaluated. Then IORD is determined. It is very important

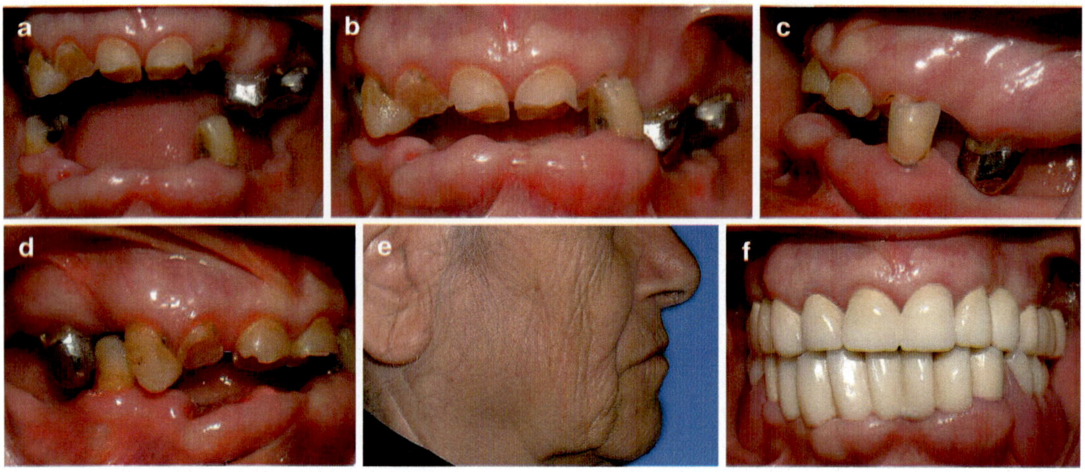

Fig. 21.9 (**a–f**) Although there is tooth loss (**a–d**), decrease in OVD may not be observed (**e**). Such patients should be treated with a minimum increase in OVD required for the restoration (**f**) and followed at short intervals by checking occlusion for possible collapse

to keep in mind that the determination of the IORD has many restrictions:

(a) Physiologic rest position or RVD occurs in a zone rather than a specific level.
(b) Physiologic rest position can change in different examination periods even during the same appointment for the same patient. Changes in muscle tonus due to aging may also affect RVD.
(c) Loss of OVD may be associated with a similar loss of RVD.
(d) Evaluation of the RVD can vary from clinician to clinician for the same patient. Accurate determination of the IORD is difficult when the landmarks are located on movable skin tissues. When skin measurements are used, the tip of the nose-chin distance appears to be more reliable than the subnasal-chin distance. The IORD of more than 2–3 mm may indicate loss of OVD.

The clinical studies showed that increasing OVD beyond IORD (approximately 4–5 mm inter-incisally) did not result in any adaptation or pathological problems. However, in these studies, distinction between the actual increasing and reestablishment of OVD has not been emphasized in general.

2. *Phonetic evaluation*: Speech, particularly the use of sibilant or "s" sounds, is a better method than using IORD for determining an acceptable OVD. The closest speaking space (CSS) is the minimum distance between the anterior teeth that occurs during the pronunciation of words containing "s," "e," and "i" sounds. Average CSS values of 1–3 mm can be used in the clinical determination of OVD of prosthetic restorations, regardless of dental and skeletal classified occlusions. The CSS does not differ between males and females and no correlation was found between the amount of vertical overlap and the CSS. The CSS of more than 1–3 mm may indicate loss of OVD.

Evaluation of the CSS is also the most effective way to assess a patient's adaptation to the new OVD. If the teeth strike each other when the patient attempts to speak, the determined OVD is excessive and should be reduced. It is necessary to hold an articulating paper between the teeth and have the patient say English words "sixty-six" or

"Mississippi" and non-English words "sessantasei," "seyis," or "seis" and adjustment are performed. After 1 month, if the patient is still experiencing speech problems, tooth contact points are adjusted again either from the maxillary or mandibular teeth, and the process is repeated until there are no contacts present during the pronunciation of these words. More time may be required for adjustment until the speech problems are resolved.

It is important to remember that while most patients protrude their mandible to the end-to-end position, others use the retruded position when producing "s" sounds and modifications in the form of the restorations would be more necessary in the former group of patients. Phonetic evaluation, along with monitoring the patient's adaptive capacity, is much more important when actual increasing of the OVD was performed. The vertical change itself may be less stable and the patient's occlusion may need more adjustment.

3. *Facial appearance and measurements*: The OVD is an important factor that affects esthetics. Sagittal and frontal facial tissue appearance, lip morphology, and teeth display are elements that need to be considered. Proportional face measurements and evaluation of the facial appearance are also used to determine OVD such as when teeth are in CRP, there should be equality between the distance from the bony shelf under the nose to the bottom of the mandible and the distance from the pupil of the eyes to the rima oris.

   Mandibular pseudo-prognathism, which may be a sign of the OVD loss, can be observed from the sagittal view. Nasolabial and mentolabial angles are also evaluated.

   From the frontal view, diminished facial contour, deep folds in the commissures of the mouth, thin lips, presence of angular cheilitis, and loss of muscle tone with the face appearing flabby instead of firm are typical facial aspects associated with the loss of OVD (Fig. 21.5c). When reestablishing OVD, it is necessary to pay particular attention to lip closure. Patients should be able to close their lips comfortably without any tension.

   As a conclusion, evaluating all the above-mentioned factors is essential to determine the amount of the loss of OVD. The movies show the sagittal and facial views of patients having normal and decreased OVD when their mandible move between OVD and RVD, and the CSS during fonation (Figs. 21.10, 21.11, 21.12, 21.13, 21.14 and 21.15).

   It is important to remember that increasing OVD should be resisted simply for esthetic reasons in patients without functional disturbances, such as severe tooth wear or chewing problems and that the patient's consent must be obtained before performing any changes in the OVD.

The ratio of patients who adapted to the increase in the OVD can be termed "the adaptation level." The time required for adaptation to the increase in the OVD is "the adaptation period." With removable prostheses, the adaptation level has been found to be 86–100% and the adaptation period varies from 2 days to 3 months. In the adaptation period, a detailed evaluation should be made. Any adjustments of the temporary restorations can then be performed according to the needs of the patient.

The use of conventional occlusal splints in the adaptation period is not indicated, except in temporomandibular disorder patients. First of all, the use of occlusal splints might expose signs and symptoms relating to occlusal splint wearing instead of increased OVD. Second, it is not possible to evaluate chewing function, speech, and esthetics with occlusal splint usage in the adaptation period.

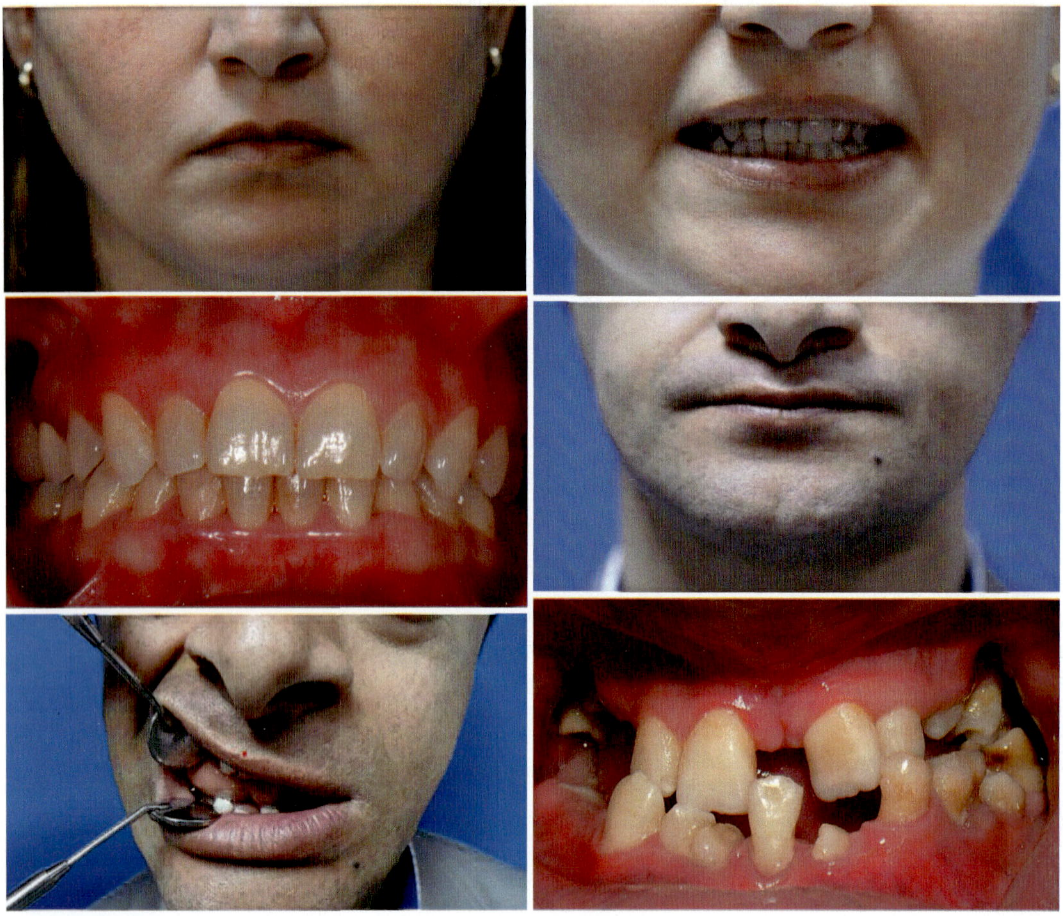

Figs. 21.10, 21.11, 21.12, 21.13, 21.14 and 21.15 As there is no exact method to determine the OVD, clinical observation of the patient is very important to determine the amount of loss of OVD. Videos show the frontal and profile appearances when the patients move their mouths between RVD and OVD in addition to CSS during speech. IORD in normal OVD (Fig. 21.10, Video 21.2); CSS in normal OVD (Fig. 21.11, Video 21.3); Intraoral view of the patient having normal OVD (Fig. 21.12); IORD in decreased OVD (Fig. 21.13, Video 21.4); CSS in decreased OVD (Fig. 21.14, Video 21.5 - the patient's lips were retracted for demonstrative purposes); Intraoral view of the patient having decreased OVD (Fig. 21.15)

21.5 Basic Clinical Steps of Increasing the Occlusal Vertical Dimension

1. The new OVD and CR are determined similarly to edentulous patients as described above. When actual increasing of OVD is performed, a sliding guide, leaf gauges, or anterior bite planes/jigs can be used to establish OVD and CR records. The minimum amount of increase in the OVD required for the restoration can easily be visualized by using the Woelfel sliding guide (Fig. 21.16). Meanwhile, it should be kept in mind that painful/mobile teeth may cause mandibular deviation while recording the CR.

   The above-mentioned procedure can be applied in patients with few missing teeth, small IORDs and/or the need for actual increasing OVDs, but in patients with numerous missing teeth, who have large IORDs and the need for reestablishing OVDs, fabrication of base plates and occlusal rims are absolutely necessary to determine new maxillomandibular relationships. If the patient also needs an anterior tooth restoration, evaluation of esthetics and the extent of anterior teeth visibility can be accomplished by intraorally fabricating a diagnostic mock-up in the first appointment. The new OVD and CR can also be determined by using this direct composite resin mock-up as an anterior jig. Unlike Class III cases, it is necessary to prepare a platform in the posterior part of the mock-up in Class I and II cases. The platform can be fabricated on the temporary base plate in partially edentulous patients (Fig. 21.17a–f). In cases that require restoration of anterior teeth, a direct mock-up can be made with composite material in the mouth. Thus, after approval of the temporary restoration, an impression obtained from the direct mock-up can be a guide that reflects the esthetic expectations of the patients for the diagnostic wax-up that is fabricated in the laboratory (Fig. 21.18a–e). In addition, the final restoration can be completed according to this guiding restoration.

If the IORD is large, esthetic verification can also be made using a base plate shaped with white autopolymerizing acrylic-resin covering the occlusal, buccal, or incisal part of the teeth (Fig. 21.8b, c).

2. Maxillomandibular records are completed (Figs. 21.17f and 21.18e). The diagnostic casts are mounted on a semi-adjustable articulator. Depending on the IORD, both temporary and final treatment options are assessed.
3. After finishing the diagnostic wax-up, an acetate splint or silicone matrix/index is fabricated in the analog workflow. Thus, temporary restorations/mock-ups can be re-made with bis-acrylic composite resin material by using this splint or silicone matrix preferably without any preparation in the mouth. ORPDs are

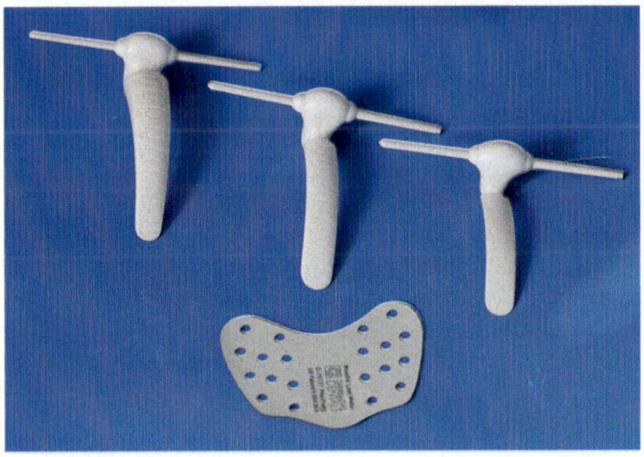

Fig. 21.16 The amount of increase in the vertical dimension required for the restoration can easily be visualized by using the Woelfel sliding guide placed between the incisors in cases having anterior teeth

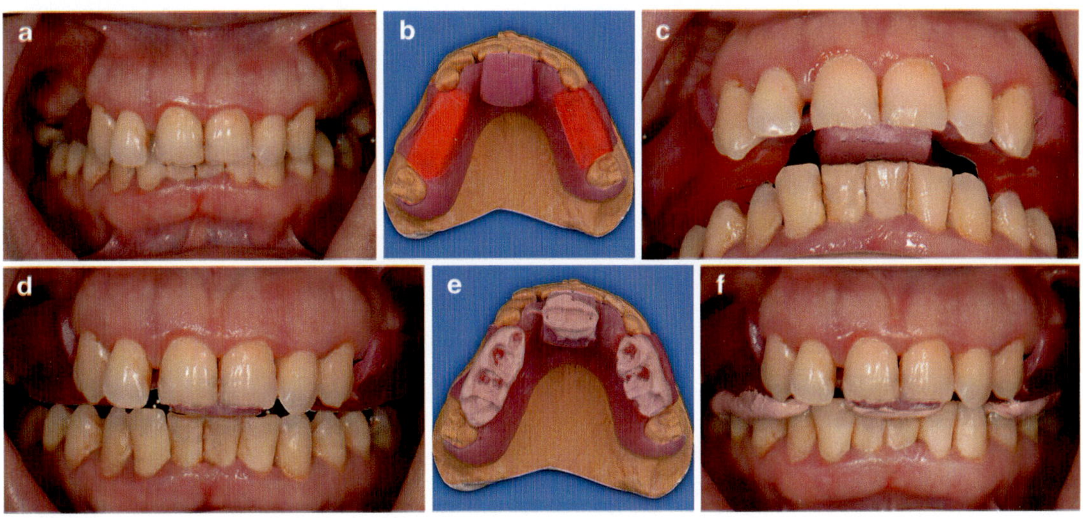

Fig. 21.17 (**a–f**) In partially edentulous cases, determining the new OVD and CRP with a platformed temporary base plate may facilitate the evaluation of IORS and CSS

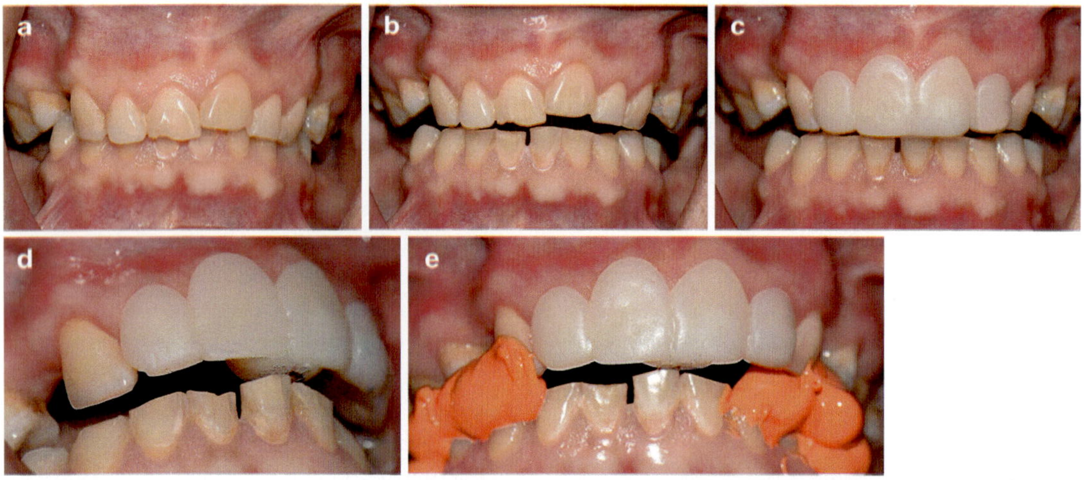

Fig. 21.18 (**a**–**e**) In cases requiring restoration of the anterior teeth, a direct mock-up allows us to obtain the new OVD and CRP and also to learn the patient's esthetic expectations

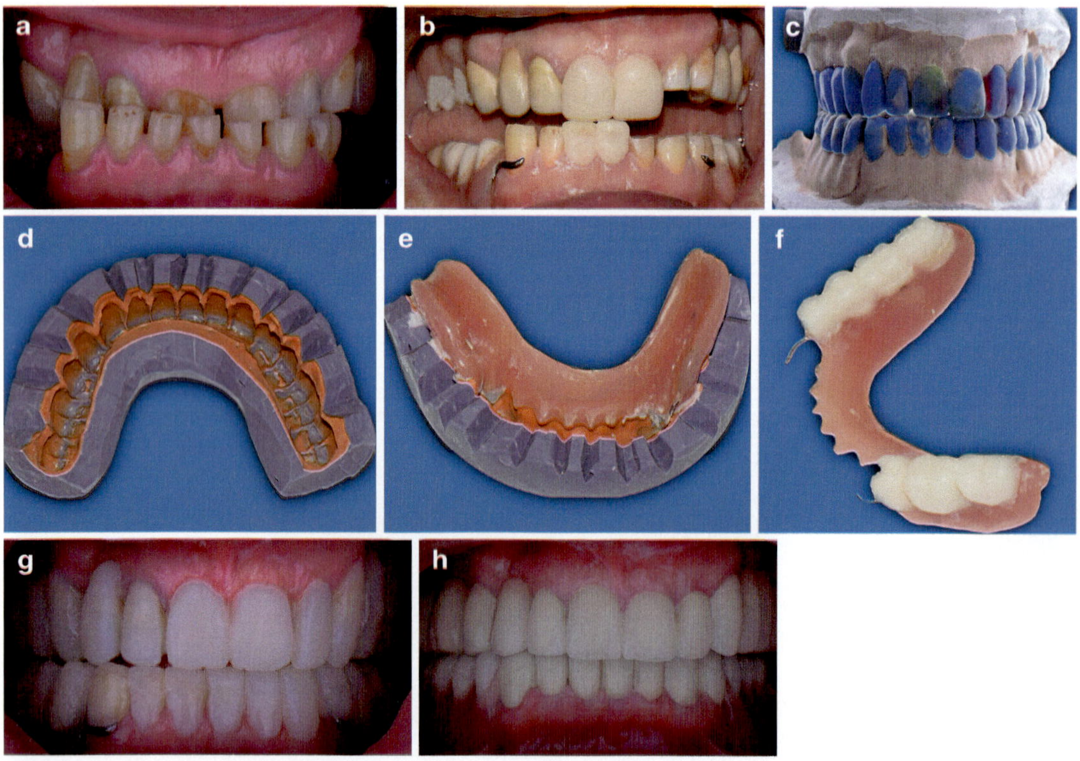

Fig. 21.19 (**a**–**h**) The patient's current dentures can be used during the adaptation period by modifying them in accordance with the new OVD and CRP records

satisfactory alternatives in cases having a large IORD. If the patient has already a removable denture, it can also be used by adding acrylic resin in accordance with the index during the adaptation period (Fig. 21.19a–h). In digital workflow, tooth-colored/shaped both removable and fixed splints are also presented.

4. Esthetic and functional evaluation should be performed before the final decision. The temporary restorations should be the same as the final restoration in terms of both static and dynamic maxillomandibular occlusal relationships (see Chap. 13) and artificial tooth shape and position. Briefly, it may be emphasized that centric relation occlusion for static and canine guidance for dynamic occlusal relationships are the first choices in cases requiring extensive occlusal rehabilitation. Finally, it should be noted that the stability of the OVD increase is closely related to stable and equilibrated both centric and eccentric maxillomandibular occlusal relationships.

21.6 Overlay Removable Partial Dentures

In partially edentulous patients, after the adaptation period of new OVD and MIP, final restoration can be performed with the fixed partial dentures, which is beyond the scope of this book. Implant-assisted RPDs or RPDs with precision attachments can also be used. These treatment alternatives are defined in the relevant chapters (see Chaps. 16 and 17).

In contemporary dentistry, emphasis should be on conservative management strategies. ORPDs, which will be discussed in this chapter, can be both provisional and definitive treatment options to reestablish OVD and MIP.

21.6.1 Advantages of Overlay Removable Partial Dentures

1. Can be a treatment alternative if the IORD is too large for metal–ceramic restorations, as well as the presence of periodontally compromised and/or doubtful endodontically treated teeth, which are unsuitable for clasping.
2. Effective and financially viable and esthetically acceptable to patients.
3. Simple treatment alternative for elder patients who are not able to tolerate invasive treatment options and also for children who are still actively growing and will need several new prostheses during maturation.
4. Noninvasive, reversible, and conservative treatment option.
5. Possible to evaluate the esthetics, phonetics, occlusion, and function with ORPDs during the adaptation period of newly established OVD and MIP.
6. Can be fabricated with minimal or no tooth preparation.
7. Rest seat preparations not needed because the entire occlusal surface of all the teeth serves as a rest seat under the cast framework.
8. Natural teeth that are not suitable for other types of restorations can be preserved under the ORPD to avoid the alveolar bone resorption.

21.6.2 Potential Disadvantages of Overlay Removable Partial Dentures

1. When dentures are removed and the color of the esthetic material is incompatible with the color of the natural teeth, esthetics may be compromised and also the presence of metal clasp retainers may negatively affect the esthetics.
2. Erosive wear may continue or dental caries may occur under the ORPDs if patients are not motivated enough to maintain good oral hygiene.
3. Esthetic material wear, fracture, debonding, or discoloration may take place.
4. Hard palate coverage with the major connector and increased size and thickness can be irritating for the patient. If there are enough abutment teeth, an ORPD can be fabricated without a major connector. But in patients with extensive hard and soft tissue defects, such as cleft plate, a major connector, should be used.

21.6.3 Occlusal and/or Esthetic Materials for Overlay Removable Partial Dentures

Composite and acrylic resins, porcelain, acrylic resin teeth, and metal occlusal surface can be used as occlusal and/or esthetic materials in ORPDs. Porcelain veneers are superior to acrylic resin regarding the color stability and esthetics. Acrylic resin and acrylic resin teeth can be easily repaired and they are cost-effective, compatible with most dental alloys, time saving, simple to produce, and may have reasonably good esthetics. The retention of the resin to the metal is mainly mechanical, but porcelain veneers need a bonding agent to compensate for different expansion coefficients between metal and ceramics and blocs escaping metal oxides. While porcelain materials are more suitable for the rigid areas of ORPD because of their low deformation at the yield point, acrylic resin materials are more suitable for the flexible areas of the denture because of their high compressive load and yield strength. Thus, if the patient is a bruxer, composite or acrylic resin should be selected as an esthetic material and a different RPD design can be used as an occlusal splint for the nocturnal usage (see Chap. 20).

21.6.4 Clinical and Laboratory Procedures for Fabricating an Overlay Removable Partial Denture

1. The determination of the new OVD and CR, the construction of the temporary restorations, and the evaluation of esthetics and function during the adaptation period are applied as described in the "basic clinical steps of increasing the OVD" section.
2. If necessary, recontouring and polishing of unsupported enamel or infrequently a "dimpling" procedure can be used to provide retention on posterior abutments that have insufficient undercut for buccal clasps. Additionally, in some instances, facial reduction of the enamel surface in the esthetic zone is required to accommodate the veneers, which would be fused to the ORPD and, in the cases of missing natural undercut for adequate retention, guide planes are placed on proximal tooth surfaces.
3. As a general rule, 2–3 mm of IORD should be present in the anterior region beyond the patient's OVD. This would allow for approximately 0.3–0.5 mm of space in the most posterior region, which is needed for the structural integrity of an all-metal occlusal surface. Metal on labial and buccal surfaces may be thinned to approximately 0.2 mm. An effort should be made to limit labial or buccal thickness to 1–1.5 mm, including metal, opaque, and composite resin, to provide proper esthetics and avoid fracture of the resin at peripheries (Fig. 21.20a–d).
4. The casts should be surveyed to determine the most desirable path of placement (see Chap. 14). If necessary, retention beads are placed for the veneering material on the occlusal and facial surfaces where it is needed. The framework is generally cast with a cobalt–chromium alloy.
5. The framework is tried in. With the framework in position, OVD and CR records are verified. If necessary, the definitive cast is remounted on the semi-adjustable articulator. Artificial teeth are arranged and veneering material is then applied.
6. New OVD and CR records and dynamic occlusal relationships during the esthetic try-in are verified in the mouth.
7. After delivery of the denture, the patient is instructed to clean ORPDs with a nonabrasive paste after every meal and especially after the consumption of acidic beverages. The importance of cleaning the internal surface of the prosthesis as well as their own teeth must be emphasized. Additionally, patients are advised to use a fluoride gel as an anticaries preventive measure. After thorough cleaning of both prostheses and teeth, the fluoride gel is placed inside the ORPD and then inserted in the mouth.

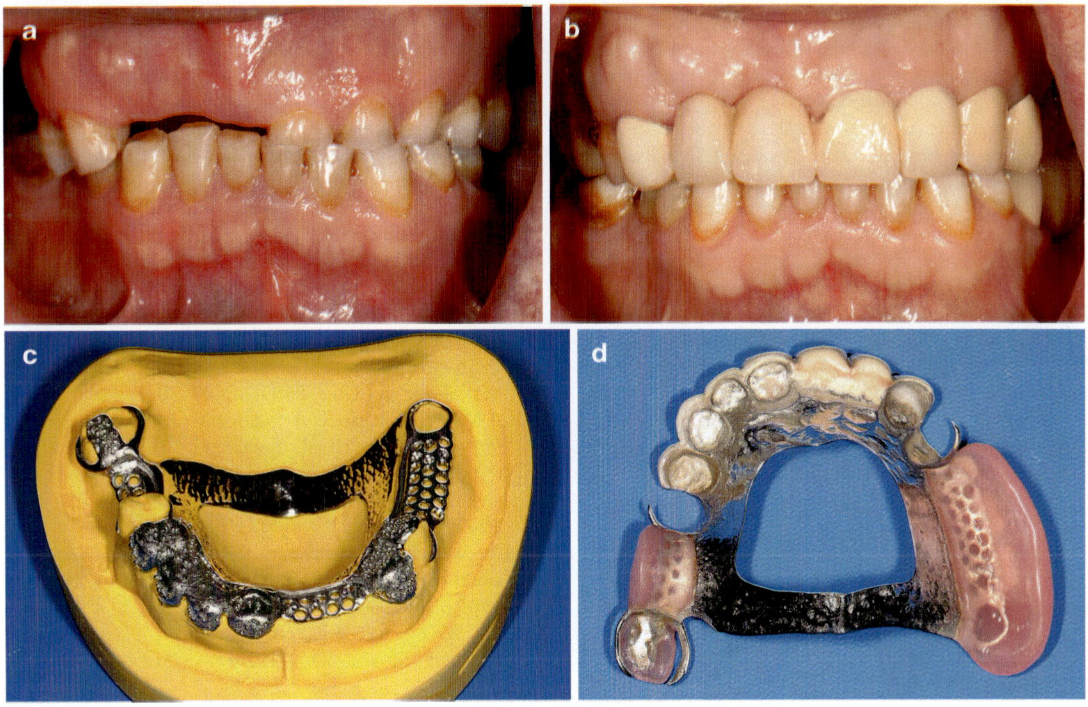

Fig. 21.20 (**a–d**) In some cases, ORPD framework may be extended to the buccal surfaces. If necessary, preparation is performed on the natural teeth and metal may be thinned to approximately 0.2 mm

Further Reading

Abduo J. Safety of increasing vertical dimension of occlusion: a systematic review. Quintessence Int. 2012;43:369–80.

Abduo J, Lyons K. Clinical considerations for increasing occlusal vertical dimension: a review. Aust Dent J. 2012;57:2–10.

Bartlett DW. The role of erosion in tooth wear: aetiology, prevention and management. Int Dent J. 2005;55:277–84.

Barzilay I, Myers ML, Cooper LB, Graser G. Mechanical and chemical retention of laboratory cured composite to metal surfaces. J Prosthet Dent. 1988;59:131–7.

Calamita M, Coachman C, Sesma N, Kois J. Occlusal vertical dimension: treatment planning decisions and management considerations. Int J Esthet Dent. 2019;14:166–81.

Carlsson GE, Ingervall B, Kocak G. Effect of increasing vertical dimension on the masticatory system in subjects with natural teeth. J Prosthet Dent. 1979;41:284–9.

Craddock HL, Youngson CC, Manogue M, Blance A. Occlusal changes following posterior tooth loss in adults. Part 1: a study of clinical parameters associated with the extend and type of supraeruption in unopposed posterior teeth. J Prosthodont. 2007;16:485–94.

Crothers AJ. Tooth wear and facial morphology. J Dent. 1992;20:333–41.

Dahl BL, Krogstad O, Karlsen K. An alternative treatment in cases with advanced localized attrition. J Oral Rehabil. 1975;2:209–14.

Dahl BL, Krogstad O. Long-term observations of an increased occlusal face height obtained by a combined orthodontic/prosthetic approach. J Oral Rehabil. 1985;12:173–6.

Dahl BL, Carlsson GE, Ekfeldt A. Occlusal wear of teeth and restorative materials. A review of classification, etiology, mechanisms of wear, and some aspects of restorative procedures. Acta Odontol Scand. 1993;51:299–311.

Dawson PE. Functional occlusion: from TMJ to smile design. 3rd ed. St Louis: Elsevier Mosby; 2007.

Del Castillo R, Lamar F Jr, Ercoli C. Maxillary and mandibular overlay removable partial dentures for the treatment of posterior open-occlusal relationship: a clinical report. J Prosthet Dent. 2002;87:587–92.

Edelhoff D, Schweiger J, Prandtner O, Trimpl J, Stimmelmayr M, Güth JF. CAD/CAM splints for the functional and esthetic evaluation of newly defined occlusal dimensions. Quintessence Int. 2017;48:181–91.

Fabbri G, Sorrentino R, Cannistraro G, Mintrone F, Bacherini L, Turrini R, Bombardelli T, Nieri M, Fradeani M. Increasing the vertical dimension of occlusion: a multicenter retrospective clinical comparative study on 100 patients with fixed tooth-supported, mixed, and implant-supported full-arch rehabilitations. Int J Periodontics Restorative Dent. 2018;38:323–35.

Fayz F, Eslami A. Determination of occlusal vertical dimension: a literature review. J Prosthet Dent. 1988;59:321–3.

Fishman LS. Dental and skeletal relationships to attritional occlusion. Angle Orthod. 1976;46:51–63.

Fonseca J, Nicolau P, Daher T. Maxillary overlay removable partial dentures for the restoration of worn teeth. Compend Contin Educ Dent. 2011;32:12,14–20.

Ganddini MR, Al-Mardini M, Graser GN, Almog D. Maxillary and mandibular overlay removable partial dentures for the restoration of worn teeth. J Prosthet Dent. 2004;91:210–4.

Garcia LT, Bohnenkamp DM. The use of composite resin in removable prosthodontics. Compend Contin Educ Dent. 2003;24:688-90,692,694.

Goldstein G, Goodacre C, MacGregor K. Occlusal vertical dimension: best evidence consensus statement. J Prosthodont. 2021;30:12–9.

Graser GN, Rogoff GS. Removable partial overdentures for special patients. Dent Clin North Am. 1990;34:741–58.

Graser GN, Rogoff GS. Overdentures for acquired and congenital anomalies: part 2. Partial overdentures. Int J Prosthodont. 1990b;3:361–7.

Grasso JE, Miller EL. Removable partial prosthodontics. St Louis: Mosby; 1991.

Gross MD, Ormianer Z. A preliminary study on the effect of occlusal vertical dimension increase on mandibular postural rest position. Int J Prosthodont. 1994;7:216–26.

Guttal S, Patil NP. Cast titanium overlay denture for a geriatric patient with a reduced vertical dimension. Gerodontology. 2005;22:242.

Hassall D. Centric relation and increasing the occlusal vertical dimension: concepts and clinical techniques—part one. Br Dent J. 2021a;230:17–22.

Hassall D. Centric relation and increasing the occlusal vertical dimension: concepts and clinical techniques—part two. Br Dent J. 2021b;230:83–9.

Johansson A, Johansson AK, Omar R, Carlsson GE. Rehabilitation of worn dentition. J Oral Rehabil. 2008;35:548–66.

Kaffaf MB, Şeşen P, Şakar O. Rehabilitation of occlusal vertical dimension in a patient with acromegaly: a clinical report. J Prosthodont. 2021;30:97–103.

Kale B, Buyukcavus MH. Comparison of three-dimensional soft-tissue evaluations between skeletal and pseudo-class III malocclusions. Sci Rep. 2020;10:14717.

Lewis GR, Munro AM. Advances in partial denture ceramics. Quintessence Int. 1995;26:617–20.

Liu C, Huang D, Zhou L, Liu G, Wang Y, Jiang T. Two-year observation of the occlusal vertical dimension after bite raising via cone-beam computerized tomography: a preliminary study. Sci Rep. 2019;9:3509.

McNeill C. Science and practice of occlusion. Chicago: Quintessence Pub. Co; 1997.

Moreno-Hay I, Okeson JP. Does altering the occlusal vertical dimension produce temporomandibular disorders? A literature review. J Oral Rehabil. 2015;42:875–82.

Nashed RR, Holmes A. A posterior open bite. Br J Orthod. 1990;17:47–53.

Ormianer Z, Gross M. A 2-year follow-up of mandibular posture following an increase in occlusal vertical dimension beyond the clinical rest position with fixed restorations. J Oral Rehabil. 1998;25:877–83.

Ormianer Z, Palty A. Altered vertical dimension of occlusion: a comparative retrospective pilot study of tooth-and implant-supported restorations. Int J Oral Maxillofac Implants. 2009;24:497–501.

Patel MB, Bencharit S. A treatment protocol for restoring occlusal vertical dimension using an overlay removable partial denture as an alternative to extensive fixed restorations: a clinical report. Open Dent J. 2009;3:213–8.

Proffit WR, Vig KW. Primary failure of eruption: a possible cause of posterior open-bite. Am J Orthod. 1981;80:173–90.

Proffit WR, White RP Jr, Sarver DM. Contemporary treatment of dentofacial deformity. St Louis: Mosby; 2003.

Rivera-Morales WC, Mohl ND. Relationship of occlusal vertical dimension to the health of the masticatory system. J Prosthet Dent. 1991;65:547–53.

Rivera-Morales WC, Mohl ND. Restoration of the vertical dimension of occlusion in the severely worn dentition. Dent Clin North Am. 1992;36:651–64.

Sato S, Hotta TH, Pedrazzi V. Removable occlusal overlay splint in the management of tooth wear: a clinical report. J Prosthet Dent. 2000;83:392–5.

Silverman MM. The speaking method in measuring vertical dimension. 1952. J Prosthet Dent. 2001;85:427–31.

Şakar O, Aren G, Mumcu Z, Ünalan F, Aksakallı N, Tolgay CG. Familial gigantiform cementoma with Ehlers–Danlos syndrome: a report of 2 cases. J Adv Prosthodont. 2015;7:178–82.

Şakar O, Beyli M, Marsan G. Combined prosthodontic and orthodontic treatment of a patient with a class III skeletal malocclusion: a clinical report. J Prosthet Dent. 2004;92:224–8.

Şakar O, Bural C, Sülün T, Öztaş E, Marşan G. Evaluation of the closest speaking space in different dental and skeletal occlusions. J Prosthet Dent. 2013;109:222–6.

Şakar O, Sülün T, Kurt H, Gençel B. Reliability and comparison of two facial measurements to detect changes of occlusal vertical dimension in complete denture wearers. Gerodontology. 2011;28:205–8.

Şakar O, Şeşen P, Kaffaf B. Occlusal veneers and rehabilitation of occlusal vertical dimension. In: Ulukapı H. Posterior Bölge Estetik Restorasyonlar. Ankara: Türkiye Klinikleri; 2019. p. 34–41.

The glossary of prosthodontic terms: ninth edition. J Prosthet Dent. 2017;117(5S):e1–e105.

Turner KA, Missirlian DM. Restoration of the extremely worn dentition. J Prosthet Dent. 1984;52:467–74.

Willis FM. Features involved in full denture prosthesis. Dent Cosmos. 1935;77:851–4.

Windchy A, Khan Z, Fields H. Overdentures with metal occlusion to maintain occlusal vertical dimension and prevent denture fracture. J Prosthet Dent. 1988;60:11–4.

Windchy AM, Morris JC. An alternative treatment with the overlay removable partial denture: a clinical report. J Prosthet Dent. 1998;79:249–53.

Woda A, Pionchon P, Palla S. Regulation of mandibular postures: mechanisms and clinical implications. Crit Rev Oral Biol Med. 2001;12:166–78.

Woelfel JB. New device for accurately recording centric relation. J Prosthet Dent. 1986;56:716–27.

Zanardi PR, Santos MS, Stegun RC, Sesma N, Costa B, Laganá DC. Restoration of the occlusal vertical dimension with an overlay removable partial denture: a clinical report. J Prosthodont. 2016;25:585–8.

Zarb G, Hobkirk JA, Eckert SE, Jacob RF. Prosthodontic treatment for edentulous patients. 13th ed. St Louis: Elsevier Mosby; 2013.

Prosthetic Treatment of Partially Edentulous Maxillofacial Defect Patients

22

Banu Karayazgan

Abstract

Maxillofacial defects may occur due to congenital or developmental anomalies or secondary to acquired conditions such as trauma or surgery. For a patient with a maxillofacial defect, getting the lost function, phonation, and aesthetics back is of great importance in terms of quality of life. The prosthetic treatment of these defects has always been a challenging approach and removable prostheses that replace the lost tissues quickly, cost-effectively, and with minimum trauma have always been a referred treatment approach in maxillofacial defects where there is loss of bone, soft tissue, and adjacent structures. The process of a prosthodontic treatment from the planning to the delivery should include all the principles that need to be carefully considered. The deterioration of the healthy structure necessitates some changes in the conventional biomechanical rules of partial removable dentures. Therefore, a maxillofacial prosthesis based on a well-designed foundation not only restores the lost function and aesthetics but also provides a significant effect on the well-being of the patient.

B. Karayazgan (✉)
School of Dental Medicine, Department of Prosthodontics, University of Pittsburgh, Pittsburgh, PA, USA

Medical Center, Department of Maxillofacial Prosthodontics, University of Pittsburgh, Pittsburgh, PA, USA
e-mail: bak139@pitt.edu

22.1 Definitions

Definitive obturator: A maxillofacial prosthesis that replaces a portion or all of one or both maxillae and associated anatomy as a result of surgery or trauma; a definitive obturator is made when tissue changes or recurrence of tumor are unlikely, and a more long-term prosthetic rehabilitation can be achieved.

Facial prosthesis: A maxillofacial prosthesis that artificially replaces a deficient anatomy of the face as a result of surgery, trauma, or congenital absence.

Interim obturator: A maxillofacial prosthesis, which is made following completion of initial healing from the surgical resection of a portion or all of one or both maxillae; this prosthesis replaces the surgical obturator, which is usually inserted at or immediately following the resection; generally, an interim obturator is made to facilitate closure of the resultant defect after initial healing has been completed.

Mandibular resection prosthesis: A maxillofacial prosthesis used to maintain a functional position for the jaws (maxillae and mandible), improve speech and deglutition following trauma and/or surgery to the mandible and/or adjacent structures.

Maxillofacial prosthesis: Any prosthesis used to replace part or all of any stomatognathic and/or craniofacial structures.

O. Şakar (ed.), *Removable Partial Dentures*, https://doi.org/10.1007/978-3-031-47083-7_22

Surgical obturator: A temporary maxillofacial prosthesis inserted during or immediately following surgical or traumatic loss of a portion or all of one or both maxillae and contiguous alveolar structures.

22.2 Etiology of Maxillofacial Defects

22.2.1 Congenital and Development Defects

Congenital and developmental defects, closely related conditions, impact the entire developmental process. They are characterized by structural and functional anomalies that originate during intrauterine life. Diagnosis of these defects is feasible before or shortly after birth. While genetic, infectious, nutritional, and environmental factors are commonly associated with these anomalies, identifying a precise cause is not always possible. Additionally, these defects may be linked with various syndromes, such as Down, Turner, Treacher Collins, and Pierre Robin syndromes, leading to clinical manifestations like facial hypertrophy, achondroplasia, hemifacial dysplasia, agnathia, micrognathia, agenesis of the condyles, and exostoses in the maxillofacial region. Cleft lip and palate are among the most prevalent congenital maxillofacial defects, with the severity ranging from a minor notch in the lip to a complete or unilateral cleft of the palate. These may present as isolated defects or in association with numerous inherited conditions and syndromes. In certain instances, despite comprehensive surgical interventions, closing the defect may be unachievable due to inadequate maxillary fusion. Prosthetic treatment of cleft lip and palate involves an integrated approach involving surgery, orthodontics, pedodontics, and prosthodontics. This multidisciplinary treatment, complemented by speech and hearing therapies, aims to restore satisfactory function, phonation, and aesthetics, thereby significantly enhancing the patient's quality of life (Fig. 22.1).

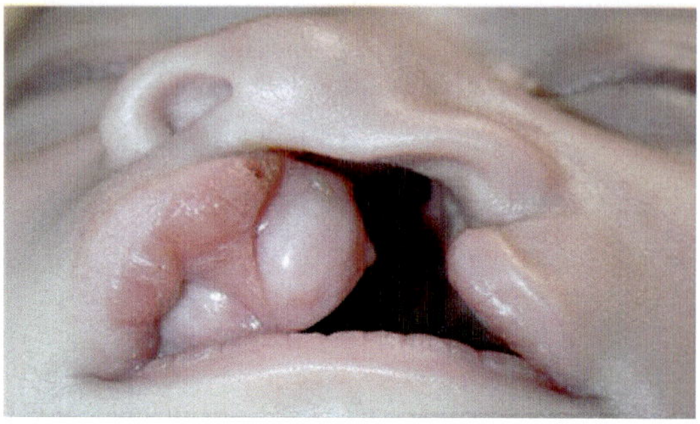

Fig. 22.1 A newborn patient with cleft lip and palate

22.2.2 Acquired Defects

Acquired defects in the maxillomandibular region can arise from various causes, including trauma, surgical resection of neoplasms, cyst formations, infectious diseases (such as fungal infections), osteonecrosis (resulting from radiation therapy or bisphosphonate use), or the long-term use of addictive substances. These defects compromise the anatomical integrity of the region, affecting the patient's aesthetics, function, and phonation. Consequently, understanding the underlying cause is crucial for the overall prognosis and treatment strategy. It necessitates a carefully planned treatment from start to finish, employing a multidisciplinary team approach to address the complexity of these conditions. Maxillofacial traumas, which can result from motor vehicle accidents, industrial injuries, gunshot wounds, falls, crashes, physical assaults, exposure to chemical agents, and burns, may damage not only the skin and soft tissues but also the underlying bone structures and vital organs. These injuries often lead to functional impairments and aesthetic concerns, necessitating comprehensive approaches to treatment that consider both soft and hard tissue losses and fractures (Fig. 22.2).

Defects in the maxillofacial region are primarily caused by head-and-neck cancers. The predisposing factors for these cancers are diverse and not entirely clear, but they generally include immune system issues, hereditary and genetic factors, diet and nutrition, habits such as alcohol

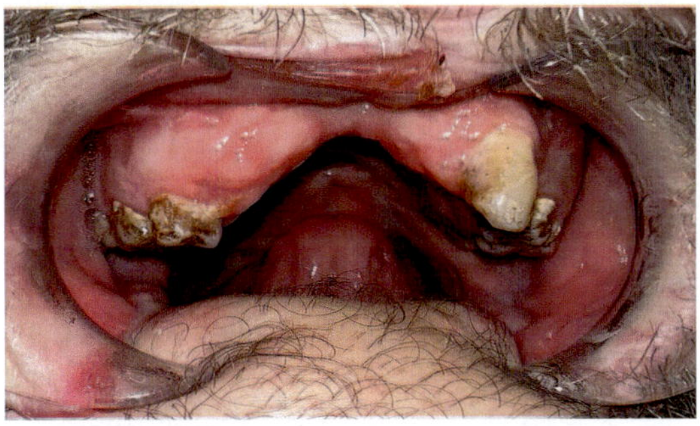

Fig. 22.2 An acquired maxillofacial defect due to gunshot injury

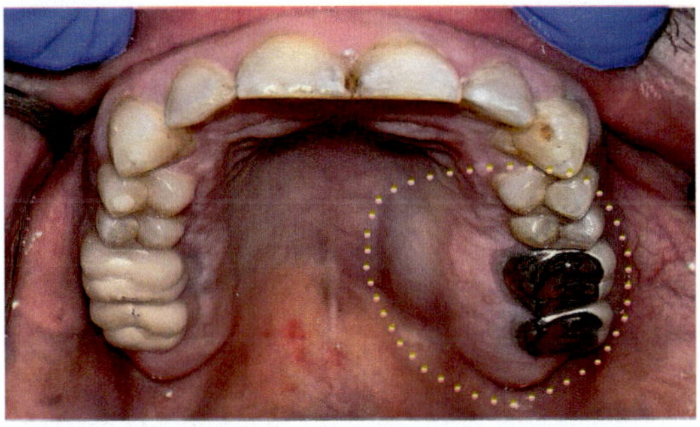

Fig. 22.3 An adenoid cystic carcinoma of the maxilla

and tobacco use, viral and fungal infections, radiation exposure, and continuous trauma. Precancerous lesions such as leukoplakia, erythroplasia, lichen planus, and exposure to certain chemicals are also significant contributors. Squamous cell carcinoma, ameloblastoma, and osseous carcinoma are among the most prevalent neoplasms affecting the mandibular region. In the palatal and paranasal areas, the most common tumors include adenoid cystic carcinoma, mucoepidermoid carcinoma, pleomorphic adenoma, lymphoepithelioma, and lymphosarcoma. Understanding the etiology and the surgical procedures involved is crucial for integrating and optimizing the overall treatment process for patients (Fig. 22.3).

Maxillofacial neoplasms often necessitate extensive surgery due to their potential for invasion and metastasis. In cases involving malignancies, prosthetic applications are frequently favored over surgical reconstructions. This preference allows for continuous monitoring of both recurrence risks and the area of the defect. Prosthetic solutions offer a quicker, less traumatic, and often more aesthetically pleasing alternative for replacing lost tissues. Factors such as the patient's age, overall health status, and reluctance to undergo major surgery further contribute to the decision to opt for prosthetic treatment. Additionally, secondary infections resulting from local and systemic disorders—beyond trauma and cancer—can lead to necrosis and destruction of bone and soft tissues, necessitating resection. These scenarios underscore the importance of a tailored approach to treatment, considering the unique circumstances and needs of each patient.

22.3 Pre-surgical and Pre-prosthetic Evaluation

A comprehensive pre-surgical intraoral and extraoral examination is crucial in treating maxillofacial defects. These preparatory steps typically include intraoral and extraoral photographs, diagnostic casts, jaw relation records, and X-rays. Prior to surgery, and potentially before radiation therapy, dental treatments such as decay removal, infection control, extractions, and periodontal care must be addressed. The preservation and restoration of existing teeth are vital for the retention of the obturator, while teeth deemed non-restorable should be extracted. Post-surgery, anatomical changes may necessitate a reevaluation of the patient before finalizing the treatment. Factors to consider during this phase include the type and size of the defect, the condition of residual hard and soft tissues and teeth, their proximity to vital structures, the patient's psychological state and general health, and their ability to utilize the prosthesis effectively. The period immediately following resection presents significant challenges for both the patient and physician, marked by psychological and functional adaptation difficulties. Given the limited time before surgery, it might not be possible to address all dental issues, and secondary dental problems may emerge post-operatively. Hence, fulfilling dental requirements and reevaluating the patient for the definitive prosthesis become essential. New intraoral and extraoral records should be taken as needed.

22.4 Maxillary Defects

22.4.1 Classification of Maxillary Defects

Classifying maxillary defects is challenging due to their complex nature, extent, and the variety of combinations that can result from maxillectomy. No single classification system ideally addresses all surgical and prosthetic needs because these disciplines prioritize different aspects of treatment. A comprehensive classification must consider various criteria, including the type and location of the defect, the condition of remaining teeth, the status of oroantral and nasal communication, and the involvement of the soft palate and adjacent structures. Given the focus of this book on 'removable partial dentures,' the Aramany Classification system is utilized to detail defect localization and plan for removable denture components. This system, which classifies post-surgical maxillary defects into six subgroups, serves as a valuable tool for research, education, and clinical communication:

Class I: Unilateral defect extending to the midline involving one half of the arch and palatal bone.

Class II: Unilateral defect posterior to the canine on one side of the arch.

Class III: Central defect in the palatal bone.

Class IV: Combination of unilateral defect and the contralateral entire premaxilla.

Class V: Bilateral defect posterior to the second premolar.

Class VI: Bilateral anterior defect (Fig. 22.4a–f).

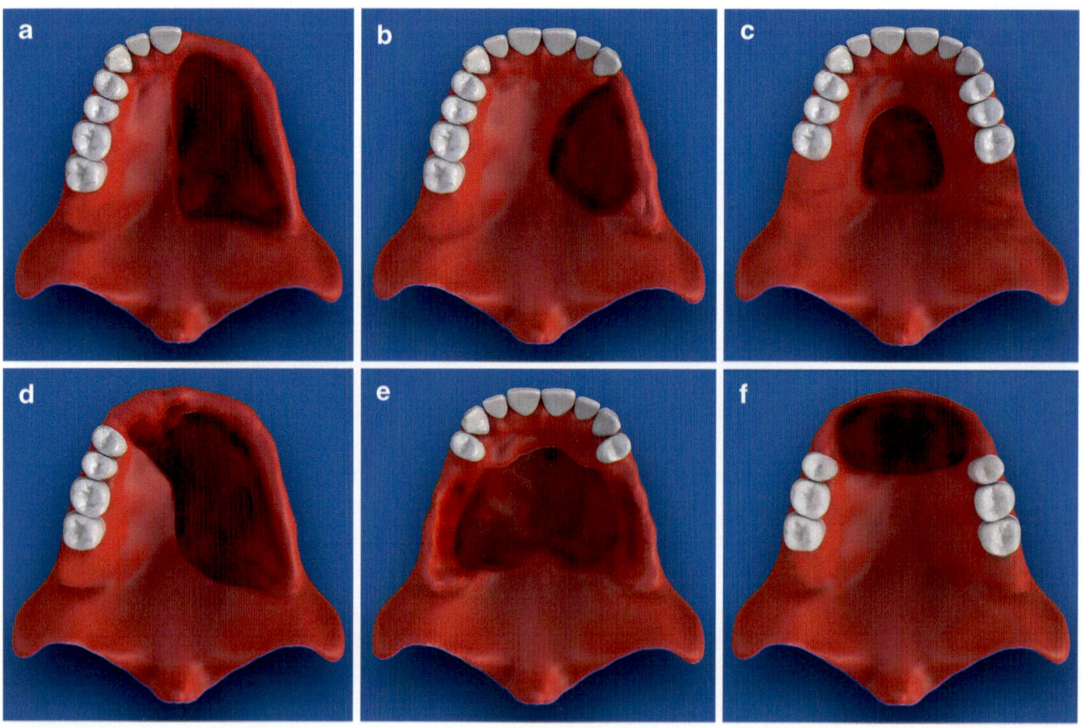

Fig. 22.4 Aramany Classification of the maxillary defects: Class I (**a**), Class II (**b**), Class III (**c**), Class IV (**d**), Class V (**e**), Class VI (**f**)

22.4.2 Surgical Resection and Reconstruction of Maxilla

In the resection of the maxilla, the choice of surgical method is dictated by the type and extent of the neoplasm. Palatectomy represents a less invasive approach, performed intraorally, suitable for certain cases. In contrast, the Weber–Fergusson technique for radical maxillectomy describes a more extensive and aggressive procedure. It involves incisions starting from the lower edge of the orbit, extending along the edge of the nose and philtrum, and into the mouth. After neoplasm removal, defect areas are covered with split-thickness skin grafts, which not only protect the resected site but also provide retention, stability, and support for prosthetic contact, particularly on the inner cheek. Restoring the defect using autologous tissue is often preferred over prosthetics, which require removal and maintenance. This approach can be concurrent with the resection or follow after healing. Various grafts and flaps, including cancellous or cortical bone grafts (from sites like the iliac, rib, tibia, fibula, and skull) and skin grafts (full or split thickness), as well as local, regional, and free flaps, can be used for reconstruction. While these methods effectively separate the oral and nasal cavities, enhancing patient comfort, they can also impact speech and chewing due to the altered tissue volumes and structures. Additionally, complications such as oronasal fistulas, tissue necrosis, and cosmetic issues can arise from autologous augmentations. Titanium mesh plates and screws, alongside or in lieu of autologous tissue augmentations, implant materials, tissue expansion, tissue engineering, stem cell applications, and digital medical modeling, represent advanced treatment options for reconstructing the maxillofacial area. Implants may also be placed to improve the retention of the obturator, either after complete healing or concurrently with surgical steps like resection or reconstruction. Although surgical closure post-resection may enhance patient comfort, the need to monitor for cancer recurrence, the invasive nature of procedures for such defects, or the patient's overall health may limit the feasibility of this approach (Fig. 22.5).

In all surgical approaches to addressing maxillofacial defects, optimizing the design to accommodate the path of insertion, restoring and preserving abutment teeth, and maintaining healthy supporting bone structures are critical for the favorable prognosis of the prosthesis. Thus, the involvement of a prosthodontist in the planning stages of these treatments, including the surgery itself, is crucial. It is essential to retain restorable teeth, conserve the hard palate and alveolar crest, and preserve the bone around teeth designated as abutments. Such multidisciplinary collaboration ensures that surgical interventions are aligned with prosthetic requirements, enhancing both the functionality and longevity of the prosthesis.

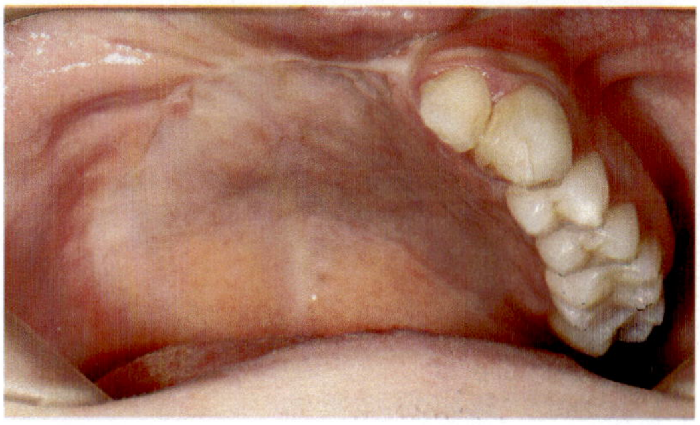

Fig. 22.5 A surgically reconstructed maxillary defect

22.4.3 Prosthetic Workflow of Maxillary Defects

22.4.3.1 Surgical Obturation

The post-surgical period poses the greatest challenge for patients undergoing maxillectomy. They encounter difficulties related to speech, swallowing, chewing, and aesthetics. Providing a prosthesis immediately after surgery significantly aids patients in overcoming these challenges, offering considerable physical and psychological relief. The initial prosthesis, known as a "*surgical obturator*" is crucial during the first 1 or 2 weeks post-surgery. The ideal preparation for a surgical obturator begins before the surgery. Impressions are taken in advance, and the surgeon and the maxillofacial prosthodontist discusses the anticipated resection margins. These margins are then marked on the dental cast. The model is adjusted by removing teeth and adding

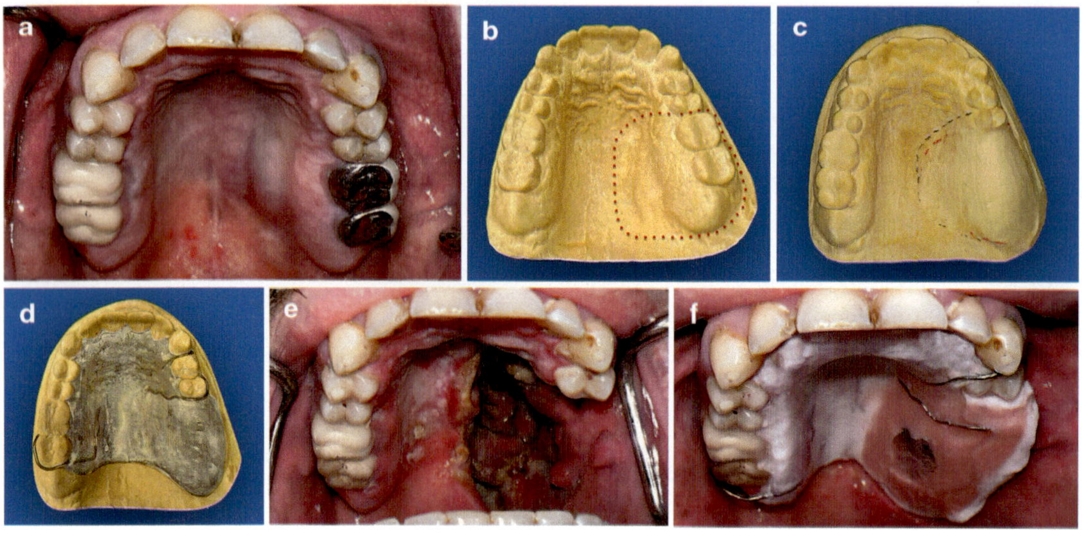

Fig. 22.6 Fabrication steps of a surgical obturator: (**a**) neoplasm identified in the left posterior maxilla, (**b**) cast obtained, (**c**) removal of the tissues and teeth affected from the surgery and reshaping the area, (**d**) fabrication of the surgical obturator, (**e**) resection of the neoplasm, (**f**) application of the relined surgical obturator

an edentulous crest on the side of the expected defect to simulate the post-surgical oral environment. If various surgical approaches are planned, several casts may be prepared. The base plate is constructed from auto-polymerized or heat-polymerized polymethylmethacrylate (PMMA). After resection, the surgical obturator is placed to close the defect, with wrought clasps anchored on existing teeth for retention. This setup not only stabilizes the surgical dressing but also secures the skin graft during the critical initial healing phase (Fig. 22.6 a-f).

In situations where the retention provided by the teeth and tissues is not sufficient, an effective strategy involves creating holes along the margins of the obturator. Through these holes, the obturator can be securely anchored in place using sutures, wires, or screws that are threaded through the holes and attached to the surrounding tissues. This method helps the obturator to remain stable within the oral cavity, supporting the surgical site effectively. Following the placement of the surgical obturator, the patient is advised to wear it continuously for the first week without attempting any adjustments or removals. This uninterrupted use is crucial for the initial healing process. The patient is instructed not to manipulate the prosthesis until the first post-operative follow-up visit, allowing for professional assessment and necessary adjustments by the healthcare provider (Fig. 22.7a,b).

The following advantages are provided with surgical obturators:

1. Direct nutrition without the need of a nasogastric tube and swallowing;
2. Ability to speak;
3. Healing and epithelization of intradefect surfaces;
4. Inhibition of contraction of unsupported defect areas;
5. Supporting of free skin grafts;
6. Prevention of the defect area from contamination and infection.

22.4.3.2 Interim Obturation

An interim obturator, also referred to as the "*therapeutic obturator*," is used for approximately 3–4 months following the surgical obturator phase. Serving as a bridge between the initial surgical obturator and the final, definitive obturator, it plays a significant role in the patient's recovery and adaptation process. The base plate from the surgical obturator can also be used in the conversion to the interim obturator. During the patient's follow-up visit, any gauze placed during

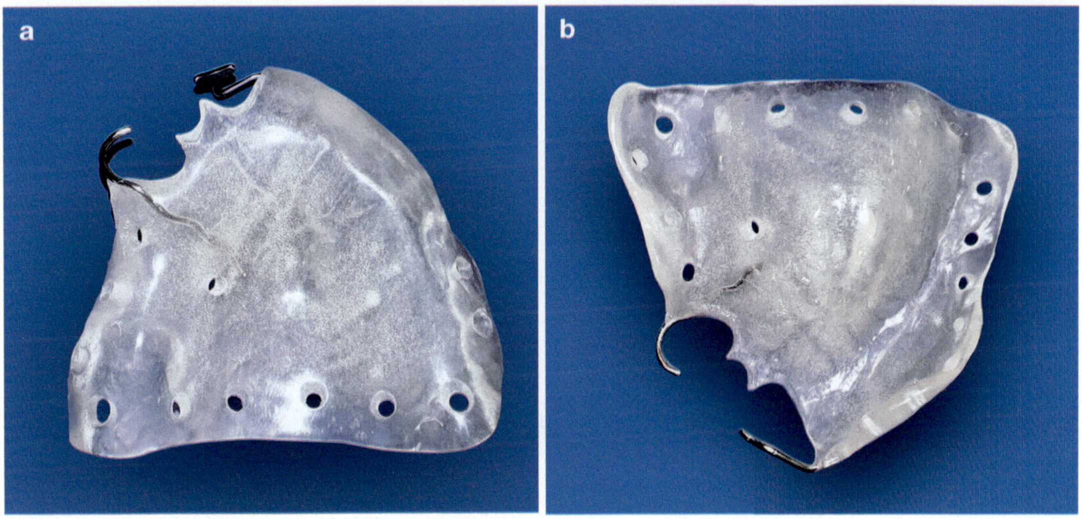

Fig. 22.7 (**a**, **b**) Surgical obturator fabricated with wrought wires and holes

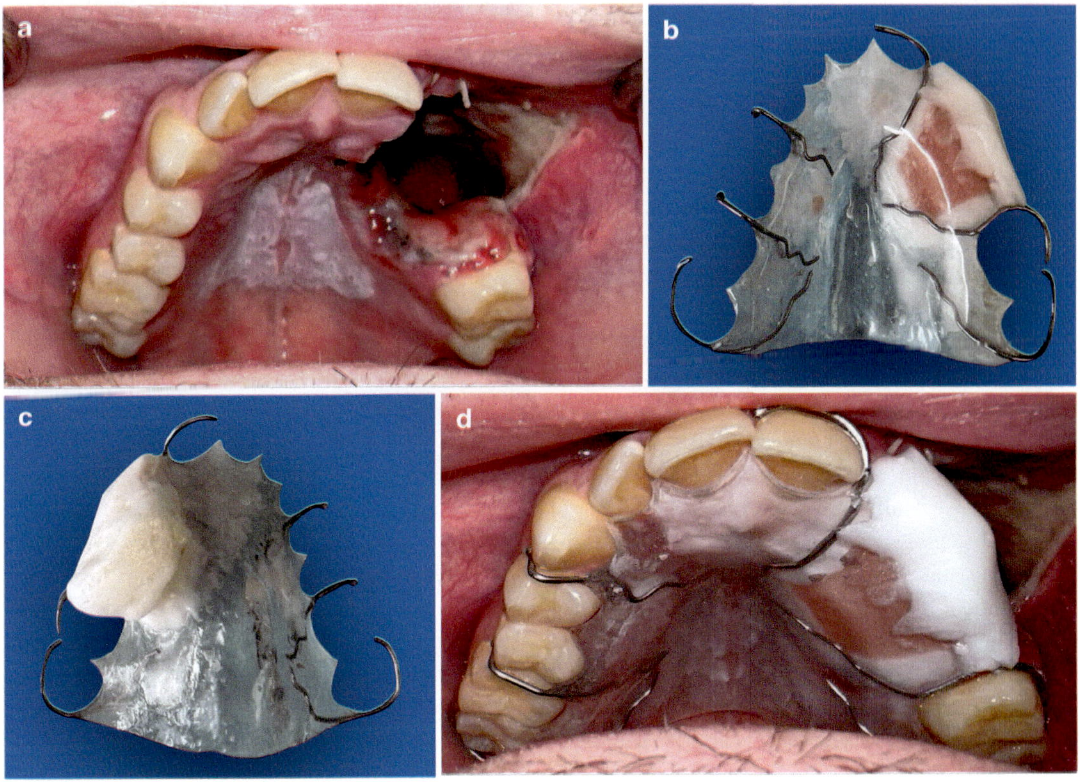

Fig. 22.8 (**a**–**d**) Soft tissue relining of a surgical obturator

surgery is removed, and comprehensive wound care is provided. To transition to the interim obturator, a soft tissue conditioner is applied as a reline material to the existing base plate. This conversion process ensures that tissues still in the healing process are protected from the potentially harmful pressure of direct impression materials (Fig. 22.8a–d).

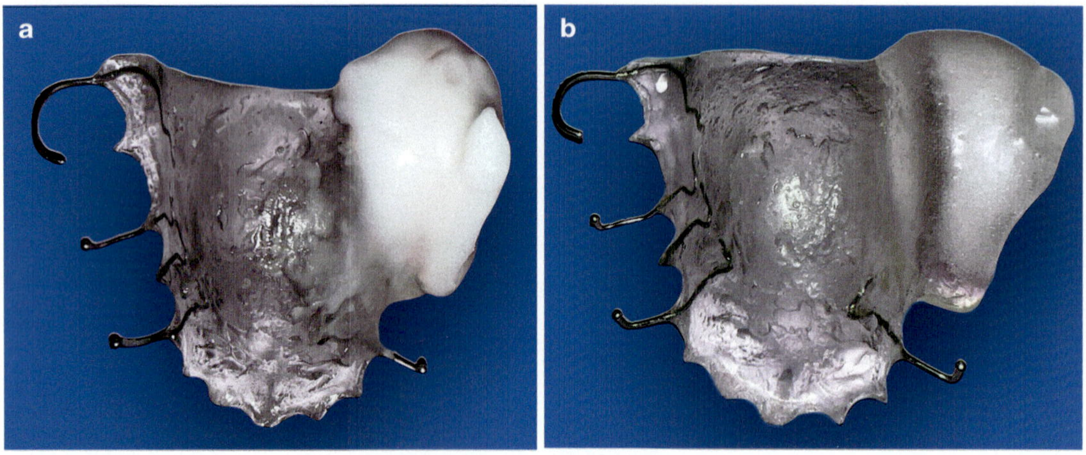

Fig. 22.9 (**a**, **b**) Conversion of the soft tissue reline (**a**) of interim obturator to PMMA (**b**)

Soft tissue reline has the capacity to adapt the contraction of the defect and a positive impact on tissue healing. By extending into the undercuts of the defect, it aids in the retention of the obturator. Interim obturator can be used for up to 6 months with adjustments made every 2–3 weeks, alongside oral hygiene control, and defect cleaning. During this period, due to changes in the defect area, achieving a satisfactory seal can be challenging, and leakage into the defect may be observed.

Clasp retention is the most effective means of securing the obturator, followed by edentulous ridges and the defect itself. However, complete engagement with the defect is often not possible due to ongoing healing. Denture adhesives can be recommended on the intaglio surface that will seat on the remaining acrylic denture-bearing areas that are not surgically approached.

During this transition, it becomes essential for the patient to actively participate in their treatment. This phase is a learning process where the patient acquires skills to place and remove the obturator and to monitor the defect area. As healing progresses, the interim obturator, initially relined with a soft material, can be converted to a hard lining material (Fig. 22.9a, b). Through the progress of healing, teeth can be added to the interim obturator after an accommodation period for a better esthetic look (Fig. 22.10).

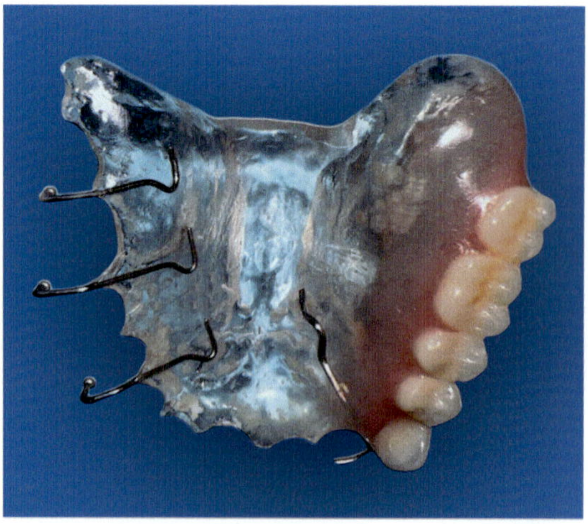

Fig. 22.10 An interim obturator with the addition of teeth

Common complications such as mucositis and xerostomia-related irritation may be encountered in the interim period, particularly in patients receiving radiotherapy and chemotherapy. Trismus may also emerge as a long-term radiotherapy complication. Therefore, the patient should be aware of the significance of engaging in physical therapies and related mouth-opening practices. Chewing on the defect side is not recommended.

22.4.3.3 Definitive Obturation

After completion of the epithelialization and scar formation of the remaining tissues, the final treatment stage, which is the "definitive obturation," starts depending on the condition of the defect. It

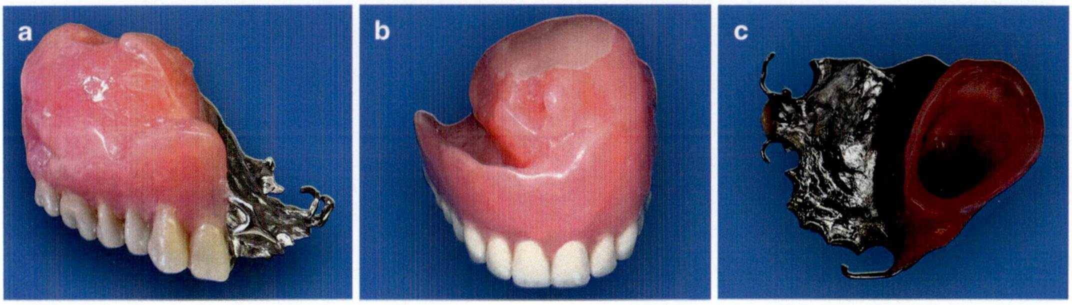

Fig. 22.11 (**a**–**c**) Various types of bulbs fabricated for maxillary defects closed (**a**), closed hallow (**b**), open bulb (**c**)

typically takes 2–6 months on average for the surgical site to be stable. However, the definitive obturator delivery may be postponed to 6–12 months in situations such as an insufficient defect healing, complication in the overall systemic condition of the patient, limited mouth opening, inadequate oral hygiene control, and the presence of radiotherapy or chemotherapy.

Condition of the remaining teeth, alveolar crest, the remaining hard palate, and the defect itself all play a significant role in the retention, stability, and support of the obturator. The extension of the obturator that is inserted in the defect is referred as the "bulb." Retention of an obturator in partially edentulous patients is partly obtained through the anatomical undercuts that the bulb is in contact. The extent and areas of retention should be decided following a survey and determining a path of insertion. These bulbs can also aid in creating a better phonation and improve speech resonance. Several obturator bulbs can be designed depending on the size of the defect and the condition of the surrounding tissues. It can be processed as a homogeneous full structure attached to the denture base or it can be designed with open and closed hallow shapes in order to obtain a lightweight prosthesis. The bulb can be processed from a completely rigid material or a soft material, depending on the requirements of the defect and surrounding tissues (Fig. 22.11a–c).

The vertical surface of the resected lateral bone, acting as a fulcrum, should be covered with a flap to provide sufficient support and to decrease the pain associated with functional contact. Also known as lateral scar band, it is formed at the junction of the mucosa and the tissue graft in the healing process, and this scar contracture provides a natural retention, support, and stability. If the extension of the obturator in this area reaches the distobuccal temporal bone, which is a more rigid structure than the remaining soft tissue support below, potential movement of the obturator is minimized. With the addition of the teeth support with a cross arch stabilization, further diminishes this movement (Fig. 22.12).

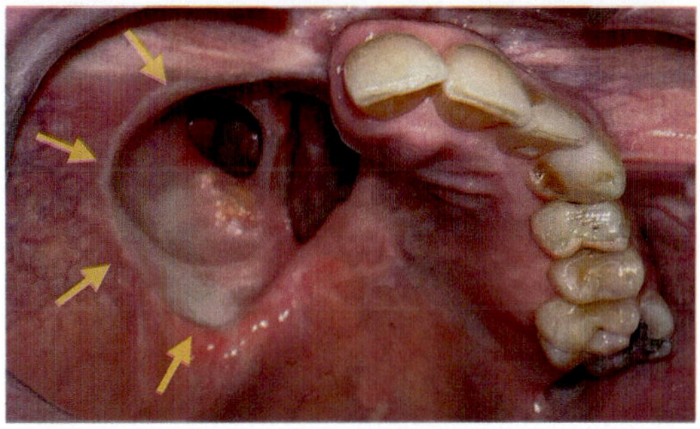

Fig. 22.12 Scar band at the junction of the mucosa and the tissue graft

The amount of remaining palatal tissue band is also important in the palatopharyngeal competence. If the resection leaves a tissue band less than one-third of the soft palate, it should be completely removed and prosthetically reconstructed (Fig. 22.13a–c).

Recording the remaining anatomical areas in combination with the existing structures play an essential role in the retention, stability, and support, and therefore a detailed impression is essential. Once the primary cast is obtained, a custom tray should be fabricated to make the definitive impression. It's important to block out undercuts

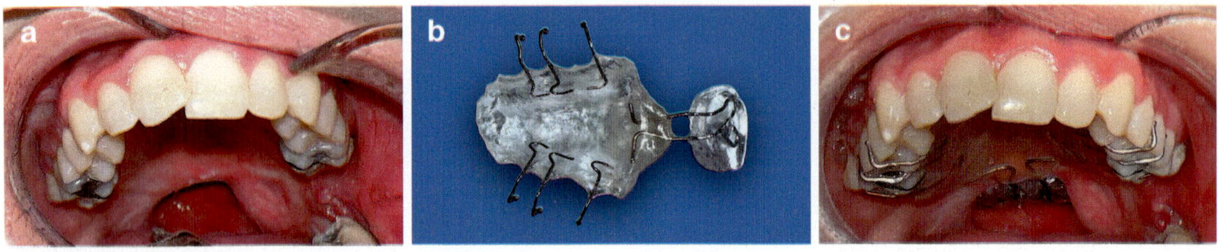

Fig. 22.13 (a–c) An interim obturator fabricated to extend and obturate a soft tissue defect

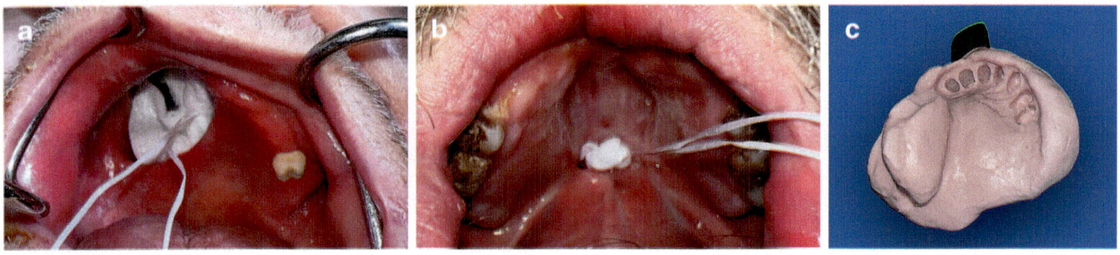

Fig. 22.14 (a–c) Block-out of a large (a) and a small (b) defect and an alginate impression (c) of a resected area

and relief areas to prepare for this process. Border molding is recommended for capturing the detailed contours of the remaining edentulous areas.

Making an impression of the defect area often presents challenges, and precautions should be taken to manage the impression material and prevent the aspiration of it. Block-out of the undercuts of the defect is essential to prevent the stuck of the impression material. For this purpose, a gauze pack is placed to block the undercuts of the defect to keep the impression material from flowing into the areas that are not required to be recorded and being torn while removing it. This impression can be formed using either hydrocolloid impression material or polyvinyl silicone, or a combination of both (Fig. 22.14a–c).

In recent years, digital impressions have become a viable option for capturing the oral anatomy of maxillectomy patients. Trismus, a common complication following surgery and radiation therapy, often limits mouth opening, making it challenging to insert traditional impression trays. In such cases, using the scanner tip of an intraoral scanner for digital impressions is notably easier and more comfortable for the patient. Digital impressions are considered a safer and more convenient method for these patients. However, it's important to acknowledge the limitations of digital impressions in accurately capturing maxillary defects. Consequently, obturators fabricated using digital impressions may require subsequent relining to achieve an optimal seal.

As the master cast is obtained, a record base is fabricated after blocking out the undercuts with wax. Excessive amount of block out may cause unstable record bases that may jeopardize the accuracy in obtaining the vertical dimension of the occlusion and centric relation. These records are obtained similar to the conventional methods.

Teeth setup must be approached with the understanding that teeth positioned on the defect side primarily serve aesthetic purposes, provide soft tissue support, and prevent the super-eruption of opposing teeth. A lingualized occlusion scheme is favored to enhance stability.

The fit and occlusion are checked at the time of delivery and necessary adjustments are made. Denture adhesives can be recommended on the remaining surface-bearing areas.

The position of the retentive and stabilizing elements and indirect retainers in a partial removable obturator help in even load distribution. Surveying the teeth as well as the defect and determination of the guide planes is essential before designing the framework. The teeth adjacent to the defect bear a significant load, leading to increased stress on these teeth. Solutions to improve long-term prognosis include avoiding retentive clasps on these heavily loaded teeth and considering splinting them together.

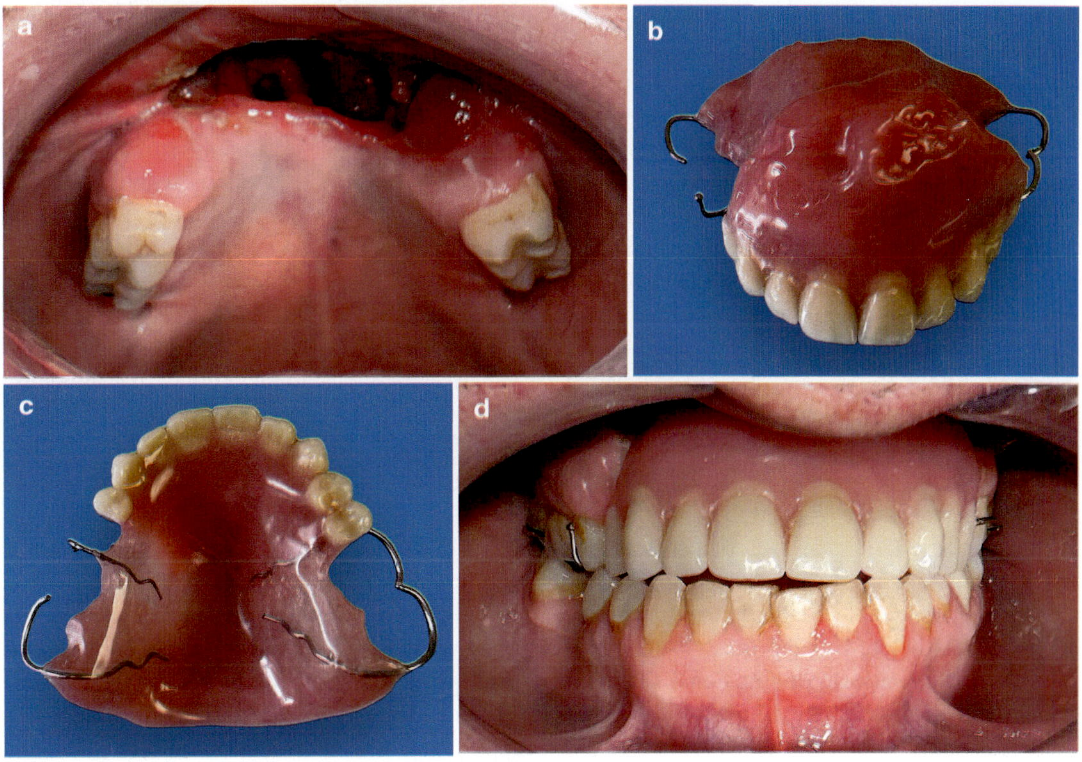

Fig. 22.15 (**a–d**) A PMMA interim denture fabricated for an anterior maxillectomy case

Removable denture designs that could be used in maxillary defects can be summarized as follows:

1. Full PMMA partial dentures.
2. Polyetheretherketone (PEEK) framework reinforced partial dentures with the clasps.
3. Cast framework reinforced partial dentures with clasps.
4. Cast framework reinforced partial dentures with precision attachments and/or implant.

Full PMMA dentures are prostheses made entirely of acrylic, without any metal reinforcement. Wrought or cast clasps are attached to this acrylic base plate to secure the denture in the mouth. Generally, these prostheses are more appropriate for temporary use. However, their lower cost, ease, and speed of processing may make them a preferred option for permanent use over more stable, metal-reinforced prostheses. Additionally, full PMMA dentures offer the convenience of easy repair and the ability to add artificial teeth in place of natural teeth that have been extracted. Despite these advantages, the lack of rigidity compared to metal-based prostheses requires that acrylic partial dentures be processed thicker, which may introduce certain challenges. These include restrictions on tongue movement, potential impacts on speech, and a period of adjustment for the patient to become accustomed to the denture (Fig. 22.15a–d).

PEEK materials have gained attention in the literature due to their strength, esthetic properties, and ease of production. However, their elastic properties result in a degree of flexibility, which is a less desirable feature in a maxillary defect, requiring a stable obturator for less trauma formation in the resection site. Polyetherketoneketone (PEKK) is often highlighted in literature for its strength, esthetic properties and straightforward manufacturing process. Since proper retention, stability and support are required in a partial denture, flexible denture materials such as nylon resins, polyoxymethylene, and polyamides are not indicated as a framework material due to their nonrigid properties.

Metal Framework Reinforced Partial Dentures with Clasps

Metal frameworks are frequently used in the partial obturators fabricated for maxillary defects. However, biomechanical considerations should be considered in determining the location of the components of the framework. Thus, the forces acting on an obturator can be distributed as evenly as possible over the primary support areas rather than just the teeth. The remaining palatal surface, alveolar crest, tuberosities, and the defect itself are reliable sources for a framework design. If a framework-supported partial obturator distributes and shares the functional forces between these tissues in an equilibrium, the prognosis of the prosthesis and the supporting tissues is mostly predictable in the long term.

Framework planning of a partial obturator is similar to the principles applicable to conventional partial removable dentures mentioned previously in this book. To keep these loads under control, a sufficient level of functional retention and stability must be provided, and overloading of the remaining teeth and other supporting tissues must be avoided. In addition to these rules, defect-specific conditions such as position, size, presence of lateral scar band, bony margin, undercuts, availability of remaining teeth, and size of the arch (curved or linear) should be taken into consideration. In a curved teeth alignment, the rests can be distributed evenly and on a wide area, helping to direct occlusal forces vertically and to eliminate the lateral forces.

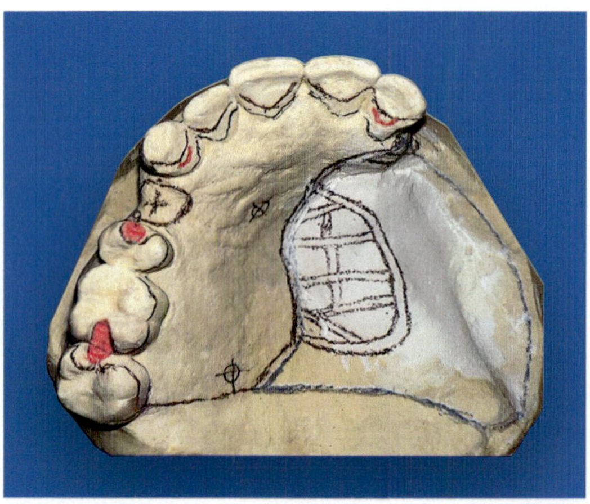

Fig. 22.16 Framework design on the study model

Diagnostic casts should be surveyed to determine guide planes and path of insertion. Undercuts in the defect should be properly examined and included in the survey for a proper path of insertion. Thus, the guiding surfaces on the supporting teeth are in harmony with the path of insertion of the obturator framework (Fig. 22.16). In cases where the crown lengths of the abutment teeth are short, the creation of guiding surfaces may require crowning. This also helps in improving retention and stability by increasing the effectiveness of the clasp, ensuring the splinting of teeth, using of precision attachments, and protecting the teeth from radiation caries.

The major connector of the obturator framework acts as a critical retentive area that extends toward the defect side. Depending on the defect's anatomy and any deformations resulting from resection, this connector may either maintain a standard design or require modifications for enhanced adaptation. Maxillary defects generally necessitate a full coverage for an increased support and seal. It has been reported that the number of rests used in obturators should be increased and they should be wider than the usual sizes to distribute the forces on as many teeth surface as possible. Guiding planes are instrumental to prevent anteroposterior movement. Retainers are the most essential components in reducing the stress via the abutment teeth and to obtain retention. It is essential to use a minimal number of clasps to achieve adequate retention and stability in a conventional framework. The obturators are relatively larger and heavier than conventional dentures and the clasps in the major connector of the obturator may apply destructive forces on the abutment teeth, especially in cases with unilateral defects, causing a progressive periodontal damage and teeth loss. Therefore, these prostheses require the use of additional clasps for these prostheses.

The rotational movement of the maxillary obturators differs from the conventional prosthesis due to the presence of additional fulcrums under varying functional loads. Not only do the teeth serve as rotational axes, but the bony margin of the defect also contributes to this dynamic. Therefore, accurately determining the prosthesis's fulcrum and ensuring an adequate level of indirect retention are

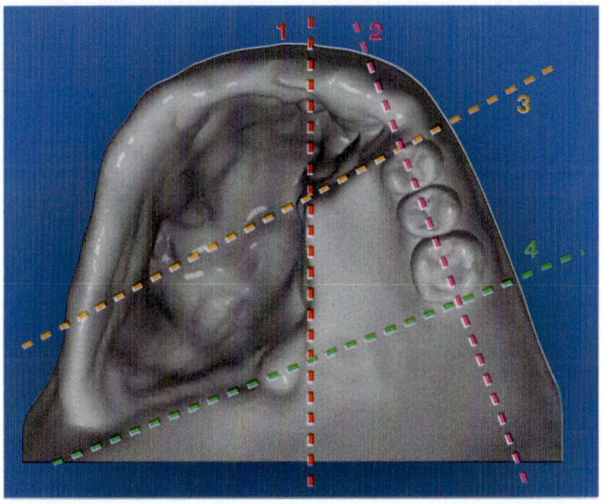

Fig. 22.17 Various rotation axes of a maxillary defect

crucial for the effective function and longevity of the obturator (Fig. 22.17).

It has been reported that the "end position effect" created by the positioning of the retainer arms on the teeth closest and furthest to the defect significantly affects the retention of the prosthesis. To mitigate the 'torque' force exerted on abutment teeth by the prosthesis, the utilization of wrought wire clasps, flexible cast clasp designs, or precision attachments should be considered.

Both the circumferential and bar clasps can be used in the framework of obturators. However, in cases where it is required to increase the number of clasps, designs such as embrasure clasps offer a viable solution.

Different defects classified by Aramany have different rotational axis and framework designs that has to be considered separately to better understand the design principles. This classification combines the remining teeth with the defect to be able to design an appropriate prosthesis based on basic principles of removable partial denture (RPD) planning. It should always be remembered that every patient is a unique case and modifications can be done on each planning approach. However, the preservation of the remaining tissues for an even load distribution is essential when planning the framework. A quadrilateral or tripodal design that provides more even load distribution is favored over a linear design.

Class I:

- The most frequent type of defect that may cause a rotational movement of the obturator.
- A tripodal design providing an evenly distributed load is favored for the support, stability, and retention of the prosthesis.
- Support is obtained from the teeth, palate, and the defect.
- More tissue-bearing surfaces are obtained in square or ovoid arch forms.
- Bone support around the tooth adjacent to the defect should be preserved.
- Rests are placed on the closest anterior teeth to the defect and the mesio-occlusal surface of the most distal abutment that may extend to the disto-occlusal surface of adjacent tooth. This can help prevent wedging and separation of these two teeth causing a periodontal problem due to food impaction.
- A rest placed on the disto-occlusal surface of the most distal tooth also provides cross arch support and stabilization in cases with several axis of fulcrum.
- Guide planes assist in ensuring proper path of insertion for more retention and stability. Guide planes on the anterior teeth should be at a minimum vertical height (1–2 mm) to prevent the torque applied on the teeth.
- Palatal surfaces of the teeth can be utilized for additional bracing and stability to reduce the torque effect.
- A fulcrum line connects the rests that are the nearest and the farthest from the defect and a perpendicular line that extends generally to a canine or a first molar provides an indirect retention and allows a maximum use of leverage to resist movement downward.
- Retention is obtained by the direct retainers. Often a cast circumferential clasp engages 0.25 mm undercut on the buccal surface of posterior teeth. Posterior double Akers (embrasure) clasps with anterior and posterior direction help retention.
- If the dental arch is curved, direct retention is obtained from the labial surface of the anterior teeth with a gate design or I bar and the buccal surface of the molar and bracing palatal.

- A wrought wire can be favored over cast metal on the labial surface of the tooth adjacent to the defect to prevent excessive torque. Splinting a couple of teeth adjacent to the defect might provide an additional protection.
- Tripodal design may be possible in some cases and linear design is considered if anterior teeth are not included. In a linear design, support is obtained from the remaining posterior teeth and the palatal tissues. Retention is obtained from the buccal surfaces of premolars and palatal surfaces of molars (Figs. 22.18a–d and 22.19a–c).

Class II:

- Premaxilla and premaxillary dentition are preserved on both sides.
- Pre-surgical consultation should be made to be able to convert a Class I situation to Class II if the tumor invasion permits. This allows to make a tripodal design with an even load distribution.
- Support and stability are obtained best in the ovoid and square forms, providing this tripodal design.

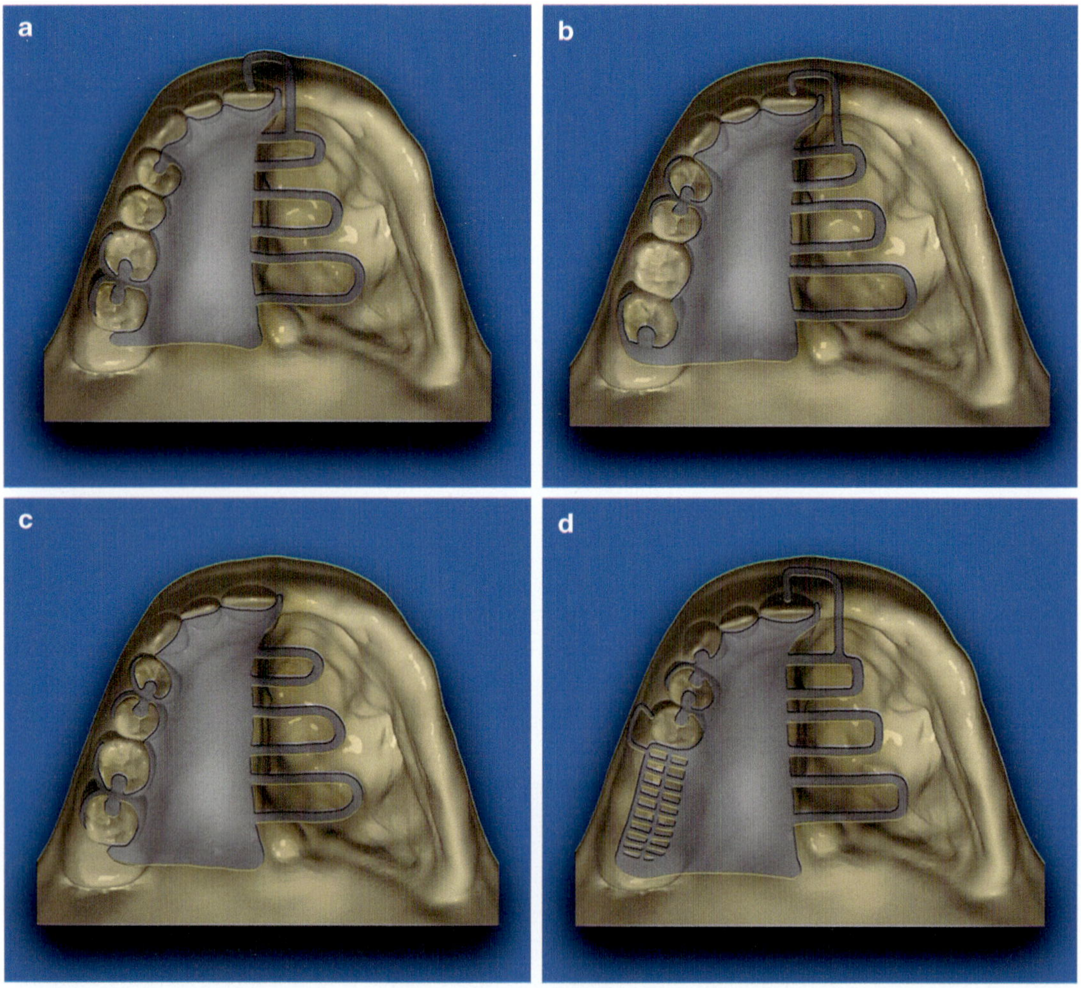

Fig. 22.18 (**a**–**d**) Various framework designs in a Class I Aramany maxillectomy defect

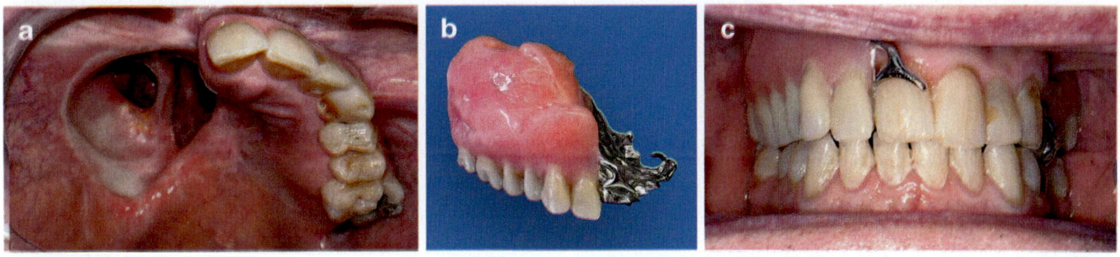

Fig. 22.19 (a–c) Prosthetic treatment of a Class I Aramany defect with a clasp-retained removable partial obturator

- The Prosthetic design is similar to Kennedy Class II design.
- Support is provided by the palate and the rests located on the nearest and farthest teeth from the defect.
- Double rests can be placed on the adjacent posterior teeth.
- The guide plane location and size are similar to Class I with full use of the palatal surfaces of the posterior teeth or distal (proximal) surfaces of the anterior and posterior teeth.
- An indirect retainer is located on a perpendicular line to the fulcrum usually on a canine and premolar and serves as an indirect retainer.
- Anterior teeth adjacent to the defect are critical for retention. This clasp needs to be resistant to displacing forces but needs to rotate, disengage, or flex in function.
- A cast circumferential clasp or an I-bar clasp is used in a 0.25 mm undercut, or a 19-gauge wrought wire clasp in a 0.5 mm or less mesiofacial undercut is also a frequent choice. If additional clasp is required on canine, it should be less flexible. Wrought wire clasps prevent the overloading of the abutment teeth.
- Anterior teeth may be splinted for additional support.
- Posterior retainer: a cast circumferential clasp using 0.25 mm distobuccal undercut. A posterior clasp assembly facing both the anterior and posterior aid in retention.
- A combination of buccal and palatal retention is not indicated (Figs. 22.20a, b and 22.21a–d).

Class III

- Dentition is preserved.
- It may or may not include the soft palate.
- The design is simple, and retention, stabilization, and reciprocation are easily obtained.
- Design is similar to the Kennedy Class III RPD design.
- Support is obtained from the teeth. Little or no support is expected from the palate and defect.
- Rests are bilaterally located (quadrilateral) on canines and molars, proving bilateral symmetry to the major connector.
- Avoidance of the rugae area is recommended.
- Proximal surfaces can be used as guide planes in the presence of any edentulous areas. Theses may be longer and physiologic adjustment is not necessary since there is little movement of the obturator.
- Short guide planes on the palatal surface of the posterior teeth are required.
- Each abutment is supported by a direct retainer, so indirect retainer is not required.
- Retention is often obtained with cast retainers in 0.25 mm undercuts using circumferential clasps, bar clasps, or combination type retainers in which retainer can engage a deeper undercut for esthetic gain (Figs. 22.22a–c and 22.23a–e).

Class IV

- Since premaxilla and a lateral resection are performed, there are often few teeth in

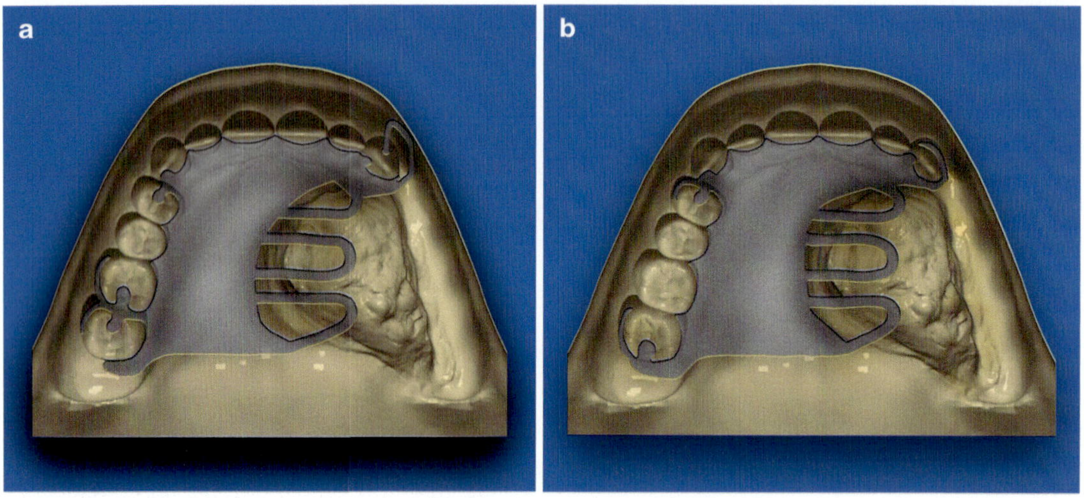

Fig. 22.20 (**a**, **b**) Various framework designs in a Class II Aramany maxillectomy defect

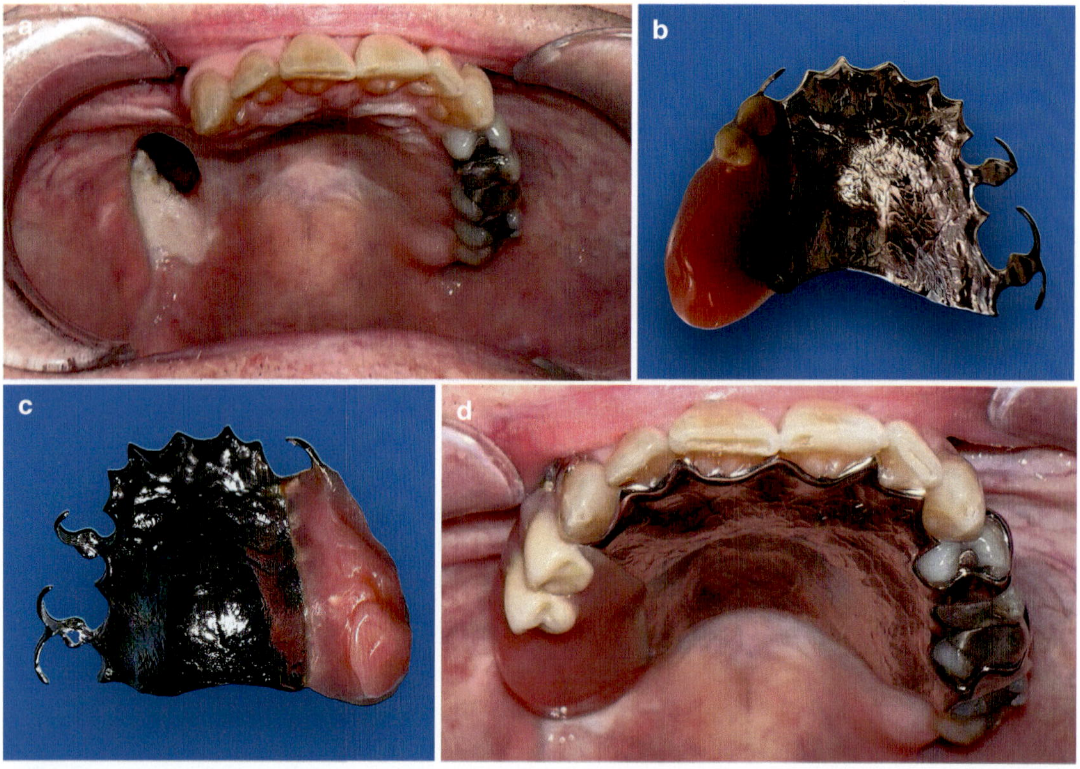

Fig. 22.21 (**a**–**d**) Prosthetic treatment of a Class II Aramany defect with a clasp-retained removable partial obturator

posterior creating a linear alignment rather than a tripodal.

- Support is obtained from the rests located centrally on almost all the remaining teeth.
- Guiding plane is placed on the proximal surface of the tooth adjacent to the defect.
- The defect should be engaged as much as possible. Therefore, creating scar tissue is essential in providing a proper denture-bearing area and obtaining a retention and stability with the help of this area.

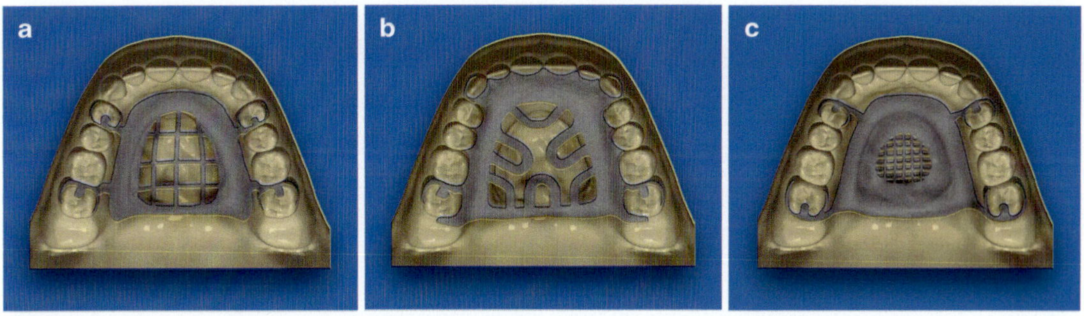

Fig. 22.22 (**a**–**c**) Various framework designs in a Class III Aramany maxillectomy defect

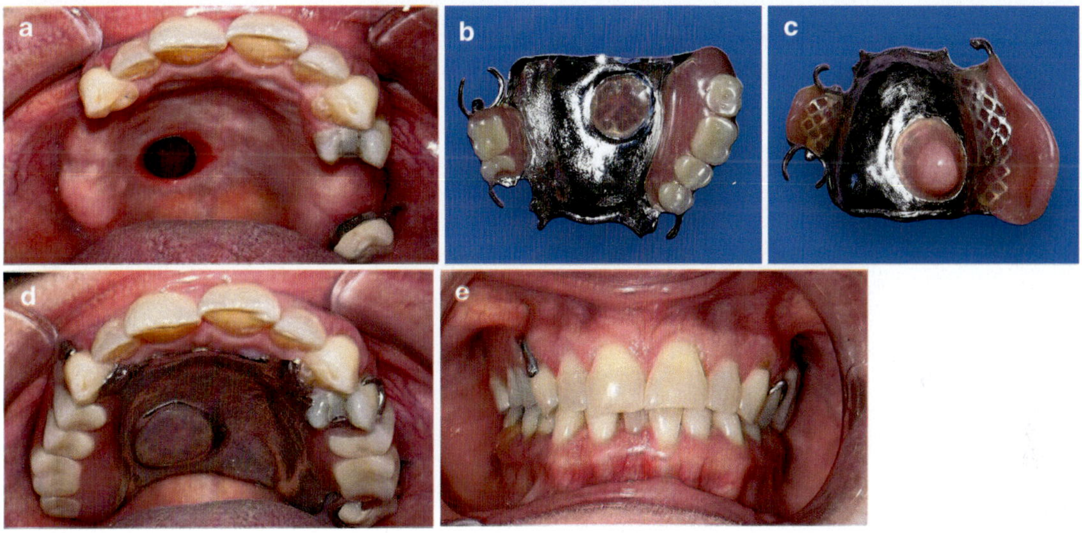

Fig. 22.23 (**a**–**e**) Prosthetic treatment of a Class III Aramany defect with a clasp-retained removable partial obturator

- A palatal major connector is mostly used due to the lever arm force created by the extension of the prosthesis and to also reduce leakage toward the defect.
- Retention in this type of design is challenging. Retention and bracing are diagonally apposed.
- Buccal and palatal retention should be avoided but need to be used if a scar band is not created surgically.
- Retention should be obtained from facial surfaces of the remaining teeth and the lateral wall of the defect.
- Occlusal load should be reduced in the posterior (Fig. 22.24a, b).

Class V:

- Similar to Class IV defects, the extent of the defect is huge and defect itself should also be utilized for the retention and stability of the prosthesis.
- Tripodal design is possible.
- Labial stabilization and splinting of the terminal teeth are necessary in most cases.
- Support is provided by rests on the mesio-occlusal surface of the most posterior teeth. Double rests can be utilized for reasons outlined earlier. Fulcrum line passes through these rests.

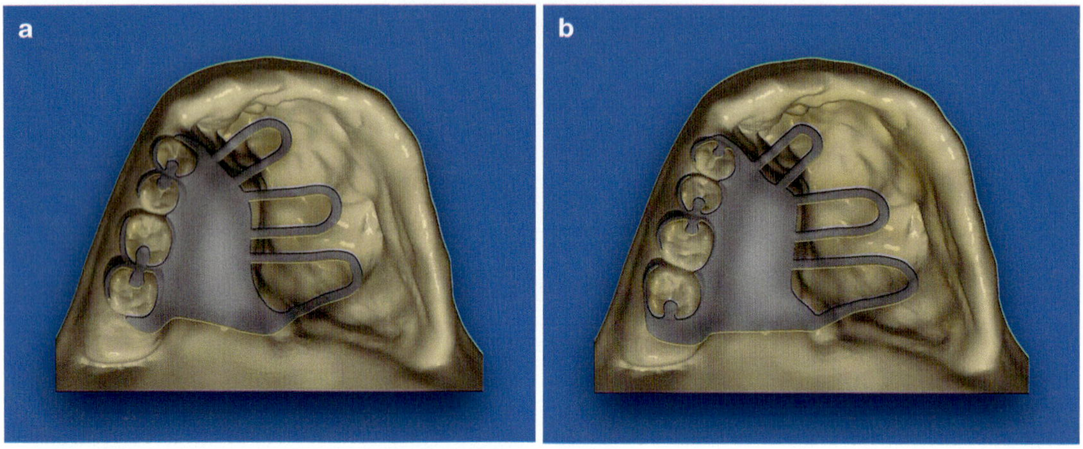

Fig. 22.24 Various framework designs in a Class IV Aramany maxillectomy defect

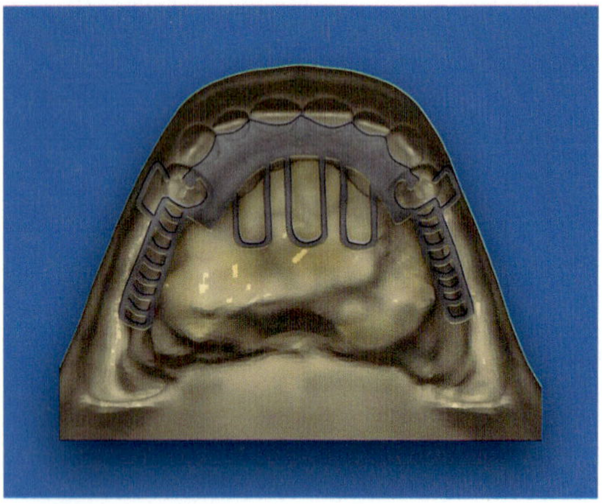

Fig. 22.25 A framework design in a Class V Aramany maxillectomy defect

- Stabilization and bracing are provided by the palatal coverage of the palatal surfaces of the remaining teeth.
- Indirect retention is located far from the fulcrum line generally the central incisors. Occlusal adjustment might be needed due to insufficient space in this area.
- An I-bar retention close to the fulcrum line provides retention.
- When the remaining palate is scarred and immobile, it also aids in retention (Figs. 22.25 and 22.26a–f).

Class VI:

- Existing teeth provide the majority of support, whereas the defect site is not effective as in other defect types. Additional retention can be achieved by extending the anterior part of the prosthesis into the nasal aperture.
- Support is provided by rests located on the mesio-occlusal surfaces of the most anterior tooth.
- Double rests are used when adjacent posterior teeth are involved.
- Additional rests could be utilized in the posterior.
- In cases with extended defect, indirect retention may not be possible.
- Guide planes are located on the proximal surfaces of the after teeth adjacent to the defect and should kept to a minimum length.
- Splinting with an across arch tissue bar might be helpful.
- Retention is often provided with cast retainers close to the fulcrum line (Figs. 22.27a, b and 22.28a–e).

As these defects extend to the soft palate, resonance and articulation is impaired, causing a functional limitation. Bilateral direct retainers placed posteriorly, and indirect retainers placed

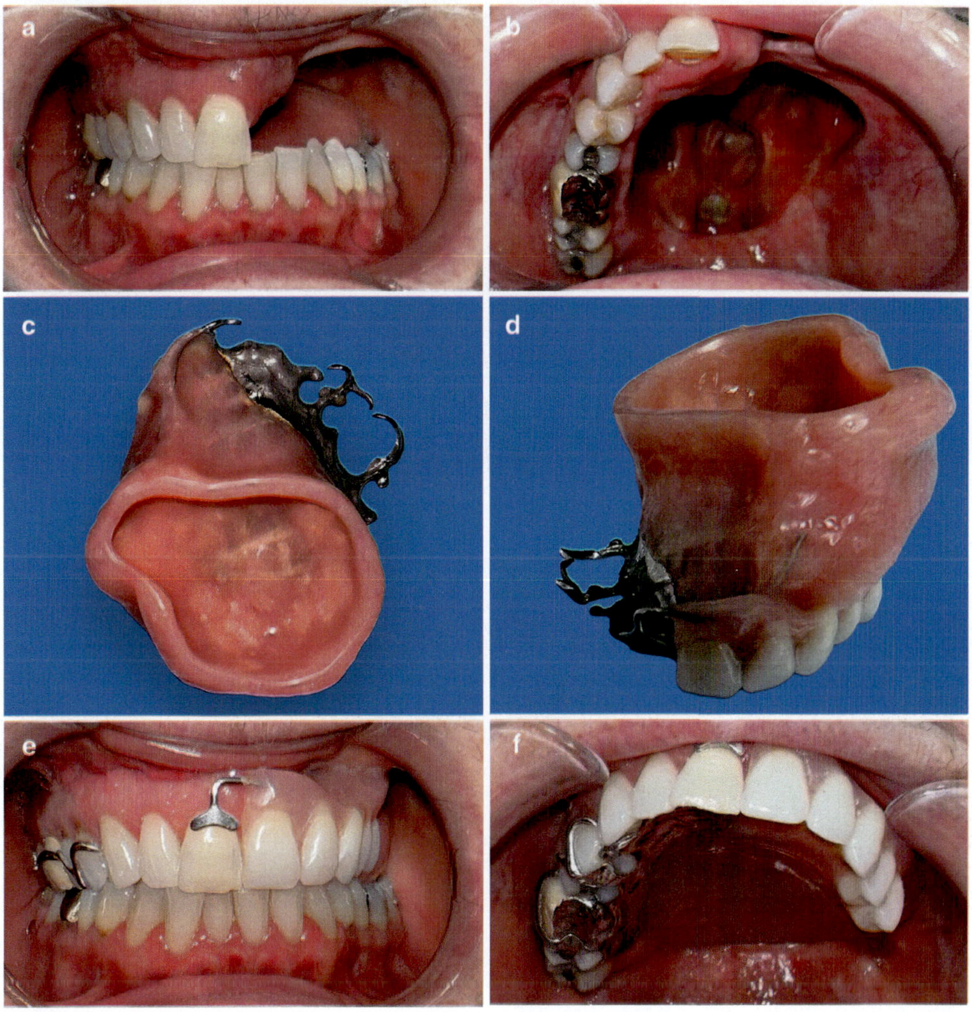

Fig. 22.26 (**a–f**) An extensive bilateral defect

anteriorly to help maintain prosthesis position against the dislodging forces (Fig. 22.29a–d).

Extra-coronal precision attachments could be utilized as they are indicated for improved aesthetics and retention in comparison to conventional clasps. The precision attachments can be used in combination with/without wrought or cast clasps (Fig. 22.30 a-d). Particularly in cases where the defect is in proximity with the anterior teeth, these teeth can be splinted, and precision attachments can be attached for a better stress distribution, preventing an overload on the tooth closest to the defect. Rest seats on the teeth supporting the extra-coronal attachments should be utilized to provide the forces along the long axes (Fig. 22.31a, b).

While these classifications facilitate identification and communication, it's important to recognize that each defect has its own unique characteristics. With this in mind, it should be remembered that every case may have more than one prosthetic treatment option.

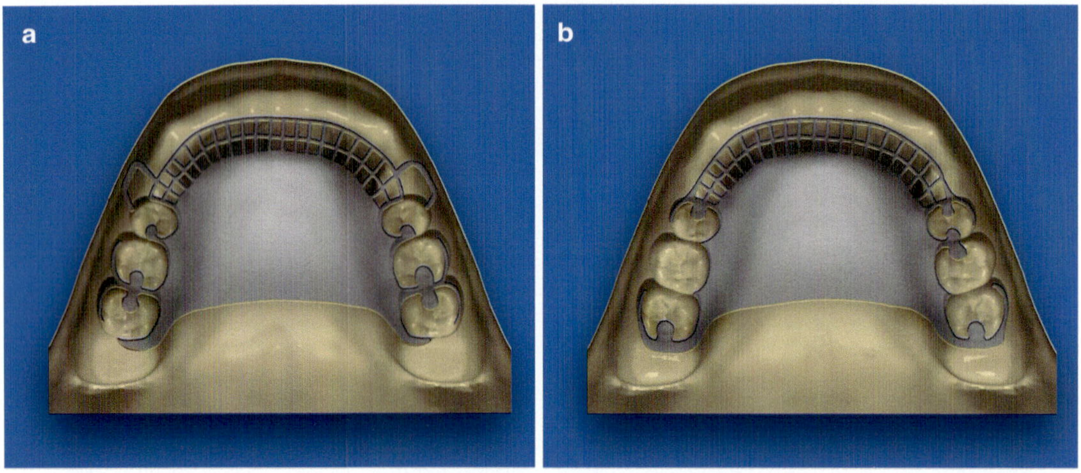

Fig. 22.27 (a, b) Various framework designs in a Class VI Aramany maxillectomy defect

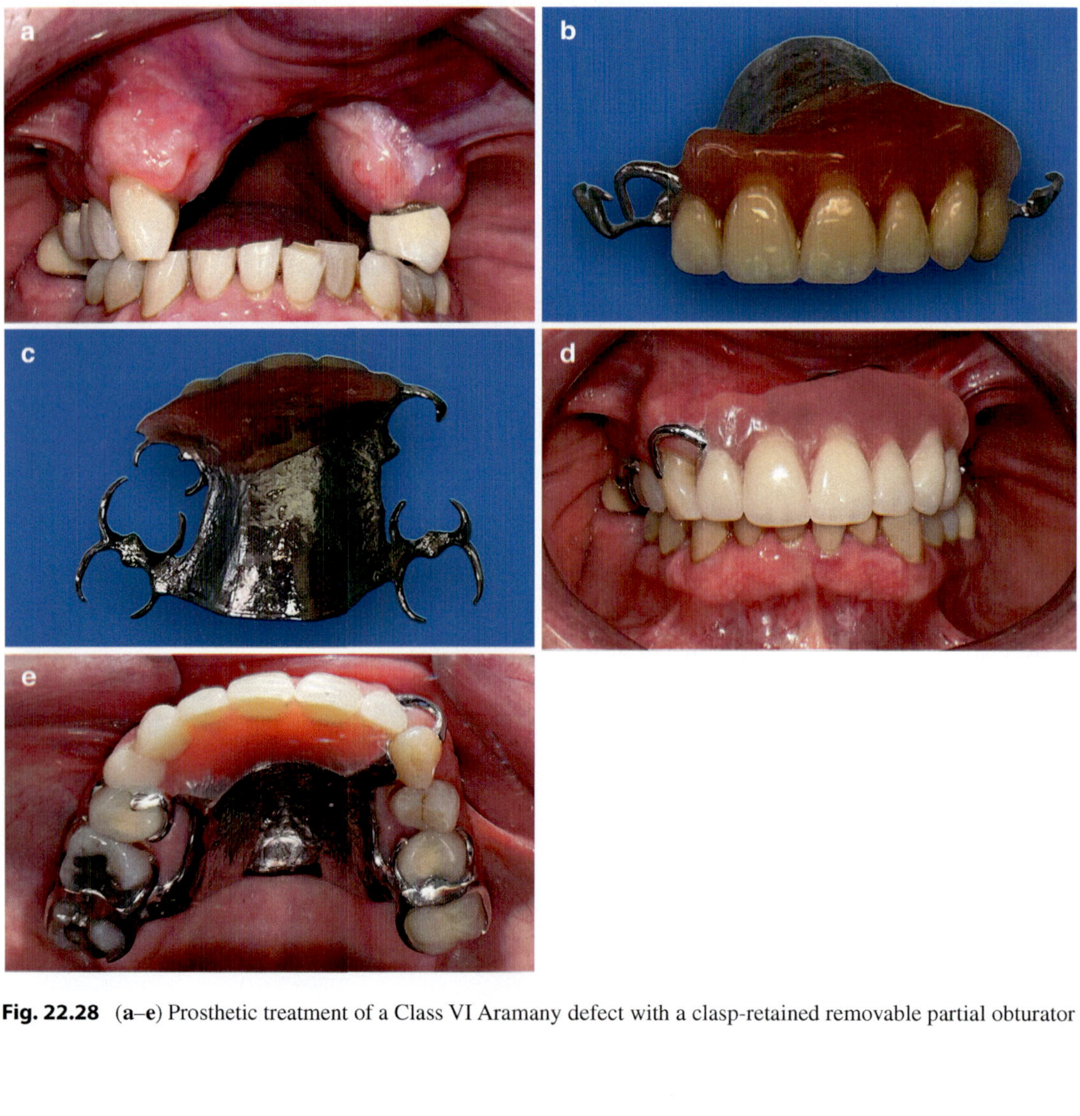

Fig. 22.28 (a–e) Prosthetic treatment of a Class VI Aramany defect with a clasp-retained removable partial obturator

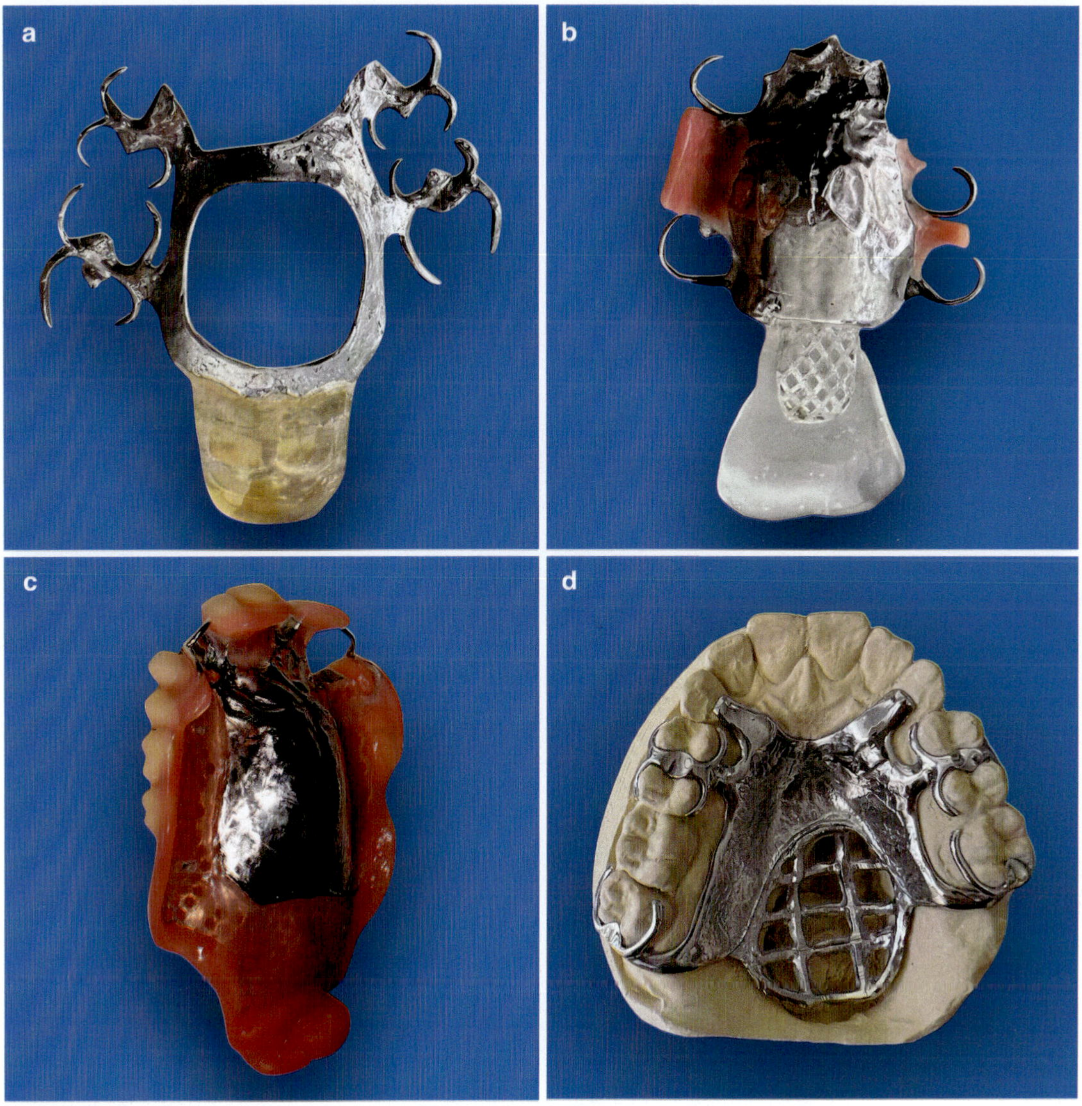

Fig. 22.29 (**a**–**d**) Various obturators that extend to the soft palate

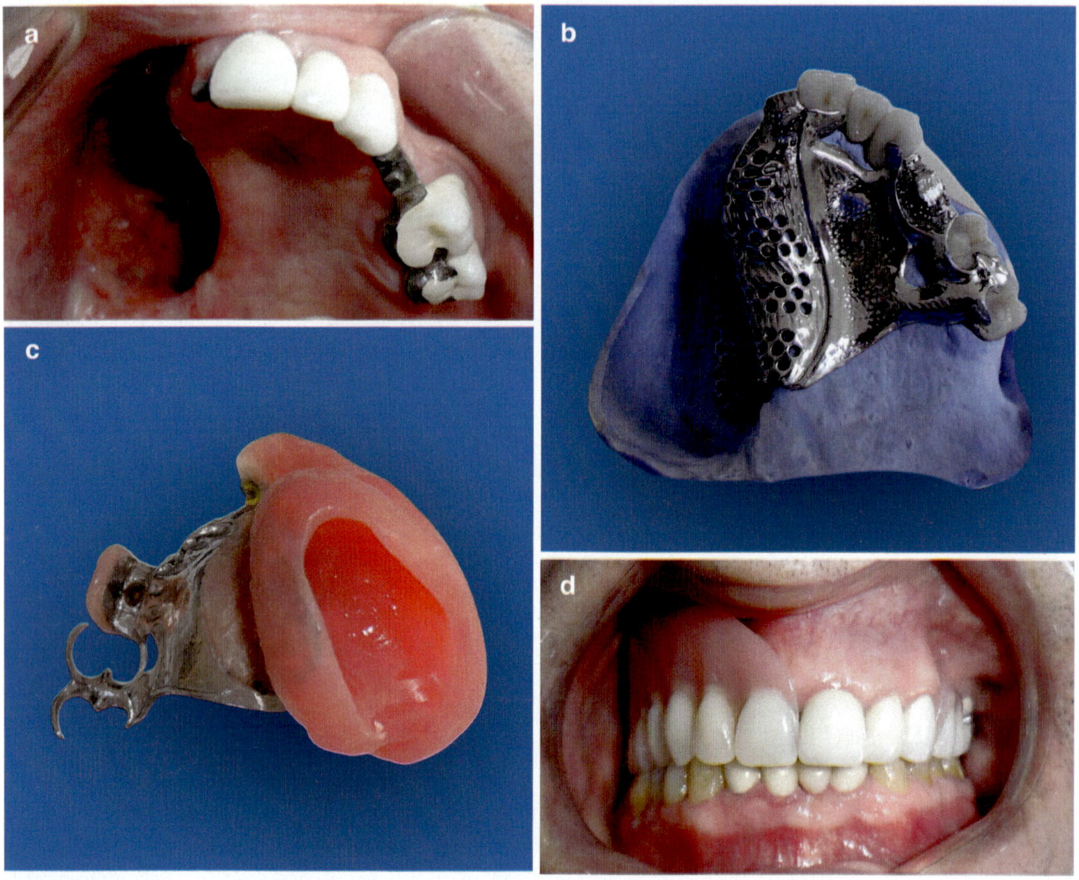

Fig. 22.30 (**a**–**d**) An obturator framework design with precision attachments

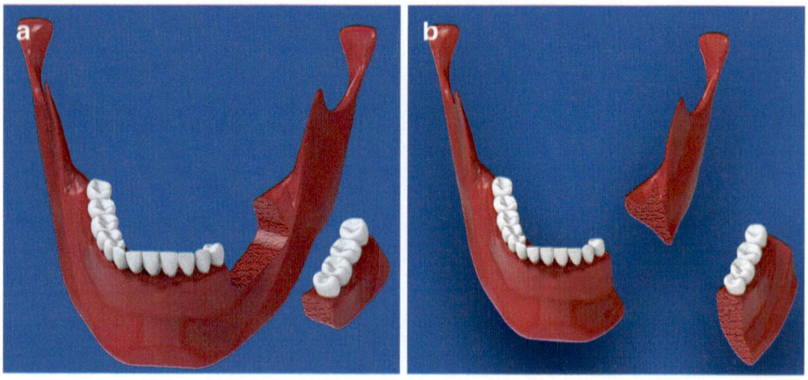

Fig. 22.31 Schematic view of a marginal (**a**) and segmental (**b**) mandibulectomies

22.5 Mandibular Defects

The mandible is a significant anatomical structure, comprising the lower third of the face. It serves essential functions in esthetics, mastication, articulation, deglutition, and respiration. A mandibular resection often leads to cosmetic disfigurement and functional insufficiency. Additional consequences may include loss of saliva control, resulting in drooling on the defect side, as well as the development of cracks and large fissures, often infected with *Candida albicans*. Many cancer patients undergo radiotherapy, which further impairs the function and health of the soft and hard tissues. Consequently, the primary goal of mandibular reconstruction is to restore continuity and stability, establish an acceptable alveolar volume and form, and regain lost function, phonation, and esthetics, ultimately enhancing the patient's quality of life.

22.5.1 Classification of Mandibular Defects

A mandibular classification distinguishes between 'marginal' and 'segmental' resections, delineating the extent of the resection and the presence of continuity in the mandible, irrespective of the surgical site. Marginal mandibulectomy preserves mandibular continuity after neoplasm removal, resulting in defects resembling normal to severely resorbed mandibles requiring similar treatments. Conversely, segmental mandibulectomy involves removing a segment of the mandible, creating a bony discontinuity necessitating additional reconstruction. Failure to stabilize and restore these non-connected segments can lead to mandibular dislocation and deviation toward the surgical site at rest, with the deviation exacerbating during jaw opening, causing functional and aesthetic issues (Fig. 22.31a, b).

There are various classification systems for defining the mandibular defects. Since Pavlov's pioneering classification in 1974, several classifications have been proposed. Among these, a classification propesed by Cantor and Curtis stands out for its relevance in the prosthetic treatment. This classification system delineates six distinct types of mandibular defects, each with its own characteristics and implications for treatment. These six types provide a comprehensive framework for understanding the complexities of mandibular reconstruction and guiding appropriate therapeutic interventions (Fig. 22.32a–f).

Class I: Marginal resection with preservation of mandibular continuity.

Class II: Segmental resection with a mandibular discontinuity distal to the canine area.

Class III: Segmental resection with a mandibular discontinuity that involves a loss up to the mandibular midline region or farther toward the contralateral side.

Class IV: Segmental resection with a mandibular continuity obtained with an augmentation of bone and soft tissue.

Class V: Anterior resection with a mandibular continuity obtained with an augmentation of bone and soft tissue.

Class VI: Similar to Class V, except that the mandibular continuity is not restored.

22.5.2 Surgical Resection and Reconstruction of Mandible

The extent of the surgical approach significantly influences the prosthetic outcome of the treatment. In marginal resections, where the existing teeth and their functionality are minimally impacted, the outcomes tend to be more consistent. However, when the grafting procedures become a part of the treatment, denture bearing tissues change to a more mobile structure. Furthermore, when it is a segmental mandibulectomy, the tongue and the surrounding tissues may be involved, complicating the restoration of function and esthetics.

Autogenous bone augmentation is accepted as the gold standard of mandibular reconstructions. In general, microvascularized free flaps, pedicled osteotomy flaps, grafts including particulate and cortical bone and reconstruction plates, distraction osteogenesis, and endoprosthesis have been considered as the major reconstruction options for the mandibular defects. Today, the majority of free flaps for mandibular reconstruction are the radial forearm, scapula, iliac crest, and fibula. When free flaps are used, tongue function is less affected and patients achieve nearly normal function.

Pectoralis major myocutaneous pedicle flaps followed by other myocutanous pedicle flaps such as deltopectoral latissimus dorsi, sternocleidomastoid, platysma, and trapezius have been frequently used for the reconstruction; however, they have complications such as scar tissue formation, limited mobility that might cause speech

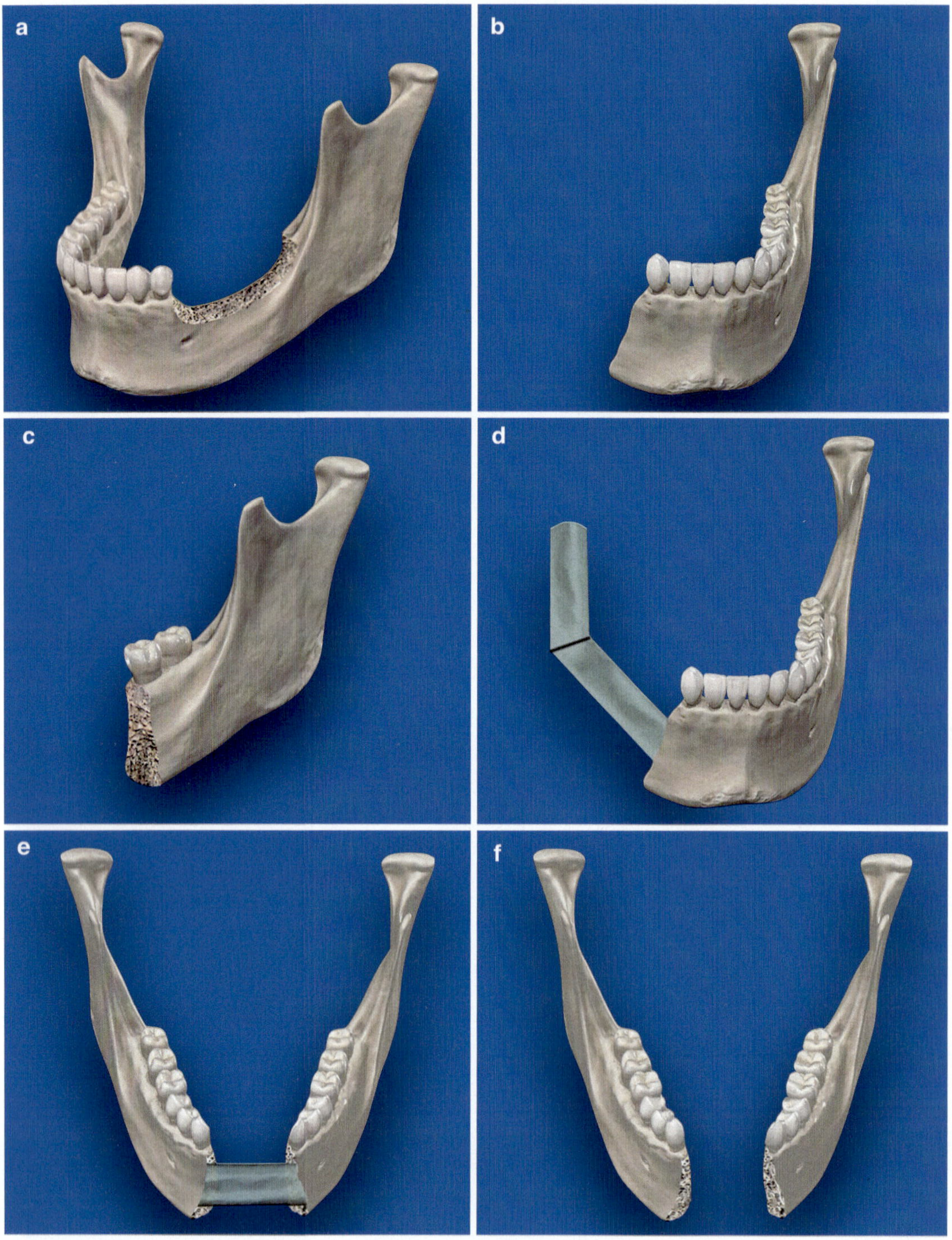

Fig. 22.32 (**a**–**f**) Schematic view of Cantor and Curtis classification

impairment as well as deglutition and swallowing problems.

An extensive resection may be required following the removal of the tumors of the tongue and the floor of the mouth. Surgical resection of the carcinoma of the lateral tongue, if extensive, may require resection of a portion of the body of the mandible. As the defect extends to a larger area, a

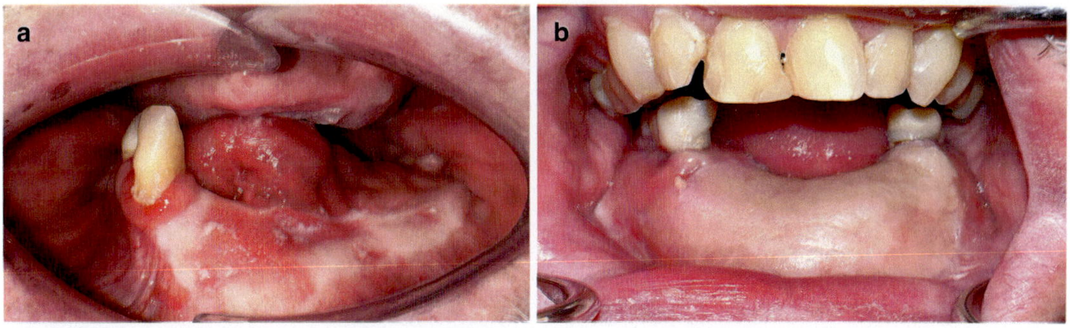

Fig. 22.33 (**a**, **b**) Various mandibular defects associated with the floor of the mouth

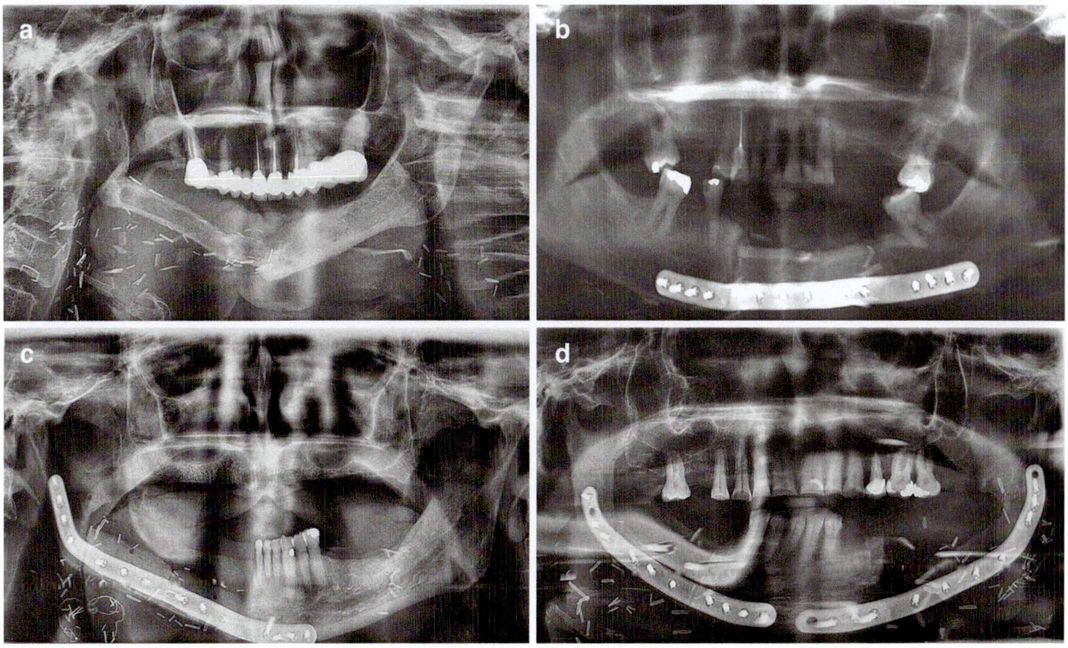

Fig. 22.34 (**a**–**d**) Panoramic X-ray of various mandibular reconstructions

more extensive reconstructive surgery is required after the resection. Moreover, the presence of bulky soft tissue components and reduced mobility of the tongue can impact the success of future prosthetic treatments. These patients may also need additional surgeries such as sulcus deepening and skin grafting. However, scar tissues between the lip and tongue also have an effect on the disengagement of the removable prosthesis (Fig. 22.33a, b).

The quality and quantity of the bone and soft tissue obtained, along with their management for reconstruction and availability for future implant placement, are critical parameters, and the design of the grafted structure and prosthetic considerations are essential for the long-term functionality of the reconstruction. Therefore, a comprehensive treatment planning is required for achieving optimum osseous construction.

Reconstruction plates, which are used to maintain the continuity of the contours of the mandible with and without the use of bone grafts, are among the reconstruction methods utilized in these patients (Fig. 22.34a–d).

Today, reconstruction plates are designed with the help of CAD–CAM techniques prior to surgery on three-dimensional models. Guides for the proper shape of the grafts are also fabricated for a more precise surgical result (Fig. 22.35a, b).

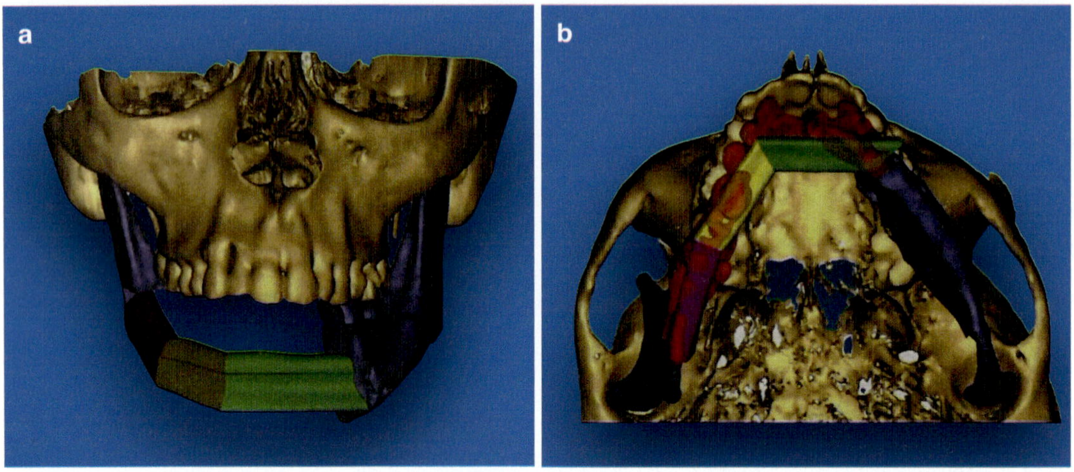

Fig. 22.35 (**a**, **b**) A digital surgical planning of a mandibular defect

In most of the cases, radical neck dissection is performed to surgically control the metastatic spread involving the removal of lymph nodes from levels 1 to 5, along with structures such as the submandibular glands, the sternocleidomastoid and omohyoid muscles, the internal jugular vein, and the spinal accessory nerve.

Following the surgery, patients are typically maintained with nasogastric tube feedings for the first 7–10 days transitioning to a mechanically soft diet to prevent fibrous union of the osteotomy site. Maxillomandibular fixation is generally not required.

Patients who undergo total or partial mandibulectomies often experience significant impacts on chewing function due to tooth and supporting tissue loss. Depending on additional treatments such as radiotherapy, clinicians may consider simultaneous or delayed implant placement to support the retention of removable or fixed prostheses.

22.5.3 Prosthetic Workflow of Mandibular Defects

Every mandibular defect case is unique, and the planning of a removable prosthesis may exhibit variations with resections of the mandible and/or surrounding tissues. The number and the condition of the teeth as well as the remaining soft and hard tissues are important for the support, retention, and stabilization of a removable partial mandibulectomy prosthesis. Mandibular defects extending to the tongue, floor of the mouth, and adjacent structures may lead to impaired phonation, function, and esthetics. Consequently, prosthetic treatment in such cases poses notable challenges.

Unlike maxillary defects, providing an immediate denture for mandibulectomy patients is not typically a priority. Instead, the primary goals include achieving proper healing and a stabilized maxillomandibular relationship after surgical reconstruction. Treatment should commence only once this stability is attained. However, it's crucial to prioritize function, and patients should be encouraged to begin functional activities once healing is underway. Therefore, the use of an interim denture plays a vital role in transitioning towards the definitive prosthesis.

As previously indicated for maxillary defects, similar removable denture options as given below can be utilized for mandibular defects.

1. Full PMMA partial dentures.
2. Cast framework reinforced partial dentures with clasps.
3. Cast framework reinforced partial dentures with precision attachments and/or implant.
4. PEEK framework reinforced partial dentures with clasps.

Full PMMA dentures with wrought wire and/or cast clasps are mostly used as interim solutions following mandibulectomy. However, this use can be extended if no discomfort is stated by the patient. Due to the common contraindications of PMMA dentures, more stable cast frameworks can be utilized for the long-term success.

While PEEK is not primarily preferred due to its flexibility and potential pressure on the defect area, advancements in its physical properties have led to considerations for its use as a framework material. Despite historical concerns, recent improvements suggest that PEEK may become a more favored option in the future, as indicated in the literature.

Metal framework reinforcement of a mandibulectomy prosthesis helps to obtain even load distribution, cross arch stabilization, and retention to prevent dislodging functional forces. Similar to conventional framework guidelines, the major connectors should be rigid, and occlusal rests are needed to direct the occlusal forces along the long axis of guiding planes. Stability and retention must be within the limits of physiological tolerance, and the components of the framework should not express excessive lateral forces on the remaining abutment teeth. Adjacent soft tissues can be utilized as an additional source of support.

A well-performed surgical reconstruction of the mandible undoubtedly enhances the predictability of prosthetic outcomes, both functionally and aesthetically. The extent of the prosthesis covering the defect area is contingent upon the underlying structural support provided by the surgical reconstruction.

From a restorative perspective, a marginal resection with mandibular continuity and protected inferior alveolar nerve can be easily restored with removable partial dentures fabricated with conventional methods. If the resection extends to the lingual and buccal mucosa, tongue, muscles, nerves, and glands, both the surgical and the prosthetic approaches to obtain retention, stability, and support can be challenging. Therefore, the condition of the remaining teeth and the surrounding tissues is essential, and implants can be helpful in cases with insufficient teeth and tissue support. If the continuity of the bone is maintained with simultaneous reconstructions with segmental resection, a conventional planning with customized modifications would be quite sufficient in the treatment of these patients. After surgery, mandibular dislocation can sometimes limit the available prosthetic space, preventing the denture from extending to the posterior. In such cases, a denture with a shorter distal extension may be fabricated.

A mandibulectomy site with continuity can resemble edentulous sites, allowing for the utilization of conventional framework designs. In case of a lateral mandibulectomy with the remaining teeth, the edentulous condition looks more like a Kennedy Class II classification. Similarly, if there is a lateral defect and the contralateral side is an edentulous ending arch, the framework resembles a Kennedy Class I, whereas if the marginal resection is in the anterior area, the design may be more like a Kennedy Class IV classification. The resection site can be more extensive if there is a combination of these groups (Fig. 22.36a–e).

It should always be remembered that framework design may require modifications due to patient-specific factors and there is not a single design for every case. Therefore, defect-specific considerations and precautions should be taken into account when designing the framework.

Retention obtained from the remaining teeth in mandibular defects is significant in terms of patient's quality of life. The number of fulcrum lines increases in cases where edentulous ending areas are present on the non-defect side. Increasing the number of direct and indirect retainers is suggested in the literature to prevent rotation around these fulcrum lines.

In the presence of abutments with questionable prognosis, the design should enable the partial denture to be modified if a tooth needs to be extracted. In such a situation, a soldered wrought wire *clasp* with adequate flexibility engaging the undercut of the anterior abutment adjacent to the defect should be used to prevent the torquing stresses (Fig. 22.37).

Retention can be achieved through various types of clasp assemblies. If the remaining teeth

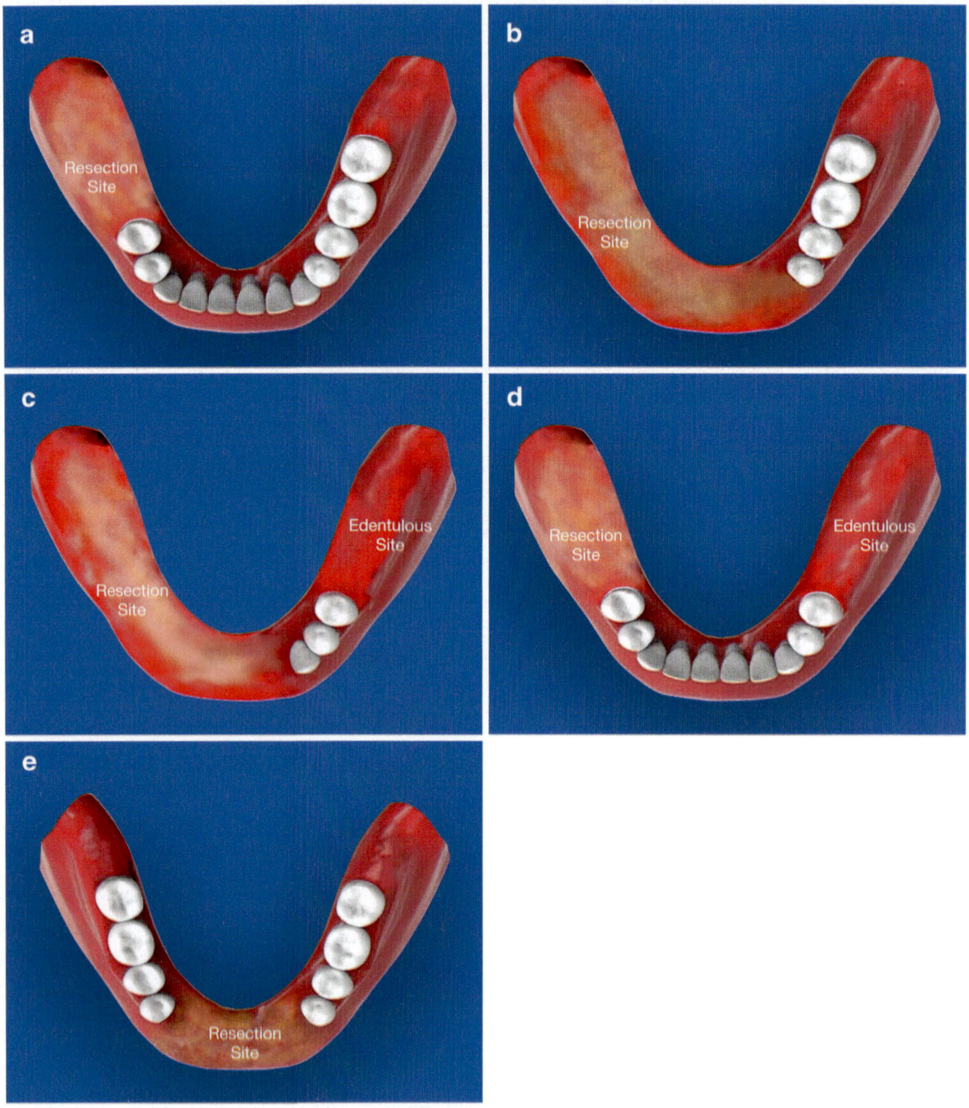

Fig. 22.36 (**a**–**e**) Several mandibular defect types

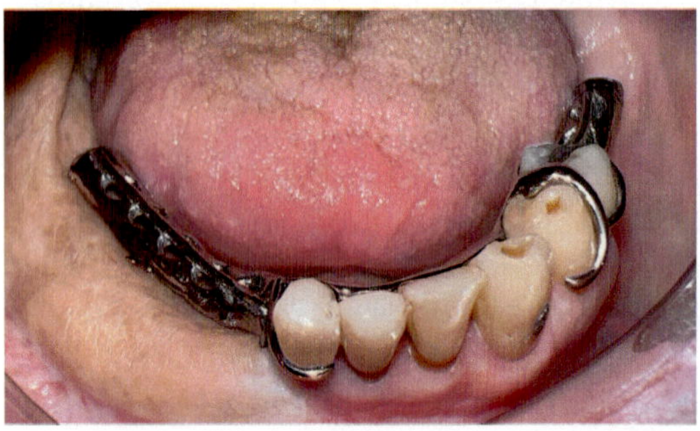

Fig. 22.37 A cast metal framework design featuring a wrought clasp on the incisor and a cast clasp on the premolars on a mandible reconstructed with a fibula graft

are aligned in a straight-line configuration, embrasure clasps on the posterior teeth and infra bulge retainers on the anterior abutment are effective obtaining this retention. Multiple rests are suggested in these defects to increase the amount of the support and stability. Swing lock type retention systems, which lock on the vestibular surfaces of the remaining teeth can also be considered. However, this decision should be made with several considerations in mind, as it may introduce additional stresses on the teeth. It is particularly challenging to manipulate these

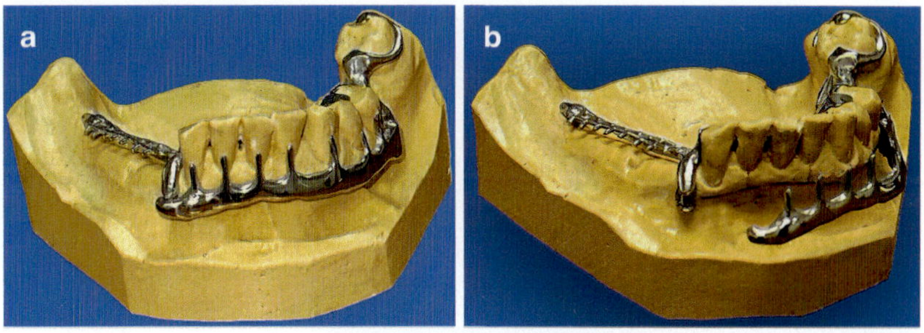

Fig. 22.38 (**a**, **b**) Swing lock type framework that can be used in a mandibulectomy case

frameworks in elderly patients (Fig. 22.38a, b). Therefore, the use of buccal and lingual retention could prove more effective in these cases. Rests should be positioned extensively and wrought wire retainers can serve as a viable alternative to bar clasps.

The selection of the major connector is related to the height of the floor of the mouth and the contact of the attached gingival margins during function. Preserving as many teeth as possible is crucial in more extensive defects, which may involve resection of a part of the tongue and floor of the mouth. The loss of the tongue's normal anatomical shape, coupled with lip pressure, may cause teeth to tilt lingually, disrupting the neutral zone. To address this issue, a labial plate major connector can be employed to maintain the position of the teeth and provide enhanced bracing (Fig. 22.39).

Unilateral defects with anterior and/or posterior teeth on the nonsurgical site are the most commonly observed defect types. The presence of existing teeth as well as denture-bearing areas highly affects the planning protocol for a framework. However, depending on the resection and reconstruction, the extent of the framework on the defect and the amount of load planned on this area should be carefully evaluated to ensure the success of the reconstruction. Excessive buccal contacts on denture teeth cause more movements, so the denture extending toward the resection site should be nearly nonfunctional. Mastication on this site should not be encouraged as it is not a denture-bearing area, and the movement of the prosthesis on the reconstructed tissues causes a significant stress on the remaining teeth (Fig. 22.40a–e).

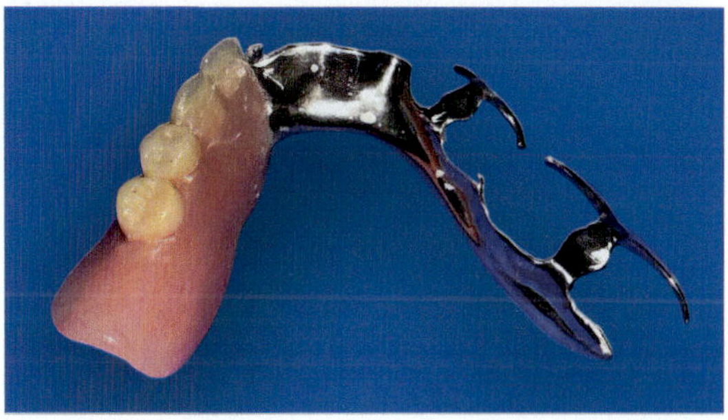

Fig. 22.39 A mandibulectomy prosthesis with a plate type major connector

In a case where the resection is done in the posterior of the premolars, a prosthesis may not always be necessary. While it may not always be required, in some instances, it can aid in supporting the soft tissue for improved chewing swallowing and saliva control. Placing occlusal rests on the mesio-occlusal surface of the nearest abutment and corporating a retainer on the distal abutment of the resection site allows the denture to disengage during posterior occlusal load. This retainer must either be placed on the height of contour or must possess adequate flexibility not to cause pathologic stresses.

Occlusal rests that are placed in a tripodal design have a significant effect on the stability and the retention of the prosthesis. Rests should be placed on the nearest and farthest teeth to the defect with an indirect retention at a rest placed on the tooth on the line perpendicular to the fulcrum line that is mostly on mesial fossae of the first premolars, the lingual surfaces of the canines, or multiple rests localized on these neighboring teeth (Fig. 22.41a–d). In some cases, the bony support of the teeth close to the defect may be insufficient and the condition of the anterior teeth

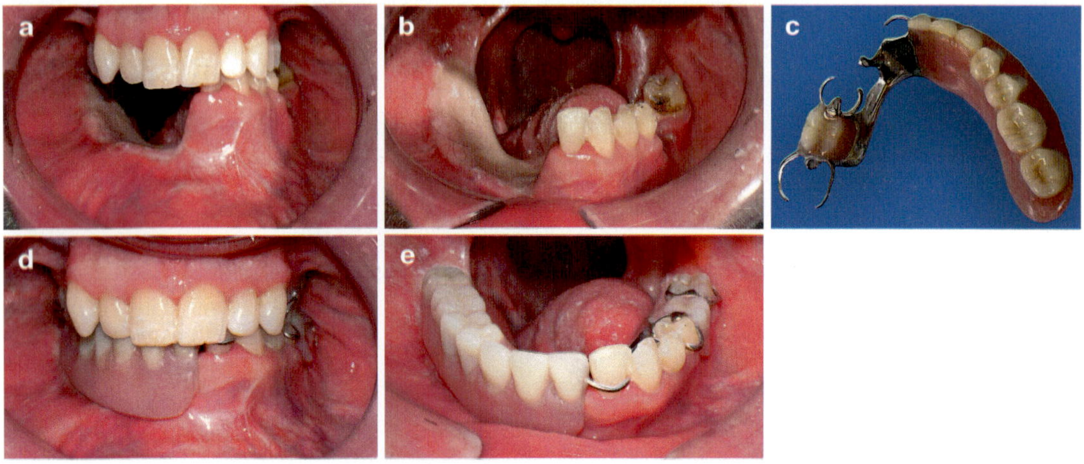

Fig. 22.40 (**a**–**e**) A mandibulectomy limited to the midline and the applied removable partial prosthesis

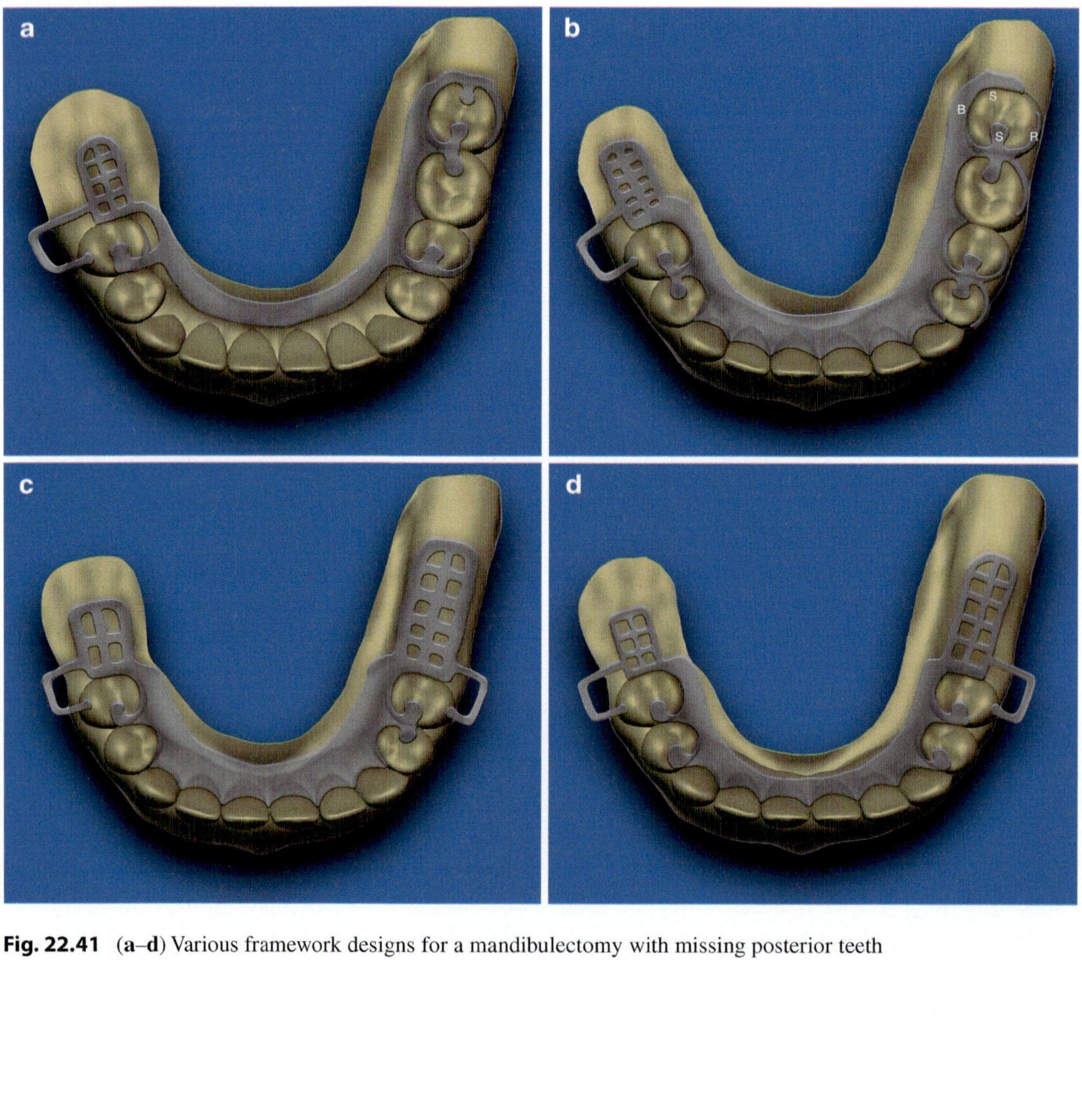

Fig. 22.41 (**a**–**d**) Various framework designs for a mandibulectomy with missing posterior teeth

may not be suitable for retention. In these cases where the anterior teeth cannot contribute to retention, excluding these teeth may cause the prosthesis design to change from tripodal to linear (Fig. 22.42a–c).

Similarly, as the defect extends to a larger area with the long lever arm of the prosthesis, the remaining teeth may not distribute a tripodal load distribution. This compromised edentulous mandibulectomy prosthesis-bearing surface contributes to excessive movement during function particularly with a linear design (Fig. 22.43a–c). In such defects, one rest should be placed on the mesial side of the tooth close to this area. Placing a rest on the disto-occlusal surface of the tooth farthest from the defect is required for retention as in conventional framework planning. In addition, this distal rest facilitates disengagement of the retainers during closure and forms one of the fulcrum lines of the prosthesis (Fig. 22.44a–c).

Anterior defects of the mandible may resemble a Kennedy Class IV edentulous patients. When continuity is preserved, the occlusion, inter-arch relations, and pattern of mandibular movement may not be affected by the muscular contraction. Therefore, prosthetic treatment of these defects with mandibular bone continuity can be predicted with confidence (Fig. 22.45a–d).

The framework design for an anterior defect with continuity closely adheres to conventional guidelines. Typically, the occlusion of the posterior teeth is not changed in these patients and mandibular movements are within normal limits except for graft contracture or inaccurate positioning of the fragments. As indirect retention, rests on the cingulum or mesial rests on both teeth adjacent to the defect with the retainers on the posterior teeth provide a tripodal or even a quadrilateral load distribution. Rests adjacent to the defect allows retainers to disengage with the posterior load. Distal retainers provide the disengagement of the retainers during maximum intercuspation (Fig. 22.46a, b). Post-processing is crucial to physiologically relieve these retainers for optimal function.

The misalignment of bone segments can lead to occlusal abnormality. Therefore, the remaining teeth may need to be crowned to maintain evenly distributed occlusal loads. Abnormal soft tissue and bone formation in the edentulous anterior region may result in the absence of attached gingiva and may need a vestibuloplasty requiring skin grafts. Resulting scar tissue can displace the prosthesis or can be traumatized by the prosthesis. Even if the movements are normal and the relationship between the jaws is within normal limits, the lack of motor and sensory innervation of the tongue affects the management of the denture and the bolus.

In a case when the mandibular discontinuity is not restored, uncoordinated movements of the mandibular segments occur due to the loss of proprioceptive sense of occlusion as well as scar contracture and tightness and the resection of neighboring structures such as the muscles and ligaments leading to a mandibular deviation. The suprahyoid muscles, tongue muscles, and the related masticatory muscles pull the mandible posteriorly, superiorly, and medially if the mandibular continuity is not restored, causing a functional and cosmetic disfigurement. Due to the limited space in this area, the tongue retrudes posteriorly, causing an obstruction in the airway. In such an anatomical change, the possibility of providing a proper occlusion and thus fabricating a functional and a stable prosthesis is low (Fig. 22.47a).

If a lateral continuity is not adequately restored, the arc of closure changes using the remaining mandibular segment to retrude and deviate towards the surgical side at the vertical dimension of occlusion (VDO). As the patient keeps opening, this deviation increases. In maximum opening, there is a 1–2 mm deviation laterally and 2–4 cm retrusion posteriorly (Fig. 22.47b). The displacement of the lower jaw toward the resected side compromises mastication, the control of saliva, and cause cosmetic disfigurement (Fig. 22.48).

The lack and impairment of neighboring muscle attachments on the surgical side result in the rotation of the mandible on the non-resected side at the closure. In the frontal plane aspect, the surgical side of the mandible moves away from the opposing maxillary teeth creating more space occurs on the defect side, This leads to a man-

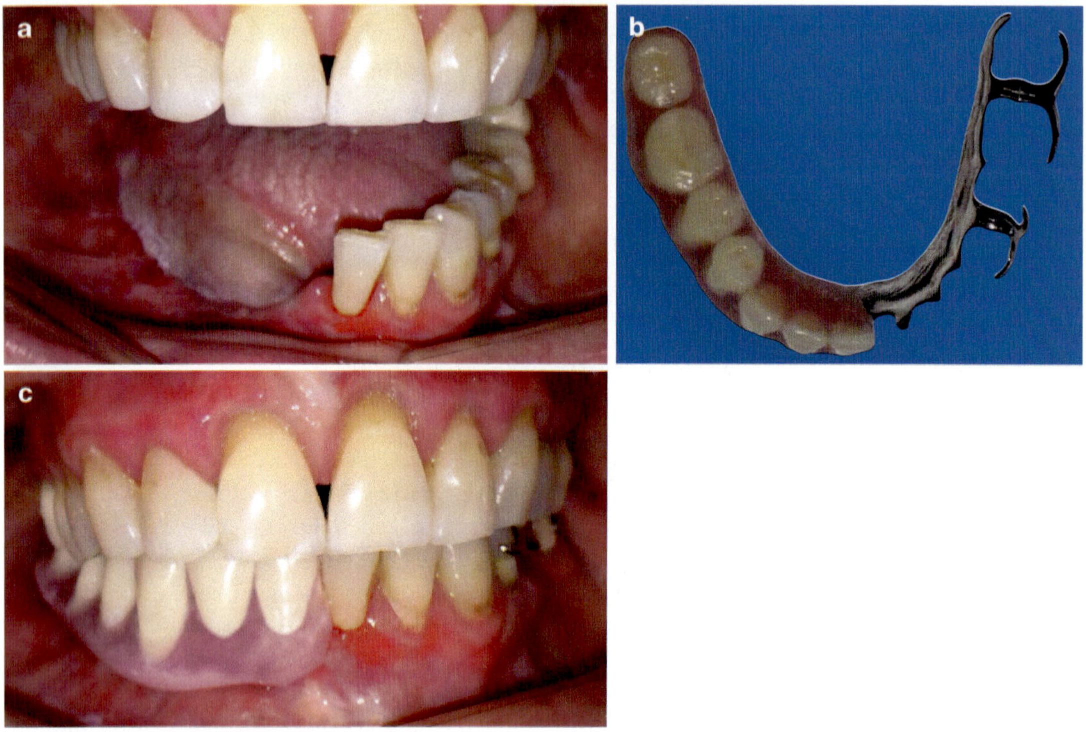

Fig. 22.42 (**a**–**c**) A mandibulectomy prosthesis with a tripodal framework design

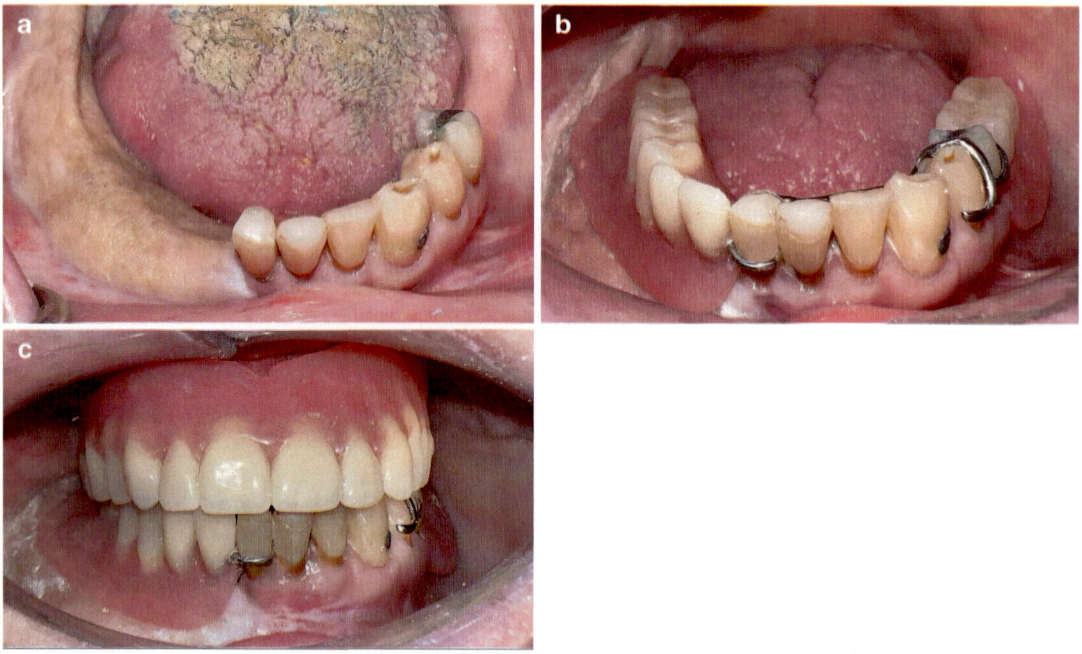

Fig. 22.43 (**a**–**c**)A mandibulectomy prosthesis with a linear framework design

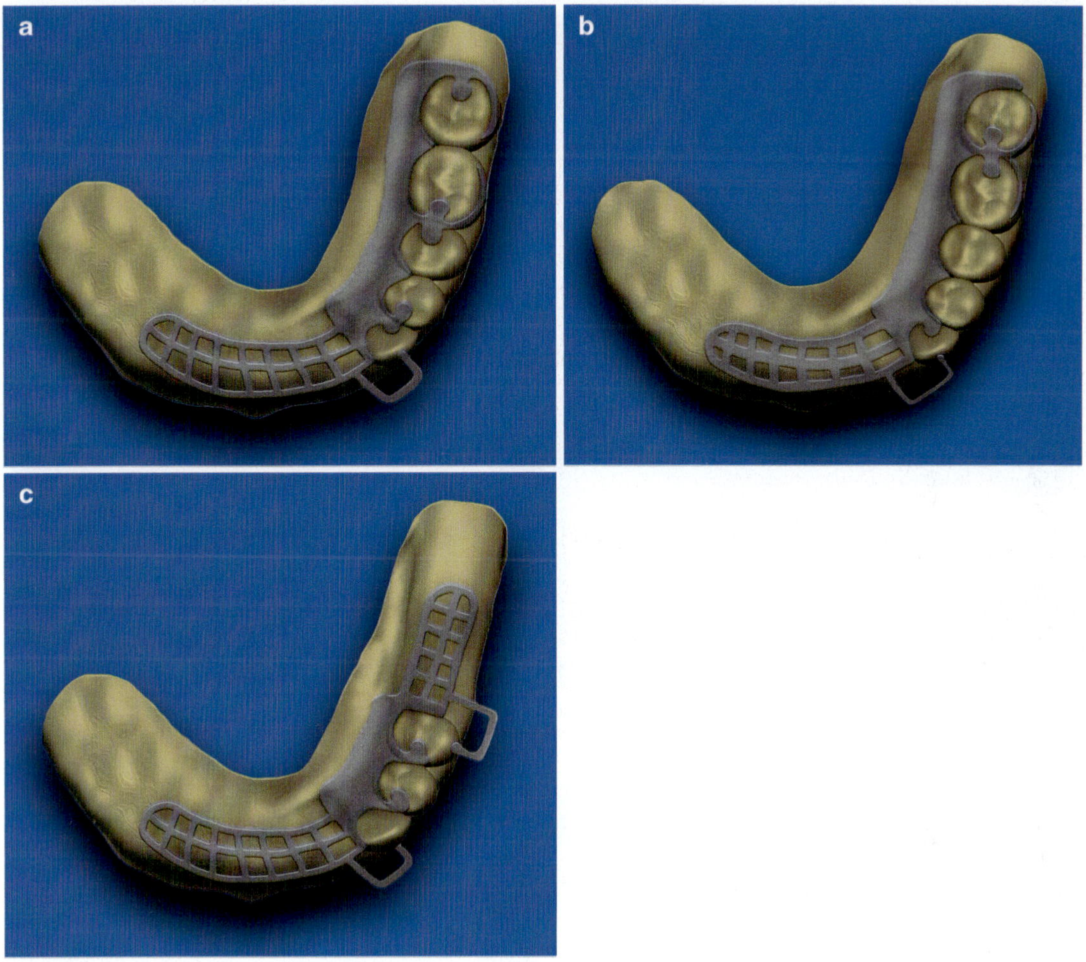

Fig. 22.44 (**a–c**) A mandibulectomy extended to the midline and the applied removable partial prosthesis

dibular rotation with the change in cuspal interdigitation on the non-resected side. Frontal and sagittal plane border movements deviate from normal, causing a severe disruption, and this causes the fulcrum line not to be easily determined.

The envelope of motion shifts towards the surgical defect side and both lateral and protrusive movements are limited. Consequently the arc of closure is angular rather than vertical (Fig. 22.49a, b).

In a discontinuity defect, the movement of the mandibular segment becomes uncoordinated. The surgical site keeps on changing during the healing process, and efforts should be made to guide these movements to maintain the movement trace and range. A guide flange prosthesis is often used in mandibular deviation patients to redirect the movements in a more midline closure pattern with the support of an exercise program during the healing period. This prosthesis is designed to encourage the patient to close in maximum occlusal contacts. Over time, this assistance may facilitate scar relaxation, allowing the patient to achieve unassisted masticatory contact. These flanges can either be attached to the mandibular dentures or designed as a palatal ramp (Fig. 22.50a–c).

In addition to our basic knowledge of removable treatment protocol, patient-related factors should be considered in the prosthetic treatment of maxillary and mandibular defects.

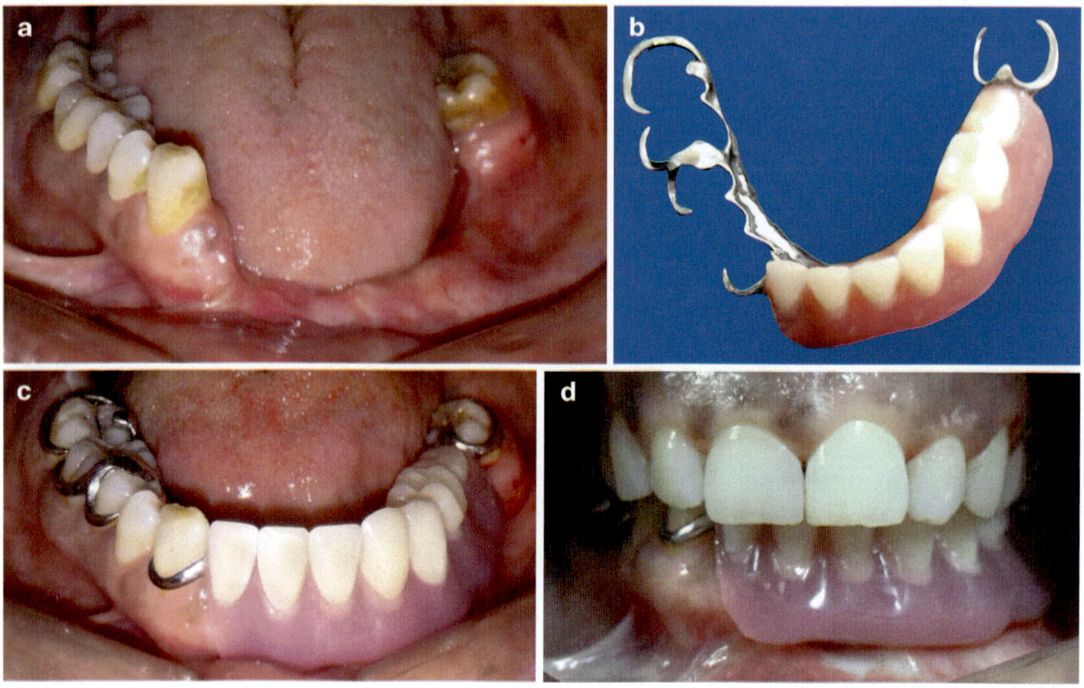

Fig. 22.45 (**a**–**d**) An anterior mandibular defect treated with a removable partial prosthesis

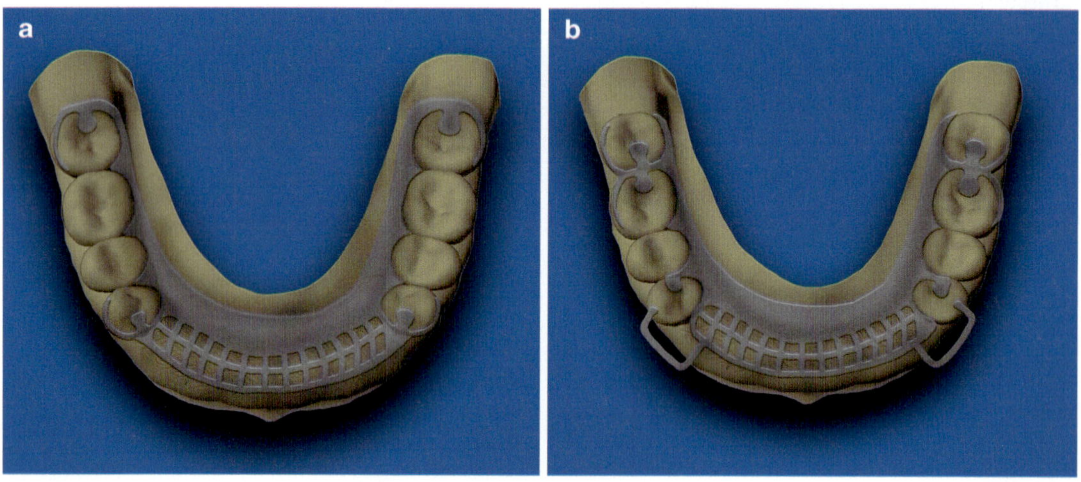

Fig. 22.46 (**a**, **b**) Various framework designs for an anterior mandibulectomy case

From a prosthetic standpoint, the biomechanics of these defect prosthesis has a significant effect on long-term success. Therefore, it is important to reconstruct the defect surgically to provide retention, stability, and support for the prosthesis that will be fabricated in the future to decrease the amount of forces on the teeth. It is essential to remember, that "the correct planning" is one of the keys to success. The following principles should always be kept in mind and integrated into the workflow for a predictable outcome:

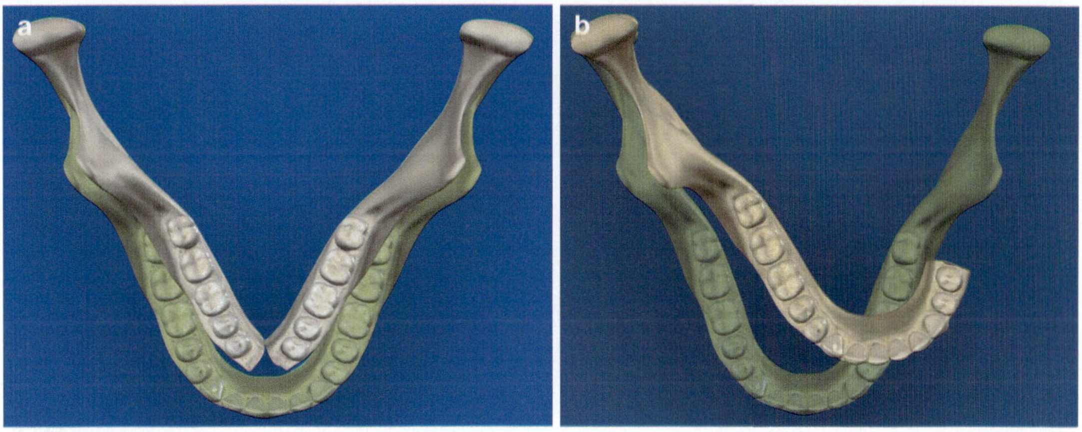

Fig. 22.47 (**a**, **b**) The medial dislocation of two disconnected bone fragments. Mandibular deviation toward the surgical side of a discontinuity defect

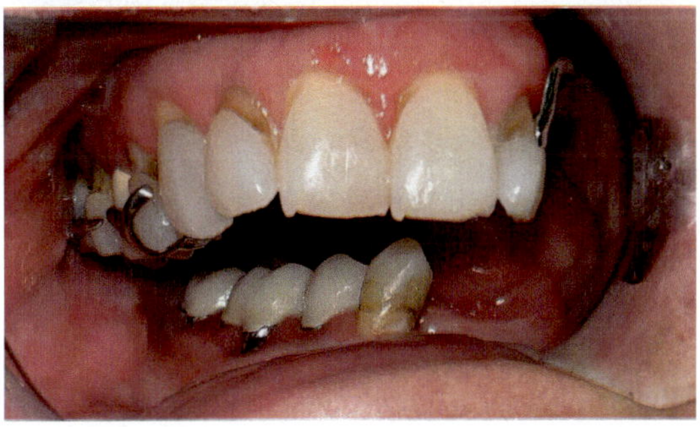

Fig. 22.48 The intraoral view of a mandibulectomy patient with discontinuity, causing a deviation toward the resection side

- The prognosis is dependent on the size of the defect, the number of remaining teeth, and the presence of denture-bearing areas.
- A detailed impression is important to record these areas. Functional impression of the borders should be obtained, and the remaining structures and defect area should be carefully recorded.
- The casts should be surveyed for the undercuts, location, guiding planes, and the path of insertion.
- Survey crowns help in getting retention, establishing guiding planes, and providing occlusal rests. Splinting certain teeth can be advantageous in protecting them from excessive forces. It's important to design the framework components in such a way that they do not exert vertical or lateral forces on the abutment teeth, particularly those in proximity with the resection line.
- The number of rests can be increased within the physiological limits of the teeth, without applying excessive torque.
- Selection of denture teeth depends on the configuration of the opposing dentition. Cusps should approximate the angulation displaced by the opposing dentition.
- The patient should be encouraged to function primarily on the non-defective side.

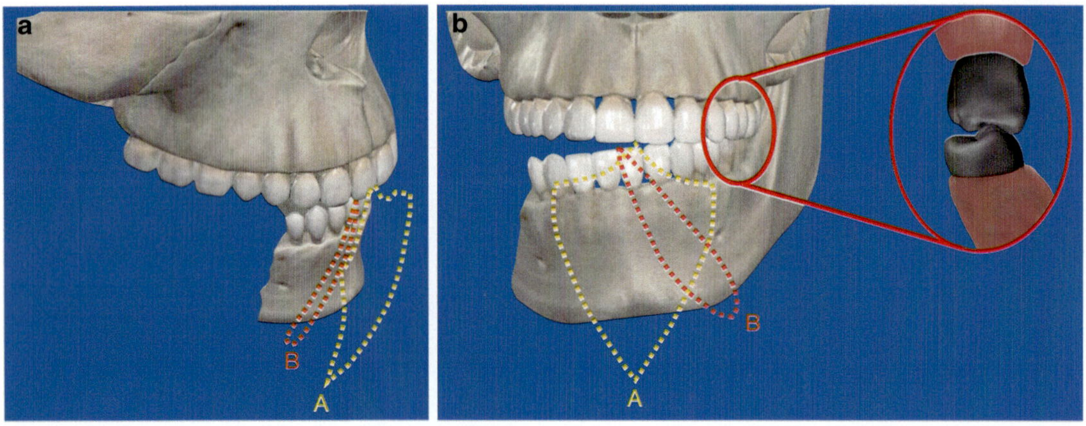

Fig. 22.49 (**a**, **b**) Frontal and sagittal view of the occlusion and moving patterns of a mandibulectomy with deviation

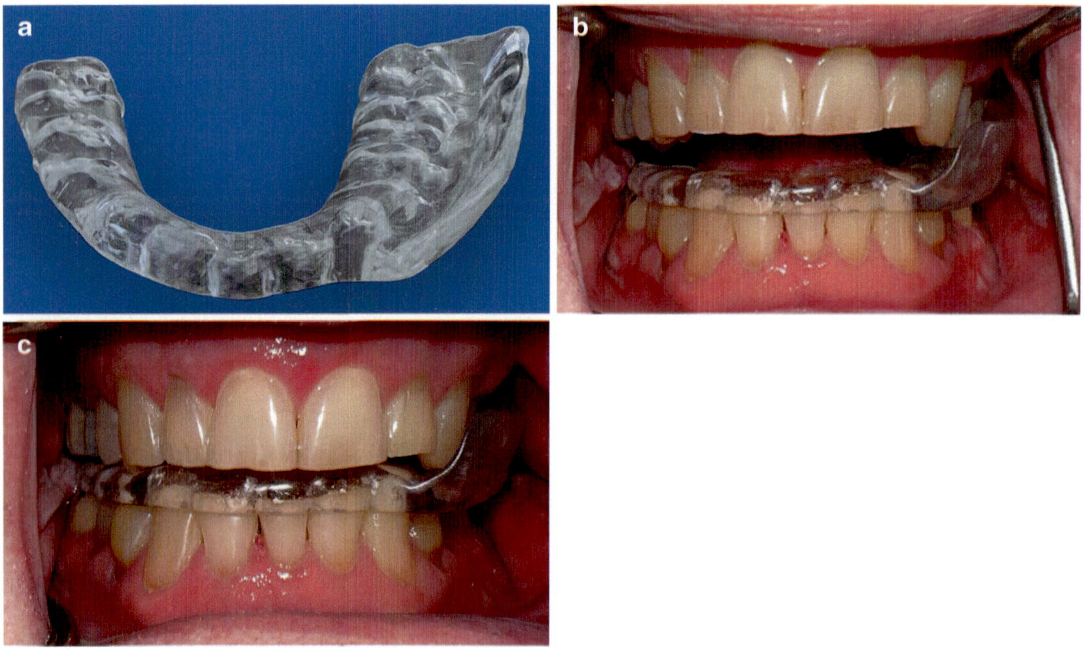

Fig. 22.50 (**a**–**c**) A mandibular guide appliance fabricated to prevent the mandibular deviation

Further Reading

Aramany MA. Basic principles of obturator design for partially edentulous patients. Part I: classification. J Prosthet Dent. 2001a;86:559–61.

Aramany MA. Basic principles of obturator design for partially edentulous patients. Part II: design principles. J Prosthet Dent. 2001b;86:562–8.

Beumer J III, Marunick MT, Esposito SJ. Maxillofacial rehabilitation: prosthodontic and surgical management of cancer-related, acquired, and congenital defects of the head and neck. 3rd ed. Hanover Park, IL: Quintessence Publication; 2011.

Brandão TB, Vechiato Filho AJ, Batista VE, de Oliveira MC, Santos-Silva AR. Obturator prostheses versus free tissue transfers: a systematic review of the optimal approach to improving the quality of life for patients with maxillary defects. J Prosthet Dent. 2016;115:247–53.

Carr AB, Brown DT, editors. McCracken's removable partial prosthodontics. 13th ed. St. Louis, MO: Elsevier; 2016.

Desjardins RP. Obturator prosthesis design for acquired maxillary defects. J Prosthet Dent. 1978;39:424–35.

Devlin H, Barker GR. Prosthetic rehabilitation of the edentulous patient requiring a partial maxillectomy. J Prosthet Dent. 1992;67:223–7.

Dos Santos DM, Caxias FB, Bitencourt SB, Turcio KH, Pesqueira AA, Goiato MC. Oral rehabilitation of patients after maxillectomy. A systemic review. Br J Oral Maxillofac Surg. 2018;56:256–66.

Jacob RF, King G. Indirect retainers in soft palate obturator design. J Prosthet Dent. 1990;63:311–5.

Jagtiani K, Gurav S, Singh G, Dholam K. A review on the classification of mandibulectomy defects and suggested criteria for a universal description. J Prosthet Dent. 2022:S0022-3913(22)00354–7.

King GE, Gay WD. Application of various removable partial denture design concepts to a maxillary obturator prosthesis. J Prosthet Dent. 1979;41:316–8.

McArthur DR, Turvey TA. Maxillary segmental osteotomies for mandibular removable partial denture patients. J Prosthet Dent. 1979;41:381–7.

Ogami K, Hagio M, Ueda T. Maxillary obturator prosthesis made with polyetherketoneketone using optical impression and CAD/CAM system. Bull Tokyo Dent Coll. 2023;64:31–7.

Parr GR, Gardner LK. Swing-lock design considerations for obturator frameworks. J Prosthet Dent. 1995;74:503–11.

Parr GR, Gardner LK. The evolution of the obturator framework design. J Prosthet Dent. 2003;89:608–10.

Parr GR, Tharp GE, Rahn AO. Prosthodontic principles in the framework design of maxillary obturator prostheses. J Prosthet Dent. 2005;93:405–11.

Petrovic I, Shah JP, Huryn JM, Ahmed ZU, Rosen EB. Intraoral rehabilitation after marginal mandibulectomy. Int J Prosthodont. 2019;32:241–7.

Rogers WA, Salinas TJ, Novoselsky A. Maxillary definitive obturators: rationale of design. J Dent Technol. 1996;13:19–26.

Schneider RL, Taylor TD. Mandibular resection guidance prostheses: a literature review. J Prosthet Dent. 1986;55:84–6.

Shifman A, Lepley JB. Prosthodontic management of postsurgical soft tissue deformities associated with marginal mandibulectomy. Part I: loss of the vestibule. J Prosthet Dent. 1982;48:178–83.

Tasopoulos T, Chatziemmanouil D, Kouveliotis G, Karaiskou G, Wang J, Zoidis P. PEEK maxillary obturator prosthesis fabrication using intraoral scanning, 3D printing, and CAD/CAM. Int J Prosthodont. 2020;33:333–40.

The glossary of prosthodontic terms: ninth edition. J Prosthet Dent. 2017;117(5S):e1–e105.

Part VII

Maintenance and Postinsertion Problems of Removable Partial Dentures and Infection Control in Practice

Postinsertion Problems

23

Onur Geçkili

Abstract

Similar to the other prosthetic treatments, treatment with removable partial dentures may also cause problems after insertion and these problems should be taken into consideration seriously. Patients should be recalled for periodic evaluations; the oral condition and prosthesis should be evaluated and their problems should be considered. Postinsertion problems may encounter more difficulties if not solved seriously as far as failure of the treatment. This chapter deals with the problems after insertion of the removable partial dentures; the possible solutions to handle these problems and the precautions the clinicians should take to avoid recurrence of these problems. The problems and solutions are classified into categories and mentioned one by one for clarification.

23.1 Definitions

Acrylic resin: Any of a group of thermoplastic resins made by polymerizing esters of acrylic or methyl methacrylate acids.

Alveolar bone: The bony portion of the mandible or maxillae in which the roots of the teeth are held by fibers of the periodontal ligament.

Articulating paper: Ink-coated paper strips used to locate and mark occlusal contacts.

Deflective occlusal contact: A contact that displaces a tooth, diverts the mandible from its intended movement, or displaces a removable denture from its basal seat.

Gag: An involuntary contraction of the muscles of the soft palate or pharynx that results in retching.

Hard palate: The bony portion of the roof of the mouth.

Incisive papilla: The elevation of soft tissue covering the foramen of the incisive or nasopalatine canal.

Occlusal prematurity: Any contact of opposing teeth that occurs before the planned intercuspation.

Occlusal reshaping: The intentional alteration of the occlusal surfaces of teeth to change their form.

Pressure indicating paste: Any substance applied to a dental prosthesis, which, when seated on a structure, demonstrates the adaptation of the prosthesis to the structure it opposes.

Remount procedure: Any method used to relate restorations to an articulator for analysis and/or to assist in development of a plan for occlusal equilibration or reshaping.

Residual ridge crest: The most coronal portion of the residual ridge.

Retention: That quality inherent in the dental prosthesis acting to resist the forces of dislodgment along the path of placement.

O. Geçkili (✉)
Faculty of Dentistry, Department of Prosthodontics, İstanbul University, İstanbul, Türkiye
e-mail: geckili@istanbul.edu.tr

O. Şakar (ed.), *Removable Partial Dentures*, https://doi.org/10.1007/978-3-031-47083-7_23

Stability: The quality of a removable dental prosthesis to be firm, steady, or constant, to resist displacement by functional horizontal or rotational stresses.

Trauma: An injury or wound, whether physical or psychic.

Patients rehabilitated with removable partial dentures (RPDs) should be recalled the day after the insertion of the prosthesis. If anything, more than a minor tissue damage is observed, they should be seen in the following 2 or 3 days to ensure the healing of the damaged tissues, 1 week after and every 6-month interval for periodic oral evaluations. The patients susceptible to caries or having periodontal problems may be recalled more often.

The recall visits should be long enough to give the patient confidence that required adjustments will be provided and to give warning that an appointment is needed for future adjustments without intruding the clinician's routine schedule.

It is not feasible to make an intraoral examination immediately after the patient is seated. The clinician should ask questions about the function, esthetics of the RPDs, and the condition of the remaining dentition prior to intraoral examination. Intraoral examination should be performed in detail with and without the RPDs even if no complaints exist afterward. It should be remembered that some minor tissue damages or premature occlusal contacts not felt by the patients can be detected and corrected by the clinician and future pain and discomfort problems may be prevented. The problems associated with wearing RPDs may be classified into six categories:

- Pain and discomfort related to soft tissues or remaining teeth
- Difficulty seating or removing the RPD
- Lack of retention and stability
- Functional problems
- Esthetic problems
- Compromised periodontal health and mucosal lesions

23.2 Pain and Discomfort Related to Soft Tissues or Remaining Teeth

Pain and discomfort may be associated with the remaining teeth, soft tissues surrounding the denture base or both and classified as one of the most usually seen RPD postinsertion problems. The areas of tissue trauma may be in the incisive papilla, hard palate, residual ridge crest, the peripheral borders of the RPDs or the mucosa not covered by the RPD such as lips and cheeks. Tissue trauma reveals as increased redness or translucency in the oral mucosa. Increased redness is the symptom of the ulcerations and the translucency occurs just before ulceration exists. Overextension of the denture bases, the pressures on the fragile tissues such as incisive papilla or occlusal prematurities are the main causes of these ulcerations. Ulcerations due to tissue trauma (Fig. 23.1) develop generally at the initial recall appointments and can be solved easily by relieving the denture base parts touching the pain area. In case of overextension, ill-fitting RPDs or acrylic irregularities, the areas can be identified by the aid of an indelible pencil or pressure indicating paste. Nevertheless, it is much better to prefer an indelible pencil because using a pressure indicating paste or cream for determining

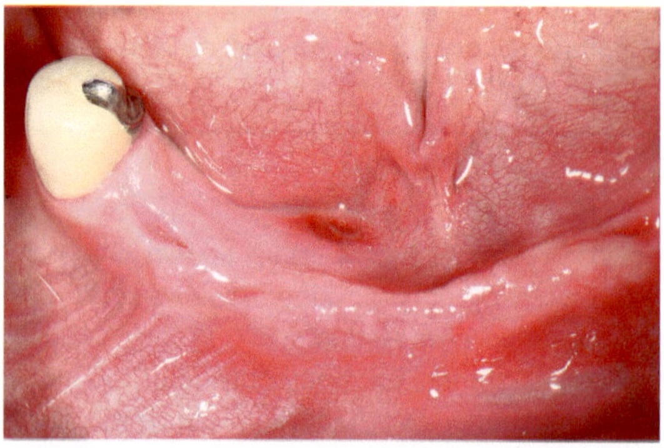

Fig. 23.1 An ulceration due to tissue trauma caused by the overextension of the lingual border of an RPD

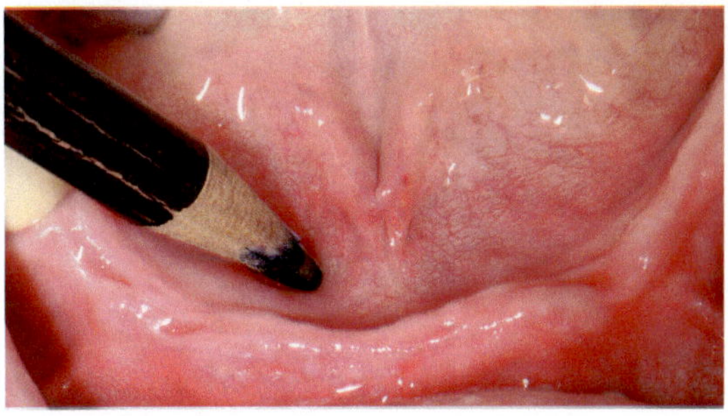

Fig. 23.2 An indelible pencil may be used to mark the ulceration area

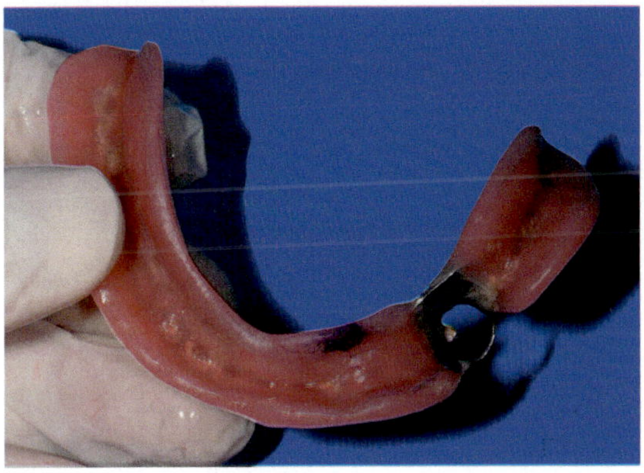

Fig. 23.3 The ulceration area is transferred to the RPD. The marked parts may be easily removed using a tungsten carbide bur afterwards

these areas may cause faulty results as the paste is easily displaced due to its softness. The indelible pencil is used to mark the ulceration area (Fig. 23.2) and after the area is transferred to the RPD (Fig. 23.3), these parts are gently removed using a tungsten carbide bur.

The ulcerations appearing on the residual ridge crests are usually due to occlusal prematurities, but they may also be because of the irregularities of the acrylic resin on the intaglio surface of the denture base. These irregularities may be recognized by the clinicians by examining the denture base with fingertips and eliminated before the delivery of the RPDs. Additionally, denture base roughness can be corrected after using a pressure indicator paste and identifying the exact areas causing the discomfort. After the adjustment, the pressure indicating paste should be reapplied for verification. Topical agents may be used to relieve pain and stimulate healing.

23.3 Difficulty Seating or Removing the Removable Partial Dentures

The difficulties in seating or removal of the RPDs are usually seen in the insertion period but this complaint may also appear after the RPD has been in use for some time. This complaint may be classified into the following three categories.

23.3.1 Incomplete Seating of a Rest and Clasp Assembly on the Related Abutment

If the rest and clasp assembly is not fully seated on the abutment (Fig. 23.4), it may apply non-axial forces to the abutment. These forces may cause significant discomfort, tooth movement, or metallurgical fatigue of the clasp arms due to being active all the time. This may usually occur because of design errors. If a proper path of insertion was not designated at the time of treatment planning, the RPD may not fully seat on the abutments. The guiding planes should be carefully examined and if there is a minor incongruity, the RPD may seat after preparing the guiding planes. If it is not possible to seat the RPD by modifying the guiding planes, refabricating procedure may be the only solution.

23.3.2 Seating Problems Due to Pronounced Soft Tissue Undercuts

Soft tissue undercuts may create problems if any component of an RPD passes over them during

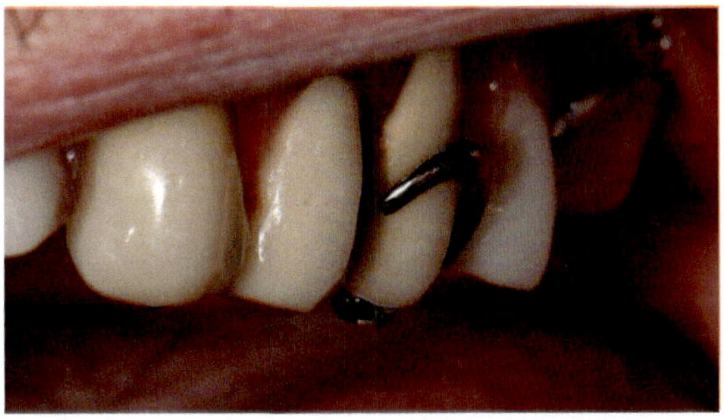

Fig. 23.4 A rest and clasp assembly not fully seated will probably apply non-axial forces to the abutment tooth

insertion or removal of the prosthesis. These problems usually involve pain and discomfort due to injuries of these soft tissues. These soft tissue undercuts should be surgically corrected prior to definitive treatment (see Chap. 6), but if they appear after the treatment, the RPDs may be rebased, relined, or refabricated according to the extent of the surgical procedure.

23.3.3 Patient-Related Factors

Patient-related factors may include the inability to manipulate or distortion of the RPD after use. Elder RPD users may have systemic neurologic disorders. Therefore, it is not feasible to use complicated RPD designs that have more than one path of insertion. It is very important to show the patient how to insert and remove the prosthesis and ask him/her to manipulate with the practitioner in the first and the following early appointments. Distortion of the RPD may occur if the patient tries to tighten the RPD or uses the clasps while inserting and removing the prosthesis. The distorted clasps may be changed with wrought wires or cast clasps by the laboratory after making an impression with the RPD.

23.4 Lack of Retention and Stability

Retention or stability loss of an RPD may originate from the following situations:

1. Broken clasps or loss of the precision attachments
2. Decrease in the function of the clasps or precision attachments
3. Overextended or underextended denture bases
4. Deflective occlusal contacts
5. Loss of the contact between the RPD and the underlying soft tissue

Retention or stability loss may be due to one or all of these situations. The clinician must examine the origin of the looseness and make the appropriate treatment.

23.4.1 Broken Clasps or Loss of the Precision Attachments

Broken clasps are usually due to fatigue of the RPD components and will be discussed in detail in Chap. 20.

23.4.2 Decrease in the Function of the Clasps or Precision Attachments

Function of a clasp may decrease after some time of usage because of multiple insertion and removal cycles of the patient and may be easily solved by bending the retentive arms into the undercut areas with the aid of an appropriate plier (Fig. 23.5). However, excessive bending should be avoided in order not to cause an accelerated fatigue of the clasp. Because in case of excessive bending, the RPD may not seat properly and the retentive clasp arm have to be rebended toward its original position. Clasps may not function properly in case of wear of the abutment teeth due to caries (Fig. 23.6), abrasion, or erosion on the facial or proximal surfaces or because of patient misuse. However, it should be underlined that these may be the reasons if only a proper design of the RPD has been carried out. The design must have been completed using a surveyor for deciding the path of insertion and for

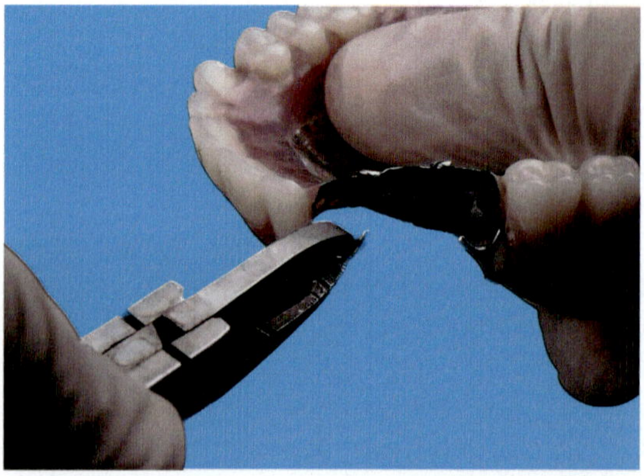

Fig. 23.5 If the function of the clasp decreases, it can be reactivated using a plier and bending the retentive arm into the undercut area

tracing the survey line to obtain efficient retentive clasps. If this procedure has not been employed before, the clasps of the RPD are obliged to be loosened every time. If wear exists on the abutments, the nonfunctioning clasps may be changed to functioning by adding composite material to the teeth surfaces and bending the retentive arm into the deepened undercut with a plier.

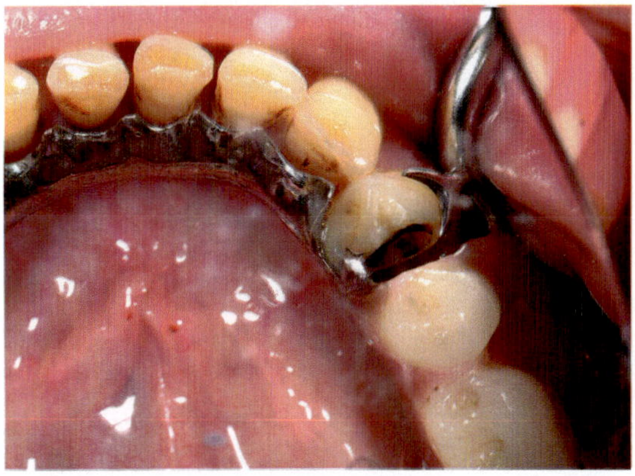

Fig. 23.6 The clasp assemblies may lose their retentive properties due to caries of the abutment teeth

The function of the precision attachments may be abridged in time because of the wear of plastic components and this should have been told to the patients prior to the insertion of the prosthesis. The consistent replacement has to be a standard process of the planned patient maintenance. The worn plastic components should be replaced with new ones regularly in accordance with the manufacturer's recommendations (Fig. 23.7). Activation of the precision attachments is also possible in some attachment types (Fig. 23.8).

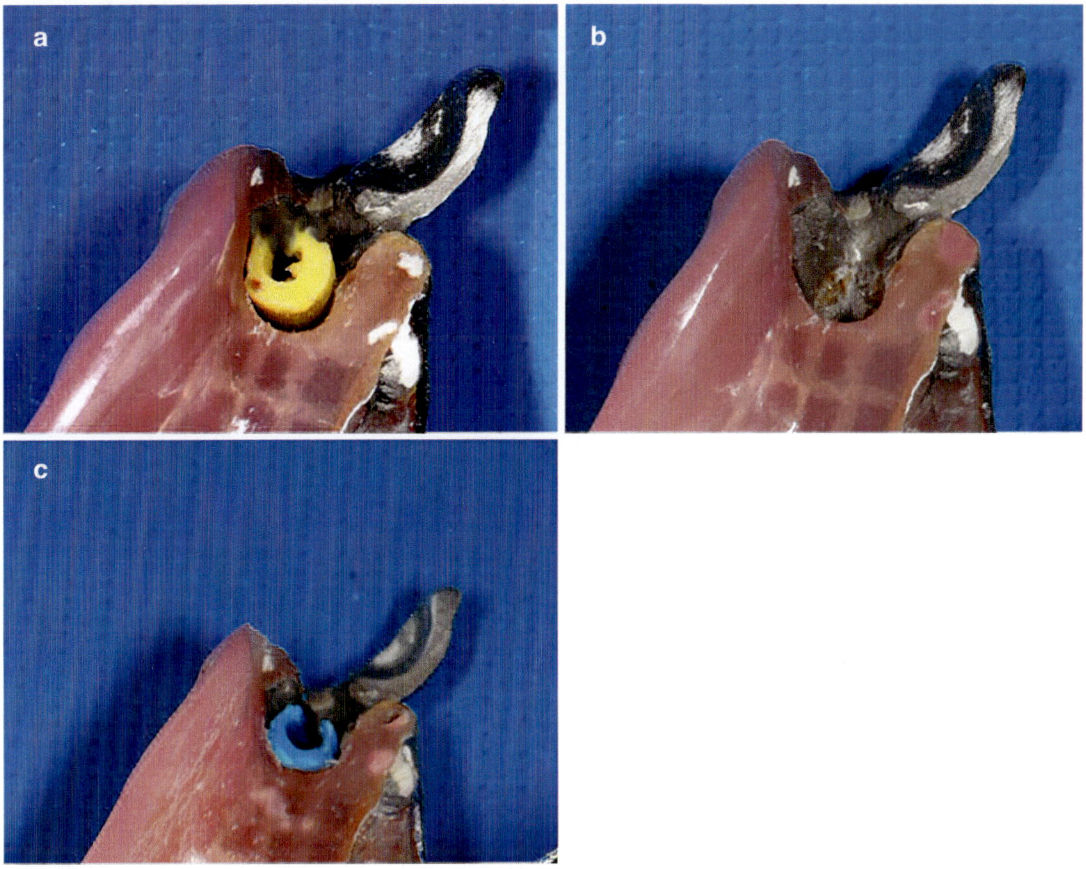

Fig. 23.7 Precision attachments may lose their retention properties due to wear of plastic components. Worn plastic components (**a**) are removed (**b**) and replaced with new ones (**c**) regularly in accordance with the manufacturer's recommendations

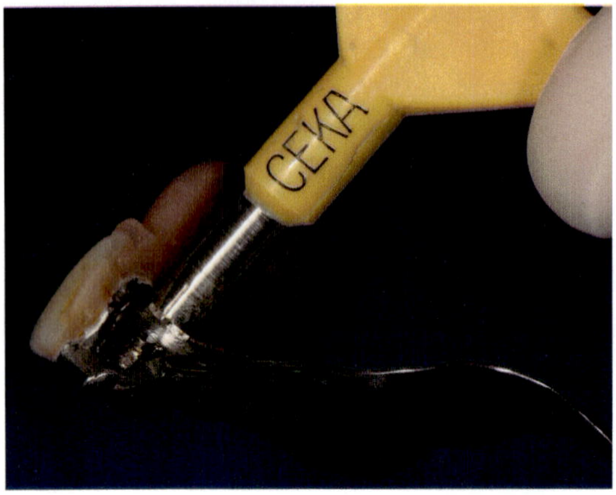

Fig. 23.8 CEKA attachments may be activated using the driver provided by the manufacturer

23.4.3 Overextended or Underextended Denture Bases

An overextended denture base (Fig. 23.9) may cause the muscles and frena to dislodge the RPD, and an underextended denture base (Fig. 23.10) may affect stability; the RPD may not be stabilized under lateral forces and may result in food entrapment.

Overextended denture base areas should be corrected with a laboratory bur and the flange must be rounded thoroughly while it is being shortened. RPDs with underextended denture bases may be relined or rebased with functional impression methods. However, if the borders are too short to be relined, the RPD can be remade by completely removing the resin and the artificial teeth if the framework exhibits a clinically acceptable fit.

23.4.4 Deflective Occlusal Contacts

Deflective occlusal contacts usually affect the stability of the RPDs and therefore should be eliminated. If the deflective occlusal contacts are minor, they can be removed by occlusal reshaping with the aid of articulating papers; however, if they are gross, the artificial teeth may be changed following a new interocclusal record. If the RPD is a tooth supported one, occlusal reshaping should be completed using intraoral methods; however, if it is a distal extension RPD,

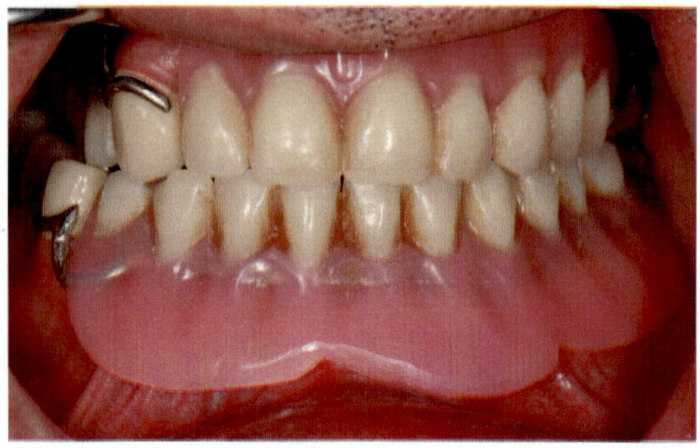

Fig. 23.9 Overextended denture bases may cause the muscles and frena to dislodge the RPDs and may also cause tissue irritation and subsequent ulcerations

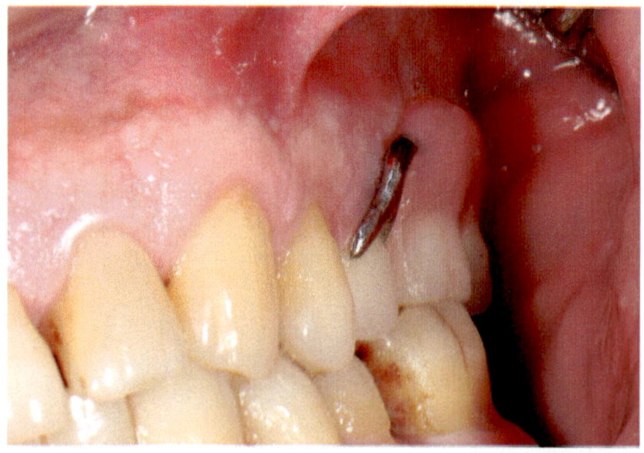

Fig. 23.10 Underextended denture bases may affect the stability of the RPDs and food entrapment is inevitable in such cases

the grinding procedures should be performed using remount procedures with the aid of an articulator. However, it should be emphasized that the final grinding procedures should be completed intraorally to compensate the resiliency of the supporting soft tissues with articulating papers having various thicknesses.

23.4.5 Loss of the Contact Between the Removable Partial Denture and the Underlying Soft Tissue

Continuing resorption of the alveolar bone resulting in the loss of denture bearing ridge is a major problem in prosthetic rehabilitation of the edentulous areas. It has been shown that alveolar bone starts to resorb rapidly immediately after tooth loss for about 10 weeks and slowly but progressively afterwards. Additionally, recent studies have shown that resorption of the edentulous alveolar bone increases with the RPD use because of more pressure delivery as compared to lack of dentures. As the bone underlying the RPD continues to resorb, the gap between the RPD and the soft tissues increases, which negatively affects the appropriate fit and the retention of the RPD. Therefore, particularly, distal extension RPDs should be relined time to time during periodic evaluations in the follow-up appointments, which will be discussed in detail in Chap. 20.

Moreover, retention of the distal extension RPDs may be enhanced by using denture adhesives, especially by patients having decreased neuromuscular control or unfavorable alveolar ridge anatomy. The fit of RPDs and the underlying tissues is very important in maintaining the chewing performance, preserving the periodontal health of the abutment teeth and the overall satisfaction of these patients. Denture adhesives not only serve as the retention enhancer but also reduce the stress on the soft tissues by improving the distribution of the occlusal load equally on abutment teeth and the mucosa.

It should be kept in mind that the recommendation of an adhesive does not negatively affect the clinician's skills, which is a common belief throughout the clinicians. Proper use of an adhesive strengthens bilateral retention and support of an RPD having long distal extension only on one side of the maxillary or mandibular arch.

Denture adhesives are mainly classified into two as soluble (pastes, powders, creams) and insoluble (wafers and pads) products. Both groups activate with hydration, which is the salivary wetness of the mucosa. Soluble products swell and become sticky and viscous, whereas insoluble products turn into sticky upon absorbing saliva.

Insoluble products are properly trimmed according to the shape of the distal extension areas by using a scissors before intraoral use. Subsequently, they are moisturized by water, applied to the RPDs, and start their intraoral use. They can be removed from the RPDs by lifting the corners and peeling away. Soluble products are applied to the intaglio surface of dry dentures and firmly seated into the mouth. For the cream or paste type adhesives, two methods can be used according to the application size as strip or spot method. It has been shown that spot method is more beneficial in the amount of the adhesive used and easier for the control of the patients. Among all the adhesives, previous research has shown the most effective one as the cream or paste type ones as well.

Although the use of adhesives is generally advised to improve the performance of complete dentures in certain situations, in vitro studies have shown their probable positive effect on retention, stability, and the fit of RPDs. However, clinical scientific data is still needed to confirm the results of in vitro studies and to evaluate the use of denture adhesives in patients with RPDs.

23.5 Functional Problems

Functional problems are classified into five parts in this section as gagging, eating or chewing difficulties, phonetic problems, tongue or cheek biting, and food impaction or collection on the RPD borders.

23.5.1 Gagging

Gag reflex is a somatic response in which the body tries to abolish foreign bodies from the oral cavity by muscle contraction at the base of the tongue and the pharyngeal wall. Unstable or poorly retained RPDs, increased occlusal vertical dimension, overextension of the mandibular RPDs in the retromylohyoid space, and the overextended or very thick borders of the maxillary RPDs in the posterior regions can intrude the "trigger zones" and produce gagging. Gagging may usually be observed as a problem of the first-time RPD users and mostly disappears after using the prosthesis for several days. However, patients with severe gagging problems present big difficulties in using the RPDs. Therefore, the RPD design and denture borders should be fabricated with caution taking into consideration the above-mentioned factors. The patient and the RPD should be examined thoroughly to find the reason of gagging. Unstable or poorly retained RPDs can be relined, rebased; clasps or precision attachments can be activated or changed or the RPD may be remade if these are not sufficient enough to maintain adequate retention. To correct the problem of overextensions, the posterior lingual and palatal borders should be shortened and thinned. Correction of the increased occlusal vertical dimension requires reestablishing of the appropriate occlusal vertical dimension and removing and rearranging the artificial teeth of the RPDs. Poor adaptation of the maxillary RPDs to the tissues because of faulty impressions may also induce gagging. If the denture base is acrylic relining may be the solution of this problem but if the denture base is metal like most of the cases, the RPD should be remade. Placement of posterior denture teeth lingually may also restrict the tongue space and induce gagging. This can be corrected after removing and rearranging the artificial teeth in correct positions. Alternative treatment options such as hypnosis may also be applied to the patients with a stubborn gagging problem.

23.5.2 Eating or Chewing Difficulties

Patients usually report chewing or eating problems before prosthodontic treatment. It should be underlined that these problems decrease rapidly after treated with fixed partial dentures but slowly after RPD treatment due to an adaptation period for the new prosthesis. Moreover, it has been shown that RPD treatment improves the ability to reduce the bolus particle size, but is not able to fully restore the masticatory function, especially if it is a distal extension one. However, it has been shown that perceived chewing ability is an important component of perceived oral health and therefore these problems should be taken into account seriously. Patients should be advised not to eat tough and sticky food during the early period of adjustment. The occlusal surfaces of the artificial teeth should be examined with an articulating paper and the occlusal prematurities should be eliminated or the teeth of one or both sides should be reset where an occlusal adjustment is not adequate to overcome occlusal problems, or if some teeth lack occluding the opposing arch. Difficulties may also be related to retention, stability, or vertical dimension. These factors should also be evaluated and corrected if necessary.

23.5.3 Phonetic Problems

Unlike complete dentures, RPDs usually do not generate speech difficulties. However, the location of the anterior teeth, especially on a maxillary RPD, should be correct in order to allow the tongue and other articulators to work accurately. Also changes in the contour of the anterior palate and vertical dimension may show phonetic difficulties. Speech problems are usually seen in the first few days after the insertion of the RPDs especially when the patient is a first-time denture user. It has been shown that most of the patients with these problems show remarkable improvements after 1 week of use. If no improvement is achieved, alterations in the RPD design or tooth arrangement should be considered. Additionally, it should be noted that since degenerative changes in auditory abilities exhibit difficulties to adapt to new prosthesis in older patients, adaptation is usually much easier to achieve in younger patients.

23.5.4 Tongue or Cheek Biting

Tongue, cheek, or lip biting is a common complaint among patients receiving prosthodontic treatment. Patients bite their cheeks mostly because of the inadequate occluding posterior teeth overlap. With the use of monoplane posterior artificial teeth, this problem is seen more often because the teeth are arranged with no horizontal overlap. The cheeks are trapped between the occluding surfaces of the posterior artificial teeth and painful ulcerations may be seen (Fig. 23.11). To overcome the problem of insufficient overlap, the mandibular posterior teeth might be gently rounded and reduced in size buccally or all the posterior teeth may be reduced buccally to move away from the soft

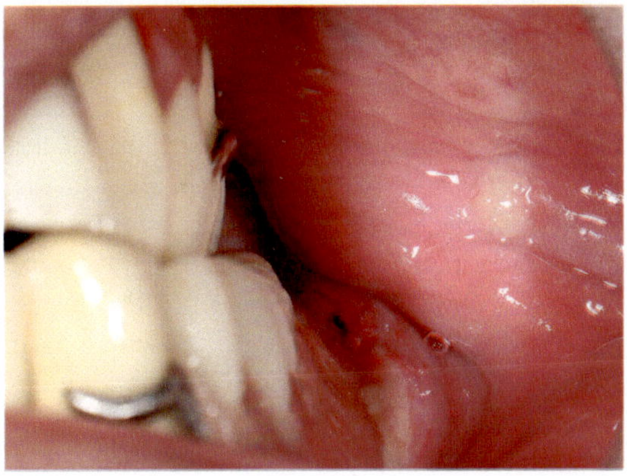

Fig. 23.11 The cheeks may be trapped between the occluding surfaces of the posterior artificial teeth and painful ulcerations may be seen in patients wearing RPDs with inadequate posterior teeth overlap

tissues. However, it should be remembered that reducing the size may reduce the chewing ability of the patients. In those circumstances, the teeth should be changed and rearranged. Cheek biting may be seen in patients who have lost their posterior teeth long time ago and have never used RPDs. In this situation, the buccinators muscle drops down to the space between the edentulous residual ridge crests. After an adaptation period, the size of the muscle turns back to original and this complaint is resolved most of the times. Additionally, if the interocclusal space between the posterior denture bases of maxillary and mandibular RPDs is too small, the patient may bite his/her cheek. Grinding the acrylic bases to lengthen the space is the only solution in those circumstances.

Tongue biting can be seen if the teeth are arranged too lingually or the mandibular posterior teeth have been missing for a long time and the tongue is broadened. The lingual cusps of the mandibular teeth should be broadened to resolve the problem. In the case of long-time missing posterior teeth scenarios, the patients stop biting their tongue after the tongue turns to its normal size if the teeth were set in correct position.

Lip biting can be seen with the presence of wrong the anterior teeth relations and usually resolved by reshaping the labial surface of mandibular canine teeth.

23.5.5 Food Impaction or Collection on the Removable Partial Denture Borders

Food impaction happens usually when the acrylic denture base is not well adapted to the abutment teeth (Fig. 23.12). The reason is usually starting the treatment without restoring the abutment teeth. Therefore, restarting the treatment with proper planning including restoring the abutment teeth rather than relining is more appropriate in these situations. However, if the food trap is because of an insufficiently extended denture base, the solution may be a relining. Food collection on the borders may occur in case of poorly contoured or not well-polished acrylic surfaces or if the patient has a reduced salivary flow. Appropriately contouring and polishing the surfaces will easily solve the problem. If a reduced salivary flow is present, medications increasing the flow rate may be prescribed or chewing gums and fluids stimulating the flow may be recommended to the patients. Some RPD designs such as lingual bar with cingulum bar, designs requiring deep reliefs because of anatomic restrictions or insufficient beading may also cause food impaction, which may only be corrected by refabricating the RPDs with an appropriate planning.

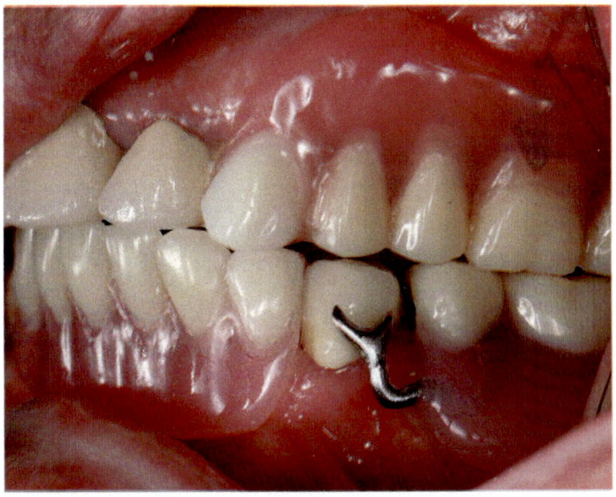

Fig. 23.12 When the acrylic denture base of the RPD is not well adapted to the abutment tooth, food impaction is unavoidable

23.6 Esthetic Problems

RPDs replacing the anterior teeth may cause esthetic problems. These problems may be related to several factors. However, before explaining these factors, it is very important to describe the esthetic zone and its effect on RPD treatment options.

23.6.1 Esthetic Zone

Esthetic zone is the observed teeth and soft tissues when a patient makes a usual smile or laugh. However; Preston describes the esthetic zone as the place wherever the patient thinks it is; meaning that even if the patient does not show metal while laughing, he or she still may believe that it is seen. Therefore, it is essential to describe the esthetic zone to the patients before the treatment because they might not want to receive any metal on the facial surfaces even if it is not in the esthetic zone. The open smiles of patients were divided into three categories as high smile, average smile, and low smile in a former study. It is easier to mask the metal components in a low smile that displays less than 75% of the anterior teeth; however, every component is visible in a high smile that shows all the anterior teeth and a contiguous band of gingiva. Therefore, it is much better to select alternative designs in these circumstances such as precision attachments or rotational path designs (see Chaps. 12 and 16), which do not show the metal components. However, it should be underlined that most of the patients have average smile in which the cervical to incisal length of the maxillary anterior teeth is displayed to either the first or second premolar. Therefore, it is very important to eliminate the metal components until the maxillary premolars for the majority of individuals. Additionally, some precautions should be considered about the maxillary denture base contours. The anterior flange should not be thick and extend to the reflection of the mucolabial fold to prevent the horizontal border of the flange from being visible during smiling.

Mandibular anterior teeth should be taken into account if they are to be replaced with an RPD. Most of the patients show 50% of the mandibular anterior teeth and less than 50% of the buccal surfaces of the premolars in the esthetic zone, similarly the occlusal surfaces of the premolars are usually displayed.

Most of the esthetic problems of RPDs are due to display of the metal components such as clasp assemblies or frameworks in the esthetic zone. These problems can be solved mostly with replacement dentures that follow the rules of the esthetic zone. Therefore, it is very important to plan the RPD before the treatment according to the esthetic zone of the patient. Additionally, the esthetic problems may be due to inappropriate axial inclination of the artificial tooth positions, discoloration or abrasion of the acrylic teeth, and too low or too high occlusal plane. These problems can be solved by replacing the artificial teeth with new ones.

23.7 Compromised Periodontal Health and Mucosal Lesions Due to Wearing of Removable Partial Dentures

The existence of the RPD in the oral cavity effects the microbial ecosystem onto both the remaining teeth and the oral mucosa because of plaque accumulation and hygienic maintenance. Although it has been publicized that if precise hygienic techniques and regular recalls are being applied, the RPDs may not cause an increase of plaque accumulation, the majority of the studies focusing on this subject reported increased susceptibility to plaque accumulation with the use of RPDs. The proliferation of Spirochaetes and Fusobacteria upsurges with the presence of RPDs.

While a rise of gingival inflammation at the marginal gingiva of the teeth in contact with the components of the RPD has been reported in a number of studies, others failed to find any difference at the gingival margin of the teeth that are in contact or not with the RPDs. Most of the studies showed an increase in the depth of the pockets in

RPD users. However, there are also investigations pointing out no changes. Bergman and Ericson showed that 3 years after RPD treatment, periodontal parameters were much better in patients who paid an annual check to a dentist as compared with those who did not. It was presented in a comparative study that both the RPD users and nonusers showed an increase in periodontal parameters after 8 or 9 years, showing that this increase should not be related directly to RPD usage. Nevertheless, there still seems to be a controversy regarding the effect of RPDs on gingival inflammation or pocket depth in the dental literature. It may be concluded that, good oral hygiene, proper RPD design, and most prominently regular recalls for RPD users are essential for controlling and preventing the occurrence of periodontal diseases.

23.8 Allergic Reactions

Allergic reactions may be seen in RPD patients due to the metal used for the framework or the resin used over the framework. All the alloys used in the RPDs release ions into the oral cavity because of corrosion and may cause allergic reactions if the patient is allergic to one of these metals used in the framework. Nickel is one of the most allergy-producing alloys and therefore the dental cast alloys are now manufactured nickel-free. The contact allergy of the oral mucosa is usually T-cell-mediated (delayed) reaction. These reactions appear intraorally as redness and edematous swelling of the mucosa underlying the RPDs (Fig. 23.13). The mucosa surface usually appears smooth and shining but sometimes ulcerations can also be seen. Lichenoid lesions and redness may also appear in the cheeks or tongue touching the RPDs. Additionally, symptoms like soreness, paresthesia, dryness, swelling, discomfort, and taste change may be seen in allergic RPD users.

It is vital for the clinician to properly diagnose the allergic reactions and differentiate the symptoms from other types. Intraoral examination, history of allergy, allergy tests such as patch or prick tests should be carried out in order to clearly differentiate and diagnose allergy.

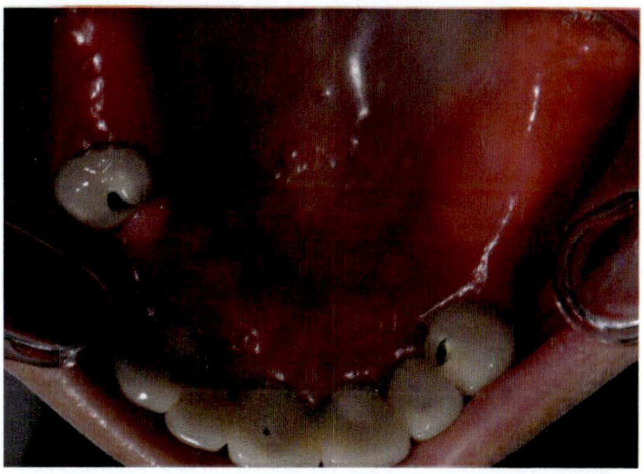

Fig. 23.13 Allergic reactions appear intraorally as redness and edematous swelling of the mucosa underlying the RPDs. Note that this patient has allergy both to the alloy and the methacrylate used in the fabrication of the RPD covering all of the area that the RPD touches

After screening with the appropriate test and diagnosing the allergy, the alloy causing the allergy should be substituted with another type such as titanium when refabricating the RPD. It should be pointed out that this alloy has some disadvantages when used as a framework material (see Chap. 14). If the patient is allergic to methacrylate, the RPD may be remade using thermoplastic base materials or CAD-CAM acrylic resins (see Chaps. 12 and 19).

Further Reading

Ancowitz S. Esthetic removable partial dentures. Gen Dent. 2004;52:453–9.

Bassi GS, Humphris GM, Longman LP. The etiology and management of gagging: a review of the literature. J Prosthet Dent. 2004;91:459–67.

Beaumont AJ Jr. An overview of esthetics with removable partial dentures. Quintessence Int. 2002;33:747–55.

Bergman B, Ericson G. Cross-sectional study of the periodontal status of removable partial denture patients. J Prosthet Dent. 1989;61:208–11.

Bergman B, Hugoson A, Olsson CO. A 25 year longitudinal study of patients treated with removable partial dentures. J Oral Rehabil. 1995;22:595–9.

Bergman B, Hugoson A, Olsson CO. Caries, periodontal and prosthetic findings in patients with removable partial dentures: a ten-year longitudinal study. J Prosthet Dent. 1982;48:506–14.

Bessadet M, Nicolas E, Sochat M, Hennequin M, Veyrune JL. Impact of removable partial denture prosthesis on chewing efficiency. J Appl Oral Sci. 2013;21:392–6.

Bezzon OL, Mattos MG, Ribeiro RF. Surveying removable partial dentures: the importance of guiding planes and path of insertion for stability. J Prosthet Dent. 1997;78:412–8.

Carlsson GE, Hedegård B, Koivumaa KK. Late results of treatment with partial dentures. An investigation by questionnaire and clinical examination 13 years after treatment. J Oral Rehabil. 1976;3:267–72.

Carlsson GE, Hedegård B, Koivumaa KK. The current place of removable partial dentures in restorative dentistry. Based on longitudinal investigations of dentogingivally supported partial dentures. Dent Clin North Am. 1970;14:553–68.

Chandler JA, Brudvik JS. Clinical evaluation of patients eight to nine years after placement of removable partial dentures. J Prosthet Dent. 1984;51:736–43.

Fletcher R, Harrison W, Crighton A. Dental material allergies and oral soft tissue reactions. Br Dent J. 2022;232:620–5.

Florêncio Costa RT, Leite Vila-Nova TE, Barbosa de França AJ, Gustavo da Silva Casado B, de Souza Leão R, Dantas de Moraes SL. Masticatory performance of denture wearers with the use of denture adhesives: a systematic review. J Prosthet Dent. 2022;127:233–8.

Geckili O, Bektas-Kayhan K, Eren P, Bilgin T, Unur M. The efficacy of a topical gel with triester glycerol oxide in denture-related mucosal injuries. Gerodontology. 2012;29:e715–20.

Geckili O, Bilhan H, Ceylan G, Cilingir A. Edentulous maxillary arch fixed implant rehabilitation using a hybrid prosthesis made of micro-ceramic-composite: case report. J Oral Implantol. 2013;39:115–20.

Grasso JE. Denture adhesives. Dent Clin North Am. 2004;48:721–33.

Hammond R, Beder OE. Increased vertical dimension and speech articulation errors. J Prosthet Dent. 1984;52:401–6.

Hatjigiorgis CG, Martin JW. An interim prosthesis to prevent lip and cheek biting. J Prosthet Dent. 1988;59:250–2.

Inukai M, John MT, Igarashi Y, Baba K. Association between perceived chewing ability and oral health-related quality of life in partially dentate patients. Health Qual Life Outcomes. 2010;8:118.

Jones JD, Garcia LT. Removable partial dentures: a clinician's guide. Iowa: Wiley-Blackwell; 2009.

Krol AJ. A new approach to the gagging problem. J Prosthet Dent. 1963;13:611–6.

Markkanen H, Lappalainen R, Honkala E, Tuominen R. Periodontal conditions with removable complete and partial dentures in the adult population aged 30 years and over. J Oral Rehabil. 1987;14:355–60.

McCord JF, Grey NJ, Winstanley RB, Johnson A. A clinical overview of removable prostheses: 5. diagnosis and treatment of RPD problems. Dent Update. 2003;30:96–7.

Olms C, Yahiaoui-Doktor M, Remmerbach TW. Contact allergies to dental materials. Swiss Dent J. 2019;129:571–9.

Oluwajana F, Walmsley AD. Titanium alloy removable partial denture framework in a patient with a metal allergy: a case study. Br Dent J. 2012;213:123–4.

Ozbek M, Tulunoğlu I, Ozkan S, Oktemer M. Evaluation of articulation of Turkish phonemes after removable partial denture application. Braz Dent J. 2003;14:125–31.

Papadiochou S, Emmanouil I, Papadiochos I. Denture adhesives: a systematic review. J Prosthet Dent. 2015;113:391–7.

Phoenix RD, Cagna DR, Defreest CF. Stewart's clinical removable partial prosthodontics. 4th ed. Chicago: Quintessence Publishing; 2008.

Preston JD. Preventing ceramic failures when integrating fixed and removable prosthesis. Dent Clin North Am. 1979;23:37–52.

Ramakrishnan AN, Röhrle O, Ludtka C, Varghese R, Koehler J, Kiesow A, Schwan S. Finite element evaluation of the effect of adhesive creams on the stress state of dentures and oral mucosa. Appl Bionics Biomech. 2021;2021:5533770.

Schwalm CA, Smith DE, Erickson JD. A clinical study of patients 1 to 2 years after placement of removable partial dentures. J Prosthet Dent. 1977;38:380–91.

Syed M, Chopra R, Sachdev V. Allergic reactions to dental materials—a systematic review. J Clin Diagn Res. 2015;9:ZE04–9.

Szentpétery AG, John MT, Slade GD, Setz JM. Problems reported by patients before and after prosthodontic treatment. Int J Prosthodont. 2005;18:124–31.

The glossary of prosthodontic terms: ninth edition. J Prosthet Dent. 2017;117(5S):e1–e105.

Tjan AH, Miller GD, The JG. Some esthetic factors in a smile. J Prosthet Dent. 1984;51:24–8.

Vanzeveren C, D'Hoore W, Bercy P. Influence of removable partial denture on periodontal indices and microbiological status. J Oral Rehabil. 2002;29:232–9.

Yusof Z, Isa Z. Periodontal status of teeth in contact with denture in removable partial denture wearers. J Oral Rehabil. 1994;21:77–86.

24 Maintenance

Onur Geçkili

Abstract

For a removable partial denture (RPD) treatment to be successful, an appropriate follow-up care is crucial. This follow-up care begins at the day of insertion and continues as the patient uses the prosthesis. Ongoing alveolar bone resorptions together with the wear of the denture materials in time or misuse by the patients necessitate a proper maintenance for RPDs. The patients should be advised about the care that should be given to the prosthesis and the possible situations that may require adjustments in time before insertion of the RPDs. This chapter focuses on the procedures used for the RPD maintenance. The techniques used for relining and rebasing, as well as advice for easy repairs that the clinicians can complete in one appointment and more complex ones that can only be completed at the laboratory, are all discussed in detail.

24.1 Definitions

Adhesive: (1) Any substance that creates close adherence to or on adjoining surfaces; (2) a luting agent.

O. Geçkili (✉)
Faculty of Dentistry, Department of Prosthodontics, İstanbul University, İstanbul, Türkiye
e-mail: geckili@istanbul.edu.tr

Border molding: The shaping of impression material along the border areas of an impression tray by functional or manual manipulation of the soft tissue adjacent to the borders to duplicate the contour and size of the vestibule.

Braze: To join with a nonferrous alloy that melts at a lower temperature than that of the metals being joined.

Elastomeric impression material: A group of flexible chemical polymers that are either chemically or physically cross-linked; generally, they can be easily stretched and rapidly recover their original dimensions when applied stresses are released.

Flask: A metal case or tube used in investing procedures.

Flasking: The process of investing the cast and a wax replica of the desired form in a flask preparatory to molding the restorative material into the desired product.

Intaglio surface: The portion of the denture or other restoration surface that has its contour determined by the impression; the interior or reversal surface of an object.

Irreversible hydrocolloid: A hydrocolloid consisting of a sol of alginic acid having a physical state that is changed by an irreversible chemical reaction forming insoluble calcium alginate.

Laser welding: The joining of metal components through the use of heat generated with a laser beam.

O. Şakar (ed.), *Removable Partial Dentures*, https://doi.org/10.1007/978-3-031-47083-7_24

Modeling plastic impression compound: A thermoplastic dental impression material composed of wax, rosin, resins, and colorants.

Polishing: The act or process of making a denture or casting smooth and glossy.

Polyether: An elastomeric impression material of ethylene oxide and tetra-hydrofluro copolymers that polymerizes under the influence of an aromatic ester.

Polysulfide: An elastomeric impression material of polysulfide polymer (mercaptan) that cross-links under the influence of oxidizing agents such as lead peroxide.

Polyvinyl siloxane: An addition reaction silicone elastomeric impression material of silicone polymers having terminal vinyl groups that cross-link with silanes on activation by a platinum or palladium salt catalyst.

Rebase: The laboratory process of replacing the entire denture base material on an existing prosthesis.

Reline: The procedures used to resurface the tissue side of a removable dental prosthesis with new base material, thus producing an accurate adaptation to the denture foundation area.

Separating medium: A coating applied to a surface and serving to prevent a second surface from adhering to the first.

Solder: To unite, bring into, or restore to a firm union; the act of uniting two pieces of metal by the proper alloy of metals.

Warp: Torsional change of shape or outline; to turn or twist out of shape.

Wrought: Worked into shape; formed, hammered.

Successful treatment with RPDs requires periodic evaluations and proper maintenance in the follow-up appointments. Especially, distal extension RPDs have a special need for maintenance, mainly relining or rebasing because of the continuing alveolar bone resorption. The disuse resorption of the edentulous alveolar crests has been continuously questioned since the 1960s and most studies focusing on this subject found more bone resorption with the use of dentures as compared to disuse. Therefore, it should be underlined that the bone underlying the RPD will undoubtedly resorb even if the RPD has been perfectly fabricated. The resorption speed of the underlying bone mainly depends on the strong pressure exerted on the mucosa because of the generated occlusal forces. The power of the occlusal forces may be predicted before the treatment by measuring the gonial angle on the panoramic radiographs. Patients with small gonial angle have more potential for powerful occlusal forces and consequently accelerated bone resorption. These patients may be recalled more often after delivery of the prosthesis. If a distal extension RPD loses the support of soft tissues and begins to move, damage to the abutments and soft tissues are unavoidable. Therefore, a maintenance plan should be made right after the delivery of the RPD and especially a distal extension RPD should be relined periodically to maintain its close adaptation to the underlying soft tissues and to avoid causing subsequent trauma to the oral cavity.

24.2 Relining and Rebasing

In case of loss of the supporting tissues, the most convenient treatment is the relining of the RPD. Rebasing is needed when the denture base has some fractures, cracks, or has become irreparably discolored. It is very important to differentiate the meanings of relining and rebasing to avoid confusion as they are frequently mixed up and used synonymously. In both situations, a new impression is necessary. However, it is also possible to complete the relining in a chairside intraoral technique, which is not possible in the rebasing procedures. To determine the need for relining or rebasing an RPD, the following evaluations may be undertaken:

1. Place a thin portion of irreversible hydrocolloid or elastomeric impression material to the intaglio surface of the RPD base; seat the RPD in the mouth and wait until the impression material sets. Remove the RPD and inspect for the thickness of the impression material. If it is more than 2 mm thick, make a reline (Fig. 24.1).
2. Seat the RPD in the mouth and apply a pressure on the most posterior part and inspect the

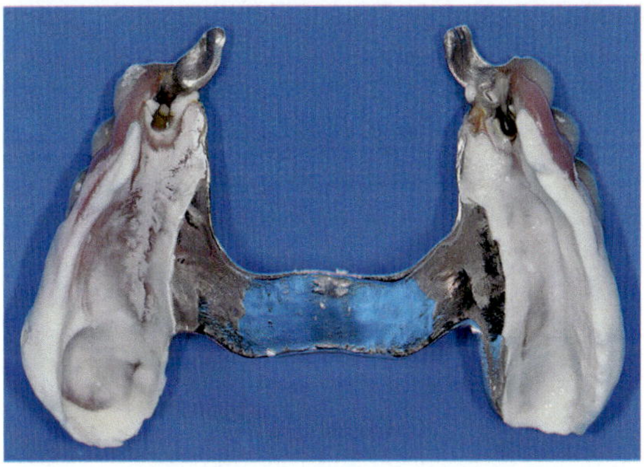

Fig. 24.1 A thin portion of irreversible hydrocolloid is placed to the intaglio surface of the RPD base to see if the RPD has to be relined. In the right extension base, the thickness of the impression material is more than 2 mm, presenting the need of a reline, whereas the impression material in the left extension base is less than 2 mm, presenting no need for relining

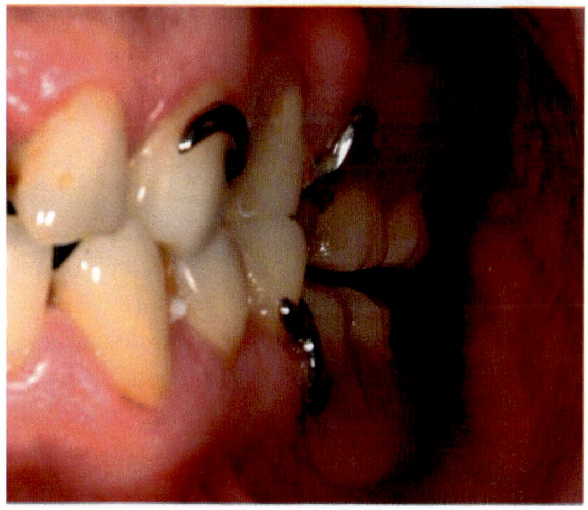

Fig. 24.3 If the occlusal contact between artificial dentition is lacking, a reline together with an occlusal correction is essential

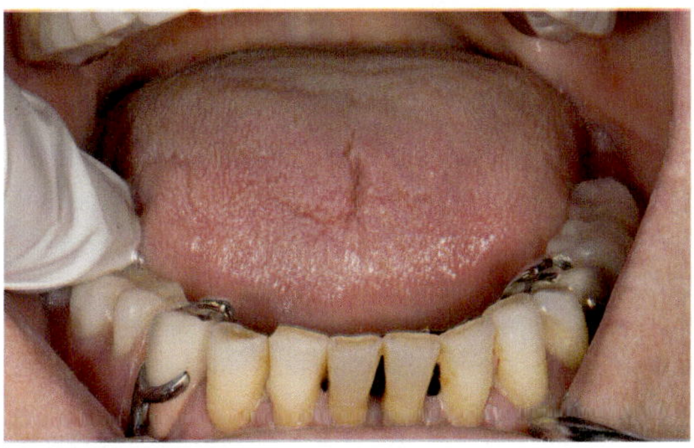

Fig. 24.2 RPD is seated and a pressure is applied on the most posterior parts. The indirect retainers lift more than 2 mm, pointing out the need of relining

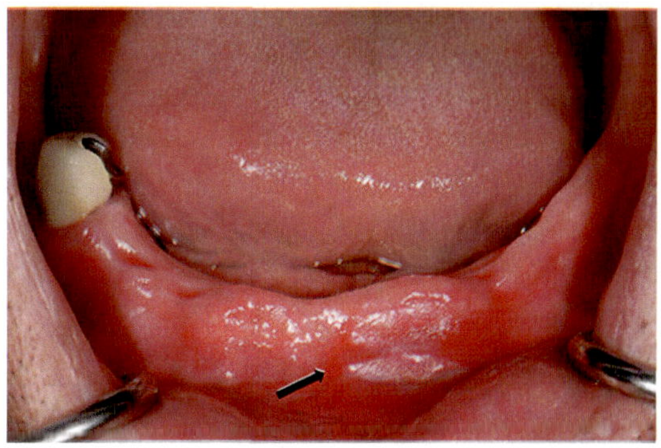

Fig. 24.4 A stubborn ulceration exists on the labial vestibule. The RPD base should be shortened and a tissue conditioner should be applied afterward to promote healing

indirect retainers. If the indirect retainers lift more than 2 mm, make a reline (Fig. 24.2).
3. Instruct the patient to close the mouth in maximum intercuspal position and inspect for the posterior contacts of the RPD. If loss of occlusal contacts on the posterior teeth is inspected (Fig. 24.3), place a wax on the occluding surfaces and instruct the patient to close. Inspect the wax, and if the occlusal contact between artificial dentition is lacking, make a reline together with an occlusal correction.
4. If there exists a stubborn ulceration, inflammation, or hypertrophy on the soft tissues underlying the RPDs (Fig. 24.4), apply a tissue conditioning material after relieving the denture base surfaces touching the irritated areas and make a reline. Instruct the patient to use the RPD with the tissue conditioner for at least 24 h. The procedure will be discussed in the following sections.

Relining procedures can be accomplished by two major techniques:

1. Direct (chairside) technique
2. Indirect technique

There are four primary criteria for an RPD reline, which are listed as follows:

1. Good chemical bond
2. Satisfactory strength

3. No warping or dimensional change in the prosthesis
4. Speed of the procedure

Despite the time and cost savings of the direct technique, the advantage of the indirect technique is a harder, denser, and more completely cured resin reline compared with direct reline materials. The materials used for direct reline procedures are more porous and flexible and less color stable. Additionally, although both the heat-cured polymethylmethacrylate (PMMA) used in the indirect technique and the direct-reline materials contain some residual monomer, which may be cytotoxic to particular patients, direct-reline materials comprise a greater risk because of less polymerization. In general, indirect method is preferred because of the above-mentioned advantages but no long-term studies have compared the outcomes of the two methods.

Before starting the relining procedures, the oral mucosa should be returned to an acceptable state of health that may require a period of function without the RPD or using the RPD with a tissue conditioner after relief of the RPD in the effected regions.

24.2.1 Relining Tooth-Supported Removable Partial Dentures

The need of relining the tooth-supported RPDs is not common because the tissue changes that arise underneath the denture bases do not distress the support of the RPDs. Since the abutments rather than the residual ridges absorb the occlusal loads, tooth-supported RPDs have the minimum amount of residual ridge resorption. Relining procedures are performed only for hygienic or esthetic reasons. It is much more practical to use an intraoral chairside technique when a tooth-supported RPD is to be relined. As making an impression requires the RPD to be flasked and processed, the vertical dimension may be increased and the RPD may be distorted during laboratory procedures. It is not feasible to take these risks for such an easy procedure if the RPD will not be rebased.

24.2.2 Relining Distal Extension Removable Partial Dentures

Distal extension RPDs require correction by relining or rebasing much more often than tooth-supported RPDs because majority of the support is from the underlying soft tissues and residual ridges and more occlusal loads are directed to the residual ridges through the prosthesis. The patient should be informed that a distal extension RPD requires periodic examination and relining due to maintaining the health of the abutments and the residual ridges before the treatment. This information has an important role in defending the rights of the clinician to charge the patient in the periodic visits.

24.2.3 Step-by-Step Procedures for Direct or Indirect Relining

No matter what technique is being used, sufficient amount of denture base (minimum 1 mm) should be relieved from the intaglio surface of the RPD to be relined. The space provided with relieving prevents the impression material to apply inappropriate pressure to the underlying tissues and potential contaminants to warrant a suitable bonding surface. Additionally, the undercuts should be removed to evade fracture of the final cast both during the separation of the impression and in the processing procedures.

24.2.3.1 Direct Relining

The procedure for direct relining an RPD is as follows:

1. Apply a separating medium to the occlusal surfaces of the remaining teeth and polished surfaces of the RPD, which are not to be modified in order to avoid new resin from adhering to these surfaces and teeth.
2. Apply a surface primer that is mostly supplied with the chairside reline product or some of the reline resin monomer if the primer is not supplied. with a small brush to enhance bonding strength of the resin reline material (Fig. 24.5).

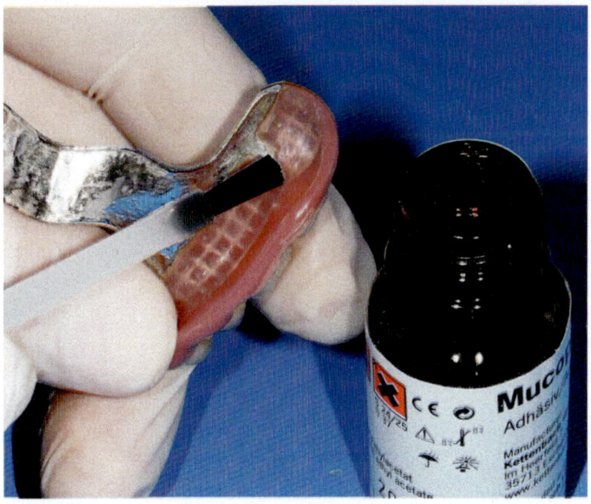

Fig. 24.5 A surface primer is applied with a small brush to enhance bonding strength of the resin reline material

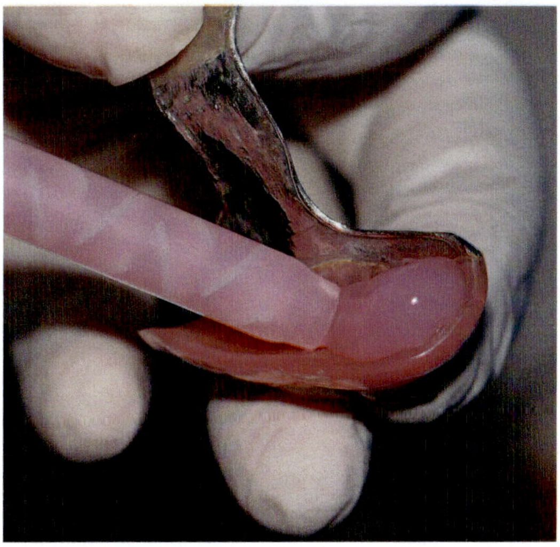

Fig. 24.6 The resin reline material is applied to the intaglio surface of the RPD

3. Mix the powder and liquid of the resin reline material in a suitable mixing container and apply to the intaglio surface of the RPD and the borders to be relined after the material begins to set but in an easily flowable stage. If the material is in a cartridge, insert the cartridge in the dispensing gun, mount a mixing tip and apply the material into the RPD base (Fig. 24.6).
4. Place the RPD in the mouth ensuring that all the rests are in their proper places and instruct the patient to close slightly into maximal intercuspal position. It is very important to avoid flowing of the material over the occlusal surfaces in order not to change the established vertical dimension of occlusion.

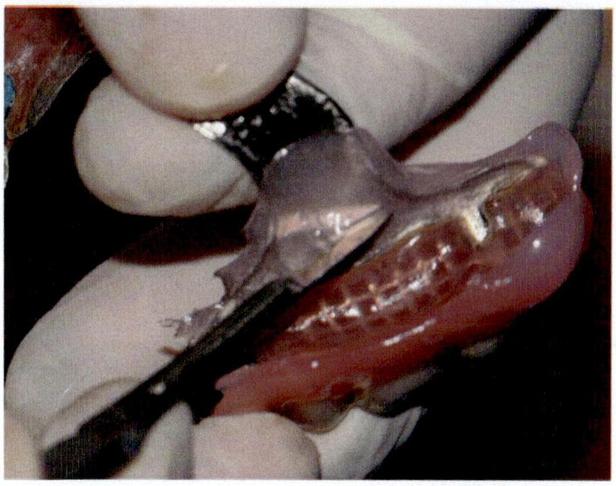

Fig. 24.7 When the resin reline material starts to be elastic, excess material is removed with a scalpel

5. Instruct the patient to open the mouth and manipulate the cheeks and the lips for border molding. If a mandibular RPD is to be relined, instruct the patient to move the tongue to the cheeks, lips, and to the anterior teeth and swallow for shaping the lingual borders. Be sure that the RPD is not displaced during border molding by applying a finger pressure on the rests.
6. Remove the RPD from the mouth when the material starts to be elastic, trim away the excess material with a scissors or scalpel (Fig. 24.7), and return the RPD into the patient's mouth afterward.
7. Instruct the patient to occlude the teeth slightly to check occlusal vertical dimension and then open his/her mouth to hold the framework against the abutments until the material totally sets. If the patient is asked to close the mouth and occlude until the material sets, the patients may rotate the distal extension base and overcompress the soft tissues if he/she does not close exactly into the desired occlusion. Therefore, it is much safer to finish the setting of the resin material with the help of the clinician and with the mouth open.
8. Remove the RPD from the mouth, rinse it in water, and examine the relined surfaces. To eliminate any tissue damage that could have

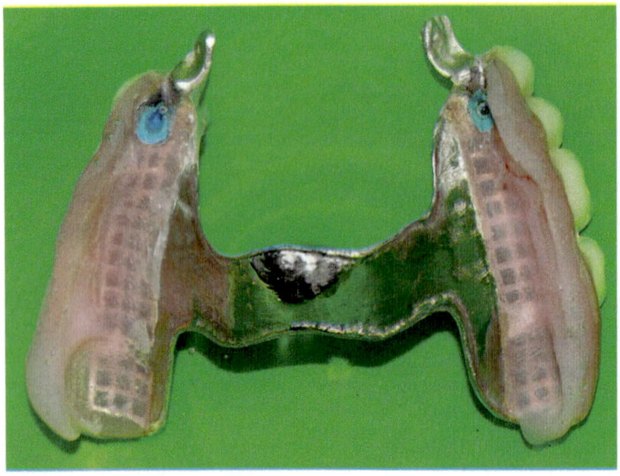

Fig. 24.8 To eliminate any tissue damage that could have resulted from the exothermic heat or prolonged contact of the tissue with unreacted monomer, the RPD is immersed in a container of 45–50 °C water for at least 15 min to polymerize

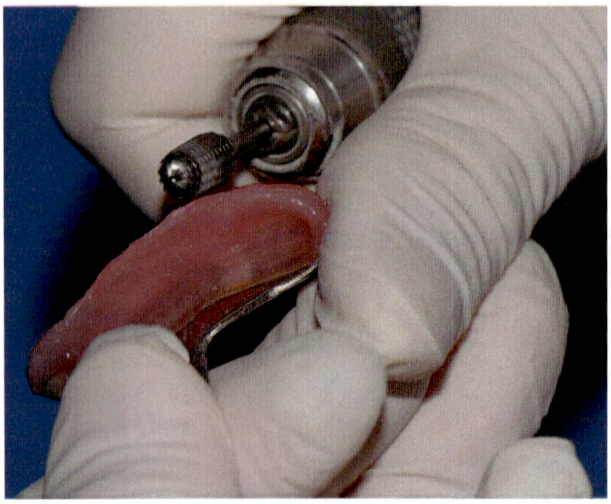

Fig. 24.9 A neat finish line is prepared between the reline material and acrylic base with the help of appropriate burs

resulted from the exothermic heat or prolonged contact of the tissue with unreacted monomer, put the RPD in a container of 45–50 °C water for at least 15 min (Fig. 24.8) or in a pressure pot for 20–30 min to polymerize.

9. After curing, trim the excess parts with appropriate burs and a rotary instrument to provide a neat finish line between the reline material and acrylic base (Fig. 24.9). If the material is a soft liner, use cross-cut steel burs for bulk reduction.
10. Finish with the polishing discs supplied with the material (Fig. 24.10) and if the material is a soft liner, apply a thin layer of silicone sealant with a brush within 90 s (Fig. 24.11) and return the relined RPD into the mouth.

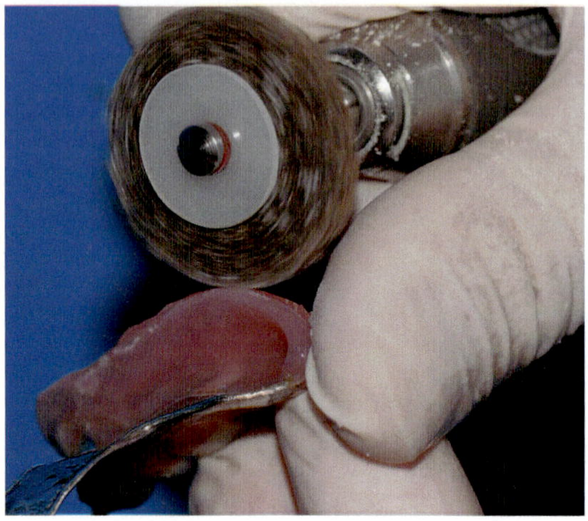

Fig. 24.10 Polishing discs are used for finishing

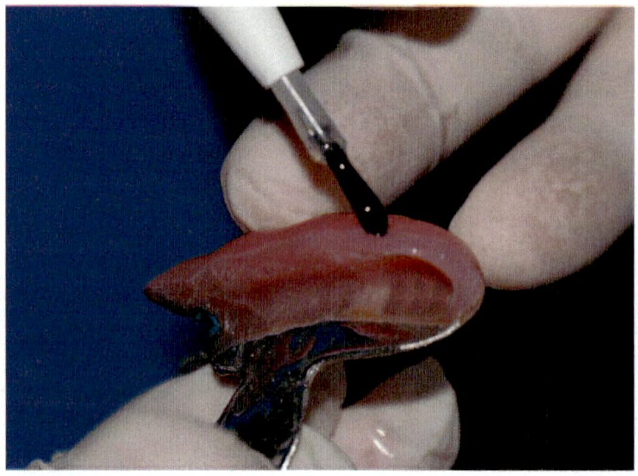

Fig. 24.11 If the material is a soft liner, a thin layer of silicone sealant is applied with a brush within 90 s

11. Check the occlusion and adjust if any change has occurred.
12. Check the borders and the intaglio surface with the help of a pressure-indicating paste to ensure they are not overextended and deliver the relined RPD to the patient.

24.2.3.2 Indirect Relining

For a successful indirect relining, it is vital to select the appropriate impression material. The impression material should not extend beyond the support of the denture base. The choice of impression material should be determined by the characteristics of the tissues. Zinc oxide–eugenol

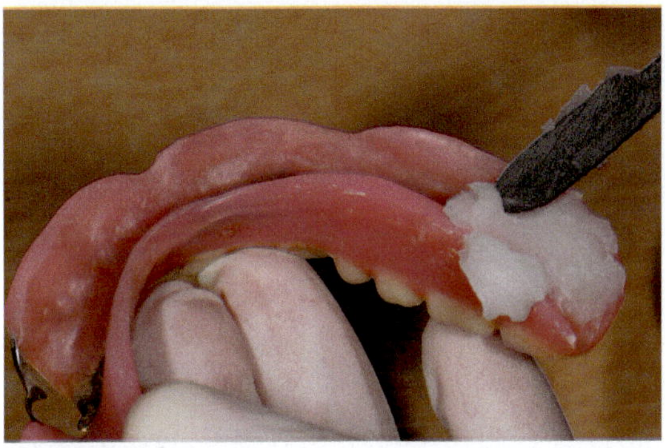

Fig. 24.12 Tissue-conditioning materials may be applied to the extension bases as a reline material

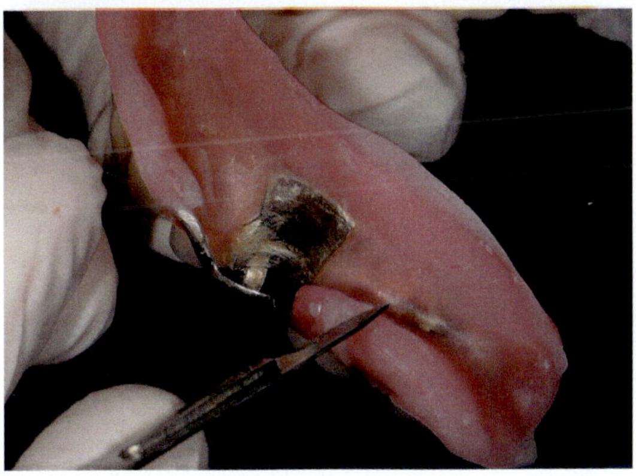

Fig. 24.13 After setting, RPD is removed and inspected and the excess borders are removed using a scalpel

impression material is indicated for most of the tissue types but strongly recommended if mobile tissues are present on the alveolar crest. If relining is to be performed on dense, firm tissues, polysulfide rubber bases, polyether, polyvinylsiloxane, and mouth-temperature waxes may similarly be used with confidence.

For indirect relining, especially if the mucosal tissues are damaged, tissue-conditioning materials may be applied to the extension bases (Fig. 24.12) and after setting, the RPD is removed and inspected. The excess borders are removed using a scalpel (Fig. 24.13) and the patient is released to use the RPD for 24 h and recalled. On the recall session, the RPD is evaluated; the excess parts are trimmed or the short borders are completed with a newly mixed tissue-conditioning material, and the patient is released again to use the RPD for a few more days. After the clinician is confident and the patient has no complaints with the RPD, it may be sent to the

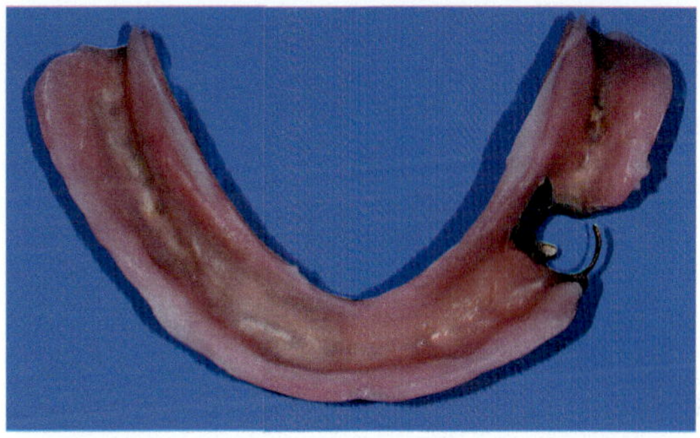

Fig. 24.14 When the patient has no complaints through the RPD with the tissue conditioning material, it may be sent to the laboratory directly for an indirect reline

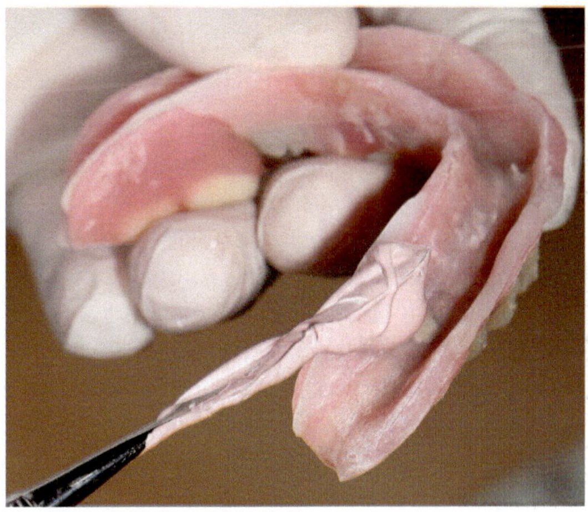

Fig. 24.15 In order to achieve better accuracy, it is preferable to apply a free-flowing zinc oxide–eugenol impression material for an additional reline impression onto the tissue conditioning material

laboratory straight for an indirect reline (Fig. 24.14). However, in order to achieve better accuracy, it is advised to apply a free-flowing zinc oxide–eugenol impression material for an additional reline impression onto the tissue conditioning material (Fig. 24.15). After setting, RPD is removed and sent to the laboratory directly for processing or an over-impression may be made using a reversible hydrocolloid (Fig. 24.16). It should be pointed out that if the over-impression extends beyond the zinc-oxide borders, these parts should be trimmed before pouring the impression (Fig. 24.16). After the processing procedures carried out in the laboratory, the relined RPD is delivered to the patient.

The procedure for indirect relining an RPD is as follows:

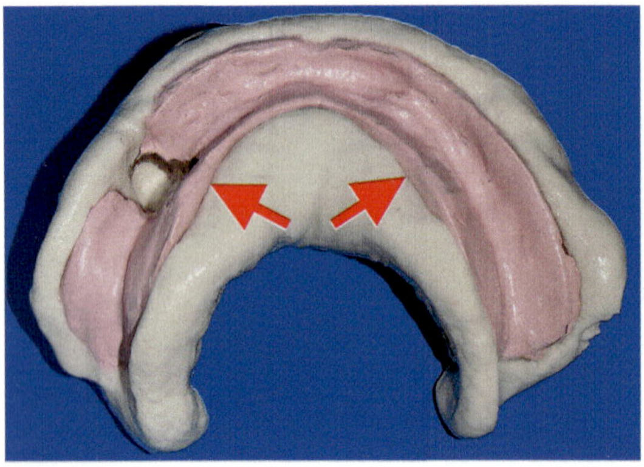

Fig. 24.16 Additionally, an over-impression may be made using a reversible hydrocolloid. If the borders of the over-impression extend to the zinc oxide–eugenol impression like shown by arrows, these parts should be trimmed before pouring the impression

1. If border molding is necessary, use a low-fusing stick-type modeling plastic impression compound: green or gray stick, for shaping the peripheral extensions step by step or a polyether impression material in one step. If a mandibular distal extension RPD is to be relined, perform border molding from the anterior extent of the buccal flange to the most posterior extent of the RPD and on the lingual and distolingual flanges. If the reline is needed for under-extended borders, border molding may be accomplished only on these surfaces to extend the missing parts (Fig. 24.17). Border molding may also be performed in one step using a polyether impression material. In that case, an adhesive should be placed to the borders of the RPD and polyether is syringed around the borders and border molding is carried out afterward.
2. Make the final impression with zinc oxide–eugenol impression material if border molding has been done with modeling sticks. If border molding is not necessary, step 1 may be eliminated and the impression may be made with one of the above-mentioned impression materials.
3. Make sure that all the rests are in their designed position on the abutment teeth and maintained in this position until the impression material sets (Fig. 24.18). An open mouth impression technique is advised for an easy observation of placement of the rests into their rest seats (Fig. 24.18).
4. Remove the impression and examine for precision (Fig. 24.19). Small defects may be corrected using a mouth temperature wax. If

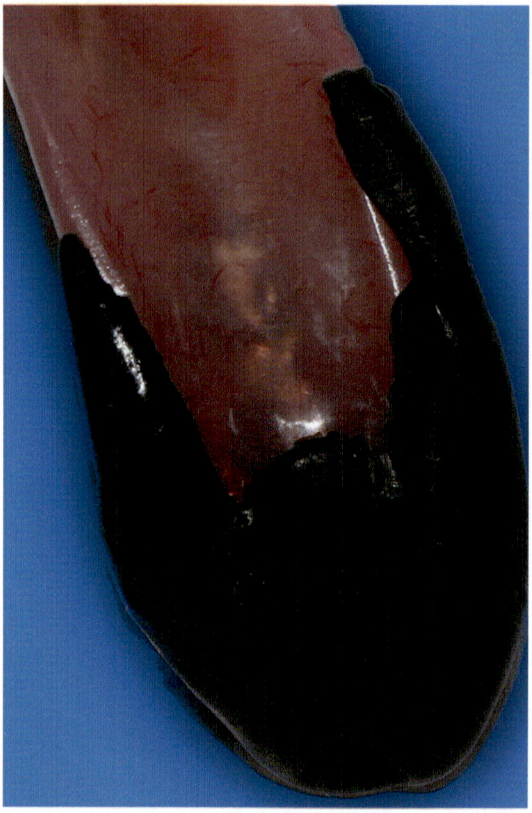

Fig. 24.17 Border molding may be accomplished to lengthen the under-extended borders during relining

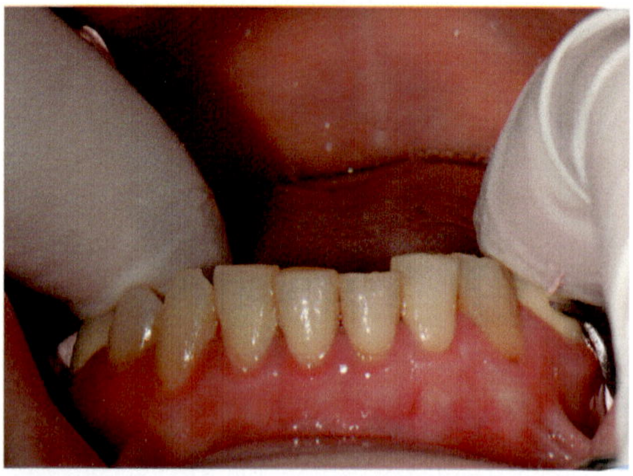

Fig. 24.18 An open mouth impression technique is advised for an easy observation of placement of the rests into their rest seats

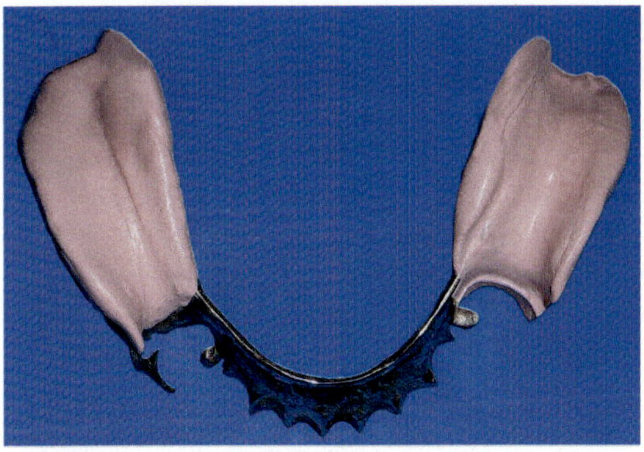

Fig. 24.19 The impression is removed and examined

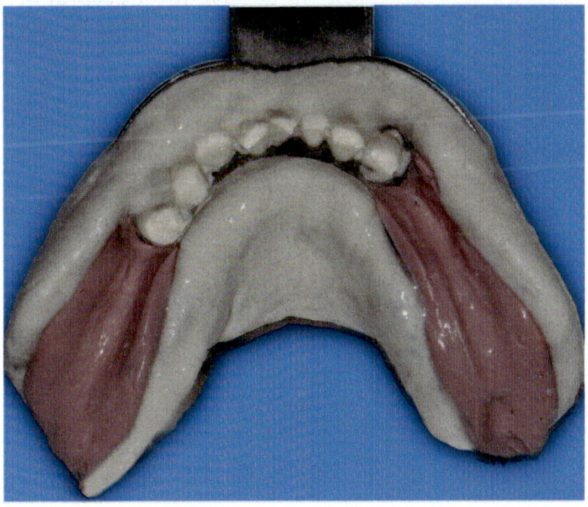

Fig. 24.20 An over-impression may be made to obtain a complete arch cast

large defects are present, impression should be repeated.

5. Return the impression to the patient's mouth and inspect for accurate placement of the rests.
6. Make an over-impression with alginate impression material to obtain a complete arch cast (Fig. 24.20). (The impression may be sent directly to the laboratory without making this over-impression.)
7. Pour the impression with Type III dental stone to make a definitive cast, but do not separate it from the cast after setting.
8. Close the spaces with wax, trim the teeth, and remove the undercut areas to prepare the impression and the cast assembly for flasking.

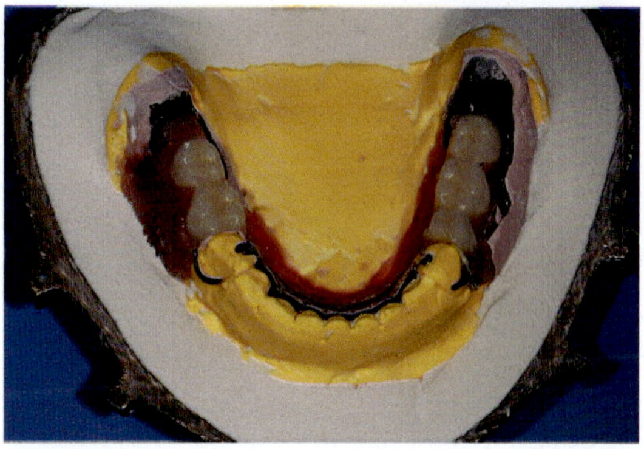

Fig. 24.21 Type II dental stone is poured into the flask; the cast is positioned and the flask is immersed in boiling water for 5 min to remove the wax and the impression from the cast

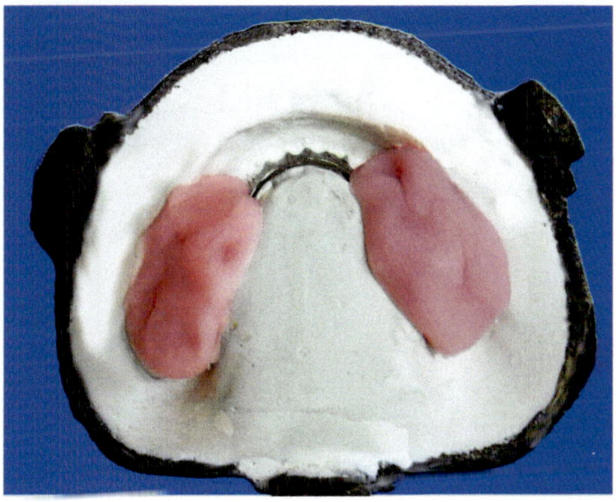

Fig. 24.22 Heat polymerizing acrylic resin is applied in the flask and polymerized using the preferred method

9. Pour Type II dental stone into the flask; position the cast and allow the stone to set completely (Fig. 24.21).
10. Place the flask in boiling water for 5 min; remove the wax, border molding material and the impression from the cast (polyether, and polyvinylsiloxane impression materials may be separated immediately after the dental stone sets without the necessity of heat). Make sure that the RPD is completely cleared from all the impression material and the wax residue.
11. Mix and place a heat polymerizing acrylic resin in the flask (Fig. 24.22), close the flask,

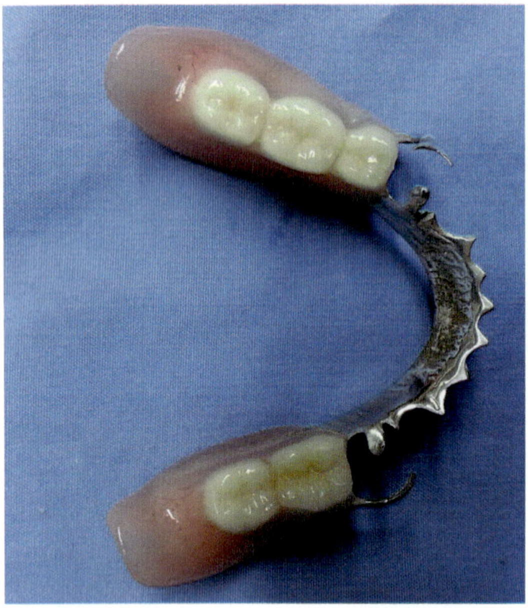

Fig. 24.23 The relined RPD is shaped and polished after removing from the flask and delivered to the patient

and polymerize the resin using an appropriate method.

12. Shape and polish the relined RPD (Fig. 24.23) using conventional techniques and deliver the RPD to the patient.

24.3 Repairs

The need for repairs to RPDs may arise after using for some time or instantly following the delivery of the prosthesis. Repairs are usually completed in the laboratory and the patients are left without their prosthesis for several days. This is generally not well tolerated by most of the patients. Therefore, it is much better to repair the RPD directly in the clinic instead of sending it to the laboratory. RPD repairs types are as follows:

1. Denture base repairs
2. Repair of major or minor connectors
3. Repair of the rests or direct retainers
4. Repair of fractured or lost artificial teeth
5. Loss of a natural tooth necessitating its replacement
6. Other repairs

24.3.1 Denture Base Repairs

A section of the denture base may be lost or fractured from the rest of the RPD usually because of careless handling by the patient. If the fractured denture base is lost or cannot be accurately positioned on the fracture site because of deterioration, a reline impression is required with the use of modeling compound to complete the fractured site. After the completed impression is poured to fabricate a master cast, the fractured segment is repaired with either autopolymerizing or heat-cured acrylic resin. However, if the fractured segment is too large, it may not be possible to reshape the tissue contours with the modeling compound and the RPD has to be refabricated.

If the fractured segment is available and can be accurately positioned on the fractured site, a simple in-office procedure is usually adequate for the repair. The fractured pieces are joined with sticky wax and dental stone is poured against the tissue side of the denture base to produce a master cast. After setting, the RPD is removed from the cast, the fractured segments are separated, and the fracture line is opened for about 1–2 mm using appropriate burs. A separating medium is applied to the cast; the opened segments are returned to the master cast and accurately positioned. Autopolymerizing acrylic resin is applied to the prepared space until the space is slightly overfilled. The resin may be left for polymerizing or the cast and RPD assembly may be placed in a pressure cooker or pressure pot for 20–30 min for less internal porosity. After polymerization, the base is trimmed, polished, and delivered to the patient.

24.3.2 Repair of Major or Minor Connectors

Major or minor connectors usually do not break because they have adequate bulk of metal. A major connector may weaken due to frequent adjustments to overcome adaptation or tissue impingement problems. Additionally, major connectors which are not rigid and indicated in only some particular situations like Kennedy bar may weaken

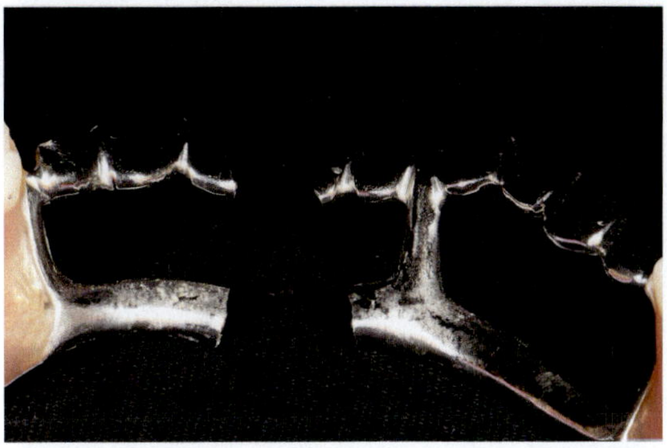

Fig. 24.24 Kennedy bar may weaken after some time, and the weakened parts cannot tolerate intraoral stresses and may break

after some time, and the weakened parts cannot tolerate intraoral stresses and may break (Fig. 24.24). Misuse of the patients may also be a reason of the distortion of the major or minor connectors. Usually, clinicians choose the option to reconstruct the RPDs when the major connectors are broken. However, there are methods to repair them at least for the interim use of the patients.

24.3.2.1 Soldering or Brazing

If the joining process is below 425 °C, the operation is called soldering and if the temperature is above 425 °C, it is called brazing. The process of bracing or torch soldering may be used for the repair of an RPD framework without acrylic resin base. A minimum space of 0.2–0.3 up to 0.5 mm should be obtained between the fractured segments by using aluminum oxide disks or fine diamond burs. An oxygen–propane torch is used for heating the segments to be joined until they are red hot, and then melted solder alloy with or without the same metal is flowed into the joint area. Once the soldering operation has initiated, it is important not to remove the flame in order not to cause cooling to overcome oxidation. The investment is left to cool slowly and then the framework is cleaned, finished, and polished with the help of appropriate instruments and burs. This method is well known by the laboratories and cheap but it has some disadvantages as follows:

1. Oxidation of the joined segments
2. Structural defects and failure of the finished framework due to porosity and overheating
3. Cannot be used to repair an RPD having a resin denture base or artificial teeth

More recently developed electric soldering involves tungsten inert gas (TIG) welding and plasma arc welding (PAW). Both systems use a torch with a tungsten electrode and a shielding gas source. The advantage of electric soldering is the ability to repair an RPD without damaging the acrylic resin base. The acrylic resin base should be protected with a wet casting ring liner during the electric soldering procedure. The main disadvantage is the presence of porosities in the soldered region because of the argon gas.

24.3.2.2 Laser Welding

Laser welding has been developed recently and successfully used in the repair of RPD framework fractures (Fig. 24.25) or clasp repair procedures and has been suggested as the best welding technique for dissimilar metals.

The technique ensures a high-intensity, concentrated light beam to reach the metal surface. As the metal absorbs its energy, it converts it into heat that takes the metal to its melting point. Before starting the laser-welding procedure, the fractured segments and adjacent areas should be sandblasted to reduce laser beam reflection.

The advantages of the laser-welding technique include higher tensile strength of the joints, permission to welding near acrylic or ceramic surfaces and less time. However, the equipment is very expensive, porosities in the region of the union may occur, and the two joining segment surfaces must have a full contact, which is very hard to achieve in some situations.

24.3.2.3 Repair with Splinting Using Metal Conditioners

It is also possible to repair a lingual plate with a cast splint and metal adhesive system. After the fractured segments are accurately positioned and a dental stone model is obtained, a groove is prepared on the lingual plate reaching the fractured denture base. A wax pattern is prepared duplicating the prepared groove and cast with a silver–palladium–copper–gold alloy. The lingual plate is air abraded and a metal conditioner is applied to the surface. The splint is positioned on the

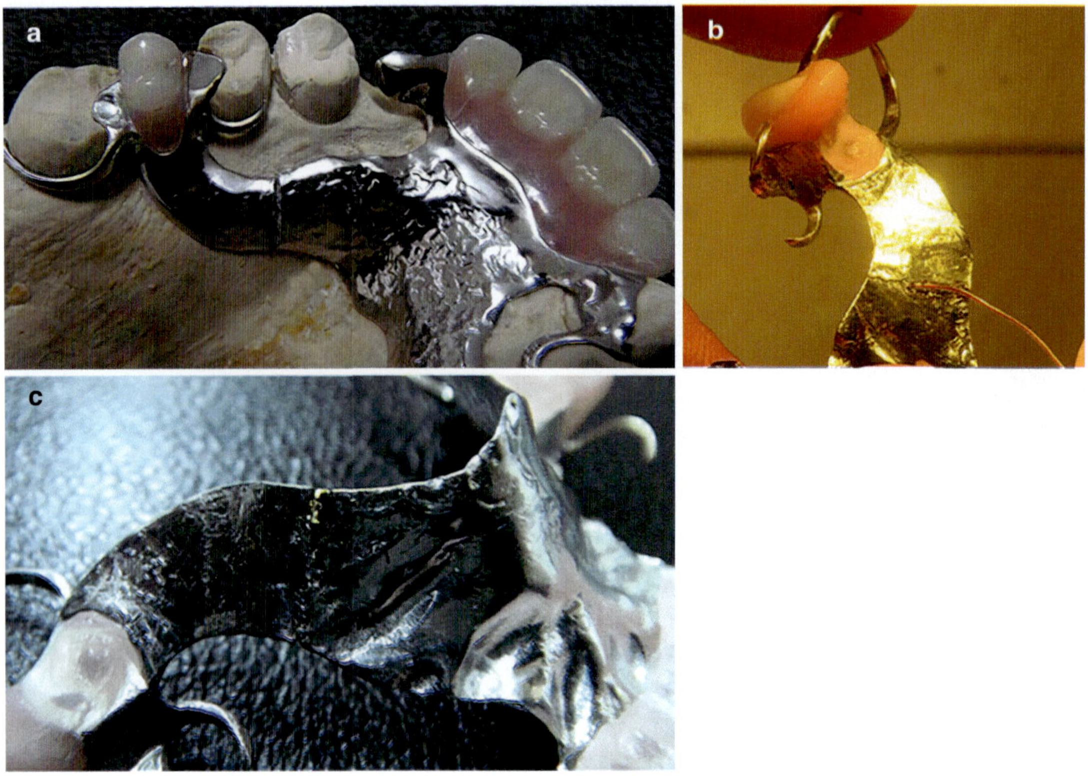

Fig. 24.25 An impression is made with the broken RPD framework and a cast is obtained (**a**). After the components are airborne-particle abraded, they are rigidly stabilized by tacking with a laser-welding machine and after stabilization welding with a parent Co–Cr wire is completed (**b**). After laser welding (**c**), the framework is finished and polished

groove and attached using an adhesive luting cement (Fig. 24.26). It should be underlined that this method may only be used for interim use until a new RPD is fabricated.

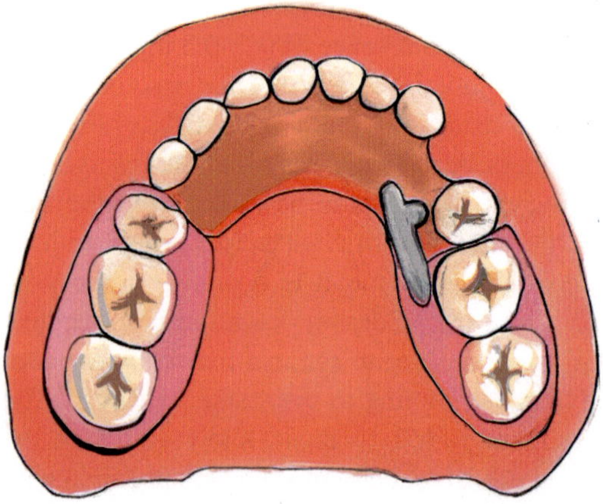

Fig. 24.26 A broken lingual plate may be repaired with a cast splint and metal adhesive system for an interim use

24.3.3 Repair of the Rests or Direct Retainers

An occlusal rest may fracture as a consequence of insufficient rest seat preparation. The rests, which have to be made too thin or have been weakened because of occlusal adjustments, may fracture. It is much better to reconstruct the RPD with appropriate seat preparations, but the rests may also be repaired by soldering or laser weld-

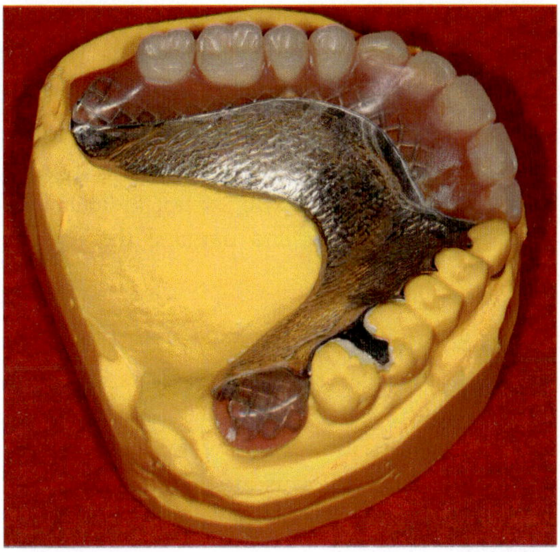

Fig. 24.27 If the occlusal rests are fractured, an impression is made with the RPDs after appropriate seat preparations have been made. The prepared rest seats are filled with impression material and the provided spaces may be observed and inspected

ing. However, in order not to cause additional fracture, the rest seat should be prepared appropriately and an impression with the RPD having the fractured rest should be made. After the completed impression is poured to fabricate a master cast, the prepared rest seat is filled with impression material and the provided space may easily be observed and inspected (Fig. 24.27).

The most common broken component of an RPD is the clasp arm because it emerges freely from the RPD. Before repairing an RPD with a broken clasp arm, the possible reasons for the breakage should be evaluated in order not to cause repeated damages. Following are the possible reasons for fracture of the clasp arms:

1. *Deep undercut*: This type of fracture is a safe one and it prevents loosening of the abutment. Undercut should be reduced before repair (see Chap. 5).
2. *Accidental dropping by the patient*: Since mostly elderly patients use RPDs, they drop them frequently because of cognitive impairments.
3. *Mechanical failure of the clasp arm*: If the metal thickness at the fracture site is less than 1.2 mm, immediate repair cannot be a solution. Proper mouth preparation in order to thicken the metal surface before repair is essential. Additionally, the clasp arms may have voids or pores that developed during casting, which may affect the fatigue resistance of clasps subjected to repetitive loads during insertion and removal of the RPDs. This may trigger mechanical failure of the clasp arms.
4. *Frequent adjustments made by the clinician*: Excessive manipulation of the clasp arm both during initial adaptation and during the follow-up visits may weaken and break the clasp arm. It is very important not to adjust the clasp arm beyond the elastic limit of the metal.

The broken clasp arms can be repaired using the following methods.

24.3.3.1 Repair with a Wrought Wire Clasp

This method is the most common one because it may be completed in the dental office without sending the RPD to the laboratory. It is a cost-effective and quick method both for the patient and the clinician. The step-by-step procedure is as follows:

1. Seat the RPD with the broken clasp in the mouth and check for fit and position (Fig. 24.28).
2. Make an irreversible hydrocolloid impression with the RPD (Fig. 24.29) and immediately pour with dental stone (Fig. 24.30). If the

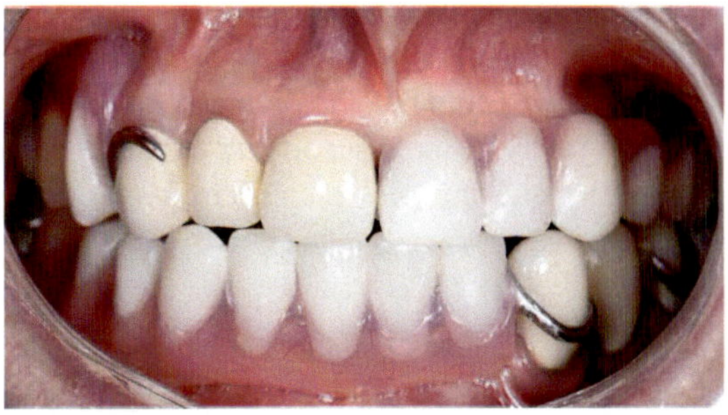

Fig. 24.28 RPD with the broken clasp is seated and checked for fit and position

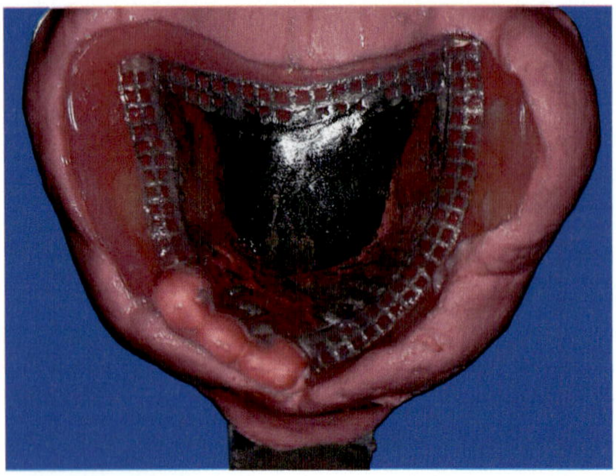

Fig. 24.29 An impression is made with the RPD using irreversible hydrocolloid

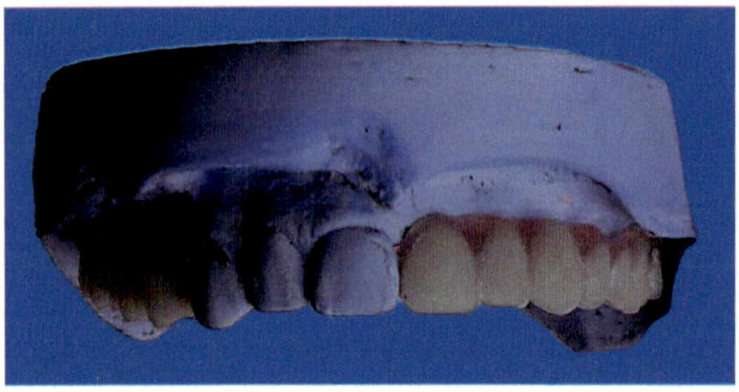

Fig. 24.30 The impression with the RPD is poured with dental stone

clasp is broken during the initial visit, a separating medium should be used before pouring the impression.

3. Remove the RPD from the cast and eliminate the fractured part of the clasp using an appropriate bur and create a space or groove in the lingual flange of the denture base just below the artificial teeth for the mechanical retention of the wrought wire to be shaped.
4. Shape and contour an 18-gauge wrought wire; adapt to the abutment and secure in place with a sticky wax on the cast and seat the RPD over the wire after preparing space on the acrylic resin.
5. Apply the autopolymerizing resin to the prepared place and final cure in a temperature- and pressure-controlled unit in warm water (about 50–60 °C) for 30 min at 30 psi.
6. Finish and polish with appropriate instruments, check intraorally (Fig. 24.31), and deliver the RPD to the patient.

24.3.3.2 Repair with Soldering a Wrought Wire Clasp

The broken clasp arms may also be repaired using electric soldering or laser-welding techniques. A precious metal high fusing wire should be used and torch soldering is not indicated in order not to overheat and damage the acrylic resin.

24.3.3.3 Repair with a Cast Clasp

A dental stone cast with the RPD is obtained and after the RPD is removed from the cast a desired type of cast clasp is fabricated in this method. The cast clasp is attached to the existing RPD using autopolymerizing resin afterward (Fig. 24.32).

24.3.3.4 Chairside Repair with a Cast Clasp

In this method, a groove is prepared in the buccal surface of the RPD where the clasp is broken. This groove should be at least 3–5 mm wide, 2–3 mm deep, and 10–15 mm long with 2 or 3 raised index islands or depressions. An impression is made with the RPD; poured after the RPD is removed from the impression, and the RPD is returned to the patient after covering the prepared space with wax. A sectional refractory model is prepared from the working area and a clasp with a temporary stabilizing arm is cast (Fig. 24.33). At the second visit, the cast clasp with the stabilizing arm is attached to the abutment and positioned to the prepared space and connected to the RPD with autopolymerizing resin afterward. The stabilizing arm is cut with an appropriate bur and the finished clasp may be prepared and modified as a T, Y, or I bar clasp (Fig. 24.34).

24.3.4 Repair of Fractured or Lost Artificial Teeth

One or more artificial teeth of an RPD may be dislodged, lost, or broken. The dislodgement of an artificial tooth may result from its insufficient bonding to the resin base. This may originate from a separating medium or wax residue that have been left between the artificial teeth and the acrylic resin base during processing of the RPD

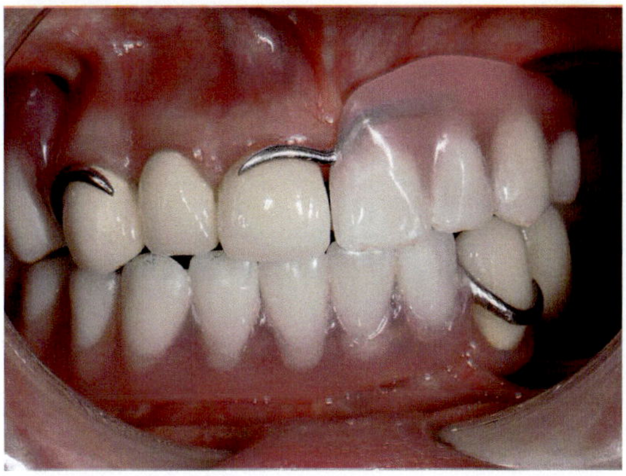

Fig. 24.31 The repaired RPD is checked intraorally and delivered to the patient

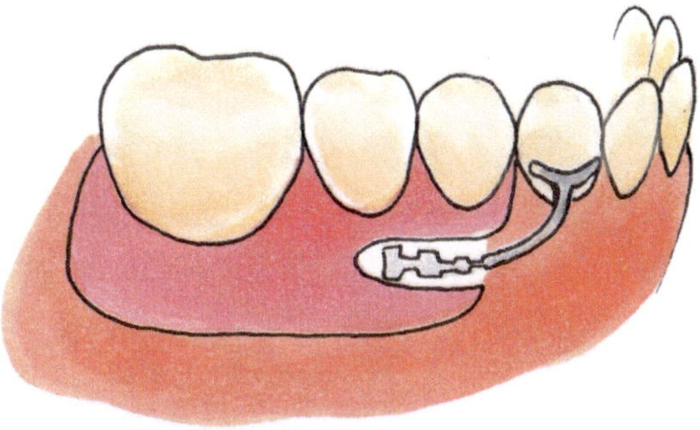

Fig. 24.32 A cast clasp may be attached to the existing RPD with a broken clasp using a cold curing acrylic resin

and may be easily repaired using autopolymerizing acrylic resin if the artificial teeth have not been lost. If any artificial tooth is lost or broken as a consequence of mishandling by the patient, it may be replaced with a new one having the same color and material using autopolymerizing resin. These procedures can be done without making an impression. However, if the lost or broken artificial tooth is adjacent to one of the abutments, an impression with the RPD is essential before replacement in order to contour the contact area.

24.3.5 Loss of a Natural Tooth Necessitating Its Replacement

If a natural tooth of the patient other than the abutment is extracted, it may be replaced by adding an artificial tooth to the RPD if an appropriate major connector has been designed. However, if the major connector is a palatal bar, strap, or a lingual bar, it is not possible to retain the artificial tooth to be replaced as the lost natural tooth to the major connector. If the major connector has a suitable design for addition of an artificial tooth like a full or U-shaped palatal plate or a lingual plate, an impression is made with the RPD (Fig. 24.34) and poured with dental stone to obtain a cast (Fig. 24.35). A loop is cast and soldered to the RPD space requiring the artificial tooth addition (Fig. 24.36). A suitable artificial tooth is shaped and contoured and retained to the existing RPD using autopolymerizing acrylic resin afterward (Fig. 24.37). If the lost natural tooth requires a distal extension denture base to be extended, the subsequent relining of the entire base is essential in order to provide favorable tissue support. If the abutment is extracted, it is still possible to retain an artificial tooth to the abovementioned RPD designs using the next adjacent tooth as an abutment, but this tooth should have a suitable retentive area, proximal guiding plane, and a rest seat. If not, a new restoration should be made to the adjacent tooth to conform these requirements. The existing clasp on the RPD is removed and an artificial tooth is added instead of the natural abutment tooth. A new clasp assembly is prepared and electrically soldered or laser welded to the RPD, and the RPD is delivered to the patient afterward. Additionally, it is possible to add an artificial tooth and a wrought wire clasp retaining the adjacent tooth to the RPD. However, this method is indicated just for an interim use because of the absence of a rest and consequent support of the RPD.

24.3.6 Other Repairs

24.3.6.1 Repair of an Abutment

When the abutment is damaged, it is possible to restore the tooth without reconstructing the RPD with the help of post-cores. After an appropriate root canal treatment, the post space is properly prepared and the post-core is made with an autopolymerizing acrylic resin (pattern resin) fitting the existing crown (Fig. 24.38). The intaglio sur-

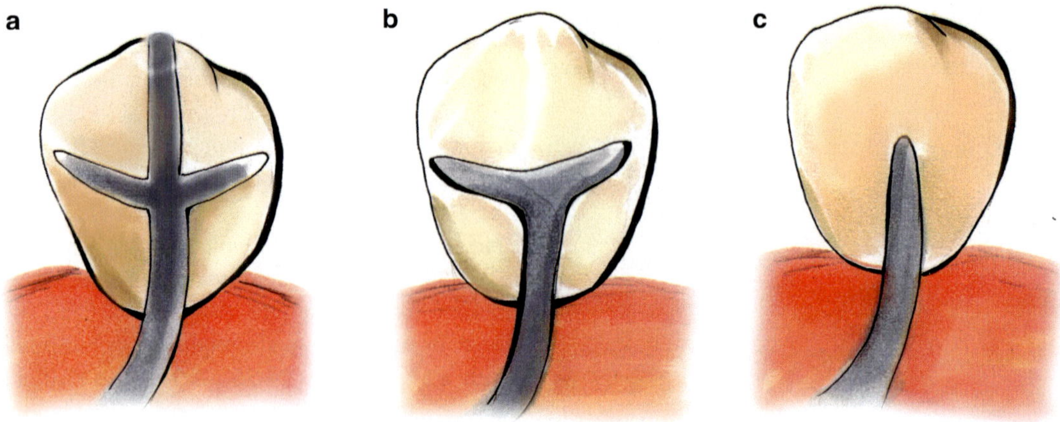

Fig. 24.33 In order to repair an RPD with a broken clasp, a clasp with a temporary stabilizing arm may be cast, fastened to the abutment tooth (**a**) and attached to the RPD with an autopolymerizing resin. After removing the stabilizing arm, the clasp may be prepared as a T, Y, or I bar clasp (**b**, **c**)

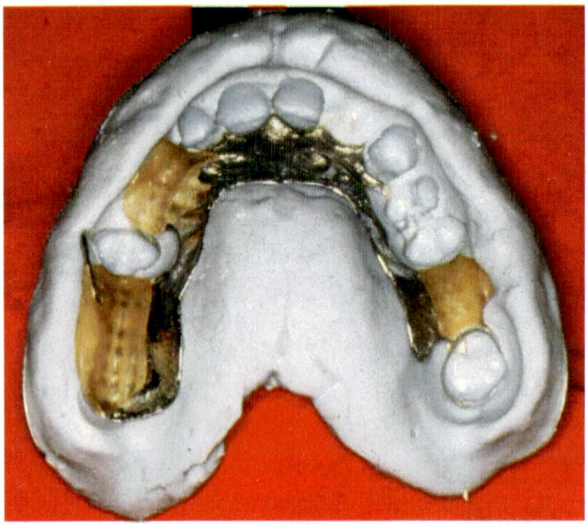

Fig. 24.34 When a natural tooth is extracted, an impression is made with the RPD in place in order to fill the space with an artificial tooth

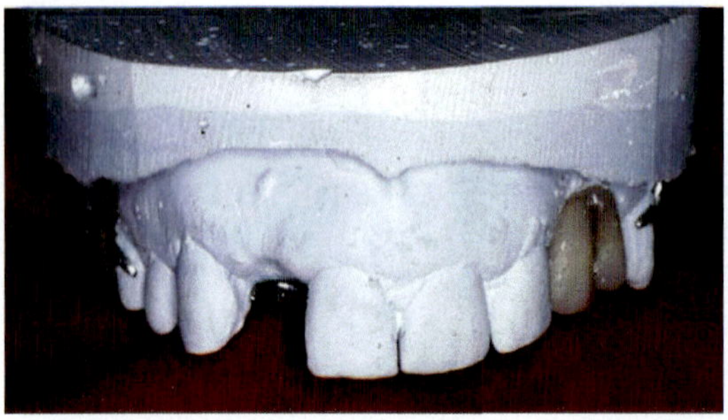

Fig. 24.35 The impression is poured with dental stone to obtain a definitive cast with the RPD

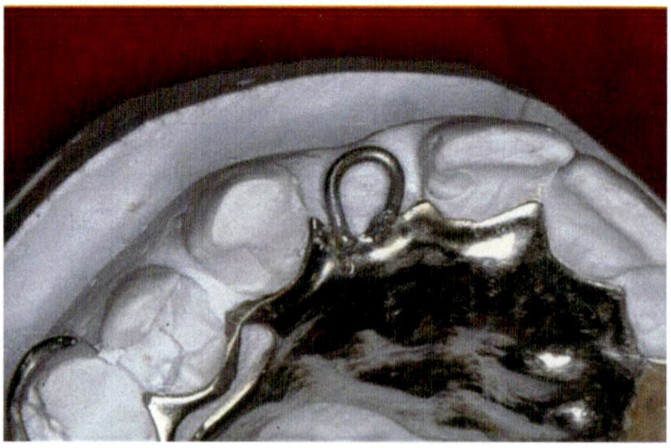

Fig. 24.36 In order to facilitate the retention of the artificial tooth, a loop is cast and soldered to the space where the natural tooth has been extracted. Besides, it is much better to make a finishing line lingually for the acrylic border

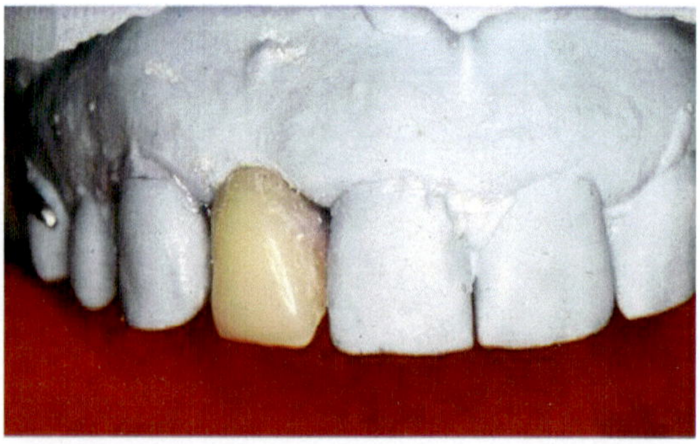

Fig. 24.37 An artificial tooth is shaped, contoured, and retained to the existing RPD using autopolymerizing acrylic resin afterward

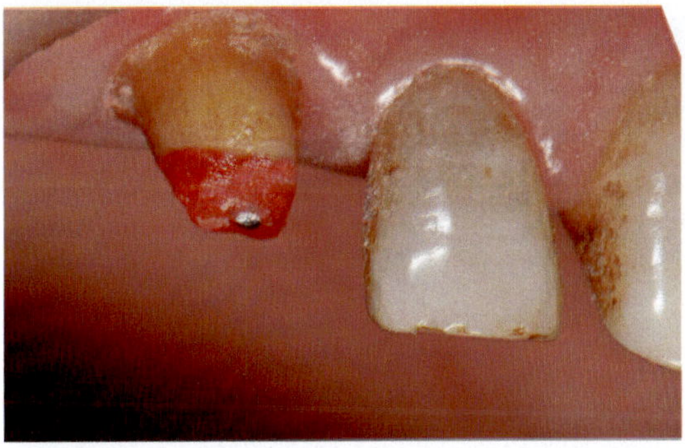

Fig. 24.38 In order to restore a damaged abutment tooth with the help of root support, a post-core restoration may be made. First, a post-core fitting the existing crown is made with an autopolymerizing acrylic resin (pattern resin)

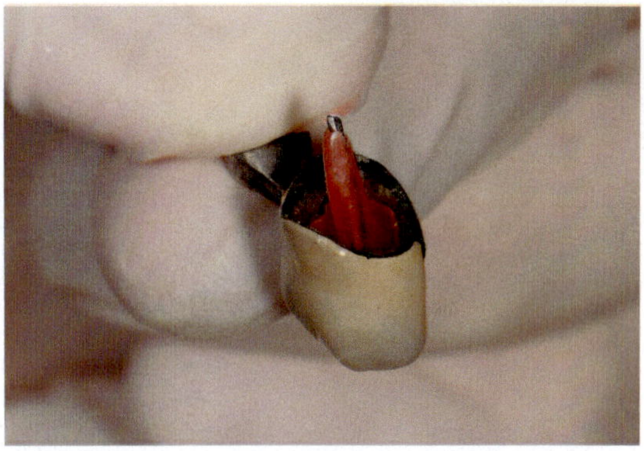

Fig. 24.39 Make sure that the acrylic core fits the existing crown exactly

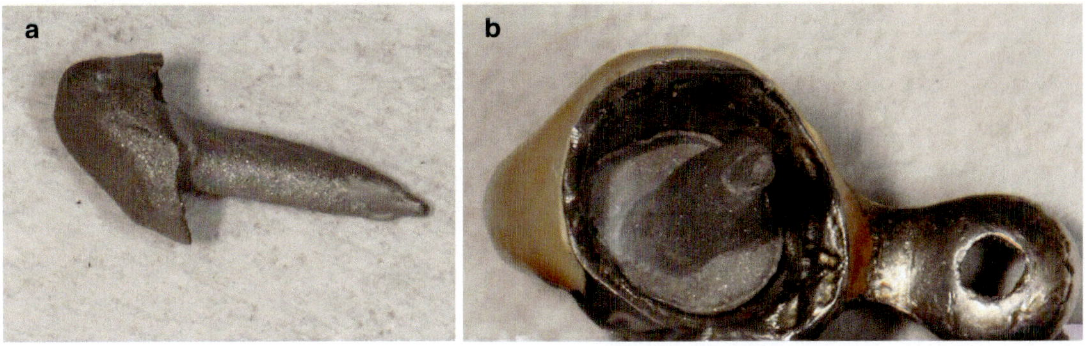

Fig. 24.40 The post-core is cast with the selected metal alloy (**a**) and checked for fitting in the existing crown (**b**) before cementation

face of the crown is isolated with a separating medium and the core part of the acrylic resin is poured into the crown. After polymerization, the acrylic post-core is separated from the crown; taken from the root in one piece and sent to the laboratory for casting procedures (Fig. 24.39). After casting (Fig. 24.40), post-core is cemented and the excess cement is cleaned with appropriate instruments after setting (Fig. 24.41). The existing crown is cemented with the RPD afterward and delivered to the patient (Fig. 24.42).

It is also possible to restore the damaged abutment in a one-appointment visit by using screw or fiber-reinforced composite post-systems following a proper root canal treatment (Fig. 24.43) with the help of the existing crown using the same method (Fig. 24.44).

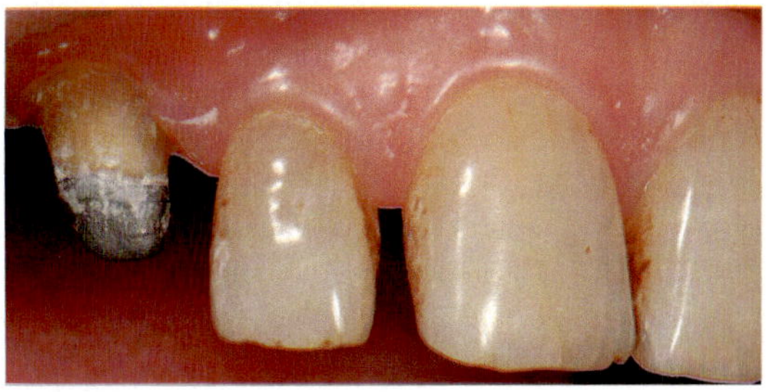

Fig. 24.41 Post-core is cemented to the damaged crown and cleaned with appropriate instruments afterward

24.3.6.2 Fabricating a New Precision Attachment Removable Partial Denture Without Changing the Crowns

When an RPD with precision attachments has to be remade because of fracture of a major compo-

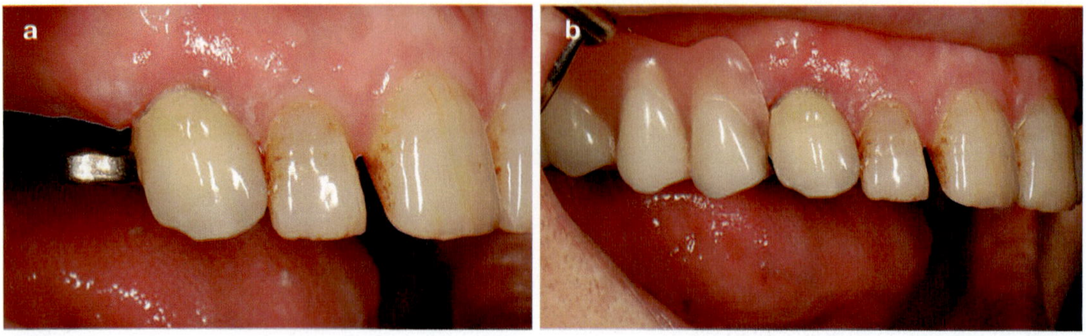

Fig. 24.42 The existing crown is cemented with the RPD; excess cement is cleaned (**a**) and the RPD is delivered to the patient (**b**)

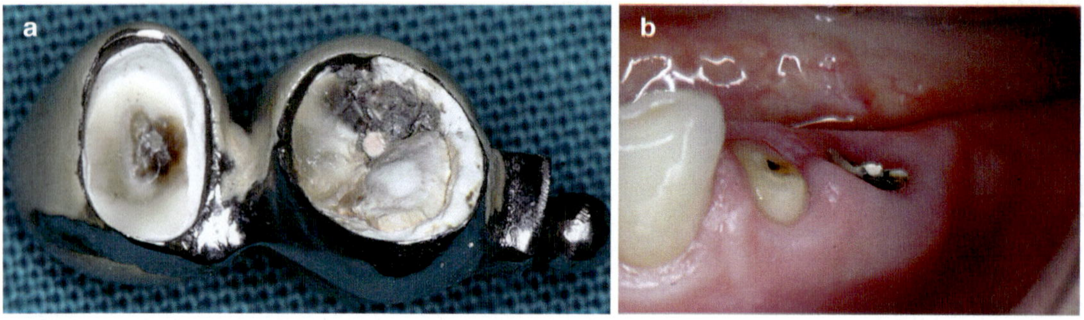

Fig. 24.43 The abutment teeth retaining a precision attachment RPD are broken (**a**, **b**)

nent or wear of the artificial teeth, the crowns fitting the RPD has to be remade because they are fabricated together to make a precise restoration. Since this procedure is time-consuming and expensive, two methods that eliminate the crown work may be recommended. If the crowns can be easily removed from the abutment teeth, an impression is made with the removed crowns in place with an irreversible hydrocolloid impression material (Fig. 24.45). The inner surface of the crowns is poured with an autopolymerizing acrylic resin and small die pins, and the rest of the impression is poured with dental stone, and the final cast is trimmed and made ready for the RPD framework fabrication (Fig. 24.46).

The other method eliminates crown removal and thus more preferable for the patients. Patients can use their existing crowns and the RPDs until the new one is fabricated. In this method, an impression is made with irreversible hydrocolloid or elastomeric impression material. The negative duplication of the male components of the precision attachments are poured with an autopolymerizing acrylic resin (pattern resin) with small die pins and the rest of the impression is poured with dental stone (Fig. 24.47). The prepared cast is sent to the laboratory for the fabrication of new RPD framework (Fig. 24.48).

24.3.6.3 Activating or Changing the Attachment Components of Removable Partial Dentures

RPDs with precision attachments require a maintenance after some period of use. The wear of the plastic attachment components may cause loosening of the RPDs and therefore should be changed and the RPD should be returned to the patient with the new attachments (Fig. 23.7) and a subsequent relining if necessary. Additionally, it is also possible to activate the components to increase retention if they permit activating like CEKA attachments with the use of suitable instruments provided by the manufacturers (Fig. 23.8). This procedure may be employed only if the retention is slightly lost. In case of larger loss of retention, the female attachment is probably

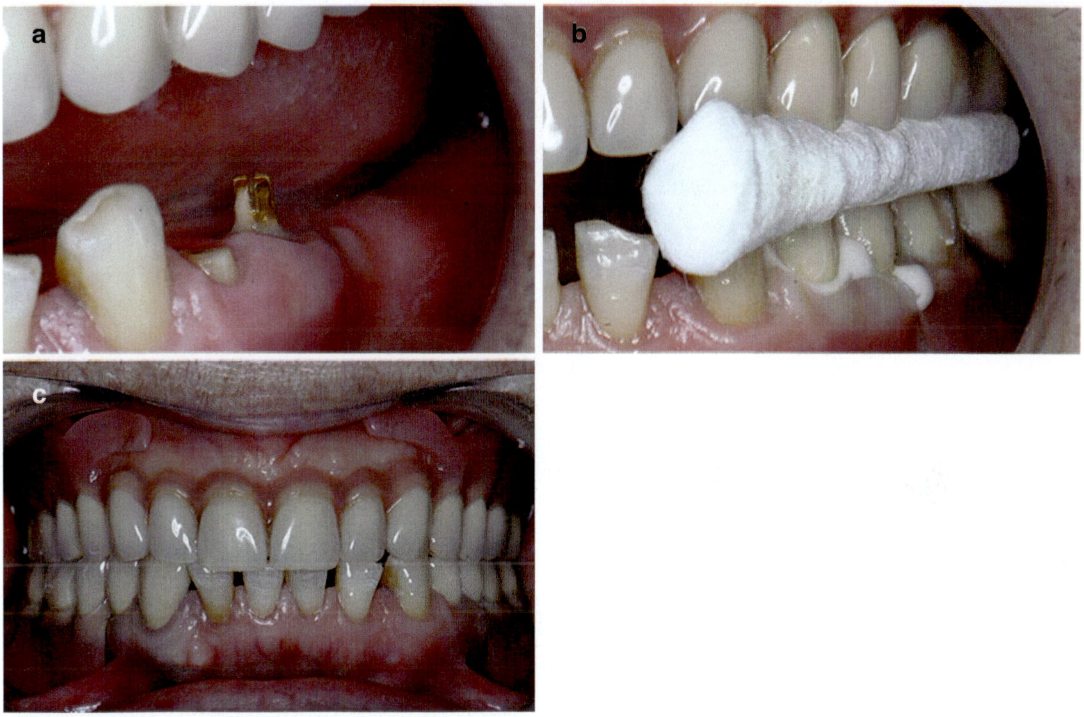

Fig. 24.44 For a one-appointment restoration of the damaged abutment teeth, the root canal is enlarged and using key, the post is dipped into cement and screwed into the root (**a**). The core part may be made with composite with the help of the existing crown. The crowns are cemented to the restorated abutment teeth with the RPD (**b**) and the RPD is delivered to the patient (**c**) after cleaning the excess cement

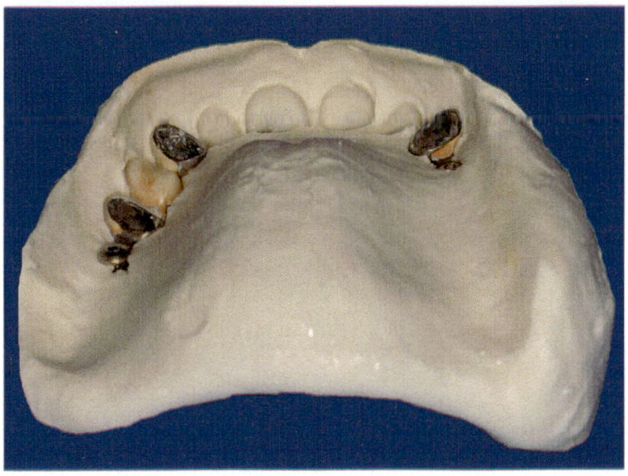

Fig. 24.45 When a precision attachment RPD has to be reconstructed, if the crowns are easily removed from the abutment teeth, an impression is made with the removed crowns in place with an irreversible hydrocolloid impression material

worn and the spring pin is removed and changed with an oversized one (Fig. 24.49).

24.3.6.4 Maintenance of the Implant-Supported Removable Partial Dentures

Maintenance of the implant-supported RPDs are similar to the maintenance of implant-retained overdentures. Mostly seen complication is the retention loss because of the wear of the plastic parts and may easily be solved by activation or replacement of the matrix in the implant-supported RPDs. Hence, it is very important for the clinicians to know the postinsertion maintenance requirements of each attachment type and choose the proper one that requires the least repairs. Plastic parts may be changed easily if no

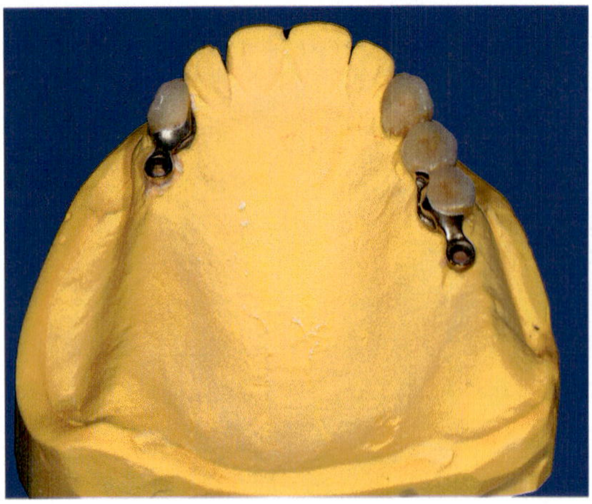

Fig. 24.46 The inner surface of the crowns is poured with an autopolymerizing acrylic resin and small die pins and the rest of the impression is poured with dental stone to obtain a definitive cast for RPD framework fabrication

damage is seen in the abutments (Fig. 24.50). If wear of the abutments is evident (Fig. 24.51), it is not sufficient to replace only the plastic parts in the prosthesis; the abutments should also be changed to newer ones.

In the situation of canine-to-canine implant-supported bridge and a distal-end RPD (see Chap. 17), some problems may also occur. The bridge may be loosened and this may become a big problem for the patients. The bridge may be decemented or screw loosening may be seen if screw-retained abutment system has been used (Fig. 24.52). Recementing with a more rigid permanent cement or tightening the screws with an appropriate torque with the help of a torque wrench according to the manufacturer's recommendation may solve the problem.

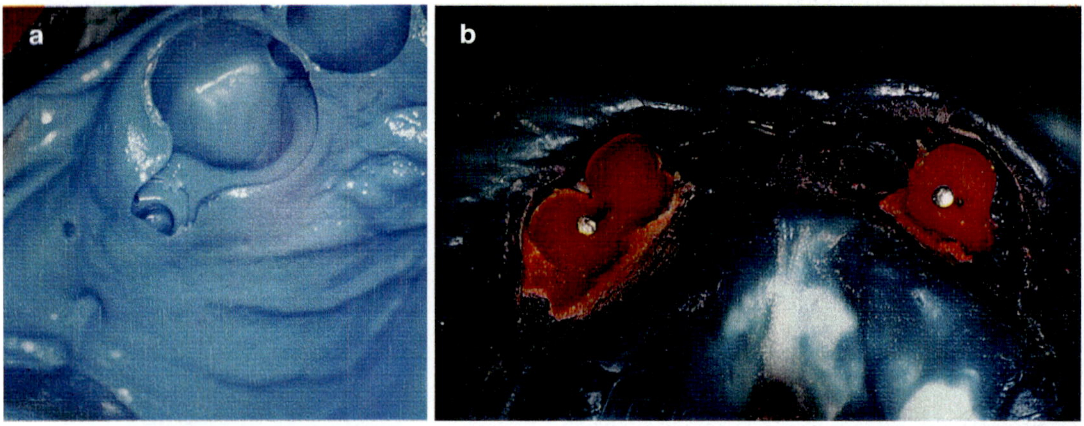

Fig. 24.47 An impression is made over the crowns with an elastomeric impression material (**a**). The negative duplication of the male components of the precision attachments are poured with an autopolymerizing acrylic resin with small die pins (**b**) and the rest of the impression is poured with dental stone

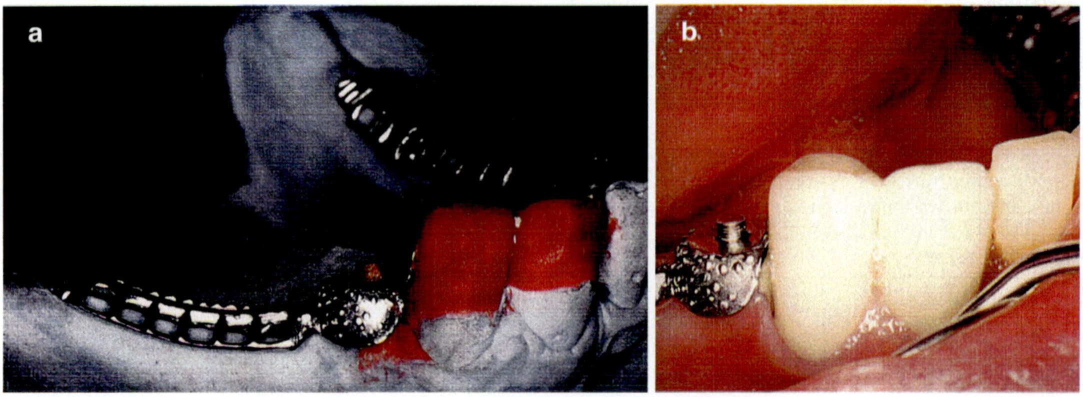

Fig. 24.48 The RPD framework is cast, checked on the cast (**a**) and intraorally (**b**)

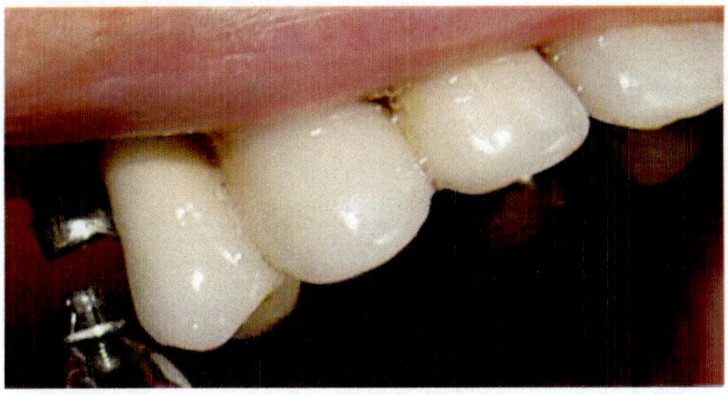

Fig. 24.49 The spring pin may be removed and changed with an oversized one to increase retention

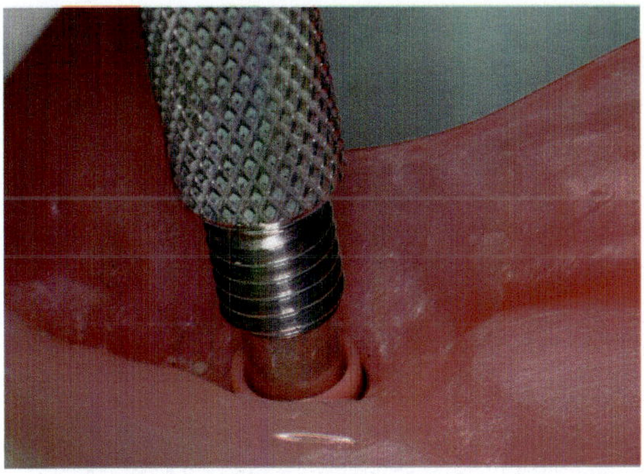

Fig. 24.50 Retention loss of implant-assisted RPDs may be recovered by changing the plastic attachment parts with the new ones

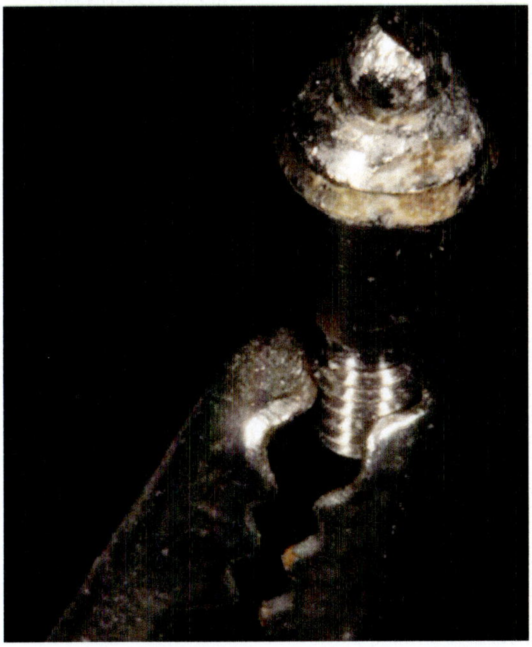

Fig. 24.51 In case of wear of the implant abutments, it is also necessary to change the male abutments

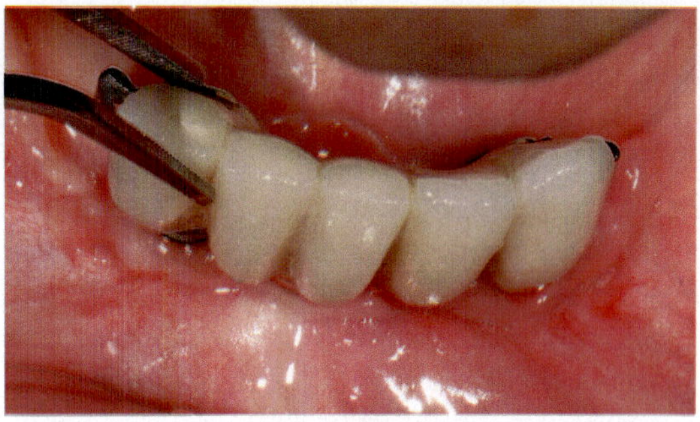

Fig. 24.52 In the situation of canine-to-canine implant-supported bridge and a distal-end RPD, the bridge may be loosened

24.4 Hygiene Maintenance of the Removable Partial Dentures

Inadequate hygiene of an RPD may lead to accumulation of plaque on both the acrylic and the metal surfaces especially when the irregular topographical surfaces exist and in turn may cause dental caries, periodontal problems, and oral diseases such as denture stomatitis. With the biofilm retention on the surface of RPDs, the oral mucosa may be at risk for the exposure of bacterial and fungal microorganisms. Especially for the physically vulnerable patients, the invasion of these microorganisms is more important because they may threaten their systemic health even by triggering the potential respiratory pathogens. Therefore, plaque accumulation on the surface of RPDs should be avoided either by the patients or the clinicians using mechanical or chemical methods or a combination of the two. Patients should be educated appropriately before the delivery of the RPDs on how to clean their prosthesis using these methods. Additional copolymer coatings containing sulfobetaine methacrylamide has been advised to increase hydrophilicity of the acrylic surfaces in order to decrease *Candida albicans* adhesion.

24.4.1 Mechanical Hygiene Maintenance

Mechanical cleaning of the RPDs includes cleaning with brushes and ultrasonic cleaning. Ultrasonic cleaning requires professional service and additional cost for the patient. Therefore, it makes sense only in the institutional environment. Most common method for cleaning the RPDs is brushing performed by the patient. Brushing is an effective, cheap, and simple method to remove the RPD biofilm. The RPD may be cleaned thoroughly using a small soft brittle toothbrush or a brush specifically designed for dentures, known as a denture brush. The patient may brush the RPD with tap water, liquid soap, or denture pastes but not toothpastes because they contain abrasives that may lead to scratches and increase the surface roughness of the acrylic resin, making it more prone to microbial colonization. Furthermore, toothpastes do not avoid antimicrobial activity but deliver fluoride to prevent caries, therefore using toothpaste to clean an RPD is not feasible. It has been shown that only mechanical cleaning does not prevent *Candida* colonization.

24.4.2 Chemical Hygiene Maintenance

Chemical cleaning of an RPD to remove the biofilm is employed by the patient using denture cleansers or household solutions. Especially for the elderly patients with a decreased manual dexterity, it is mandatory to advise chemical cleaning methods. Denture cleansers can be found as liquid form solutions or effervescent tablets. The solutions involve agents as alkaline peroxides, diluted acids, hypochlorites, disinfectants, and enzymes. While it has been shown that sodium hypochlorite is superior to all types of cleansers for removing biofilm, it should not be used because of its bad taste and odor, which can lead to bleaching of acrylic and corrosion of metal. However, since it is capable of removing *Staphylococcus aureus*, if it has to be used in hospitalized patients, RPDs should not be soaked in hypochlorites more than 15 min in order not to cause the above-mentioned adverse effects. Denture cleansing effervescent tablets are the most frequently used chemical agents that are composed of peroxides and oxygen radicals and are manufactured for antimicrobial efficacy. No adverse effect has been shown on cobalt–chromium surfaces, and therefore they can be safely used in the cleaning of RPDs. Moreover, these tablets additionally provide micromechanical cleaning by releasing percarbonate oxygen. However, these tablets do not remove *Candida* species effectively. Moreover, most commercially available tablets do not remove *Streptococcus mutans*, which is the primary etiologic agent causing dental caries from the metal surfaces of the RPDs. It has been shown that only tablets with sodium lauryl sulfate are capable of removing this microorganism. Moreover, they should be used in combination with mechanical methods for proper cleaning of the RPDs.

Further Reading

American Welding Society. Committee on brazing and soldering. Soldering manual. 2nd ed. Miami: American Welding Society; 1978. p. ix.

Amin BM, Aras MA. Repair of extracoronal direct retainers. Int J Prosthodont Restor Dent. 2012;2:42–6.

Axe AS, Varghese R, Bosma M, Kitson N, Bradshaw DJ. Dental health professional recommendation and consumer habits in denture cleansing. J Prosthet Dent. 2016;115:183–8.

Bolouri A, McCarthy SL. A procedure for relining a complete or removable partial denture without the use of wax. J Prosthet Dent. 1998;79:604–6.

Carlsson GE. Responses of jawbone to pressure. Gerodontology. 2004;21:65–70.

Carr AB, Brown DT, editors. McCracken's removable partial prosthodontics. 13th ed. St. Louis, MO: Elsevier; 2016.

Craig RG, Powers JM. Restorative dental materials. 11th ed. St. Louis, MO: Mosby, Inc.; 2002. p. 636–67.

Curylofo PA, Raile PN, Vasconcellos GLL, Macedo AP, Pagnano VO. Effect of denture cleansers on cobalt-chromium alloy surface: a simulated period of 5 years' use. J Prosthodont. 2020;29:142–50.

Dawes C. Laser welding. Cambridge: Abington Publishing Ltd., In Association with The Welding Institute; 1992.

Duymus ZY, Aydiner SF. Evaluation of methods of denture cleaning. Online J Dent Oral Health. 2021;4:OJDOH.MS.ID.000590.

Felton D, Cooper L, Duqum I, Minsley G, Guckes A, Haug S, Meredith P, Solie C, Avery D, Deal Chandler N, American College of Prosthodontists. Evidence-based guidelines for the care and maintenance of complete dentures: a publication of the American College of Prosthodontists. J Prosthodont. 2011;20(Suppl 1):S1–2.

Hill EE, Rubel B. Direct chairside hard reline at delivery of a newly fabricated distal extension removable partial denture: considerations and techniques. J Can Dent Assoc. 2011;77:b84.

Hirasawa M, Tsutsumi-Arai C, Takakusaki K, Oya T, Fueki K, Wakabayashi N. Superhydrophilic co-polymer coatings on denture surfaces reduce Candida albicans adhesion-an in vitro study. Arch Oral Biol. 2018;87:143–50.

Jones JD, Garcia LT. Removable partial dentures: a clinician's guide. Iowa: Wiley-Blackwell; 2009.

Kiesow A, Sarembe S, Pizzey RL, Axe AS, Bradshaw DJ. Material compatibility and antimicrobial activity of consumer products commonly used to clean dentures. J Prosthet Dent. 2016;115:189–98.

Knechtel ME, Loney RW. Improving the outcome of denture relining. J Can Dent Assoc. 2007;73:587–91.

Lopes Vasconcelos GL, Curylofo PA, Targa Coimbra FC, de Cássia Oliveira V, Macedo AP, de Freitas Oliveira Paranhos H, Pagnano VO. In vitro antimicrobial activity of effervescent denture tablets on the components of removable partial dentures. Int J Prosthodont. 2020;33:315–20.

NaBadalung DP, Nicholls JI. Laser welding of a cobalt-chromium removable partial denture alloy. J Prosthet Dent. 1998;79:285–90.

Ozan O, Orhan K, Aksoy S, Icen M, Bilecenoglu B, Sakul BU. The effect of removable partial dentures on alveolar bone resorption: a retrospective study with cone-beam computed tomography. J Prosthodont. 2013;22:42–8.

Phoenix RD, Cagna DR, Defreest CF. Stewart's clinical removable partial prosthodontics. 4th ed. Chicago: Quintessence Publishing; 2008.

Rodrigues RC, Faria AC, Orsi IA, Mattos Mda G, Macedo AP, Ribeiro RF. Comparative study of two commercially pure titanium casting methods. J Appl Oral Sci. 2010;18:487–92.

Shimizu H, Takahashi Y. Repair of fractured lingual plate with a cast splinting device and metal conditioners: a clinical report. Int Chin J Dent. 2006;6:79–81.

Silveira C, Castro M, Resende L, Domínguez F, Resende V, Simamoto P. Welding techniques in dentistry. In: Kovacevic R, editor. Welding processes. Rijeka: InTech; 2012.

Smith DE, Toolson LB, Bolender CL, Lord JL. One-step border molding of complete denture impressions using a polyether impression material. J Prosthet Dent. 1979;41:347–51.

Türk PE, Geckili O, Türk Y, Günay V, Bilgin T. In vitro comparison of the retentive properties of ball and locator attachments for implant overdentures. Int J Oral Maxillofac Implants. 2014;29:1106–13.

The glossary of prosthodontic terms: ninth edition. J Prosthet Dent. 2017;117(5S):e1–e105.

Wada M, Mameno T, Kani M, Miwa S, Ikebe K. Association between gonial angle on orthopantomogram and reline frequency in removable partial denture wearers. J Prosthodont Res. 2022;66:83–6.

Disinfection and Hygiene Protocols

25

Süleyman Çağatay Dayan, Pınar Şeşen, and Mehmet Berk Kaffaf

Abstract

Clinicians should take precautions to prevent the spread of germs from patient to dental staff. Although dental staff and patients have been concerned about contagious diseases for a long time, dental infection control has received increased attention among patients after the COVID-19 pandemic. The demand for infection control in the modern world is greater than ever. The safety of both dental clinical personnel and patients depends on managing bacterial, viral, and fungal contamination by sterilization and disinfection, which have traditionally been regarded as the most crucial steps in the infection control process. This chapter provides a concise overview of a clinically useful approach to sterilization and disinfection protocols in the field of removable partial denture (RPD) practice. Specifically, it covers the cleaning and decontamination of various items used in clinical environments, including impressions, stone casts, occlusal rims, registration materials, burs, and prostheses. By following these guidelines, practitioners can ensure that their RPD procedures are conducted in a safe and hygienic manner, minimizing the risk of cross-contamination and infection transmission.

S. Ç. Dayan (✉)
Dental Laboratory Technology Program, İstanbul University-Cerrahpaşa, İstanbul, Türkiye
e-mail: suleyman.dayan@iuc.edu.tr

P. Şeşen · M. B. Kaffaf
Faculty of Dentistry, Department of Prosthodontics, İstanbul Kent University, İstanbul, Türkiye
e-mail: pinar.sesen@kent.edu.tr;
; mehmetberk.kaffaf@kent.edu.tr

25.1 Definitions

Asepsis: Free from infection; the prevention of contact with microorganisms.

Aseptic: Free of infection or septic material; sterile; free from pathogenic microorganisms.

Antiseptic: Refers to the disinfectant's use of very low doses on the body's surface.

Decontamination and cleaning: Decontamination is the process of removal of pathogenic microorganisms from objects so that they are safe to handle. Cleaning is defined as the removal of visible soil (e.g., organic and inorganic materials) from surfaces and objects.

Disinfection: A process of the complete elimination of vegetative forms of microorganisms except the bacterial spores from inanimate objects.

Disinfectants: The substances used in the disinfection process.

Ethylene oxide: A bactericidal agent occurring as a colorless gas with a pleasant ethereal odor; the chemical in gas sterilization systems used for many items that cannot be sterilized in a high heat system.

O. Şakar (ed.), *Removable Partial Dentures*, https://doi.org/10.1007/978-3-031-47083-7_25

Sterile: Free from living microorganisms; aseptic.

Sterilization: The process of completely eliminating microbial viability.

25.2 Understanding the Aspects of Sterilization and Disinfection

Cross-infection during clinical practice can occur when infectious agents are transmitted between patients and oral health professionals in a clinical environment. To avoid cross-infection, it is essential to first identify the necessary transmission pathways. Due to direct patient contact, exposure to biological fluids, and aerosol/droplet generation during prosthodontic procedures, dental health professionals are very sensitive to microbial infection and at risk. Hepatitis B, hepatitis C, Human Immunodeficiency Virus (HIV), herpes, *Staphylococcus*, *Streptococcus*, *Candida albicans*, tuberculosis, and Severe Acute Respiratory Syndrome Coronavirus 2 (SARS-CoV-2) are examples of dangerous microbial infections. Microorganisms that cause disease may be transmitted not only via direct contact but also through indirect contact with contaminated dental instruments and materials. Pathogenic bacteria may be transmitted from patients to dental health professionals or vice versa through dental materials and equipment.

The purpose of sterilization is to kill any and all germs, including the hardy bacterial spores. Every method that kills bacterial spores also kills viruses, including HIV, hepatitis C, and hepatitis B. An instrument is either sterile or not; there are no semi-sterile instruments. Before sterilization, it is advised to brush or use ultrasonic cleaning to remove any remaining residue. If dental professionals use ultrasonic cleaning equipment instead of brushing by hand, they are much less likely to get a puncture wound. While it cannot eliminate all contamination, ultrasonic cleaning is an efficient and time-saving method for cleaning instruments. Cleaning equipment of any sort necessitates a thorough rinse to get rid of any remaining chemical. The instruments are then ready for sterilization.

Disinfection is the process of eliminating germs that can infect humans with disease. The substances used in the disinfection process are called disinfectants. These are usually chemicals, and a variety of chemical disinfectants are used nowadays. Modern disinfectants, on the other hand, are produced without aldehyde and are frequently used. Aldehyde-free disinfectants have great user tolerance as their key benefit. The disinfectant is applied to the body surface in very low concentrations. The term "antiseptic" refers to the disinfectant's use of very low doses on the body's surface. It is critical to understand the distinction between disinfection and sterilization since both processes may eliminate microorganisms from the treated surface. Disinfection is the process of eliminating pathogens while leaving the spore, whereas sterilization is the process of removing both pathogens and spores.

Unfortunately, studies have shown that the dental team, i.e., the dentist, dental assistant, and dental technician, have limited knowledge of asepsis and aseptic techniques. All members of the dental team must improve their compliance with approved infection control procedures. Engaging in continuing education programs and workshops focused on containing and preventing the spread of infections is a suitable approach for enhancing the expertise of dental teams.

In dental offices and labs, it is a common practice to clean and decontaminate the clinic environments, disinfect impressions, stone casts, occlusal rims, registration materials, burs, and other tools. According to a study, items received from labs are often contaminated, so there is a need for periodic disinfection of such items before use, as well as storage practices that should be evaluated. The best clinical practice would be to use consistent disinfection procedures at a number of clearly defined stages, such as before the lab work leaves the clinic, when it arrives at the lab, before it leaves the lab, and before it is delivered to the patient. This would greatly reduce the risk of cross-infection. For infection control, techniques including spray and immersion disinfection for RPDs, dental materials and equipment, and the addition of antibacterial compounds to laboratory materials like gypsum or pumice may be used. Immersion disinfection is a common method that reduces the risk of cross-contamination. However, as the disinfectant might get contaminated and lose its efficacy after repeated uses, immersion disinfectants should not be reused and should be destroyed after each use. The frequency of replacement may depend on the type of disinfectant, its concentration, and the manufacturer's recommendations, among other factors. Clinicians should remember that the purpose of sterilization and disinfection is not only to eliminate dental equipment and materials of pathogenic organisms but also to protect the items' original qualities. The spray method of disinfection uses fewer disinfectant solutions and lowers the danger of deterioration of dental tools and materials. It may not, however, reach the undercut sections, and air is released as a result, increasing occupational exposure.

25.3 Classification of the Disinfectants

The effectiveness of chemical disinfectants can be divided into three categories:

- *High-level disinfectants*: glutaraldehyde (≥2%), *ortho*-phthalaldehyde (0.55%), hydrogen peroxide (7.5%), hypochlorite (650–675 ppm), and hypochlorous acid (400–450 ppm).
- *Intermediate-level disinfectants*: ethyl and isopropyl alcohol (70%), formaldehyde (0.7–1%), chlorine compounds (10%; 500–5000 mg/L), iodophors (0.1–0.2%), and phenolic compounds (3%).
- *Low-level disinfectants*: hydrogen peroxide (≤3%), quaternary ammonium compound (0.5%), diluted glutaraldehyde, phenolics (0.5%), and detergents.

25.4 Heat Sterilization in the Dental Office

To prevent the spread of infectious agents, dental instruments such as handpieces, impression trays, burs, glass slabs, hand instruments, dental dishes, polishing wheels, and disks must be sterilized before use on each patient. Various techniques can be employed to achieve sterilization of dental instruments, including:

- Dry heat sterilization
- Unsaturated chemical-vapor sterilization
- Moist/steam heat sterilization (autoclave)
- Ethylene oxide sterilization
- Chemical sterilization (e.g., peracetic acid (0.2%), glutaraldehyde (≥2.4%), and hydrogen peroxide (7.5%))

Each approach for sterilizing dental instruments, whether through heat or chemical methods, possesses its own set of advantages and disadvantages, in addition to varying wrapping requirements that must be considered in the sterilization process. Moist/steam heat sterilization (autoclave) is one of the most popular sterilization processes. Autoclaving is a dependable and efficient method for sterilizing dental tools by producing moist heat in a confined chamber that rapidly destroys pathogens. At 121 °C and 15 psi, the required time is 15–20 min, but at 134 °C, the required time is 3–4 min. The primary disadvantages of this approach are that it causes carbon steel burs and other sharp devices to become dull and rusty and that it damages heat-sensitive materials like plastics and rubber. Even though ethylene oxide sterilization is expensive, it can be done at a lower temperature, so it can be used on materials that are sensitive to heat like rubber and plastic. Its typical concentration range for in-use is 450–800 mg/L. When using chemical solutions for sterilization, a longer time period is required, often between 3 and 12 h, to kill all possible kinds of bacteria and other microorganisms. In addition, there are less frequently used sterilization methods in the literature such as ultraviolet (UV) light, radical vapor reactor, direct current glow discharge, gamma-ray, argon radio frequency glow discharge, and microwave irradiation.

25.5 Infection Control in Removable Partial Denture Practice

As previously stated, instruments must be cleaned and debris removed before sterilization and high-level disinfection. To prevent debris from drying out, instruments must be immersed in water or a disinfectant or detergent as soon as possible after use. Debris can be removed using enzymatic solutions, manual brushing, ultrasonic equipment, or washing machines. The Spaulding classification categorizes the instruments, materials, and equipment used in the medical field and in patient contact into three categories (critical, semi-critical, and noncritical) based on the risk of infection they pose and the sterilization and disinfection requirements. Objects that penetrate sterile tissues are considered critical and must be sterilized; those that come into contact with the mucosa are considered semi-critical and require high-level disinfection; and those that come into contact with intact skin are considered noncritical and require only low-level disinfection.

During the fabrication process of RPDs, impression, stone cast, occlusal rim, and interocclusal record material are frequently transported from one location to another, posing a risk of cross-contamination among patients, clinical staff, dental technicians, and dentists. Therefore, they are at risk of developing an infection from contaminated items. Infectious pathogens such as SARS-CoV-2, hepatitis B virus, hepatitis C virus, HIV, mycobacteria, and *Pseudomonas aeruginosa* can be transmitted to health-care workers working in dental clinics and laboratories who are exposed to these microorganisms. As a result, it is essential that dental staff members take universal precautions to prevent the transmission of communicable diseases. Cross-contamination concerns will be considerably reduced by constant disinfection processes carried out at predetermined points, including before items leave the clinic, after they are sent to the laboratory, before they leave the laboratory, and before they are delivered to the patient. Consequently, dental clinic staff and technicians must protect both themselves and patients by implementing effective sterilization and disinfection procedures in daily practice.

25.5.1 Infection Control for Impressions and Impression Trays

Dental impressions represent a moderate to semi-critical risk to laboratory personnel and dentists, necessitating moderate to high disinfection. If the right precautions are not followed, dental impressions that come in contact with the patient's saliva, blood, or bacterial plaque can spread infection and cause serious problems. The most prevalent microorganisms on dental impression materials include *Streptococcus* spp., *Staphylococcus* spp., *E. coli*, *Actinomyces* spp., *Antitratus* spp., *Pseudomonas* spp., *Enterobacter* spp., *K. pneumonia*, and *Candida* spp. Before being delivered to the laboratory, the impressions must be disinfected. Even though there have been a lot of studies on how disinfectants affect dental impression materials, there is still no agreement on how to disinfect all impression materials. This is related to the considerable variance in the chemical composition of disinfectants and impression materials, as well as the varied methods used to evaluate the antibacterial activity of disinfectants and their impact on the physical

Table 25.1 For impression materials, chemical disinfectants with varying disinfection levels are used (* indicates preferred disinfection solutions for impression materials, + indicates disinfection solutions that are suitable for impression materials, – indicates disinfection solutions that are not suitable for impression materials)

	Irreversible hydrocolloid	Impression compound	Zinc oxide–eugenol paste	Polysulfide	Polyether	Addition and condensation silicone
Glutaraldehyde	+*		+*	+	+*	+*
Sodium hypochlorite	+*	+*	+*	+*	+	+*
Phenols	+	+	+	+	+	+
Iodophors	+*	+*	+*	+*	+*	+*
Chlorhexidine	+	+	+	+	+	+
Alcohols	+	+	+	+	+	+
Quaternary ammonium compounds	–	–	–	–	–	–
Detergents	–	–	–	–	–	–

properties of impression materials. Table 25.1 summarizes the chemical disinfectants with varying disinfection levels utilized for impression materials.

The American Dental Association (ADA), which has strict rules about how to clean and disinfect all dental tools and materials, recommends that all dental impressions be washed and cleaned well with water to remove any traces of blood, saliva, or food before being chemically disinfected with glutaraldehyde, sodium hypochlorite (NaOCl), iodophor, or phenol. Microorganisms can sometimes be difficult to eliminate from the surface of an impression. Particularly challenging is the thorough purification of blood and saliva from undercut regions. As a solution, it is suggested to clean the impression using a very soft brush. But it is important to keep in mind that the above-mentioned disinfectants are not suitable for all types of impressions, and they may change the surface properties and stability of the impression materials. For effective disinfection, it is very important to follow the manufacturer's instructions for how long the disinfectant should be in contact with the impression, to rinse the impression right after disinfection, and to remove the disinfectant.

The immersion method guarantees that all surfaces of the impression are in contact with the disinfectant, but as disinfectants have a limited shelf life, they must be produced fresh, which takes more time and costs more money. Immersion methods can be applied to hydrophobic impression materials like polyvinyl siloxane and polysulfide. It causes the water absorption phenomenon of hydrophilic impression materials and chemical interactions between impressions and disinfectants. Prolonged storage of the alginate impression in the disinfectant solution may result in dimensional changes, and spraying would be a more appropriate approach. In contrast to hydrocolloids, studies reported that the immersion method could improve elastomeric impression accuracy by compensating for its polymerization shrinkage. Moreover, it has been demonstrated that it has greater antibacterial efficiency on elastomeric impressions. However, the use of the immersion method in polyethers has caused controversy due to its hydrophilic nature.

There are differences in how bacteria adhere to and grow on dental impression materials with different chemical compositions and surface properties. For instance, alginates are very easy to contaminate because they are hydrophilic, and it is known that microbial growth in alginate impressions is about five times higher than in elastomeric materials. Based on this evidence, the effectiveness of disinfection that should be used on impression materials should be clearly defined based on the materials. To disinfect alginate, only quick immersion or spraying techniques are utilized. Since the spray method results in minimal dimensional change and distortion in alginate, it is frequently utilized for such impression materials. Although the ADA recommends spraying the irreversible hydrocolloid impression material, placing it in a sealed bag, and allowing 10 min for disinfection, a recent study found that 15 min of activation with an ultrasonic device had no significant effect on dimensional stability.

In vitro tests showed that the quantity of colony-forming unit per milliliter (CFU/mL) on the surface of alginate impressions could be reduced by disinfecting them with chlorhexidine, alcohol, glutaraldehyde, or NaOCl. Effective disinfection for alginate impressions can be achieved by the following procedures:

- 10 min by spraying 0.5% NaOCl,
- 10 min of immersion in iodophor (1:213),
- 20 min of immersion in 2% glutaraldehyde, and
- 20 min of immersion in phenols.

To avoid the adverse effects of disinfectants, antimicrobial agents can be added to the impression material or antimicrobial solutions can be substituted for water in the mix. When an antimicrobial agent is added to alginate, it is crucial to ensure that it does not adversely affect the impression qualities and stability. For this purpose, mostly water-soluble antimicrobial compounds (quaternary ammonium compounds, bisguanidine compounds, substitute phenols, chlorhexidine, etc.) are used. Moreover, antimicrobial nanosilver particles are added to impression materials for disinfection. The addition of nanosilver particles to alginate makes it effective against *S. aureus*, *L. acidophilus*, *A. viscosus*, and *P. aeruginosa*. The addition of more than 1% by weight of silver nanoparticles affects the gelling time and strength of the alginate.

Immersion in 2% glutaraldehyde, 0.5–1% NaOCl, and iodophors (1:213) solutions for 10 min is the recommended method for disinfection of polyvinyl siloxane and condensation silicones. Glutaraldehyde disinfectants improve wettability by acting as a surface energy-reducing agent on polyvinyl siloxane and polyether impressions. In addition, there are autoclavable polyvinyl siloxanes available on the market. Autoclaving of polyvinyl siloxanes at 121 °C for 15 min is the recommended method. Alternatively, after waiting 10 min after the spray method, glutaraldehyde showed the same antimicrobial properties and did not affect the dimensional stability of the polyvinyl siloxane silicones. Polyvinyl siloxane is hydrophobic and extremely resistant to disinfection solutions, regardless of the duration of exposure. Nevertheless, modern impression material contains surfactants to improve its ability to replicate details, which can increase water absorption when impressions are immersed in disinfectants for extended periods of time. Hence, long-term disinfection is not suggested from a clinical standpoint. Studies showed that the use of quaternary ammonium compounds, ammonium chloride, and alcohol-based disinfectants did not change the surface properties of polyvinyl siloxane and condensation silicones; however, their antimicrobial efficacy still requires further investigation.

For polyether impression material, immersion in 2% glutaraldehyde and iodophors (1:213) solutions for 10 min is the recommended method. However, the duration of the immersion period in 2% glutaraldehyde should never exceed 30 min. An extended immersion period can negatively affect the properties of the impression. Since the spray method does not cause dimensional change and distortion in polyether, only quick immersion or spraying techniques are recommended for disinfection of the polyether, like using alginate. For the spraying method, ADA's suggestion can be followed: placing impression material in a sealed bag and waiting the required amount of time for disinfection. There are contradictions in the literature on the disinfection of polyether with NaOCl. While several studies reported that NaOCl adversely affects the dimensional stability of polyether, others demonstrated it does not.

Zinc oxide–eugenol impressions can be chemically disinfected with 0.5–1% NaOCl, 2% glutaraldehyde, or iodophors (1:213) solutions for 10 min by the immersion method. This is a safe and effective way to eliminate microorganisms. Several studies have shown that the impression's dimensional stability and surface properties do not suffer during a prolonged immersion duration due to its nature, which is not affected by evaporation and absorption of water. Even so, 30–60 min must be the maximum safe time for prolonged immersion.

Herbal disinfection, microwave irradiation, and ozone are alternative methods for disinfecting impression materials. Previous studies have investigated aloe vera, neem bar extracts, and apple cider vinegar as disinfectants, yet there is insufficient evidence to evaluate whether they are effective. Celebi et al. evaluated the antibacterial activity of ozone and NaOCl on polyvinyl siloxane samples, as well as their effects on wettability. Ozone has both excellent antibacterial activities against polyvinyl siloxane and a beneficial effect on wettability. Finally, gaseous ozone therapy has been found to be a viable approach for disinfecting polyvinyl siloxane impression materials. A study also showed that using ozonated water caused less dimensional change than using 0.5% NaOCl and that it may be used as a backup disinfectant in clinical practice. Moreover, using microwave irradiation plus hydrogen peroxide for 3 min to disinfect polyvinyl siloxane impressions showed strong antibacterial activity against *E. coli*, *S. aureus*, and *S. mutans* without altering the mechanical qualities of the impressions.

Before using prefabricated metal impression trays, they must be autoclaved. Custom acrylic immersion trays should be immersed in a 5.25% NaOCl solution for 10 min.

25.5.2 Infection Control for Stone Cast

A dental stone cast should be disinfected after each clinical and laboratory procedure. According to the ADA, a 1:10 solution of NaOCl (0.525%), calcium hypochlorite (0.5%), or an iodophor should be used to immerse stone casts in order to disinfect them. Casts should be immersed in disinfectant for at least 30 min. Studies immersed die stone models in a range of disinfectants and reported that the unfavorable physical effects on cast die stone ranged from none to minimal with 1:10 NaOCl and 1:213 iodophor. Hypochlorous acid (HOCl), a cleaner that the U.S. Environmental Protection Agency (EPA) has suggested for fighting COVID-19, could be used instead of regular disinfectants. A study examining the impact of immersion or spray solutions of HOCl on the surface hardness of type III dental stone revealed a decrease in hardness levels. Specifically, the effects of a 1:10 NaOCl solution and a 200 ppm HOCl solution were compared on dental stone casts. Interestingly, the reduction in surface hardness was found to be lower after immersion in HOCl compared to NaOCl. Notably, no significant difference in surface hardness was observed between HOCl and NaOCl when the spray technique was employed. The efficiency and potential negative impacts of HOCl in disinfecting dental stone cast and other dental materials are not yet fully established. Further study is required. In addition, some researchers have advised incorporating different disinfectants into the dental stone. Unfortunately, this procedure may alter the dental stone cast's physical characteristics, dimensional stability, and surface porosity. By adding 0.5% NaOCl to distilled water, the setting time of stone cast may be shortened and the compressive strength increased; however, the setting expansion of the stone models was not significantly altered. As well, adding 1–4% chlorhexidine to dental stone did not influence its dimensional stability or detail reproduction capabilities while being worked with. Several manufacturers produce self-sterilizing gypsum as an alternative to integrating various disinfectants into dental stone. Maciel et al. conducted a study to investigate the antibacterial activity against *Streptococcus aureus* and *Candida albicans*, as well as the compressive strength and surface roughness of self-disinfecting gypsum and gypsum supplemented with 2% chlorhexidine added at 1 h and 24 h after pouring the gypsum. The researchers compared these groups to a control group consisting of dental stone mixed with sterile distilled water. The findings indicated that the addition of 2% chlorhexidine to the gypsum formulation exhibited superior antibacterial activity against *S. aureus* compared to the self-disinfecting gypsum group. However, neither group demonstrated a significant impact on *C. albicans*. It is worth noting that the incorporation of 2% chlorhexidine in the gypsum formulation resulted in a noticeable reduction in compressive strength and an increase in surface roughness. These observations provide valuable insights into the potential advantages and limitations of employing self-disinfecting agents in gypsum materials for dental applications. In contrast, the utilization of self-disinfecting gypsum resulted in comparable surface roughness to the control group, while exhibiting a decline in compressive strength solely during the 1-h observation period.

Some research has also investigated the effect of microwave irradiation on the characteristics of gypsum casts. The studies showed an increase in mechanical characteristics but a detrimental influence on compressive strength. When the gypsum casts were subjected to high-power microwave irradiation, cracks or porosities appeared on the surface. Therefore, the microwave irradiation that is applied at 900 W at 2450 MHz for 5 min seems appropriate according to current knowledge. Additionally, ozonated water (OZW) has been investigated for its efficacy in disinfecting stone casts. OZW has various advantages over standard chemical disinfectants, as it is environmentally friendly and will not pose a subsequent risk to the environment after its administration. Although OZW is a useful candidate for a relatively safe disinfection material for dental stone casts, there is no agreement on several factors, such as what the ideal concentration is, how much OZW to use, and how long it takes to disinfect.

25.5.3 Infection Control for Removable Partial Denture

Disinfection of RPDs can be achieved through mechanical, chemical, physical, or combined methods. Mechanical cleaning can be accomplished using brushing techniques with liquid soap or chemical agents and ultrasonic devices. Chemical cleaning can be achieved with a variety of disinfectants, which may differ in their effectiveness against different microorganisms and their possible interactions with prosthetic materials. Chemical disinfectants can be applied through spraying or immersion techniques. While spraying is more economical, it also increases the risk of exposure to hazardous chemicals among dental staff. Immersion techniques are generally more effective in reaching critical areas within the complex components of RPDs, such as clasps or minor connectors, which may be missed when using the spray method.

Clinicians should disinfect dentures prior to delivery to patients to prevent infection, instead of relying on infection control by the laboratory. Three highly recommended options for RPD infection control include: rinsing under running water, cleaning for debris in an ultrasonic cleaner, and storing for 12 h in an alkaline glutaraldehyde disinfection solution; rinsing under running water, scrubbing with 4% chlorhexidine for 15 s, and exposing to chlorine dioxide for 3 min; or sterilizing with ethylene oxide gas at concentrations between 450 and 800 mg/L. Furthermore, metal frameworks should be stored in a 5.25% NaOCl solution for 3 min before and after try-in, and then washed with water.

The effectiveness of chlorhexidine with both the spray and immersion methods at different concentrations has been investigated and has been shown to have antimicrobial effects against various bacterial and fungal species. A concentration of 4% chlorhexidine is effective in reducing the number of microorganisms in dentures within 10 min. However, chlorhexidine has minimal activity against SARS-CoV-2. Frequent use of chlorhexidine digluconate has the potential to cause staining in acrylic resin. It has been reported that chlorhexidine does not have any adverse effects on the physical properties of acrylic bases, such as roughness, bending strength, and hardness. However, prolonged use of chlorhexidine for denture disinfection may increase the cytotoxic effect of acrylic resins over time. No negative effects of chlorhexidine have been detected on the cobalt chromium (CoCr) metal surface. Chlorhexidine can be recommended for the disinfection of RPDs contaminated with *C. albicans*, especially in patients with denture stomatitis, due to its advanced antifungal properties. However, it should be kept in mind that long-term use of chlorhexidine may cause color changes in the denture.

The use of 2% glutaraldehyde as a disinfectant does not appear to have any negative effects on the physical properties of acrylic resins, likely due to its low concentration. Studies have shown that disinfecting artificial teeth with 2% glutaraldehyde does not significantly affect microhardness. Glutaraldehyde solutions with concentrations ranging from 0.5 to 3% can rapidly inactivate SARS-CoV-2 with a disinfection time of 2 min. Therefore, glutaraldehyde has been recommended for use during the COVID-19 outbreak when repeated disinfection lasting longer than 30 min is necessary. While 2% glutaraldehyde may not have a significant antifungal effect on the adhesion of *C. albicans*, it can still reduce the number of microorganisms. However, it is important to use glutaraldehyde with caution due to its toxicity, pungent odor, and potential to cause skin irritation, dermatitis, and asthma.

Although NaOCl has good antimicrobial activity, it may have adverse effects on acrylic, metal, and artificial tooth components of RPDs, depending on the exposure time. When the concentration and immersion time increase, the acrylic base may be affected, such as by an increase in surface roughness and a whitening of its color. Studies have also reported a decrease in the hardness of artificial teeth and a reduction in the bond strength between the artificial teeth and the microwave-cured acrylic denture base. The concentrated amount of NaOCl used successfully in the acrylic resin base may have detrimental effects on the CoCr framework. These undesirable effects can include tarnishing (surface discoloration), reduction in surface gloss, increase in ion release, increase in surface roughness, weight change, decrease in microhardness, and spot corrosion (surface pitting). Its taste and smell may also disturb patients, and it may cause skin irritation if the denture is not thoroughly rinsed with water after disinfection. Moreover, it is contraindicated in patients with NaOCl allergies. While clinicians or dental staff can use

NaOCl to clean the dentures after they have been delivered from the laboratory, before they are customized and repaired for the patient, and before sending the try-in dentures back to the laboratory, it is not advised for patients to use this chemical at home, as the concentration and exposure time might be exceeded.

The mechanism of antimicrobial action of acetic acid, a component of vinegar, is not fully understood. However, it is known that the alcohol in its composition acts on the cell wall, resulting in antimicrobial activity. Acetic acid is used in diluted form as an antibacterial, antifungal, and antiprotozoal agent. Recently, vinegar has been used in denture disinfection because it is cost-effective, easily accessible, and effective against a wide range of microorganisms. It has been found that 50–100% white vinegar is effective in inhibiting the growth of *C. albicans* in thermosetting and autopolymerized acrylic resin. Soaking the dentures in a 50% vinegar solution for 10 min was as effective as 1% NaOCl and 2% chlorhexidine digluconate against *C. albicans*, *E. coli*, and *S. mutans* in the disinfection of heat-cured acrylic resin. However, long-term studies are required on the effects of vinegar on acrylic resin and other RPD components. Daily disinfection of RPDs in homemade vinegar solutions overnight has been reported to adversely affect the surface hardness of artificial teeth. Additionally, the cytotoxic effect of acrylic resin was prolonged over time by the daily soaking of dentures in vinegar-based solutions. However, when used for short-term disinfection, they do not cause mucosal irritation, unlike other chemical disinfectants, even if they are not completely removed from the dentures. The mixture of vinegar and hydrogen peroxide was found to be very successful in eliminating *C. albicans* and *S. aureus* from the acrylic surface. The recommended formula for this mixture is to use white vinegar containing 4% acetic acid and hydrogen peroxide in a ratio of 1:1, 1:3, or 3:1. All three formulas were found to be equally effective as NaOCl. To achieve effectiveness, keeping the dentures in the mixture for 10 min was sufficient. However, due to the mixture's strong cytotoxic effect, it is recommended to rinse thoroughly with water. Additionally, this mixture may interact with the metal components of RPDs.

Patients who use RPDs may need to visit a dental office for repairs or adjustments. Unfortunately, RPDs can easily become colonized by bacteria, viruses, and fungus, which can be challenging to eliminate due to the complex structure of RPDs. RPDs are composed of different materials such as acrylic resin, artificial teeth, and metal alloys, making it difficult to clean them with a single disinfectant. The framework of RPDs is usually made of CoCr alloys, which may corrode or become discolored as a result of surface contact with disinfectants. It is important for RPD users, clinicians, and dental technicians to be educated on selecting the correct cleaning agent for disinfection. Acrylic resin is particularly sensitive to surface changes, and its interaction with various disinfection methods has been studied extensively. However, the available literature on metal alloy surfaces is still insufficient, and the best disinfection protocol for these materials is still up for debate. Regarding artificial teeth, only a limited number of studies have investigated the interaction of disinfecting agents with certain brands of teeth. Unfortunately, there is no definitive disinfection protocol that has been proven safe for RPDs.

Table 25.2 provides information on effective disinfectants that can be used to clean RPD components, including their recommended concentration percentages, the length of time they should be used, the microorganisms they eliminate, and how they affect RPD components. For more detailed information on the care and hygiene procedures that patients should follow for RPDs, refer to Chap. 24.

25.5.4 Infection Control for Burs and Handpieces

Burs, regardless of type, should be discarded after use or sterilized. Careful cleaning to eliminate dental material, blood clots, or saliva residues is a requirement before sterilizing a bur. The most popular cleaning technique for burs and other microinstruments is the use of ultrasonic equipment with proper solutions and the addition of proteolytic enzymes. Burs are vibrated at a frequency of 60–80 kHz for at least 15 min in an

Table 25.2 Effective disinfectants that can be used for RPD disinfection, recommended concentrations, duration of use, the microorganisms they are effective, and their effects on RPD components

Disinfectant	Percentage (%)	Duration	Microorganism	Effect on the RPD
Sodium hypochlorite	0.1, 0.5, and 1	10–15 min	*S. aureus, P. aeruginosa, C. albicans, B. subtilis, E. coli, S. mutans, E. faecalis,* and *C. glabrata*	Sodium hypochlorite causes diffuse surface changes and dark spots that indicate corrosion in CoCr alloys. It also results in increased ion release, surface roughness, weight change, and decreased microhardness. Moreover, it causes a significant decrease in the hardness values of artificial teeth
Chlorhexidine digluconate	1, 2, and 4	10–15 min	*E. coli, S. aureus, S. mutans,* and *C. albicans*	Frequent use of chlorhexidine digluconate has the potential to cause staining on acrylic resin
Glutaraldehyde	2	15 min	*C. albicans, S. oralis,* and *S. aureus*	The toxicity of glutaraldehyde is a significant limitation to its clinical use. It should be used cautiously due to its pungent odor and the risk of skin irritation, dermatitis, and asthma
Acetic acid (vinegar)	50 and 100	10–15 min	*C. albicans, E. coli, S. mutans,* and *S. aureus*	Prolonged and repeated use of homemade solutions made with vinegar can have negative effects on the surface hardness of the different layers of cross-linked artificial teeth. Additionally, daily exposure of dentures to disinfectant solutions containing vinegar may increase the cytotoxic effects of acrylic resins over time
Thyme oil	0.05	15–20 min	*C. albicans, A. flavus,* and *S. mutans*	Thyme essential oil has been found to have minimal or no adverse effects and can be used for cleaning dentures without affecting their flexural strength
Tea tree oil	1	5–10 min	*E. coli, C. albicans, S. aureus,* and *S. mutans*	This chemical causes minimal wear when used for brushing denture base resin
Lemongrass oil	1	5 min	*C. albicans*	There is minimal wear when denture base resin is brushed with this chemical
Grapefruit seed extract	0.1 and 1	5 min	*C. albicans*	There are no adverse effects on the acrylic resin
Ricinus communis (castor oil)	2, 8, and 10	10–20 min	*C. albicans, C. glabrata, S. aureus, E. coli, P. aeruginosa,* and *S. mutans*	R. communis solutions resulted in clinically acceptable roughness values and did not cause any detrimental effects on the CoCr surface. It was also found that there were nonsignificant changes in the surface roughness, hardness, and color of the artificial teeth and acrylic resin

Table 25.2 (continued)

Disinfectant	Percentage (%)	Duration	Microorganism	Effect on the RPD
Peroxymonosulfate	2	15 min	*C. albicans*	Disinfecting Valplast with peroxymonosulfate has been found to increase its impact strength and theoretical hardness. However, immersion disinfection with peroxymonosulfate did not have a significant effect on Sunflex
Sodium perborate	3.78	10 min	*S. mutans*	Disinfection with solutions containing sodium perborate may cause discoloration of the lining material. Moreover, an increase in surface roughness values of acrylic and CoCr alloy was observed after disinfection with sodium perborate
Cinnamaldehyde	0.27	20 min	*Candida* spp. and *S. mutans*	There were clinically acceptable minor changes observed in the Vickers microhardness, surface roughness, and color of the acrylic resin after prolonged immersion
Caffeine	6	24 h	*C. albicans*	Disinfecting with caffeine solution has been shown to have comparable effects to standard chlorhexidine therapy on acrylic surfaces. However, further studies are necessary to evaluate its effects on the surfaces of RPD materials

ultrasonic device, utilizing the appropriate solution at a temperature of around 65 °C. The burs need to be dried using hot air and absorbent paper once they have been removed from the ultrasonic bath. Depending on the substance they are composed of, burs then need to be put in a suitable device for sterilization. Burs made of common carbon steel, for instance, should not be put in the autoclave since they will oxidize. Stainless steel and tungsten carbide burs are not, however, affected in the same way. All types of burs can be sterilized using dry heat ovens, chemical vapor sterilization ovens, and ethylene oxide ovens. Dry heat ovens, on the other hand, can adversely harm the cutting edge of the burs due to the extended heating involved. For a satisfactory sterilization, different aldehydes and phenols can be used for at least 30 min; after 12 h, chemical sterilization is achieved. However, they might jeopardize the durability of rotating cutting tools.

Studies have demonstrated that patients' blood and saliva can get on the inside surfaces of handpieces, even though handpieces are only considered semi-critical category equipment. Failure to adequately clean and sterilize these instruments using an autoclave can increase the risk of subsequent patient infections. Although the recommended protocol for effective decontamination entails a thorough process involving sterilization, detergent washing, water rinsing, and mechanical friction, it has been observed that some health-care practitioners only rely on friction using 70% (w/v) alcohol for hand hygiene, without ensuring proper cleaning of the handpieces between patient encounters. This practice deviates from the prescribed guidelines and raises concerns regarding its potential impact on infection control. Researchers previously found that the processes currently used in clinical practice are not safe after examining handpieces that had been reprocessed only utilizing 70% water-to-alcohol ratio alcohol for 30, 60, and 90 s. Consequently, it is desirable to perform routine sterilization of handpieces between different patients. In addition, external micromotors should be covered with a disposable handpiece sleeve protector and discarded after use.

25.5.5 Infection Control for Occlusal Rims and Interocclusal Record Materials

0.5% chlorhexidine, 1% NaOCl, and 2% glutaraldehyde and iodophor can be used for the disinfection of occlusal rims and interocclusal recording materials. In addition, the ADA recommends the spray-wipe-spray technique to disinfect occlusal rims and interocclusal recording materials. Occlusal rims and interocclusal record materials need to be left in place for the required amount of time for disinfection to be effective. They may be contained in a plastic bag that is sealed for the advised period of time following the second spray. After disinfection, they should likely be rinsed one more time to remove any disinfectant residue. In a conducted study, the researchers investigated the comparative effects of 0.5% chlorhexidine, 1% NaOCl, and 2% glutaraldehyde on the linear dimensional stability of silicone and wax, both commonly used as interocclusal recording materials. The disinfection process employed both spray and immersion methods, with durations of 30 and 60 min. The study findings revealed that there were no statistically significant differences in the linear dimensions observed among any of the tested groups, irrespective of the disinfection method employed. These results held true for both the 30- and 60-min exposure periods. In another related study, the researchers focused on evaluating the linear dimensional changes of various materials commonly used in dental practice, including wax, zinc oxide–eugenol impression paste, polyether, polyvinyl siloxane, and bisacryl bite registration materials. These materials were subjected to immersion in 2% glutaraldehyde and 5% NaOCl disinfection solutions for 10 and 60 min, respectively. The immersion of bisacryl bite registration material in both disinfection solutions for the specified time periods did not significantly affect the material's dimensional stability. Additionally, the study recommended a specific disinfection approach for the other materials. Polyether and polyvinyl siloxane were advised to be immersed in a 5% NaOCl solution for 60 min, while wax and zinc oxide–eugenol were recommended to maintain their dimensional stability by immersing them in a 2 or 5% glutaraldehyde solution for 60 min.

25.5.6 Infection Control for Pumice

Commonly, brushes, wheels, and pumice are used to finish polishing RPDs. As the last phase in polishing an RPD, pumice may be a source of cross-contamination among technicians, dentists, and patients, as well as a transmission source for many oral and non-oral pathogens. According to a study, it was found that 61% of dental technicians did not engage in disinfection practices for pumice, while a staggering 93% neglected to disinfect their polishing equipment. The pumice can be sterilized with low-temperature gas or plasma sterilization techniques. Polishing the RPDs with sterile pumice or pumice that has been treated with disinfectants can help prevent the spread of infection, as can the daily substitution of the polishing paste and the sterilization of containers after each use. Numerous different possible disinfectants include 0.2% chlorohexidine gluconate, octenidine hydrochloride, benzoic acid, and 5% NaOCl.

25.5.7 Infection Control for Dental Chair

When each patient has been treated and the day's activities have been completed, the dental chair and the benches around it should be cleaned using a paper towel and an appropriate cleanser. In addition, the dental chair should be cleaned with disinfectants, including chlorine and 75% ethanol, after each patient visit. Alternatively, intermediate-level disinfectants such as iodoform, phenol, and chlorine compounds or high-level disinfectants such as NaOCl solution with a concentration of 1:100 can be used. In addition, NaOCl solution is used for cleaning and washing the surrounding surfaces and removing obvious stains. When left in this solution for an extended period of time, metal dental equipment, particularly those made of aluminum, corrodes. The EPA-approved low-level disinfectants are used for wall, floor, or room cleaning. If contamination is suspected, clean all surfaces at least twice a day with disinfectants.

25.5.8 Recommendations for the Cleaning and Decontamination of Clinic Environments

- Before entering the operation room, the patient should get instructions on how to wash their hands properly, use hand sanitizer, and use mouthwash containing chlorhexidine.
- Detergents and disinfectants should be prepared fresh every day and diluted as directed by the manufacturer.
- Plasma devices that do not require extra filters can be utilized for air disinfection.
- After each patient, disinfectants such as chlorine and 75% ethanol should be used to disinfect the dental chair.
- A disposable sheath should be placed over the dental chair and removed after treatment.
- Separate and clearly marked areas for sterilization and practice are essential.
- High-level disinfectant should not be used on the surfaces of the work area and waiting rooms for patients.
- Detergent should be used to wipe down the surfaces in the clinic.
- It is recommended to use just detergent when routinely cleaning table tops and countertops.
- Personal protective equipment, such as disposable gowns, gloves, and face masks, should be worn by all dental staff. A designated area for taking off protective clothing is required.
- Prior to patient interaction, the materials should be given by a noncontaminated dental assistant.
- To disinfect the clinical environment, fogging devices might be employed. It works by spraying hydrogen peroxide, which provides the greatest disinfectant properties with the least side effects. Moreover, a short period is required to reenter the dental office after disinfection.
- Dental clinic floors should be mopped with water and detergent instead of dry mopping, which creates dust aerosols.
- The dental staff must be aware of how to properly clean and decontaminate the surfaces in the clinic.

Further Reading

AlEraky DM, Abuohashish HM, Gad MM, Alshuyukh MH, Bugshan AS, Almulhim KS, Mahmoud MM. The antifungal and antibiofilm activities of caffeine against Candida albicans on polymethyl methacrylate denture base material. Biomedicines. 2022;10:2078.

Alfaifi AA, Lin WS, Aldhaian BA, Levon JA, Gregory RL. Impact of caffeine on metabolic activity and biofilm formation of Candida albicans on acrylic denture resin in the presence of nicotine. J Prosthet Dent. 2020;123:875–9.

AlHamdan EM, Al-Saleh S, Nisar SS, Alshiddi I, Alqahtani AS, Alzahrani KM, Naseem M, Vohra F, Abduljabbar T. Efficacy of porphyrin derivative, Chlorhexidine and PDT in the surface disinfection and roughness of Cobalt chromium alloy removable partial dentures. Photodiagnosis Photodyn Ther. 2021;36:102515.

Alkhtani F. Disinfection of polyvinyl siloxane impression material using ozone gas, 0.1% riboflavin, glutaraldehyde, and microwave irradiation and their effect on physical properties. Photodiagnosis Photodyn Ther. 2023;41:103242.

Alqahtani MA. Decontamination of a siloxane impression material by using 5-aminolevulinic acid activated by photodynamic therapy, microwave irradiation, and hydrogen peroxide. Photodiagnosis Photodyn Ther. 2022;38:102867.

Amin WM, Al-Ali MH, Al Tarawneh SK, Taha ST, Saleh MW, Ereifij N. The effects of disinfectants on dimensional accuracy and surface quality of impression materials and gypsum casts. J Clin Med Res. 2009;1:81–9.

Anjum R, Dhaded SV, Joshi S, Sajjan CS, Konin P, Reddy Y. Effect of plant extract denture cleansing on heat-cured acrylic denture base resin: an in vitro study. J Indian Prosthodont Soc. 2017;17:401–5.

Arruda CNF, Salles MM, Badaró MM, de Cássia Oliveira V, Macedo AP, Silva-Lovato CH, de Freitas Oliveira Paranhos H. Effect of sodium hypochlorite and Ricinus communis solutions on control of denture biofilm: a randomized crossover clinical trial. J Prosthet Dent. 2017;117:729-34.

Azevedo MJ, Correia I, Portela A, Sampaio-Maia B. A simple and effective method for addition sili-

cone impression disinfection. J Adv Prosthodont. 2019;11:155–61.
Badaró MM, Salles MM, de Arruda CNF, Oliveira VC, de Souza RF, Paranhos HFO, Silva-Lovato CH. In vitro analysis of surface roughness of acrylic resin exposed to the combined hygiene method of brushing and immersion in Ricinus communis and sodium hypochlorite. J Prosthodont. 2017;26:516-21.
Bustos J, Herrera R, González U, Martínez A, Catalán A, González U. Effect of inmersion desinfection with 0.5% sodium hypochlorite and 2% glutaraldehyde on alginate and silicone: microbiology and SEM study. Int J Odontostomatol. 2010;4:169–77.
Celebi H, Büyükerkmen EB, Torlak E. Disinfection of polyvinyl siloxane impression material by gaseous ozone. J Prosthet Dent. 2018;120:138–43.
Chidambaranathan AS, Balasubramanium M. Comprehensive review and comparison of the disinfection techniques currently available in the literature. J Prosthodont. 2019;28:849–56.
Craig RG, Powers JM, Wataha JC. Dental materials properties and manipulation. 7th ed. St Louis: Elsevier; 2000. p. 138–84.
Dalwai S, Rodrigues SJ, Baliga S, Shenoy VK, Shetty TB, Pai UY, Saldanha S. Comparative evaluation of antifungal action of tea tree oil, chlorhexidine gluconate and fluconazole on heat polymerized acrylic denture base resin - an in vitro study. Gerodontology. 2016;33:402-9.
de Almeida MAL, Batista AUD, de Araújo MRC, de Almeida VFDS, Bonan PRF, Nóbrega Alves D, da Costa TKVL, Nóbrega DF, de Castro RD. Cinnamaldehyde is a biologically active compound for the disinfection of removable denture: blinded randomized crossover clinical study. BMC Oral Health. 2020;20:223.
Demajo JK, Cassar V, Farrugia C, Sango DM, Sammut C, Valdramidis V, Camilleri J. Effectiveness of disinfectants on antimicrobial and physical Properties of Dental Impression Materials. Int J Prosthodont. 2016;29:63–7.
Dulaimi SF, Kanaan SM. The effect of microwave oven drying on the compressive strength of type III and IV dental stones at different time intervals. Open Dent J. 2018;12:494.
Elyassi Gorji N, Salehabadi N, Zakariaei Z, Yazdani Cherati J, Delavaryan L, Ebrahimi Saravi M. Viral contamination of acrylic resin removable denture bases in patients with COVID-19: a cross-sectional study. J Prosthet Dent. 2021:S0022-3913(21)00693-4.
Estafanous EW, Palenik CJ, Platt JA. Disinfection of bacterially contaminated hydrophilic PVS impression materials. J Prosthodont. 2012;21:16–21.
Gounder R, Vikas BV. Comparison of disinfectants by immersion and spray atomization techniques on the linear dimensional stability of different interocclusal recording materials: an in vitro study. Eur J Dent. 2016;10:7–15.
Hardan L, Bourgi R, Cuevas-Suárez CE, Lukomska-Szymanska M, Cornejo-Ríos E, Tosco V, Monterubbianesi R, Mancino S, Eid A, Mancino D, Kharouf N, Haikel Y. Disinfection procedures and their effect on the microorganism colonization of dental impression materials: a systematic review and meta-analysis of in vitro studies. Bioengineering (Basel). 2022;9:123.
Infection control recommendations for the dental office and the dental laboratory. ADA Council on Scientific Affairs and ADA Council on Dental Practice. J Am Dent Assoc. 1996;127:672–80.
Ismail HA, Mahross HZ, Shikho S. Evaluation of dimensional accuracy for different complete edentulous impressions immersed in different disinfectant solutions. Eur J Dent. 2017;11:242–9.
Iwasaki Y, Hiraguchi H, Iwasaki E, Yoneyama T. Effects of immersion disinfection of agar-alginate combined impressions on the surface properties of stone casts. Dent Mater J. 2016;35:45–50.
Jasim ZM, Abass SM. The effect of hypochlorous acid disinfectant on the reproduction of details and surface hardness of type III dental stone. Cureus. 2022;14:e32061.
Kang YS, Rueggeberg F, Ramos V Jr. Effects of chlorine-based and quaternary ammonium-based disinfectants on the wettability of a polyvinyl siloxane impression material. J Prosthet Dent. 2017;117:266–70.
Karimzadeh F, Sajedi SM, Taram S, Karimzadeh F. Comparative evaluation of bacterial colonization on removable dental prostheses in patients with COVID-19: a clinical study. J Prosthet Dent. 2021:S0022-3913(21)00252-3.
Koseki Y, Tanaka R, Murata H. Development of antibacterial denture cleaner for brushing containing tea tree and lemongrass essential oils. Dent Mater J. 2018;37:659–66.
Latib YO, Owen CP, Patel M. Viability of Candida albicans in denture base resin after disinfection: a preliminary study. Int J Prosthodont. 2018;31:436–9.
Lopes Vasconcelos GL, Curylofo PA, Targa Coimbra FC, de Cássia Oliveira V, Macedo AP, de Freitas Oliveira Paranhos H, Pagnano VO. In vitro antimicrobial activity of effervescent denture tablets on the components of removable partial dentures. Int J Prosthodont. 2020;33:315–20.
Macêdo LO, Campos DES, da Nóbrega Alves D, Carreiro ADFP, de Castro RD, Batista AUD. Effects of long-term cinnamaldehyde immersion on the surface roughness and color of heat-polymerized denture base resin. J Prosthet Dent. 2022;128:e1–521.e8.
Maciel PP, de Lima Gouveia C, Marques IL, Maciel PP,Lima JM, Castellano LRC, Bonan RF, Bonan PRF, Batista AUD. Antimicrobial effect and the mechanical and surface properties of a self-disinfecting and a chlorhexidine-incorporated Type IV dental stone. J Prosthet Dent. 2023;129:e1–365.e8.
Masetti P, Arbeláez MIA, Pavarina AC, Sanitá PV, Jorge JH. Cytotoxic potential of denture base and reline acrylic resins after immersion in disinfectant solutions. J Prosthet Dent. 2018;120:155.e1–7.

Matos AO, Costa JO, Beline T, Ogawa ES, Assunção WG, Mesquita MF, Consani RX, Barão VA. Effect of disinfection on the bond strength between denture teeth and microwave-cured acrylic resin denture base. J Prosthodont. 2018:27:169–76.

Michael J, Khamas AM, Al-Azzawi S. Compressive strength and surface roughness of die stone cast after repeated disinfection with sodium hypochlorite solution. J Bagh College Dentistry. 2010;22:27–33.

Muscat Y, Farrugia C, Camilleri L, Arias-Moliz MT, Valdramidis V, Camilleri J. Investigation of acrylic resin disinfection using chemicals and ultrasound. J Prosthodont. 2018;27:461–8.

Nautiyal M, Jyothi KS, Muttagi S, Pallavi NT, D'Almeida AU, Shah CP, Kaur H, Singh N. Effect of hypochlorites on the compressive strength and surface hardness of Type V dental stone: an in vitro study. J Contemp Dent Pract. 2022;1:215–20.

Nishikiori R, Sawajiri M, Okuda T, Otoshi A, Watanabe K, Hirata I, Nishijima W, Okazaki M. Effect of ozonated water on the surface roughness of dental stone casts. Dent Mater J. 2018;30:740–5.

Papadiochou S, Polyzois G. Hygiene practices in removable prosthodontics: a systematic review. Int J Dent Hyg. 2018;16:179–201.

Patel RK, Pai SA, Nagaraj T, Kohli A, Kj MJ, Bg S. Linear dimensional changes of five interocclusal recording materials when immersed in two disinfectants for different time intervals. J Contemp Dent Pract. 2019;20:732–7.

Pinto FM, Bruna CQ, Camargo TC, Marques M, Silva CB, Sasagawa SM, Mimica LM, Graziano KU. The practice of disinfection of high-speed handpieces with 70% w/v alcohol: an evaluation. Am J Infect Control. 2017;45:19–22.

Polychronakis N, Polyzois G, Lagouvardos P, Andreopoulos A, Ngo HC. Long term microwaving of denture base materials: effects on dimensional, color and translucency stability. J Appl Oral Sci. 2018;26:20170536.

Qiu Y, Xu J, Xu Y, Shi Z, Wang Y, Zhang L, Fu B. Disinfection efficacy of sodium hypochlorite and glutaraldehyde and their effects on the dimensional stability and surface properties of dental impressions: a systematic review. PeerJ. 2023;11:14868.

Rathod P, Pustake S, Hasban S, Jadhav M. Evaluation of the anti-microbial properties of prepared herbal solution on dental impressions with irreversible hydrocolloid—an ex vivo study. Int J Appl Dent Sci. 2021;7:216–23.

Sahoo AR, Oswal P, Jagadeesh KN, Ramaiah PT. Comparative evaluation of glutaraldehyde, UV radiation, herbal and autoclave for disinfection of impression materials. Int J Dent Oral Sci. 2020:S2:02:006:21–23.

Sequeira AL, Narayan AI, George VT. Effects of nonaldehyde immersion disinfection on the mechanical properties of flexible denture materials. J Prosthet Dent. 2019;121:843–7.

Sharif RA, Abdelaziz KM, Alshahrani NM, Almutairi FS, Alaseri MA, Abouzeid HL, Elagib MFA. The accuracy of gypsum casts obtained from the disinfected extended-pour alginate impressions through prolonged storage times. BMC Oral Health. 2021;21:296.

Sorrentino R, Basilicata M, Ruggiero G, Mauro MID, Leone R, Bollero P, Zarone F. A review on risk management of Coronavirus Disease 19 (COVID-19) infection in dental practice: focus on prosthodontics and all-ceramic materials. Prosthesis. 2022;4:338–52.

Soto AF, Mendes EM, Arthur RA, Negrini TC, Lamers ML, Mengatto CM. Antimicrobial effect and cytotoxic activity of vinegar-hydrogen peroxide mixture: a possible alternative for denture disinfection. J Prosthet Dent. 2019;121:966.e1–6.

Spaulding E. The role of chemical disinfection in the prevention of nosocomial infections. Proceedings of the International Conference on Nosocomial Infections, 1970. Chicago, IL: American Hospital Association; 1971:247–54.

The glossary of prosthodontic terms: ninth edition. J Prosthet Dent. 2017;117(5S):e1–e105.

Timbó ICG, Oliveira MSCS, Regis RR. Effect of sanitizing solutions on cobalt-chromium alloys for dental prostheses: a systematic review of in vitro studies. J Prosthet Dent. 2022:S0022-3913(22)00627-8.

Trivedi R, Sangur R, Bathala LR, Srivastava S, Madhav S, Chaubey P. Evaluation of the efficacy of Aloe Vera as a disinfectant by immersion and spray methods on irreversible hydrocolloid impression material and its effect on the dimensional stability of resultant gypsum cast—an in vitro study. J Med Life. 2019;12:395–402.

Tsutsumi-Arai C, Takakusaki K, Arai Y, Terada-Ito C, Takebe Y, Imamura T, Ide S, Tatehara S, Tokuyama-Toda R, Wakabayashi N, Satomura K. Grapefruit seed extract effectively inhibits the Candida albicans biofilms development on polymethyl methacrylate denture-base resin. PLoS One. 2019;14:0217496.

Ud Din S, Sajid M, Saeed A, Chaudhary FA, Alam MK, Sarfraz J, Ahmed B, Patel M. Dimensional changes of commercial and novel polyvinyl siloxane impression materials following sodium hypochlorite disinfection. PeerJ. 2022;10:12812.

Ueda T, Kubo K, Saito T, Obata T, Wada T, Yanagisawa K, Sakurai K. Surface morphology of silicone soft relining material after mechanical and chemical cleaning. J Prosthodont Res. 2018;62:422–5.

Vasconcelos GLL, Curylofo PA, Raile PN, Macedo AP, Paranhos HFO, Pagnano VO. Effect of alkaline peroxides on the surface of cobalt chrome alloy: an in vitro study. J Prosthodont. 2019;28:337–41.

Wezgowiec J, Paradowska-Stolarz A, Malysa A, Orzeszek S, Seweryn P, Wieckiewicz M. Effects of various disinfection methods on the material properties of silicone dental impressions of different types and viscosities. Int J Mol Sci. 2022;23:10859.

Index

O. Şakar (ed.), *Removable Partial Dentures*, https://doi.org/10.1007/978-3-031-47083-7

I

K

L

Printed by Printforce, the Netherlands